# Pharmaceutical Practice

book is to be
the last date s

*For Churchill Livingstone:*

*Commissioning editor:* Mike Parkinson/Ellen Green
*Project manager:* Valerie Burgess
*Project editor:* Barbara Simmons
*Project controller:* Derek Robertson
*Design direction:* Eric Bigland/Judith Wright
*Copy editor:* Sue Beasley
*Indexer:* Tarrent Ranger Indexing Agency
*Promotions manager:* Hilary Brown

# Pharmaceutical Practice

Edited by

## A. J. Winfield BPharm PhD MRPharmS ACPP

Head of Pharmacy Practice, School of Pharmacy,
The Robert Gordon University, Aberdeen, UK

## R. M. E. Richards OBE BPharm PhD DPharmSc FRPharmS PhC(Thai) PhC(Zimb)

Professor and Head of School, School of Pharmacy,
The Robert Gordon University, Aberdeen, UK

SECOND EDITION

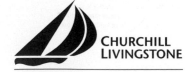
CHURCHILL
LIVINGSTONE

EDINBURGH LONDON NEW YORK PHILADELPHIA SAN FRANCISCO SYDNEY TORONTO 1998

CHURCHILL LIVINGSTONE
An imprint of Harcourt Publishers Limited

© Longman Group UK Ltd 1990
© Harcourt Brace and Company Limited 1998
© Harcourt Publishers Limited 2000

 is a registered trademark of Harcourt Publishers Limited

First edition 1990
Second edition 1998
  Reprinted 1999
  Reprinted 2000

Standard edition ISBN 0443 05729 X

International edition ISBN 0443 05730 3
  Reprinted 1999
  Reprinted 2000

**British Library Cataloguing in Publication Data**
A catalogue record for this book is available from the British Library

**Library of Congress Cataloging in Publication Data**
A catalog record for this book is available from the Library of
Congress

Medical knowledge is constantly changing. As new information
becomes available, changes in treatment, procedures, equipment and
the use of drugs become necessary. The editors, contributors and
publishers have, as far as it is possible, taken care to ensure that
the information given in this text is accurate and up to date.
However, readers are strongly advised to confirm that the information,
especially with regard to drug usage, complies with the latest
legislation and standards of practice.

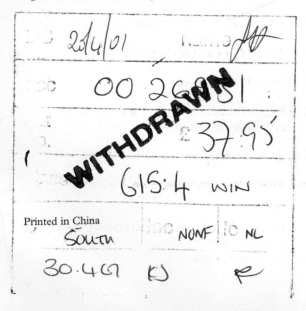

The
publisher's
policy is to use
paper manufactured
from sustainable forests

Printed in China

# Contents

# Contributors

**Derek G. Chapman** BSc(Pharm) PhD PRPharmS
Lecturer in Pharmacy Practice,
School of Pharmacy,
The Robert Gordon University,
Aberdeen, UK

*Ch. 6    Packaging*
*Ch. 24    Clean rooms for the production of*
*pharmaceutical products*
*Ch. 25    Parenteral products*
*Ch. 29    The principles of quality assurance*

**Diana M. Collett** BPharm PhD MRPharmS
Department of Pharmaceutical Sciences,
De Montfort University,
Leicester, UK

*Appendix 3    Medical abbreviations*
*Appendix 4    Latin terms and abbreviations*

**John A. Cromarty** BSc MSc(Pharmacol.) MSc (Clin.
Pharm.) Cert Ed MRPharmS
Professor, National Specialist in Clinical Pharmacy
(Scotland),
School of Pharmacy,
The Robert Gordon University,
Aberdeen, UK

*Ch. 1    The contribution of pharmacy to today's health*
*care provision*
*Ch. 31    Clinical pharmacy practice*
*Ch. 35    The evaluation of medicines*

**Gillian Cunningham** BSc(Hons) PhD MRPharmS
European Project Coordinator/Administrator,
School of Pharmacy,
The Robert Gordon University,
Aberdeen, UK

*Ch. 32    Adverse drug reactions*

**David Graham** BSc(Pharm) MSc MRPharmS
Radiopharmacist and Quality Assurance
Pharmacist,
Foresterhill Hospital,
Aberdeen Royal Hospitals NHS Trust,
Aberdeen, UK

*Ch. 26    Specialized services from a hospital pharmacy*

**John G. Hamley** BSc(Pharm) MSc MRPharmS
Principal Pharmacist (Clinical Pharmacy),
Ninewells Hospital and Medical School,
Dundee, UK

*Ch. 31    Clinical pharmacy practice*

**Sandra L. Hutchinson** BSc MRPharmS
Lecturer in Pharmacy Practice,
School of Pharmacy,
The Robert Gordon University,
Aberdeen, UK

*Ch. 3    Communication skills for the pharmacist*
*Ch. 26    Specialized services from a hospital pharmacy*
*Ch. 27    Hospital at home: the alternative care setting*
*Appendix 6    Homoeopathy and other complementary*
*therapies*

**Emily J. Kennedy** BSc PhD MRPharmS
Boots' Teacher Practitioner,
School of Pharmacy,
The Robert Gordon University,
Aberdeen, UK

*Ch. 1    The contribution of pharmacy to today's health*
*care provision*
*Ch. 2    Social and behavioural aspects of pharmacy*
*Ch. 3    Communication skills for the pharmacist*
*Ch. 11    Solutions*
*Ch. 12    Suspensions*

Ch. 13  Emulsions
Ch. 16  Powders and granules
Ch. 17  Oral unit dosage forms
Ch. 33  Responding to symptoms
Ch. 42  Substance misuse and harm reduction

**Janet Krska** BSc PhD MRPharmS MCPP
Reader in Clinical Pharmacy,
School of Pharmacy,
The Robert Gordon University,
Aberdeen, UK

Ch. 31  Clinical pharmacy practice
Ch. 32  Adverse drug reactions
Ch. 34  Formularies
Ch. 35  The evaluation of medicines
Ch. 43  Professional and clinical audit

**Märta M. Moody** BSc ARCST MRPharmS
Lecturer in Pharmacy Practice,
School of Pharmacy,
The Robert Gordon University,
Aberdeen, UK

Ch. 3  Communication skills for the pharmacist
Ch. 4  Dispensing techniques (compounding and good practice)
Ch. 5  Pharmaceutical calculations
Ch. 8  Labelling of dispensed medicines
Ch. 9  The prescription
Ch. 10  Routes of administration and dosage forms
Ch. 15  Suppositories and pessaries
Ch. 18  Aerosols and other dosage forms
Ch. 37  Counselling
Ch. 38  Health promotion and health education
Appendix 1  Current UK pharmaceutical legislation
Appendix 2  National Health Service dispensing

**Jean H. Musset** BPharm PhD MRPharmS
Lecturer in Pharmaceutical Sciences,
School of Pharmacy,
The Robert Gordon University,
Aberdeen, UK

Ch. 19  Wound management, stoma and incontinence products

**R. Michael E. Richards** OBE BPharm PhD DPharmSc
FRPharmS PhC(Thai) PhC(Zimb)
Professor and Head of School,
School of Pharmacy,
The Robert Gordon University,
Aberdeen, UK

Ch. 1  The contribution of pharmacy to today's health care provision
Ch. 21  Principles of sterilization
Ch. 22  Methods of sterilization
Ch. 23  Aseptic technique
Ch. 28  Ophthalmic products
Ch. 30  Sterility testing

**Jonathon Silcock** BPharm MSc PhD MRPharmS
Boot's Teacher Practitioner,
School of Pharmacy,
University of Bradford,
Bradford, UK

Ch. 35  The evaluation of medicines

**Derek C. Stewart** BSc MSc
Lecturer/Practitioner in Clinical Pharmacy,
School of Pharmacy,
The Robert Gordon University,
Aberdeen, UK

Ch. 36  Drug information
Appendix 7  Sources of information

**Arthur J. Winfield** BPharm PhD MRPharmS ACPP
Head of Pharmacy Practice,
School of Pharmacy,
The Robert Gordon University,
Aberdeen, UK

Ch.1  The contribution of pharmacy to today's health care provision
Ch. 7  Storage and stability of medicines
Ch. 14  External preparations
Ch. 19  Wound management, stoma and incontinence products
Ch. 20  Medical gases
Ch. 39  Patient medication records
Ch. 40  Residential care
Ch. 41  Compliance
Ch. 42  Substance misuse and harm reduction
Appendix 5  Systems of weights and measures
Appendix 8  The development and organization of pharmacy in the UK

# Acknowledgements

The editors would like to take this opportunity to thank the many people who have helped to make this second edition possible.

The contributing authors, mostly from within the School of Pharmacy at Robert Gordon University, have spent a great deal of time and effort in researching the subjects, preparing text and revising it as necessary. This has been achieved at a time of many extra pressures from course developments, internal and external reviews, implementing semesterization and preparing for the Teaching Quality Assessment. The willing cooperation of all authors at such a time has been a great encouragement to the editors who would like to record their grateful thanks.

We as a group of authors must also acknowledge out thanks to our students who have encouraged us over the years. We are indebted to them for their constructive criticism of and enthusiastic participation in the teaching/learning process.

Our families have also been involved, not least in their patience and support during the time we have taken working on the book. In particular, AJW wishes to remember his first wife Janet, who though terminally ill, gave her encouragement on the undertaking of the project. This work is dedicated to her memory.

At various places in the book there are acknowledgements to particular companies and other sources for permission to use or modify material. We are indebted to them for their cooperation. Robert Gordon University library staff have been very helpful in providing support when required and many companies and organizations have assisted in answering queries and providing information which has been used by the authors.

Thanks are also due to Tandy Stalker in the School office for always being prepared to assist and by so doing helping things to progress smoothly.

Throughout the project, there has been support from the editorial staff of Churchill Livingstone. Our thanks go to them for steering us through some of the practical problems and always being available to answer questions when they arose.

AJW
RMER

# Preface

The second edition of *Pharmaceutical Practice* has been produced by new editors and a predominantly new team of authors. However, the overall philosophy of the book – to produce a sound base for all aspects of good pharmaceutical practice – is unchanged. A considerable amount of new material has been introduced in order to provide the knowledge and skills necessary for the developing role of the pharmacist. This is particularly pertinent in the area of primary care where the health care professions, including pharmacy, are seeking to maximize their contribution to the well being of the patient. The pharmacist's role is particularly concerned with the many aspects which interplay in achieving the goal of maximizing patient benefit from their medications. The unique 'pharmaceutics' core of applied pharmaceutical science has been carefully selected in order to provide the sound knowledge base necessary for the competent practice of pharmacy both in the UK and internationally.

The scientific principles which underlie dosage form design in particular are covered in greater detail in the companion volume *Pharmaceutics: The science of dosage form design* (edited by Aulton ME) and further aspects of clinical practice are considered in another companion volume *Clinical pharmacy and therapeutics* (edited by Walker R and Edwards C).

October 1997                                      AJW
                                                  RMER

# About this book

Since the publication of the first edition of this book there have been many advances both in the practice of pharmacy and in the way in which it is taught in the Schools of Pharmacy in the United Kingdom. In considering the contents of this edition, these changes have been taken into account. However, given the limited space in the book, it has also been necessary to omit some material. Thus a compromise has been made in which some but not all of the more traditional material is retained and most but not all of the recent developments are included.

The book has been divided into four sections, each dealing with a different aspect of practice and called:

- The pharmacist in society
- Dispensing
- Sterile products
- From theory to pharmaceutical care.

Part 1, The Pharmacist in Society, begins with an overview of the way the profession of pharmacy has changed and developed over recent years. Chapter 2 then deals with the general area of social and behavioural science, including some of the more important aspects of the sociology and psychology of patients. The important requirement for effective communication skills in the pharmacist is also dealt with in Chapter 3 of this section of the book.

Part 2, Dispensing, covers aspects of extemporaneous dispensing together with some aspects of dispensing practice. Extemporaneous dispensing is less common in current practice, but is unique to pharmacists amongst health care professionals. It is a very broad subject which requires an acute awareness of the principles which are employed, the ability to perform arithmetic functions accurately and to carry out practical manipulations. This section of the book deals with background requirements first in Chapters 4 to 8 – the basis for compounding medicines and good practice, how to carry out calculations, consideration of containers and closures, storage, stability and labelling. The details of the prescription and the routes which are available for administering medicines are covered in Chapters 9 and 10. The main types of extemporaneous preparation are then dealt with in chapters 11 through to 16. In doing this, very little of the relevant physical chemistry has been dealt with. Students are advised to consult other relevant textbooks, such as the companion volume to this book *Pharmaceutics, the science of dosage form design* if they wish to understand more of the underpinning science involved. Chapters 17 to 20 consider a number of other medicines, dressings, appliances and products which may be prescribed or sold to the public through a pharmacy.

The third part of the book deals with sterile products. The first two chapters (Chapters 21 and 22) deal with the principles of and methods for sterilization of liquids and solids. The techniques for aseptic production are considered in Chapter 23 and the principles of clean room design and operation are the subject of Chapter 24. Chapters 25 through to 28 deal with different types of sterile product. These include general parenteral products (Chapter 25) and the more specialized products containing intravenous additives, cytotoxic drugs, radiopharmaceuticals, and those used for parenteral nutrition, dialysis and for treatment of the eye and surrounding surfaces. The next chapter deals with the principles of quality assurance, which apply to all medicines, but which can be appreciated most clearly with sterile products. Finally this part has a chapter dealing with sterility testing and the problems which are associated with this.

Part 4 of the book has been give the title 'From Theory to Pharmaceutical Care'. Pharmacists are becoming increasingly involved in clinical practice and in direct patient care. This is a rapidly changing area. The aim has been to give background information, cover the main principles which are used in practice today and, where possible, indicate the direction in which practice may move in future years. The latter is always a potentially hazardous process, so those using this book are reminded of the necessity for keeping up to date with the relevant literature in order to find out about recent trends. Pharmacists are becoming more involved in the clinical aspects of the use of drugs. The actual clinical use is dealt with in more detail in the companion volume to this book *Clinical Pharmacy and Therapeutics*. This book is concerned primarily with the processes involved. After the general survey in Chapter 34, a series of clinical topics are dealt with – adverse drug reactions, responding to symptoms in community pharmacy, formulary development and management, pharmacoeconomics and sources of drug information. The more direct services which pharmacists provide to patients are covered in the chapters dealing with patient counselling, health promotion, patient medication records, services to residential homes, patient compliance and the misuse of drugs, including the principles of harm minimization. The book ends with a chapter dealing with the principles and practice of professional and clinical audit – a technique which helps to demonstrate the quality of service provided.

A number of appendices are added for reference. The first two deal with current United Kingdom pharmaceutical legislation and the processes involved in National Health Service dispensing. Two short appendices give lists of common medical and pharmaceutical abbreviations. For reference purposes there is also a listing of weight and measure systems. Many community pharmacists sell homoeopathic medicines and other alternative therapies to customers. Appendix 6 gives a brief outline of some of those commonly used. Appendix 7 complements Chapter 36 in giving a list of important sources of information. Finally, there is an appendix which looks briefly at the development of the profession of pharmacy and how it integrates with current patient care.

No book of this size can be comprehensive. At the end of each chapter there are a number of suggestions for further reading. When these are to the standard reference works, students should be aware that these, such as the pharmacopoeias, BNF, guidelines etc., change with time. Therefore it is important to check in the latest edition, which includes any addenda which may have been published. As suggested previously, pharmacy is currently in the process of change. During the anticipated lifetime of this book new developments are to be expected. Every effort has been made to ensure that the information is current at the time of going to press. However, regular consultation of journals will be required in order to keep your knowledge up to date. This is a challenging, but enjoyable, task which rewards those who spend the time carrying it out.

# PHARMACY IN SOCIETY

# 1

# The contribution of pharmacy to today's health care provision

*A. J. Winfield, J. A. Cromarty, R. M. E. Richards and E. J. Kennedy*

---

After studying this chapter you will know about:

**An outline of the position of pharmacy within the National Health Service in the UK**
**Recent developments in the services being provided by pharmacists**
**The need for lifelong learning.**

---

## Introduction

Pharmacists are experts on the action and uses of drugs. There are many facets to this expertise, including the chemistry of drugs, the formulation of medicines and the way in which drugs are used to manage diseases. Pharmacists are often in close contact with patients so that they also have a role in assisting patients to make the best use of the medicines, to advise on matters concerning health and to supply medicines for use with minor conditions. They are also in close working relationships with other members of the health care team – doctors, nurses, dentists and others – where they are able to give advice on a wide range of issues surrounding the use of medicines.

Pharmacists are employed in many different areas of practice. However, the two main areas of work are in hospital and community practice. Additionally, pharmacists are employed in the pharmaceutical industry, in academia, as pharmaceutical advisors, and as community facilitators amongst others. The general public are most likely to meet pharmacists in high street pharmacies or on a hospital ward. However, pharmacists also visit residential homes, make visits to patients' homes and are now involved in a number of clinics. In addition, pharmacists will also be contributing to the care of patients through their dealings with other members of the health care team. This has been the case in the hospital setting for many years. In community pharmacy, pharma-

cists are increasingly working with general practitioners (GPs), nurses and health visitors.

With the advent of the National Health Service (NHS) in the UK in 1948, people had free access to medical services. In the previous 35 years, the pharmacist had provided medical advice to some members of the public as an alternative to them paying to see a doctor. This advisory function of the pharmacist then decreased. As a result pharmacists spent more of their time in the dispensing of medicines – and derived an increased proportion of their income from it. There has also been a radical change in the nature of dispensing itself over the 50 years of the NHS.

In the early years, many prescriptions were for extemporaneously prepared medicines, either to recipes from the standard formularies such as the *British Pharmacopoeia* (BP) or *British Pharmaceutical Codex* (BPC), or to recipes written by the prescriber. The situation was similar in hospital pharmacy, where prescriptions were prepared on an individual basis. There was some small-scale manufacture of a range of commonly used items. In both situations, pharmacists required the manipulative skills to produce the medicines. Thus a wide range of types of preparation were made, including liquids for internal and external use, ointments, creams, poultices, plasters, eye drops and ointments, injections and solid dosage forms such as pills, capsules and moulded tablets.

Scientific advances have greatly increased the effectiveness of drugs available to medical science. These same materials are more complex, potentially more toxic, and require a more sophisticated usage. This produced a growth of the pharmaceutical industry. As it developed, so the use of manufactured medicines increased. This had a number of advantages. For one thing, there was an increased reliability in the product, which could be subjected to suitable quality assessment. This led to improved formulations, modifications to drug availability and increased use of tablets which have a greater convenience for the patient. Some doctors did not agree with the loss of flexibility in prescribing which resulted from having to use predetermined doses and combinations of materials. From the pharmacist's point of view there was a reduction in the time spent in the routine production of medicines, which many saw as an advantage. Others saw it as a reduction in the 'mystique' associated with the professional role of the pharmacist. (Refer to Ch. 2 for a more detailed discussion on the professional roles of pharmacists.) There was also an erosion of the skill base of the pharmacist. A look through copies of the BPC in the 1950s and 1960s to the 1970s will show the reduction in the number and diversity of formulations included in the Formulary section. That section was omitted from the most recent editions.

Some extemporaneous dispensing is still required and pharmacists remain the only professionals trained in these skills. For this reason, Part 2 of this book deals with the types of medicine used, the ingredients employed in them and describes some of the practical skills required to make products suitable for use by patients.

The changing patterns of work of the pharmacist, in community pharmacy in particular, led to an uncertainty about the future role of the pharmacist. If the pharmacist was not to require skills in compounding medicines, and was not required to give general advice on diseases, what was the pharmacist to do?

## THE NUFFIELD REPORT

In October 1983, the Nuffield Foundation appointed a Committee of Enquiry with the following terms of reference: 'To consider the present and future structure of the practice of pharmacy in its several branches and its potential contribution to health care and to review the education and training of pharmacists accordingly'. The Committee presented their report in January 1986. Prior to the Report, developments were taking place. The Report endorsed many of these and led the way to many new initiatives, both by the profession and by the Government. Some of the issues and developments are dealt with in Chapter 31.

The Report, which extends to 150 pages, is divided into 11 chapters, as shown in Table 1.1, including nearly 100 recommendations. It is not appropriate to deal with all aspects in this chapter,

| Table 1.1 | The chapters in the Nuffield Report |
|---|---|
| Chapter 1 | Introduction |
| Chapter 2 | The pharmacy profession |
| Chapter 3 | Community pharmacy |
| Chapter 4 | Hospital pharmacy |
| Chapter 5 | Industrial pharmacy |
| Chapter 6 | Undergraduate education |
| Chapter 7 | Pre-registration training |
| Chapter 8 | Continuing education |
| Chapter 9 | Higher degrees and research |
| Chapter 10 | The Pharmaceutical Society of Great Britain |

but some of the main findings are relevant, because they laid the foundation for the recent developments in the practice of pharmacy, which are reflected in this book.

## Community pharmacy

The Report recognized the special knowledge which pharmacists possess on the formulation and action of medicines. The Committee did not expect a reduction in the volume of prescriptions to be dispensed, but did see these becoming increasingly available in the form of 'original pack dispensing'. Information technology was seen to have its place in community pharmacy, although limited by the essential incompleteness of any patient records in the absence of patient registration. The report noted the closer working together of medical and pharmaceutical staff in the hospital sector. It suggested that a closer working together between GPs and community pharmacists would lead to a more efficient use of NHS resources. This could take the form of a working relationship in which prescribing and dispensing would be discussed regularly and naturally (as compared to the more usual 'criticism' of a GP when an error occurred on a prescription). The Report also suggested a change in the way pharmacists interact with the public. A series of possibilities were suggested, including:

- *Advice on symptoms*. This would be renewing the traditional role which the pharmacist had carried out prior to the advent of the NHS.
- *Responding to special needs*. At the time of handing over the dispensed medicine, the pharmacist can give advice to the patient. It is important to ensure that medicines are used properly, particularly by the elderly who take a proportionately larger share of the medicines consumed.

- *Domiciliary services*. Pharmacists have traditionally delivered oxygen to a patient's home. This could be extended to include other situations where patients could benefit, such as on discharge from hospital, where they have special needs, during terminal care, for parenteral feeding. They might also have a role in helping patient compliance with drug regimens.

- *Health education*. A large number of people pass through the nation's pharmacies in any one day. In appropriate situations, these people could be in receipt of health education. One example is giving out patient information leaflets on diet, which may reduce the development of disease which would otherwise occur and lead to the need for expensive treatment.

- *Sale of medicines*. Pharmacies have been able to sell general sales list (GSL) and pharmacy (P) medicines under the personal supervision of the pharmacist. The report indicated two possible changes. The first was that more drugs be classified as P medicines from their prescription-only medicine (POM) status. The second was for a reconsideration of the extent of supervision required for such sales to take place.

- *Remuneration*. The remuneration of pharmacies was based on a practice allowance, plus the number of prescriptions and the cost of the medicines involved. The Report suggests that remuneration should be changed to allow for specific remuneration of services provided.

## Hospital pharmacy

The Report included a strong recommendation for the development of clinical pharmacy. Some of the issues surrounding this are dealt with in Chapter 31 and will not be discussed further here although they are of great importance. There was a call for a greater working together of the professions in the hospital setting including pharmacists' involvement in medication history taking, for pharmacists to be more actively involved in research, and for the provision of 24-hour services.

## Undergraduate education

Teaching of pharmacy has traditionally been under three (or four) subject headings: pharmaceutical chemistry, pharmaceutics, pharmacology (and pharmacognosy). This could be seen as a restraint on the development of new ideas of teaching to make the course more relevant to the profession. The Committee saw the need to have a firmly science-based course, with involvement in practical work. However, advances in school education meant that knowledge of some material could be assumed. The suggestion was that this time be used for teaching social and behavioural science and pathology and therapeutics. Law and ethics, whilst being introduced, could be left until the pre-registration year. Emphasis was laid on the need to develop communication skills in students and to make the course as relevant to practice as possible by making teacher–practitioner appointments. The possibility of a regrouping of subject matter under new titles should also be considered.

## Pre-registration training

The Report highlighted that the development of the pre-registration training had been independent of the changes which had taken place in the schools of pharmacy. They should be developed together. More radical suggestions were that the pre-registration year should be divided between hospital and community pharmacy, with health authorities being paid for hospital pre-registration students in the same way that community pharmacists are paid. The Report recommended the introduction of a test of competence at the end of the pre-registration period with the emphasis on practical work and oral skills. It noted that it should not be assumed that all candidates would be successful!

## Continuing education

The need for continuing education of pharmacists was accepted, but a coordinated approach was required, concentrating in the first instance on existing pharmacists. The Committee did not support the idea that participation in continuing education be made a requirement for continued registration as a pharmacist. They did, however, suggest that an assessment of practice should eventually be considered as a requirement for continued registration.

## Higher degrees and research

Taught Masters' courses should be continued and should include some research. There was a recognized difficulty in carrying out research towards a PhD in pharmacy. The Report encouraged hospital and industrial pharmacists to undertake such studies, and further highlighted the need to undertake research in pharmacy practice and publicize the findings.

## PHARMACY AFTER THE NUFFIELD REPORT

The Committee highlighted that the Royal Pharmaceutical Society of Great Britain (RPSGB) had a crucial role in implementing the findings. The Government also was required to make changes, both to the law and to the form of remuneration in order to enable some of the changes to occur. It is interesting, when writing this chapter some 11 years after the Report was published, to see how many of the changes have actually occurred or are in the process of occurring. There have also been other changes which were not envisaged in the Report. Some of the main developments will be briefly outlined and reference made to the appropriate chapters in this book.

## Changes in community pharmacy

### Original pack dispensing

The suggestion of an increasing use of 'original pack dispensing' was generally welcomed by the profession. However, its introduction has been very slow. At the time of writing there are still regular calls for manufacturers to be more proactive in introducing the packs which have potential benefits for the patients and pharmacists. Some further information is included in Chapter 6.

### Increasing use of computers

Apart from the almost universal use of computers for label production (Ch. 8), computers are widely used for keeping patient medication records (PMRs; Ch. 39). There are no moves towards patient registration, so the records tend to be incomplete. Nevertheless, computers have many uses and are considered beneficial. Pharmacists are now paid for keeping these patient medication records, provided they have completed appropriate training.

### GP–pharmacist links

Government White Papers have been increasingly forthright in moving towards an integration in the provision of health care in the community. This is seen as being centred on the general medical practitioner. The White Paper 'Choice and Opportunity. Primary Care: the Future' published in October 1996 highlights community pharmacy for further development. It foresees community pharmacy: facilitating better use of prescribed medicines; as the first port of call for minor ailments; providing health promotion; and providing advice on medicines to the rest of the primary health care team and others.

Links between pharmacists and GPs were slow to develop. However, during the 1990s there has been increasing evidence of a coming together. Some early studies placed pharmacists in GP surgeries to evaluate their contribution. Many doctors realized that pharmacists had many possible additional roles and began to make use of their services. More recently there has been an extension of 'clinical pharmacy' into the community, with many pharmacists now providing doctors with advice on GP formulary development (Ch. 34) and undertaking patient medication reviews and taking responsibility for specific clinics following agreed protocols. Anticoagulant and *Helicobacter pylori* assessment clinics are examples. It appears that there is scope for much more development in this area of activity.

### Responding to symptoms

Advertising campaigns, particularly those by the National Pharmaceutical Association (NPA), have brought to the public attention the advice which is available from the pharmacist. Despite some adverse publicity, notably arising from Consumer Association reports, the public seem to respond positively. Provision of advice is now an accepted part of the work of a pharmacist. It has also extended to the counter staff, who require special training and must adhere to protocols. Some of the principles of responding to symptoms are dealt with in Chapter 33.

### Patients with special needs

The range of 'special needs' now recognized by pharmacists has expanded beyond those envisaged in the Nuffield Report. Chapters 40 and 41 deal with some aspects of this area. In particular, aiding patients to comply with and maximize the benefits of their medicine regimen is recognized as an important contribution of pharmacy to health care.

### Domiciliary service

Some pharmacists do make regular visits to patients' homes, but this is the exception rather than the norm. However, the development of services to residential homes has meant a high level of involvement by pharmacists as reviewed in Chapter 40. In addition, a few pharmacists are involved in specialized services, often called the 'hospital at home', where patients may be on palliative care, cytotoxic agents, intravenous antibiotics or artificial nutrition.

## Health education

The provision of health education material has become part of the pharmacist's NHS contract. In many instances this has been limited to the provision of a range of leaflets and there have been relatively few examples of extensive health promotion in pharmacies. Nevertheless, there are many opportunities, some of which are discussed in Chapter 38.

## Personal control

This issue is unresolved. The key difficulty is how aware the pharmacist should be of the transaction of providing a medicine to a member of the public in order for it to be called 'supervision'. One argument suggests that the pharmacist should be fully aware of all transactions and be able to intervene if deemed necessary. An opposite view is that pharmacists require to be involved in other activities. They cannot be involved in all sales in a busy shop and so should ensure that all the staff are adequately trained to know when a referral to the pharmacist is necessary. The Statutory Committee has considered the situation a number of times and has suggested that it is a matter of degree.

## Prescription-only to pharmacy medicines

There has been an acceleration of the re-regulation of medicines. Early examples were loperamide and hydrocortisone. There is no obvious end to the process. The Nuffield Report also suggested that there should, for safety reasons, be a move of some GSL medicines to P status. This has not happened. Indeed, ibuprofen in small packages has been re-regulated from P to GSL.

## Remuneration

There has been a change in the basis of remuneration. Recognition is now given to the general and specific provision of professional services. Pharmacies receive a practice allowance, which represents a substantial proportion of their NHS income. There have also been payments to encourage the development of specific services, such as PMR usage and health education provision. These are now being subsumed within the practice allowance, although there remain differences between England and Wales and Scotland. As new services are provided, so new forms of remuneration will need to be devised, a fact which has been recognized by the Government.

## Hospital pharmacy

The development of clinical pharmacy services has extended since the time of the Nuffield Report. In 1988, the NHS Circular 'Health Services Management: the Way Forward for Hospital Pharmaceutical Services' laid down the government policy aim as 'the achievement of better patient care and financial savings, through the more cost effective use of medicines, and improved use of pharmaceutical expertise obtained through the implementation of a clinical pharmacy service'. The hospital service has been considering its response to this. Two main components can be identified. One is the overall management of medicines on the hospital ward. This is achieved through the provision of advice to medical and nursing staff, formulary management and ensuring the safe handling of medicines. The other component is the development of individual patient care plans. This is achieved through the provision of drug information and assisting patients with problems which may arise. In practice there are many stages and activities involved in these processes. A working group in Scotland published 'Clinical Pharmacy in the Hospital Pharmaceutical Service: a Framework for Practice' in July 1996 (Steering Group and Working Group 1996). The framework advocates a systematic approach to enable the pharmacist to focus on the key areas and optimize the pharmaceutical input to patient care. Some of the thinking behind this document is discussed in detail in Chapter 31.

Other developments suggested by the Nuffield Report have taken place. For example, a 24-hour service is available in most large hospitals, with a pharmacist on call. Research into aspects of the hospital pharmaceutical service has noticeably increased, as has research into community pharmaceutical services.

There is a growing awareness of the problems which arise at the interface between community (primary) and hospital (secondary) care. Patients move in both directions. Their medical and pharmaceutical problems also move with them. There is, therefore, a need for effective transfer of information, say from hospital pharmacist to community pharmacist. Many of the issues are now being identified. Over the next few years it is hoped that a large proportion of the current problems will have been resolved.

With increasing technological developments, the

move of patient care away from hospital towards the community and the introduction of more sophisticated treatments, a number of specialized services have been developed. These include the use of cytotoxic drugs, radiopharmaceuticals, parenteral nutrition (both in hospital and at home), centralized intravenous additives services and various types of dialysis. Pharmacists are involved with these. The topics are discussed in more detail in Chapters 26 and 27.

## Undergraduate courses

There have been many changes to the undergraduate course since the Nuffield Report, some of which are reflected in the contents of this book. The Report called for schools of pharmacy to consider regrouping subjects. Most have done so to some extent. For example, Clinical Pharmacy is now accepted as a subject and is an important part of the course. The RPSGB requested that schools include social and behavioural sciences in the undergraduate programme. This is a broad subject area which covers many sociological and psychological aspects of disease and patients. It can also embrace communication skills. In this book chapters have been included dealing with social and behavioural science (Ch. 2), communication skills (Ch. 3) and counselling skills (Ch. 37). Many courses have developed techniques for assisting students to develop their communication and counselling skills. These skills are of a practical nature. They cannot be 'learned' by studying a book. Rather they have to be acquired by experience, but are based on recognized practices.

The Report called for the expansion of pharmacy practitioners' involvement in undergraduate teaching and for teachers to be involved in practice. The aim of utilizing teacher–practitioners was to ensure that the university course was related to current pharmacy practice. Initially the teacher–practitioners were established between hospitals and schools of pharmacy. When Boots the Chemists, the retail pharmacy group, agreed to provide a teacher–practitioner for each school of pharmacy, then community pharmacy practitioners also became a part of the teaching team. Other companies have started to provide teaching support for the schools of pharmacy in a similar way. Other ways of fostering current practice as part of course provision are also used – such as visiting lecturers, making GP practice and hospital visits, using part-time teaching staff, staff secondment to practice and joint academic/practice research studies. The changes mentioned above – use of practitioners, restructuring of subjects, intro-

duction of new material – have gone a long way to meeting the recommendations that university pharmacy courses should produce not only competent pharmaceutical scientists, but also graduates with a knowledge of practice.

One recommendation which has not produced a change was that the teaching of law and ethics should be moved into the pre-registration year. Many arguments can be made to support the present situation. Not least of these is that the teaching of dispensing practice without the necessary detailed legal and ethical knowledge is impractical. Concurrent teaching also ensures that students have an adequate working knowledge when they enter the world of pharmacy practice for their pre-registration period. Legal and ethical considerations can then be consolidated in practice.

There have been two important, partly interlinked, changes affecting the undergraduate course which were not foreseen in the Nuffield Report. The most obvious of these has been the introduction of the 4-year degree course. The Report 'accepted that there can at present be no lengthening of the academic course'. Some of the imperative for the extension of the course came from the European Union (EU). There is a desire to harmonize the undergraduate courses across the EU as far as possible. The minimum requirement was for an academic course of 4 years followed by a year of structured training in a practice situation. Courses in the UK, with the exception of those in Scotland, were a year shorter. The 3-year courses were initially accepted as being equivalent to the 4-year Scottish courses because of the generally higher level of entry to the 3-year courses. Over the years this difference in standard of entrant was eroded. This, together with the great pressure to include additional highly relevant material in the course, meant that representatives of the schools of pharmacy believed that there was a need to extend the course. This was necessary in order to meet the two aims of producing scientists and practitioners. The government funding Councils accepted the proposals to extend the course length. Thus, as from the intake into the schools in autumn 1997, all courses in the UK will be of 4 years' duration.

## Pre-registration training

The chapter of the Nuffield Report on preregistration training was relatively short, with only seven recommendations. However, there has been a major overhaul of the training. It is now carried out on a much more structured basis than was the case previously. The pre-registration examination has been running for a number of years. This has been designed as a test of professional competence. The recommendation to include both hospital and community practice in the pre-registration year has not yet been acted upon. Some of the differences between community and hospital practice are becoming less distinct as pharmacists in the community take on roles which in the past have been common in hospital practice, such as prescribing advice to doctors. In the future, it may be that interchange between the two will become easier to achieve than it is at present.

## Continuing education

In such a rapidly changing profession, there is a need for continual updating of knowledge. The Report recommended that the RPSGB should take the initiative in opening discussions to coordinate the provision of continuing education. The College of Pharmacy Practice (CPP) was mentioned as capable of development for this purpose. This has, to some extent, happened with the CPP requiring members to undertake continuing education. The RPSGB, through *The Pharmaceutical Journal*, have established a regular pattern of continuing education (CE) articles on a wide range of topics. Some of these now include assessment questions in collaboration with the CPP. The Council of the RPSGB has also decided to recommend that all pharmacists undertake at least 30 hours of continuing education each year. A core syllabus has been agreed and each pharmacist receives a 'planner and record' in January to improve motivation.

The greatest development in continuing education has come with the formation of the Centres for Postgraduate or Postqualification Pharmaceutical Education (CPPE). These were established to meet the call for coordinated education for pharmacists. They are located in Manchester (England), Glasgow (Scotland), Cardiff (Wales) and Belfast (Northern Ireland). Each operates in a slightly different way, but all base their provision on the RPSGB core syllabus together with responding to new needs which may be identified, either nationally or locally. Courses are provided free to pharmacists who are employed in the provision of pharmaceutical services to the NHS.

There is, therefore, an increased provision for continuing education. Pharmacists appear to be making use of this provision. Some innovative approaches have also been used, for example joint evenings at which GPs and pharmacists receive their continuing education together. Such events have

many advantages, helping to break down the barriers between professions and increasing mutual understanding of knowledge and expertise. However, the recommendation that an assessment of competence should become a requirement for continued registration has not yet been implemented.

## Higher degrees and research

In 1986 only a few taught MSc degrees were available. A wide range of such 'taught' courses are now available. Some are relatively short, others offer a postgraduate diploma, others a Master of Science. Subject matter may be very specialized or more general. Study may be full time or part time. There are also distance learning courses for those who have limited opportunity to be away from their place of work. Research has also developed. In 1986, there was very little published research into pharmacy practice in the UK. Now research articles appear regularly in *The Pharmaceutical Journal*, which also has research supplements, there are practice research sessions at the British Pharmaceutical Conference each year, the *International Journal of Pharmacy Practice* has been established and many students are now graduating with a doctorate for studies undertaken in aspects of pharmacy practice.

## The pharmaceutical society

The Nuffield Report ends with the recommendation: 'The role of the RPSGB in implementing this Report is crucial. The Report gives the Council of the Society an opportunity which it must not fail to take'.

It is obvious from the previous sections, that pharmacy has undergone many changes since the Nuffield Report. The RPSGB has been involved in many of these. However, when such radical and rapid changes are taking place, there are those who question the direction which is being taken. Some members of the RPSGB also have some reservations.

The Council decided that it was necessary to allow all members to contribute to a radical appraisal of the profession, what it should be doing and how to achieve it. The 'Pharmacy in a new age' consultation was launched in October 1995, with an invitation to all members to contribute their views to the Council. These were correlated and a follow-up document produced by the Council in September 1996 called 'Pharmacy in a New Age: the New Horizon'. This indicated that there was an overwhelming view amongst pharmacists that the profession cannot stand still. Four main areas in which pharmacy should make a major contribution to health outcomes were identified:

- *The management of prescribed medicines*. This covers drug development, provision of medicines, information and support, and ensuring patient needs are met safely, efficiently and conveniently so that they can get maximum benefit from their medicines.
- *The management of chronic conditions*. Here the need is to improve the quality of life for the patient. Pharmacists may help by supplying medicines and advice, helping to develop local 'shared care' protocols, by ensuring that patients are taking or using their medicines properly and by helping to improve the outcomes of treatment.
- *The management of common ailments*. Patients require reassurance and advice, with or without the use of non-prescription medicines, and referral to other professionals if necessary.
- *The promotion and support of healthy lifestyles*. Pharmacists can help people protect their own health through health screening, giving advice on healthy living and providing educational materials.

During the consultation process, pharmacists expressed their views on the way the profession should change. These, too, may be summarized under four main headings.

- *The strengths of pharmacy*. There was a high level of consensus that the knowledge base of pharmacy was very important. This is based on both the study of and experience with medicines and also in managing the medicines and handling relevant information. A second strength which was seen as important was pharmacists' availability and accessibility in a wide range of different locations, such as conventional business premises, health centres, supermarkets, hospitals and in people's homes. This accessibility is strengthened by easy communication with both patients and other professionals, giving pharmacists a pivotal position. The growth of information technology could be a potential threat to this, although pharmacists are noted for their adaptability.
- *Demonstrating the value of pharmacy*. Pharmacy must claim its rights as a profession and accept the responsibilities which come with this. Thus high standards must be set and achieved. Additionally, evidence must be produced which demonstrates clearly the value of pharmacy in health care. This will require research and professional audit (this is dealt with in Ch. 43). Further support for this development will come from increased continuing educa-

tion and recognition achieved by effective promotion of the profession.

- *Changes in practice*. Three main areas where there could be an increase in services were identified. These are the enhancement of services to patients (advice, counselling, domiciliary visits, health promotion and non-prescription medicine sales), improved relationships with other health care professionals (closer support for prescribers, medicine management, liaison between hospital and community pharmacy and different community pharmacists, training for other professionals and carers), practice research and audit, continuing education and better use of information technology (all required to support the other developments). There was also a high level of support for a reduction in the mechanical aspects of dispensing, sale of non-health-related products and routine paperwork associated with the NHS and business activities.
- *A sustainable future*. These elements could make up a sustainable future for the profession. In particular, pharmacy would be concerned with advice and counselling, dispensing, health promotion, the sale of non-prescription medicines, medicines management and as a 'first port of call' for health care. Some of these may require changes in the setting of pharmaceutical provision and others may require different types of employment for pharmacists. Other changes which would be required included changes to the system of payment under the NHS, a rationalization of pharmacy distribution and at least two pharmacists being employed per community pharmacy.

In conclusion, the Council of the RPSGB agreed to a programme of action over the following 12 months. As this chapter is being written the process is under way. What the outcome will be cannot be predicted. However, it can be seen that there are common threads running through the changes which were recommended by Nuffield and desired by pharmacists. This suggests that progress will be made.

## THE 'EXTENDED ROLE' OF PHARMACISTS

Following the Nuffield Report, many changes have taken place in pharmacy practice. New services have been devised and implemented, often described as the 'extended role'. Some of these have been on an experimental basis, others have been on a larger scale. Part 4 of this book is designed to reflect some of these developments.

Other developments have also occurred. Professional audit was adopted by the medical profession a quarter of a century ago. Pharmacy has now also moved into professional audit. Chapter 43 aims to give the background to the need for audit and the different ways in which it may be carried out. Audit is also an important tool in the raising of standards of service delivery.

The use of guidelines and protocols has increased over recent years. An overview of this is provided in Chapter 31. Again they are a way of increasing the quality of service because they make use of 'best practice' and so pool the knowledge and experience of leading practitioners.

Health services are expensive to run. Governments try to reduce the expenditure as far as possible. Pressure in this respect has increased over recent years. In the UK some medicines have been identified as being ineligible for prescribing on the NHS. The so-called 'Black List' was introduced in 1984 to reduce the size of the NHS bill. Furthermore the introduction of computer technology into prescription pricing has enabled far more data to be produced than was previously possible. Doctors now receive a regular breakdown of their prescribing costs. Chapter 34 considers the use of prescribing data (PACT or SPA) by pharmacists when advising doctors about reducing their prescribing costs.

Unfortunately, there are those in society who wish to misuse drugs. This has been an increasing problem. Pharmacists may be involved in a number of ways, as discussed in Chapter 42. In particular, pharmacists have become involved in needle exchange schemes and in instalment dispensing of methadone. These are important services, but also create a number of potential problems for those offering them.

## CONCLUSION

During the 20th century, pharmacy has undergone major changes. This process has accelerated since the introduction of the NHS in 1948 and further accelerated since the Nuffield Report. Thus pharmacists now deal with more potent and sophisticated medicines, requiring a different type of knowledge than was previously the case. At the same time, the public have become more aware of the services which are available from pharmacists. They are making increasing use of the pharmacist as a source of information and advice about minor conditions and non-prescription medicines. This is now extending to the general public regarding pharmacists as a source of information and advice about their prescribed medicines and seeking help from pharmacists with any medication problems which they may encounter. This process is likely to develop further as society moves into the 21st century. Pharmacists need to have the knowledge and adaptability to take a lead in these processes, so that they can have a key role in ensuring that the health care of the public can be delivered as efficiently as possible.

### Key Points

- The UK NHS came into being on 5 July 1948.
- Early developments in the NHS were in hospital services, but this has gradually changed to focus on community practice.
- Publication of the Nuffield Report in 1986 marked a watershed for pharmacy in the UK.
- Nuffield made nearly 100 specific recommendations for change in all aspects of pharmacy practice, many of which have been implemented.
- In community pharmacy, use of IT, links with GPs, responding to symptoms, health education, meeting patients' needs, re-regulation of POM to P medicines have all developed.
- Clinical pharmacy has developed strongly in hospital, together with a 24-hour cover, increased research and development of specialized services.
- Schools of pharmacy have restructured courses, introduced social and behavioural science, extensively use teacher–practitioners in order to produce pharmacists who are both scientists and practitioners.
- The pre-registration examination at the end of a structured pre-registration year is now well established.
- Continuing education has expanded with the Centres for Postgraduate or Postqualification Pharmaceutical Education being established.
- Practice research is now well established.
- A variety of courses designed to update or develop pharmacists are readily available.
- The RPSGB has sought the views of members on the future development of the profession.

- 'Pharmacy in a new age' identified four areas of contribution to health care – management of medicines, management of chronic conditions, management of common ailments and health promotion.
- The process has produced a vision for the future of the profession.
- Professional audit is a tool to improve the quality of service provided by pharmacy.

## FURTHER READING

Committee of Inquiry 1986 Pharmacy: A report to the Nuffield Foundation. Nuffield Foundation, London

Department of Health 1996 Choice and opportunity. Primary care: the future. Department of Health, London

Medicines, Ethics and Practice – a guide for pharmacists, current edn. Royal Pharmaceutical Society of Great Britain, London (Updated twice yearly)

Royal Pharmaceutical Society of Great Britain 1996 Pharmacy in a new age: the new horizon. RPSGB, London

Steering Group and Working Group of Clinical Resources Audit Group 1996 Clinical pharmacy in the hospital pharmaceutical service: a framework for practice. Scottish Office Health Department, Edinburgh

Weller P J (ed) Pharmacists' directory and yearbook, current edn. Royal Pharmaceutical Society of Great Britain, London (Updated annually)

# 2
# Social and behavioural aspects of pharmacy

*E. J. Kennedy*    *This chapter draws heavily on Harding et al (1990)*

---

After studying this chapter you will know about:

**The importance of social and behavioural sciences to pharmacy**
**Concepts of health and illness**
**Patients' responses to ill health**
**Ideas about the causes of illness**
**Social class and health**
**Compliance, change of behaviour and the placebo effect**
**The nature of and relationships between professions**
**The pharmacy–medicine interface**.

## Introduction

There has been an increased interest in aspects of social and behavioural science, and how these subject areas relate to the practice of pharmacy. The aims of this chapter are to give an understanding of the nature of behavioural sciences and their application to pharmacy and to enable the reader to appreciate sociological factors in relation to provision of health care, including pharmacy.

The topics of interpersonal skills and communication are covered in Chapter 3.

## DEFINING SOCIAL AND BEHAVIOURAL SCIENCES

The social sciences are very different from the more traditional sciences of chemistry and biology that are associated with pharmacy and medically related subjects. They are often viewed as a 'soft' science with no relevance to pharmacy, but there are, in fact, many important applications. Behavioural science describes the scientific study of human behaviour and is associated with disciplines such as psychology and sociology. The teaching of aspects of behavioural science, such as interpersonal and communication skills, has a significant part to play in the training of pharmacists. These skills when acquired equip the pharmacist to deliver a professional service that is patient orientated.

Sociology attempts to explain an individual's actions and relates this to the society in which the individual lives. It is a broad-ranging discipline and involves interpreting and understanding behaviour in various contexts. Sociology when applied to medicine is concerned specifically with those aspects of the relationship between society and the individual which influence the experiences of health and illness. This includes the way individuals respond to health and illness and to other people, including relatives, doctors, nurses and pharmacists. Our attitudes to health and illness are socially derived. An important part of the study of sociology in health is to investigate how they arose, how they are maintained and their implications for health and the health services. An appreciation of sociology in relation to pharmacy will help us to meet patients' needs, for example understanding that not all individuals will take the same action following the occurrence of symptoms. Medical sociology can give an insight into the individual's responses to illness through an appreciation of how patients' feelings about their health and illness arise, the motivations and constraints that have an influence on their using or not using of medicines and the health care services.

Psychology studies human behaviour. Many aspects of psychology are relevant to pharmacy and medicine, including understanding the patient's response to illness and treatments, and relationships between doctors and pharmacists and patients. Psychological factors can also play a large part in some physical and psychological disorders. For example, smoking can result in serious medical disorders, yet this is something that people will choose to do themselves. There are also illnesses which are seen to arise from the adverse way in which people respond to environmental factors, for example stress can be linked to incidence of heart disease. Psychological approaches to treatment are currently being explored, not just in psychiatric illness, but in, for example, attempts to alter eating behaviour in the treatment of cardiovascular disease.

## HEALTH AND ILLNESS AS SOCIAL CONCEPTS

There is a wide diversity in what lay people perceive as being 'healthy'. Many factors will affect these perceptions, such as age, physical disabilities and socioeconomic status. To one person, being healthy might mean feeling happy and getting on well with other people most of the time. To another person it might mean hardly ever going to the doctor and having a body that is in good working condition. Comparing what is important to different people about being healthy can often be the start of interesting debate and discussion. It all stems from differing expectations and perceptions of 'health'. Perceptions are directly related to previous experiences and therefore can become an assumptive process. This is illustrated by examining individual differences in response to pain. Parental responses to pain can determine how a child reacts to and copes with pain. Changes in mood or motivational state can affect perception. For example, anxious or depressed patients will selectively attend to and notice more anxiety-related stimuli than control subjects, indicating that underlying emotional state biases processing of incoming information. Perceptions of health will be affected by what an individual perceives as normal. Anything that upsets this, such as illness, upsets this state of normality that is unique for each individual.

An understanding of health as a social concept will help us to appreciate who will be most likely to seek help from the pharmacist when they suffer from symptoms and also has implications for implementing effective strategies on health promotion and education.

Health is commonly described as the absence of disease. This definition is narrow and ignores the social contribution to health. The World Health Organization (WHO) defines health as 'a state of complete physical, mental and social well-being'. This definition recognizes that health is far more than medical well-being and that social factors contribute an important part to being healthy. Public health is aimed at ensuring that the conditions in which people can be healthy exist. This includes, for example, standards of housing and food as well as health issues when travelling.

Illness is not easy to define. In a social context, illness may be described as the experience of feeling unwell (irrespective of medical diagnosis or intervention). A disease is an organic or biological phenomenon, such as a cancerous growth or chickenpox. The relationship between health and illness has been stated by Helman (1981) as 'Disease is something an organ has: illness is something a man has'. This illustrates that a person may be diagnosed as suffering from a disease, but may not regard him- or herself as 'ill'. Sociologists have carried out further research into illness and illness behaviour, which will be described in more detail later in this chapter.

## RESPONSES TO ILL HEALTH

When people experience symptoms, they may act in a number of ways. Essentially they may consider a range of actions, including ignoring the symptoms, consulting friends and family, self-medication and so on. They do not always seek help from a health care professional and when they do, it may be a pharmacist, general practitioner, dentist or other professional. There are a large number of factors which influence whether a person seeks professional help or not. Patients, when deciding whether to consult a health care professional will compare the relative costs and benefits of such an action. Pharmacists, for example, are often consulted when patients have decided to self-medicate, or to sanction a visit to a doctor.

### The symptom iceberg

The decision to seek the help of health care professionals is not always related to the severity of symptoms. A group of patients has been identified who fail to go to the doctor, or attend at very late stages, even when experiencing symptoms of serious disease. Those symptoms that are not reported to health care professionals are described as the 'symptom iceberg'. At the other extreme, there are patients who report trivial and minor complaints to the doctor which they could probably self-treat effectively.

Many studies have been carried out to determine how often people suffer from symptoms. Results range from symptoms being suffered on 1 day in 3, through to at least one symptom in a 2-week period. Symptoms are therefore commonly experienced and most are transient or forgotten. Action in response to symptoms varies and includes taking no action, consulting family or friends, taking a remedy that is already at home (prescription medicine, over-the-counter (OTC) medicine or a home remedy), buying an OTC remedy or seeing a doctor or dentist. What, then, makes a person decide to seek help from a health care professional? 'Illness behaviour' is a concept used to describe the steps that people go through in order to decide that they are 'ill'.

## Illness behaviour

People interpret their symptoms in terms of the perceived danger to them. We have already established that people frequently suffer from background symptoms, so it is the unusual or atypical symptoms which might precipitate action in an individual. Illness behaviour describes the way in which given symptoms may be differently perceived, evaluated and acted upon (or not acted upon) by different kinds of persons. According to Zola (1973), people's assessment of symptoms may be broken down into five 'social triggers':

1. Perceived interference with vocational or physical activity. If symptoms interfere with normal life, then they are abnormal.

2. Perceived interference with social or personal relations. If symptoms interfere with a person's normal pattern of social interaction, which will vary according to lifestyle, then they are likely to cause concern.

3. The occurrence of an interpersonal crisis. A change in personal relationships or a domestic crisis may change the perception a person has of a symptom.

4. A kind of temporalizing of symptomatology. The symptom may not interfere with normal life, but may still be seen as unusual and something that the person wants to investigate further. People will often set time deadlines or frequency deadlines; for example, 'If this does not clear up by next week, I'll see the doctor'. The pharmacist can help to advise on deadlines for when to seek further help.

5. Sanctioning. This refers to pressure from friends or relatives to visit the doctor. The pharmacist is also often called upon to sanction a visit to the doctor.

A visit to a doctor or pharmacist may fulfil a number of functions:

1. *Therapeutic benefit*. People often have their own perception of the treatment that the pharmacist or doctor can offer and this can influence their decision about whether and whom to consult.

2. *Recognition of the sick role*. A visit to a health care professional often legitimizes an 'illness' making it recognizable and socially acceptable.

## Sick role behaviour

A well-recognized theory, defined by Parsons (1951), suggests that, when suffering from an illness, an individual behaves in order to facilitate recovery. These behaviours may include absence from work, avoiding normal social contacts and responsibilities and seeking medical help. This social state is named the 'sick role'. There are certain criteria which must be met before society will accept that it is appropriate for the individual to behave in such a way:

- Society must recognize the disorder as an illness. A consultation with a doctor or pharmacist will help to legitimize this.
- There should be something to validate the difficulty, for example a physical symptom or an expert opinion.
- It has to be accepted by the individual concerned.

Individuals do not always assume the sick role in response to illness. There are various ways in which people respond in terms of the sick role:

- They may adopt the sick role readily, and surrender it on recovery.
- They are reluctant to adopt the sick role, but when they do they are reluctant to surrender it.
- They do not adopt it at all.
- They adopt the sick role and do not give it up.

Many factors are involved in the adoption of the sick role, including family commitments and work pressure. When people accept the sick role, they gain two benefits but are expected to fulfil two obligations. These are:

### Benefits

1. The person is temporarily excused from his/her normal role in society.

2. The patient is not responsible for the illness. Society places no feeling of failure or guilt on someone who has to seek help from a doctor about an illness. This may change in the future, as the emphasis on preventive medicine and health promotion continues. People are being encouraged to take responsibility for their own health. Therefore, people may

feel guilty about visiting the doctor about illnesses which could be perceived as being self-inflicted, for example lung cancer from a lifetime of cigarette smoking.

### Obligations

1. The patient must want to get well; that is, the sick role is a temporary status. It is easy to see members of society offering sympathy and support to those who communicate a desire to get well.

2. The patient must seek and cooperate with technically competent help; that is, the medical services.

There are two dimensions to the sick role: vulnerability and deviance. Patients must be protected in society because of their weakness. On the other hand, society needs to guard against the risk that the sickness is a device for evading social obligations. The sick role could be interpreted as being a means of stabilizing society as it emphasizes an individual's obligations and duties in society. In this interpretation, medical staff would take on a social role in monitoring and controlling the sick role and guiding people back to their customary social roles. This, however, does not seem to be the case in the social concept of medicine. Physicians still emphasize the organic origins of illness and motivating patients to get better is not always a priority in the National Health Service of today. The sick role does not apply very well to chronic illnesses as sufferers are often unable to meet all the obligations.

## Help-seeking behaviour

A lay referral system, which refers to the network of colleagues, relations and friends which a sufferer may consult, is often used when deciding whether or not to seek help from professionals about health problems. The extent of close-knit social relations and the attitudes of the lay referral system to the professional help available will influence the help-seeking behaviour. High users of health care professionals' services are likely to have views that are compatible with those of the health care professionals and to come from stable communities. Research has shown that the social environment can play a significant role in determining the frequency with which health care professionals are consulted. For example, women who live close to friends rather than family will be more frequent users of health care services than women who live close to their families. A person is likely to consult a health professional when the perceived benefits outweigh the perceived costs.

### The 'health belief model'

Health care professionals assume that people will seek help when they are suffering from symptoms which cause them discomfort or anxiety. However, good health is not always a priority for an individual who, for example, may have children to look after or ill relatives to care for. The 'health belief model' attempts to bring together all the demographic and psychological factors which will influence an individual's assessment of costs and benefits involved in seeking help. These factors are:

- Health motivation – the level of interest an individual expresses in health issues
- Susceptibility – the individual's perceived vulnerability to illness
- Severity – the perceived seriousness of certain illnesses
- Benefits and costs – the perceived value of taking health actions.

As health educators, pharmacists can use this model to assess perceptions and identify ways in which behaviour can be changed. However, this assumes that people will follow a health care professional's advice about behaviour change.

A visit to a doctor will often result in treatment or therapy, which the sufferer hopes will reduce the symptoms. However, a diagnosis is not always possible and treatments are not always available. A second reason for a visit to the doctor is that the doctor has the social and legal authority to legitimize the status of the patient, for example by issuing a 'sick note' to enable an employee to take sick leave from employment and receive Sickness Benefit. The doctor becomes an agent of social control, helping to maintain social order. A visit to a doctor may also allow the person to seek advice and reassurance about physical or mental states. Doctors are regarded as having a high status in society and are often called upon to give advice on emotional and social issues.

It is important to appreciate that people will often seek help from a pharmacist before they seek help from a doctor. Pharmacists, therefore, have an important potential impact to make on the symptom iceberg. They can help to treat the minor, self-limiting symptoms and refer the more serious symptoms to the doctor. People may also feel that they can ask the pharmacist about symptoms that have been bothering them but which they feel would be 'troubling' the doctor. The profile of the pharmacist as a source of health advice and for treatment of minor ailments has been emphasized to the public with publicity campaigns such as those introduced by the National Pharmaceutical Association (NPA). Symptoms that are presented to a community pharmacist are most likely to be perceived by the patient as trivial and self-treatable. More severe or particularly acute symptoms will most likely present to a GP or a hospital-based medical practitioner. Pharmacists are readily available and accessible, without the need to make an appointment. This gives people a more opportune way to obtain health care advice than making an appointment with a doctor, often during work time, leading to loss of earnings and other inconveniences. Therefore, people may choose to self-medicate and obtain relevant advice from the pharmacist on the most appropriate treatment. In some instances the pharmacist can reassure people that the symptoms that they are suffering from do warrant a visit to a medical practitioner, thereby sanctioning the initial transition to a sick role. Instructions from the pharmacist on how to take medicine which might help them to 'get better', also contribute to the obligations of the sick role that patients take on after seeking medical help and obtaining treatment. Patients can also seek clarification on medication-related matters from pharmacists.

## THE DOCTOR–PATIENT RELATIONSHIP

There are different types of doctor–patient relationships (based on the degree of control exercised by both doctors and patients). In the sick role the patient is passive and obedient. However, Szasz & Hollender (1956) suggested three different types of relationship:

1. *Activity–passivity*: the doctor is active and the patient is a passive recipient of medical treatment and advice
2. *Cooperation–guidance*: the doctor guides the patient, who cooperates
3. *Mutual participation*: where both doctor and patient negotiate and share the crucial decisions.

The last of these three models is probably the most applicable to community pharmacy, because the patient is usually seeking help in order to practise self-care. It should be noted that the above models have a 'consensual' approach, with the doctor and the patient sharing a common agenda. However, conflict models also exist to explain doctor–patient relationships. Freidson has pointed out that conventional doctor–patient consultations are doctor cen-

tred, with the doctor treating another clinical case. This might differ from the perspective of the patient, to whom the illness is a unique, personal experience. Community pharmacists may encounter similar conflict in their interactions with patients when the agenda is not the same. For example, a pharmacist may recognize that a patient needs to be referred to a doctor for further investigation of treatments, but the patient may not want to go to a doctor and intends to self-treat. Doctors are now trying to elicit the patients' views of their illness so that their perspectives can be addressed. Community pharmacists can also usefully utilize this approach, establishing the reason why someone has chosen to consult them in order to meet the person's needs. This could be regarded as a negotiation model and derives from the conflict model. In summary, the nature of the doctor–patient relationship is strongly related to the way in which illness is defined; that is, whether the social and psychological aspects of the illness are taken into account as well as the biological effects.

## SOCIAL CAUSES OF ILLNESS

In some cultures a sinful life or weak moral character was believed to result in disease. In the western world, from the 18th to the early 20th centuries, disease was believed to arise as a direct consequence of specific causal agents. This was known as the 'doctrine of specific aetiology' (Dubos 1959). It has become increasingly evident, however, that social factors have a strong influence on the biological causes of many illnesses. Claims that the decline in death rate that occurred in the 18th and 19th centuries was wholly due to medical intervention have been disputed. Critics state that access to other interventions such as better housing, food and hygiene have a significant influence. These are the environmental and social factors which result in improvements to health. Two approaches to health and disease have consequently been described: the medical model and the socioenvironmental model.

### The medical model of health and disease

The 'germ theory' of disease arose as a result of the discovery of the microbiological origins of some diseases. This theory is loosely termed the 'medical model'. The assumptions are that a disease can be traced to a specific aetiology and that the patient's body can be treated like a machine, made better through medical 'engineering' (Harding, Nettleton and Taylor 1990). This monocausal approach still dominates medicine, especially in medical research.

## The socioenvironmental model of disease

This model emphasizes the environmental and behavioural changes which can help production and maintenance of good health. People are, therefore, not regarded as passive victims of disease as in the medical model, but can themselves contribute to their good health. It is a multicausal model of disease, approaches within which include the 'epidemiological triangle' and the 'web of causation'. The epidemiological triangle approach sees disease as the product of an interaction between an agent, a host and the environment. The concept of the web of causation states that disorders such as arthritis or heart disease develop through complex interactions of many factors, which may be social, physical or psychological. Thus both models emphasize that health cannot be separated from the social environment in which a person lives.

## Causal models

It is important to understand the concept of cause in the relationships between factors. Causality is a complex idea which in its simplest form, states that if change in one variable brings about change in another then the former causes the latter. This could be expressed as $A \rightarrow B$, where A is the cause and B the effect; for example, wearing a watch causes a contact dermatitis on the wrist. For the vast majority of diseases the actual causal system is much more complex where a whole sequence of events may be linked to a final cause. Consider heart disease, where a poor diet could lead to a high cholesterol level which in turn could lead to heart disease. This will not be the only factor, as hereditary factors and exercise are two other recognized factors.

Establishing a causal relationship can be difficult, because a simple correlation of variables alone will not establish a causal relationship. They must occur in a temporal sequence. That is, the independent variable, A, must precede in time the dependent variable, B. This is not always easy to prove. For example, it may be suggested that an individual has become depressed as a result of losing his* job, or an equally plausible suggestion would be that depres-sion resulted in an inability to work and therefore, loss of job. Also, there must not be a third spurious variable. This often complicates the establishment of a causal relationship.

## Locus of control in health

The extent to which individuals have control over their health depends on a number of interrelated elements. The first element depends on their theories about disease and causation, and the extent to which their actions, or actions of others, have an effect on their health. The second element is the extent to which they feel they have control over the activities which are claimed to cause disease states, such as the individual's ability to give up smoking. Thirdly, there are beliefs and feelings about responsibility in the protection of health. Lay beliefs on these three elements need to be addressed for successful health education and health promotion programmes.

## Social inequalities in health

As Britain became more industrialized in the 19th and 20th centuries, the death rate declined and the life span increased. It was the social and economic changes that industrialization brought which resulted in the improvement in health. The examination of how health is distributed in the population, and linking these observations with socioeconomic factors, gives an insight into how health is a product of society.

### Defining social class

Statistics from the early 19th century illustrate that health varied with social class, with the average age of death of gentlemen being 45 years, tradesmen being 26 years and that of mechanics, servants and labourers being 16 years. This relationship between mortality and social class still remains, but before further consideration, it is important to understand what is meant by social class.

Social class refers to the form which social stratification takes in society. It can be defined in a number of ways; one of these divides the population into a series of layers representing different social and economic power. An example that is quoted commonly in research reports is the Registrar General's classification system in the UK which is based on occupation. The population is divided into five social classes, I to V, with social class III being further sub-divided into non-manual (IIIN) and manual (IIIM). Table 2.1 gives examples of the

---

* The masculine pronoun is used here and hereafter to refer, where appropriate, to both sexes.

social class classifications, from which it can be seen that there are three non-manual and three manual classes. The non-manual classes are often referred to as the middle classes or white collar workers and the manual classes as working class or blue collar workers. The allocation to a class is based on a man's occupation and married women are allocated to a particular social class on the basis of their husband's occupation, children on their father's and the retired and unemployed on that of their last significant period of employment. Single women are classified on the basis of their own occupation. There are problems with this method of classification. One example is that inadequate account is taken of women's employment. The classification is also based on status rather than on economic standing, for example social class II includes the manager of a small local shop as well as the manager of a large multinational company.

Inequalities in health are related to social class from birth through to adulthood. A standardized mortality ratio (SMR) indicates the incidence of mortality for each social class. It is a measure of the extent to which the mortality rate of each social class deviates from the average (100) of the age group as a whole. Mortality rates increase as one moves from social class I to social class V. This trend can be shown for various causes of death, as illustrated in Table 2.2. The life expectancy of a male infant born to parents in social class I is 72.19 years compared to 65.02 years for his counterpart in social class V.

The use of data which are based on causes of death is useful because it is a complete and reliable measure. Health, however, cannot be accurately measured by examining mortality rates alone, especially since many chronic conditions, such as arthritis or depression,

**Table 2.2  Social class and main causes of death in England and Wales (1979–80, 1982–83): standardized mortality rations (OPCS 1986)**

| Causes of death | I | II | IIIN | IIIM | IV | V |
|---|---|---|---|---|---|---|
| **Males 20–64 years** | | | | | | |
| Ischaemic heart disease | 69 | 81 | 102 | 106 | 110 | 137 |
| Lung cancer | 42 | 62 | 78 | 117 | 125 | 175 |
| Cerebrovascular disease | 61 | 70 | 88 | 105 | 114 | 171 |
| Bronchitis | 34 | 49 | 84 | 109 | 134 | 208 |
| Motor-vehicle accidents | 64 | 75 | 79 | 101 | 114 | 175 |
| Pneumonia | 34 | 49 | 80 | 89 | 121 | 211 |
| Suicide | 86 | 78 | 94 | 84 | 110 | 190 |
| **Females 20–59 years** | | | | | | |
| Ischaemic heart disease | 41 | 55 | 69 | 106 | 119 | 152 |
| Breast cancer | 107 | 103 | 105 | 100 | 99 | 94 |
| Cerebrovascular disease | 58 | 69 | 79 | 105 | 117 | 144 |
| Bronchitis | 33 | 54 | 71 | 100 | 119 | 165 |
| Motor-vehicle accidents | 76 | 89 | 102 | 63 | 94 | 114 |
| Pneumonia | 37 | 51 | 67 | 86 | 110 | 140 |
| Suicide | 77 | 81 | 99 | 55 | 76 | 84 |

rarely cause death. Morbidity (illness) measures, which are often less reliable but are a more valid measure of health, are beginning to be employed to study the relationship of health with social class. Researchers into heart disease have found that manual workers are more likely to experience angina than non-manual workers and that similar differences appeared with obesity and, to a lesser extent, blood pressure.

## Dimensions of social inequality

Dimensions of social inequality in the UK include working conditions, living conditions and wealth and income. Differences in wealth and income result in differences in, for example, diet, possessions and housing. The diet of those on low wages contains less fresh fruit and vegetables and fresh fish but contains more processed foods, white bread and fats when compared to the diet of those with higher wages. Poor housing, such as lack of basic hygiene facilities, lack of gardens or poor repair, is strongly related to income. Working conditions will also differ according to social class and will also have implications for health. Manual work is usually more physically demanding, noisy and dangerous than non-manual work. There is also the increased likelihood of the physical and mental disruption of shift

**Table 2.1  The Registrar General's classification of social classes**

| Social class | | Examples of occupation |
|---|---|---|
| I | Professional | Doctor, lawyer, pharmacist |
| II | Intermediate | Teacher, sales manager, nurse |
| IIIN | Skilled non-manual | Secretary, shop assistant, clerical worker |
| IIIM | Skilled manual | Bus driver, carpenter, electrician |
| IV | Semi-skilled manual | Postman, bus conductor |
| V | Unskilled | General labourer, cleaner, porter |

work, shorter holidays and repetitive work offering little variety which leads to close supervision and stricter discipline for manual workers.

Unemployment can have various effects on well-being. There are both psychological and material effects of unemployment. For a few, unemployment will release them from potentially hazardous work and stress and give them sufficient income to live, producing effects beneficial to health. For the vast majority, unemployment results in a loss of income and loss of self-esteem, causing anxiety and harmful effects on health. There is a relationship between ill health and unemployment, although this may not be a causal relationship. A large proportion of those who are unemployed are likely to be working class, who are already more likely to have health problems than those from a higher social class. Comparisons between those who are employed and unemployed in social class V have been carried out to investigate this (so that mortality differences found will be independent of social class). When this is done, there is still a 20–30% excess mortality in the unemployed. Alternatively, ill health may actually result in unemployment, which would indicate a causal link. Conclusive evidence for this does not exist, as it is extremely difficult to disentangle all the many variables which will have an effect on ill health and unemployment. The relationship between ill health and unemployment, however, cannot be ignored. The needs of the unemployed should be taken into account when planning provision of health care and health promotion activities.

## Poverty and health

Comparing the health of the members of the different social classes, or manual and non-manual workers ignores the fact that there are considerable differences in income and living conditions within each class. The term 'poverty' can be used in two ways. Absolute poverty refers to a standard of living which is incapable of sustaining life. This definition does not state how long people can live before they are incapable of sustaining life. This is important as periods of malnutrition will not kill a person instantly, but can have implications for mortality rates later on in life. Relative poverty refers to a standard of living below that which is considered normal or acceptable by the members of a particular society. This is the type of poverty which is referred to in reports and research in the western world. The term 'poverty line' is often used to describe what is considered normal or acceptable in society. Alternatively, an income below the State's Supplementary Benefit

rate can be used to establish relative poverty. A sizeable proportion of the UK population is classed as living in relative poverty, the largest groups of whom have been identified as those on low wages, in casual work, the disabled and long-term sick. There is a general pattern to a person's life stage and standard of living. It is lowest during childhood, active parenthood and old age and highest during the intervening stages. This pattern highlights the fact that there is usually an association between childhood and poverty. Further, a child who is reared in poverty is educationally disadvantaged and subsequently will usually enter the unskilled sector of the labour market. This will in turn give low wages and probably lack of financial provision for retirement, predisposing to poverty at this life stage.

The patterns of poverty during the life cycle overlap considerably with the patterns of health problems. This is clearly illustrated by examining the numbers of prescriptions which are exempt from charges. These can be between 75 and 90%, depending on the area. Children under 16 years of age, men and women over 60 years of age and those on income support or family credit are the largest groups who are exempt from prescription charges. Problems that arise due to poverty can cause medical problems, and these include:

- Poor nutrition: low birth weights, abnormal growth and development of children
- Lack of hygienic facilities: infestations of head lice and scabies
- Damp housing: upper respiratory tract infections and complications arising from this such as deafness or absence from school and work, hypothermia
- Lack of play facilities: poor psychological development, increased risk of accidents
- Attempts to maximize income: hazardous jobs, exhaustion from second job or overtime, disruption of family life, stress, depression.

Doctors are likely to treat many people for the same problems who are classed as being in relative poverty.

## Gender and health

There are gender differences in health in our society. There are higher morbidity rates amongst women than men although mortality rates are higher for men. In summary, this means that women get ill, but men die. This contradictory state of health has been investigated by sociologists, as the difference is likely to be a social one. One possibility is that men and women suffer from different types of illnesses, with those that cause death being more common in men, such as heart disease. Another is that women may report illness more often than men, who tend to view illness as a sign of weakness, which would lead to visits to the doctor and days off work. Men are more likely to take risks with their health, whereas women are more likely to adopt preventive measures to promote good health. Men may be more likely to indulge in activities which may harm their health (such as smoking and drinking alcohol) which, combined with possible stress caused by their lifestyle (which tends to be more competitive and aggressive), can lead to a higher incidence of fatal diseases. Women are susceptible to different stressors as a result of their traditional role in society and will be more likely to suffer from psychiatric illness. These gender roles are not fixed, but their effects are evident in today's society.

## Ethnicity and health

Each ethnic group pursues its different lifestyle, which can lead to different aetiology of illness when comparing different ethnic groups to the white population in the western world. The ethnic origin of a person may affect his/her life chances owing to possible discrimination or prejudice. This will result in restricted opportunities and lifestyle, demonstrating that social factors have a major part to play in determining the health of the ethnic population. Whilst research has focused on particular diseases, it is important to realize that the everyday health problems suffered by black people are the same as those suffered by white people (Donovan 1984). There are some illnesses which are a product of inheritance, and therefore more common in particular ethnic groups, for example sickle cell anaemia. Other illnesses which are particularly associated with ethnic groups can be more clearly associated with material factors, for example rickets is linked to diet and tuberculosis to poor housing conditions.

## Age and health

Overall mortality is linked to age, with rates being relatively high in infants under 1 year of age, then declining rapidly before rates increase again after middle age, with a steep increase in the elderly. Specific diseases can be associated with deaths at particular ages, for example leukaemia is a disease causing death in childhood, whilst cancer and ischaemic heart disease are more likely to cause death in old age in the western world. Ageing brings

about physiological changes which will result in an increased incidence of illnesses, but social factors in old age also have a significant role to play in determining health. Some of the changes that occur are accepted as biological in origin, such as cancers and increase in blood pressure. Environmental and cultural conditions may, however, have an effect on the existence of these, as with smoking. Diet and exercise are regarded as activities which could delay the onset of certain cancers or help to maintain normal blood pressure. The reaction of society to old people may also have an effect. It is often assumed that as people get older they want to 'disengage' from life's normal activities and society will treat old people accordingly. This may have a damaging effect on health, particularly mental health, as loneliness and bereavement are often encountered by older people.

Elderly patients may have more problems with compliance as there is a gradual decline in normal cognitive processes with age. Poor memory and reduced ability to read and understand text on medicine bottles are possible results which will not help compliance with medical treatment.

## The relationship between social inequalities and health

What causes these differences in health amongst the different social classes? It is a difficult relationship to explain, as there are many possible causal links. Also, correlations which seem to exist may be incidental and so false assumptions should not be made. The relationship between health and social class can be explored by looking at four possible explanations, first developed by the Department of Health's Working Party report on inequalities in health (known as the 'Black Report'):

1. *Artefact*. This suggests that social class differences in mortality rates can be explained by the difference in precision when describing semi-skilled and unskilled manual occupations on death registration compared to the descriptions on the census form. This explanation has been subsequently rejected, although such variations in accuracy of reporting may have some small effects on the social class differences recorded.

2. *Social selection*. This hypothesis states that health determines social class through a process of health-related social mobility. In this the healthy are more likely to move up the social hierarchy and the unhealthy to move down. This explanation is potentially applicable during the first half of life,

when social mobility is more likely, but the contribution of health to social class differences is probably small.

3. *Behavioural/cultural.* This explanation emphasizes social class differences in behaviours which damage, or fail to promote, health and are, in theory, subject to individual choice. Examples include consumption of highly processed food and alcohol, tobacco smoking and use of preventive medical services, such as family planning and immunizations.

4. *Materialist.* This explanation concentrates on the hazards which are inherent in society and to which people have no choice but to be exposed, given the present distribution of income and opportunity. Examples include damp housing and hazardous working conditions as discussed previously.

The influence of the behavioural/cultural effects combined with the materialist effects are probably the most important when considering the relationship between health and social class. The chapter on health promotion (Ch. 38) deals with the ways in which some of these problems are being addressed in society today.

## COPING WITH ILLNESS

Illness tends to be defined as a physical problem, but there can be profound psychological and social effects. Major health problems can lead to stress and anxiety in individuals and their families. The way in which the illness is perceived will be important in the psychological handling of the problem and how it is subsequently dealt with. Acute illness tends to be the least difficult to cope with as it is, by definition, a temporary situation.

Chronic illness will tend to require more readjustments to life by the patient and any immediate carers, because a chronic illness is long term. People with chronic illness will tend to be on regular medical treatment designed to control their symptoms. The pharmacist can develop supportive relationships with sufferers of chronic illness and offer advice and reassurance on their medical treatments, so that this potential worry is alleviated for them. Other problems that they face are:

- *Uncertainty.* Diagnosis is often delayed, and uncertainty may also follow with respect to the course and outcome of the disease.
- *Family relations.* Strain on relations can be caused by the high level of support and care often required.

- *Biographical work and reconstitution of self.* Chronic disabling conditions pose a threat to identity and self-concept. Individuals will often try to identify the cause of the disease in their life, as part of the process of coming to terms with it.
- *Managing medical regimens.* Daily life is often adapted to cope with the demands of the disease. This often includes the management of treatment, which may be drugs, diet or other interventions, such as the physiotherapy employed in cystic fibrosis management or dialysis machines in renal failure.
- *Information, awareness and sharing.* Information reduces uncertainty and helps the individual come to terms with the illness. Self-help groups are often important sources for sharing information.

## Labelling and stigmatization

A diagnostic label can lead to a behaviour change. For example, once children receive a diagnosis of asthma from their doctor, research has shown that they receive adequate treatment to manage their condition. Diagnostic labels can also bring unwelcome consequences for patients, especially when the condition is personally or socially stigmatizing. Stigmatizing conditions can be defined as those that set their possessors apart from 'normal' people. This marks them as socially unacceptable or inferior beings. Examples of such conditions are acquired immunodeficiency syndrome (AIDS), psoriasis and mental illness. Deviance can be defined as non-conformity to a norm or set of norms, which is accepted by a significant proportion of local citizens. Sometimes the deviant state becomes the dominant state for an individual. For example, a person may be regarded as a diabetic rather than a teacher.

There are various methods with which people attempt to cope with stigmatizing conditions. A stigma may be obvious immediately, in which case it is described as 'discredited'. Alternatively a stigma may be hidden with relative ease and is described as 'discreditable'. People with such a stigma will often have to cope with tension, for example when encountering people for the first time. They may try to avoid situations where their stigma will be emphasized, possibly leading to a withdrawal from social life. Attempts may also be made to disguise the stigma, for example by using make-up to cover an obvious skin disfiguration. Those who have a discreditable stigma will have to manage information; that is, censoring what other people know about them. Sometimes they will try to pass themselves as 'normal', but this can cause considerable psychological tension. For example, someone suffering from epilepsy, who does not disclose the condition to work colleagues, lives with the fear of a seizure whilst at work.

## Stress

In a lifetime everyone faces many difficult situations and personal crises. People learn to adapt, in order to cope with such difficulties and attempt to find a solution to the problems. Different events will evoke varying amounts of stress in different people. Some life events, such as the death of a spouse or close family member, divorce and personal illness, are widely recognized as important potential stressors.

The term 'stress' is used to cover many meanings. It can be used to describe events or situations that are considered to be stressful. Alternatively it can be used to describe behavioural or physiological responses which occur in response to a threatening situation or stressor. Another view is that stress is a reflection of an incompatibility between the individual and his or her environment. There are physiological and psychological responses to stress. The James–Lange theory attempts to explain the relationship between physiological events and emotional feelings. It states that emotional feelings consist of the perception of the physiological changes initiated by the emotional stimulus. Physiological correlates of behaviour are being researched widely in psychology and may lead to more successful treatment of some psychiatric disorders.

Response to stress will vary greatly from person to person. Factors that influence an individual's response to stress include:

- *Prior experience*. If people have experienced a stressful environment during their childhood development, they are more likely to be able to cope with a stressful situation later in life. Specific experiences of stressful situations also lead to an improved ability to cope with that situation if experienced again.
- *Information*. Information allows the individual to develop adaptive reactions. For example, information about surgical procedures can aid the patient's recovery process.
- *Individual differences*. The underlying personality of a person will be important in determining his or her specific reactions to stress. A personality measure that can be used is the concept of 'locus of control'. This refers to the degree of control individuals see themselves as having over a situation. Those with an internal locus of control are less likely to be emo-

tionally disrupted than those who have an external locus of control.
- *Perceived control*. Distressing situations are likely to be those where individuals feel they can do nothing to alter the outcome and therefore have a lack of control.
- *Social support*. Support from the family or community can help individuals cope with stressful situations and reduce the impact of the stressor on them.

## Stress and illness

In some people, the response to stress may result in illness. The term 'psychosomatic' disease is often used to describe this type of stress-induced illness (although it is often in the wrong context). Psychosomatic illnesses are often not regarded as real, or are used to cover a whole range of illnesses which may be linked to emotion. A study, entitled 'Broken Heart', demonstrated that in the year following the death of their wives, widowers were subject to an increased risk of dying themselves. The authors of the study concluded that the stress of losing their wives was a serious risk factor for heart disease and therefore there may be some truth in the myth that some people die of a broken heart. Theories surrounding this and similar research have claimed that social variables such as marital status and personal support are important for a person's physical well-being.

The relationship between stress and illness is a complex one. There have been certain psychosocial situations which have been identified as leading to an increased vulnerability to illness as a consequence of stress. These include the following:

- *Social class*.
- *Occupational factors*.
- *Lifestyle*. Work has centred on the links between the Type A/B personality dimension and coronary heart disease. The Type A personality, who is competitive, striving and has a time-pressured lifestyle, is more likely to suffer coronary heart disease than Type B individuals who are more relaxed and calm.
- *Life change or 'events'*. High levels of life changes, especially those which have a negative effect, can be correlated to the onset of illness.
- *Bereavement and loss*. The way in which individuals cope with the loss of a close friend or relative will be important in determining their vulnerability to subsequent illness.

Psychological treatments are often used to help people cope with stress-related illnesses, such as teaching relaxation techniques and stress management training. As pharmacists it will be important to recognize the effects of stress on health. Advice on lifestyle and relaxation within the context of health promotion will be significant.

## Personality

Personality differences will lead to differing responses to illness and treatment. In psychology, there are many theories which attempt to explain human behaviour and personality.

Each of us will act instinctively as well as acquiring learned behaviour. Behavioural theories of personality attempt to explain the various learning and conditioning processes that shape and determine behaviour. The behavioural approach alone is accepted as being simplistic, and cognitive factors, that is, an individual's thoughts, anticipations and expectations are being increasingly incorporated into more flexible explanations of behaviour.

A well-known cognitive theory is that our behaviour is determined by our perception and interpretation of our interactions with others, rather than the interactions themselves. Each person behaves according to a system of construing, based on how he or she interprets the particular situation. This is referred to as the 'personal construct' theory.

According to the 'locus of control' theory, an individual's perceptions can be seen as dividing people into those who see their actions as having a significant influence over their lives (internal locus of control) and those who see outside influences as having the major impact (external locus of control). The direction of our locus of control has been seen as one of the determinants of health behaviour.

## Motivation

A psychological theory of motivation which adapts well to interpreting health needs is Maslow's 'hierarchy of needs' (see Fig. 2.1). This theory puts forward the suggestion that human needs are hierarchical. Physiological needs are the most basic, and an individual striving for self-actualization is manifesting the highest need. Some human needs will remain relatively unimportant until other needs

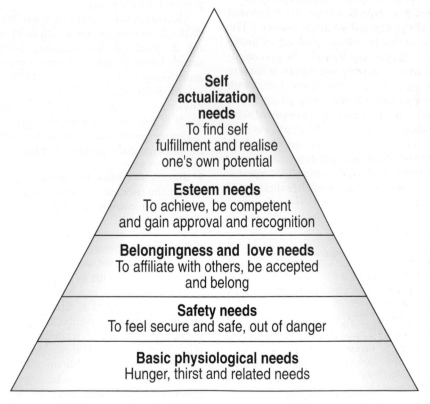

**Fig. 2.1** Maslow's hierarchy of needs.

have been satisfied. An understanding of the hierarchy of needs can help those who are planning and prioritizing health care, as long as the complexities of an individual's experiences and circumstances are taken into account.

An understanding of what affects motivation can also be useful as a manager. The equity theory is useful in this context. This suggests that an individual's motivation is largely influenced by how the individual feels he or she is being treated by colleagues. The degree of equity is defined in terms of a ratio of an individual's input into a job to the outcomes from it, as compared to that of another person. Some examples are given in Table 2.3 and most of us will be able to add to the list. Individual perceptions will be important in this and an effective manager should be able to address the equity between input and outcomes where needed. This is not always possible, but regular appraisal and communication should at least prevent problems from becoming unmanageable.

## COMPLIANCE

Patient compliance has various definitions, one of which is the extent to which a patient's behaviour coincides with the intended medical advice. The definition should embrace both the taking of medicines and changes in diet and lifestyle. Non-compliance can be defined as a situation where failure to comply is sufficient to interfere appreciably with attaining therapeutic goals. It is recognized that non-compliance with drug treatment is widespread with implications for the health of the individual as well as wasting money. The pharmacist has an important role to play in encouraging patient compliance through appropriate communication and interpretation of the patient's perceptions of his/her illness and its treatment.

Poor compliance may be affected by various factors. Poor communication to the patient about the treatment regimen is one important rectifiable factor. Other factors may be:

- volitional non-compliance: the individual decides rationally not to follow advice
- accidental non-compliance: the individual may forget or misunderstand the instructions that have been given
- circumstantial non-compliance: the treatment may be prematurely ended by severe or unpleasant side effects.

Treatment-related factors which have been associated with non-compliance are length of treatment and the complexity of the regimen, including the number of medicines being taken and the frequency of dosing. People who feel well after a period of time, may stop taking therapy because they feel that they do not need it. Conversely, people who do not feel any better may stop taking treatment because they feel that it is not working. Once- and twice-daily dosing produces the best levels of patient compliance and multiple drug therapy regimens should be coordinated so that doses are taken at one or two points during the day.

Measurement of patient compliance is extremely difficult because of the multiplicity of factors affecting it. Methods for assessing compliance include simple tablet counts, patient interviews, prescription monitoring and measurement of the drug or a 'tracer' in body fluids. Traditional methods such as physician assessment and tablet counts may be unreliable at determining patient compliance.

Before promoting compliance with treatment to the patient, three points must be confirmed:

- that the diagnosis is correct
- that the treatment is appropriate
- that the treatment is likely to do more good than harm.

The main strategy for improving patient compliance is to educate and inform the patient. These issues are dealt with in more detail in Chapter 41.

The pharmacist can help to influence prescribing so that the regimen is simple to follow in order to enhance patient compliance. This may sometimes mean rationalizing prescribing to a compromise situation between the ideal medication regimen for the patient and a manageable one. The number of medicines prescribed needs to be kept down to a realistic minimum, preferably four or less, with once or twice-daily dosing if possible.

| Table 2.3 Equity theory – inputs and outcomes | |
|---|---|
| Inputs | Outcomes |
| Education | Positive |
| Experience | Salary |
| Training | Satisfaction intrinsic to the job |
| Skill | Seniority benefits |
| Age | Fringe benefits |
| Gender | Job status and status symbols |
| Social status | Negative |
| Job effort | Monotony |
| | Poor working conditions |

## Bringing about change

In taking steps to improve compliance, the pharmacist is attempting to change the behaviour of the patient. Already in this chapter there have been a number of references to similar changes, such as stopping smoking or improving diet or lifestyle to a more healthy one. Similar processes are involved in helping people with addictive behaviour. Psychologists have been interested in how individuals come to make such a change in their behaviour. Prochaska & DiClemente (1982) proposed the 'stages of change' model to describe the stages in bringing about change. They identified five stages in the process:

- Precontemplation: no intention to make a change
- Contemplation: considering that change might be needed
- Preparation: making small changes, but avoiding the main change
- Action: decision taken and actively following a new behaviour
- Maintenance: keeping to the new behaviour through time.

An individual may not go through all the stages. However, it does indicate some of the ways in which people will weigh up the costs and benefits of making a change. For example at the precontemplative stage, a smoker is likely to focus on the problems – 'It will make me anxious and irritable'. When the action or maintenance stage is reached, the smoker will focus on the benefits – 'It will make me healthier'.

It is also recognized that relapse to the original behaviour may well occur. When this happens, the person can be reassured that this is quite normal, particularly when a difficult change, such as stopping smoking, is being attempted. Despite the setback, encouragement can be given to help start the process again. Sometimes, to help visualize this process, and reinforce the model, it is shown as a 'cycle' – the so-called 'cycle of change' (see Fig. 2.2).

It is important for a pharmacist, when dealing with someone who is trying to change, to be aware of the stage which the person has reached. In this way, the support given can be relevant to the way the person is thinking. The use of empathetic language (see Ch. 3) can be used to give encouragement. Where appropriate, the person may be urged to move to the next stage.

## THE PLACEBO EFFECT

A placebo effect is a when a treatment has an effect due to the expectations of the patient. Many pain-killing medicines are thought to have a strong placebo effect. The actual mechanisms of placebo effects are not fully understood, although theories are suggested which involve the natural opiate mechanisms in the brain. There can be considerable variability between individuals, and in the same individual in different treatment situations. Expectations of the treatment, behaviour of the doctor, the mode of administration and appearance of the medication will all influence this variability. If a doctor is authoritative and enthusiastic about a treatment then there is evidence that greater placebo effects are found. That placebo effects do exist may be useful to remember when recommending non-prescription medicines to customers in community pharmacies. Many customers want something to alleviate symptoms of a self-limiting condition. A placebo may be a useful treatment option. The placebo effect will also have important implications for clinical trials of new drugs, hence the use of 'controls' in well-designed studies.

## THE NATURE OF PROFESSIONS

An awareness of the nature of professions, and pharmacy's role and position amongst other health care professions, is important in understanding the professional relationships of the pharmacist within the primary and secondary health care team. The nature and extent of communication and collaboration between, say, community pharmacists and general medical practitioners may be affected by the perceived status of the two professions.

The nature of the concept of professions, or what constitutes a profession has been the subject of much sociological debate over the years. Various theories have been put forward to explain why some occupations are classed as professions. Some sociologists have suggested that professions achieved their status because they carried out functions that were essential for the modern industrialized society. This is referred to as the 'functionalist explanation' (Turner 1987; Harding, Nettleton and Taylor 1990). Professions provide the function of applying their specialized, expert knowledge for the benefit of the community and maintenance of the social system. The functionalist approach therefore explains the privileged position that professions attain in society.

A different theoretical perspective sees professionalization as an accumulation of attributes. These

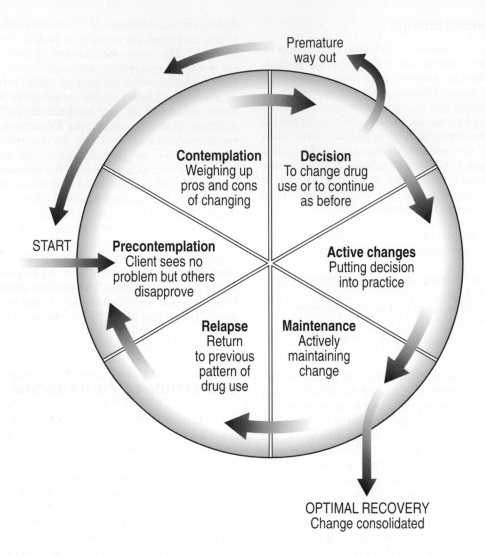

**Fig. 2.2**   The cycle of change (based on the stages of change model of Prochaska & DiClemente 1982).

attributes, or traits, are defined characteristics of an occupation, which are special or peculiar to the professions and lead to professional status. This is regarded as the 'attribute' or 'trait' approach (Hugman 1991). Harding, Nettleton and Taylor (1990) give a summary of the core features that are possessed by all professions, referred to as traits or attributes, which are:

'1.  specialized knowledge and lengthy training
 2.  service orientation
 3.  monopoly of practice
 4.  self-regulation.'

Professions may also be defined by an ethic of ser-

vice to the wider society. This develops one of the 'traits', that of service orientation. The element of power in professions, therefore, becomes important, as professions have to convince non-professionals, the State and other professions of their service ethic. Other concepts of the trait approach may also be regarded in this way, such as professions convincing society of their special expertise and knowledge. Power is, therefore, an important aspect of professionalization.

If the trait theory is rejected, power can be explored as the key element of professionalism. The specialist knowledge that professions have must also be accompanied by a distinctive mystique, suggesting a certain attitude and competence which allows professionals to interpret the knowledge they have acquired. A social distance is, therefore, established between the professional and the client, which provides the basis for a power relationship. An occupation also achieves professional status through occupational control and autonomy as a result of power struggles with the State and other interest groups. Power relationships among clients, other occupations and the State help to determine the professional status of a relationship (Johnson 1972).

## Is pharmacy a profession?

Harding, Nettleton and Taylor (1990) pose this question and combine the two views of the trait approach and the functionalist approach, that 'professions (a) possess important characteristics or traits, and (b) fulfil important societal functions'. Pharmacy appears to exhibit a number of the characteristics suggested as features of a profession, as defined by the 'trait' theory. It also fulfils a service to society in dispensing medicines and offering advice on health-related matters. Entry onto the Register of Pharmaceutical Chemists is restricted to those who have attained a degree in pharmacy at an approved school of pharmacy or who have passed the pharmaceutical chemist qualifying examination, are at least 21 years of age, and have successfully completed a pre-registration year of training in an approved establishment. Except for dispensing doctors, therefore, pharmacists have a monopoly in the dispensing of drugs, and sale of 'pharmacy medicines'. The undergraduate degree course lasts for 4 years, and is followed by 1 year of pre-registration training, except where the pre-registration year is offered as part of an undergraduate sandwich course degree. This provides pharmacists with their unique knowledge and skills. Postgraduate education is also recommended for all pharmacists by the Royal Pharmaceutical Society of Great Britain (RPSGB). A target of a minimum of 30 hours of continuing education per year has been set by the Council of the RPSGB (Medicines, Ethics and Practice 22, 1998). Pharmaceutical services are provided, including the supply of medicines and appliances, and self-regulation of pharmacy exists. This takes the form of the Statutory Committee of the RPSGB, which was formed as a result of The Pharmacy and Poisons Act 1933, and acts as the disciplinary body for members of the pharmaceutical profession (see Ch. 1).

Pharmacy is not fully acknowledged as a profession within sociological literature, with statements that pharmacy is underdeveloped as a professional group. There are many references in sociological literature to pharmacy as an incomplete or marginal profession. The reasons for these arguments are based on a number of factors.

The incorporation of the conflicting goals of business and professionalism are seen by some to distinguish pharmacy as a marginal profession. This commercialism has been recognized by community pharmacists as hindering the development of their clinical role and the acceptance of the extended role by GPs. GPs also express concern about the commercial influences in community pharmacy. It has been found that the two role orientations of profession and business do not correlate. Thus, whilst they do not necessarily have to do so, they can coexist without conflict. It has also been found that there are beneficial occupational practices related to a high professional role orientation. However, a high business role orientation could be detrimental to the beneficial practice behaviour. There is, however, little evidence of a detrimental effect to the client of a high business orientation.

A second reason is the dependence on the medical authority of the doctor. The pharmacist's reason for existence, the dispensing of medicines, is within the power of another profession. There has also been a reduction in the specialized compounding skills that were required of pharmacists, owing to industrialization of formulation and packaging. Both these factors hinder the professional autonomy of pharmacy.

Changes in the economic and technological environment have given rise to a threat to pharmacy's occupational identity, status and autonomy. This has led to the establishment of new roles, such as clinical pharmacy, which has been described as reprofessionalization. This term has been queried with the claim that professionalization is a dynamic, interactive group process. The term 'occupational imperialism', used by Larkin (1983), describes the advancement of medical occupational groups, by overcoming boundaries of responsibility and gaining skills of neighbouring medical disciplines. He suggests that there is a complex division of labour within modern medicine, so that the boundaries of competence and responsibility are continually challenged and refined. The dominance of the doctor is still maintained, but other medical occupations have acquired more prestigious functions and delegated menial tasks to subordinate occupations. An example of occupational imperialism can be seen in pharmacy. As pharmacists develop their clinical pharmacy skills, dispensing technicians take over the routine dispensing functions, supervised by the pharmacist.

## Professions and power

Professionalization is likely to be regarded as a recognition of power and status in today's society (Turner 1987; Johnson 1972). Specialized knowledge in the professions leads to dominance and power in society. Three types of professional structure have been identified, in which different power structures exist:

• The collegiate profession, where members of the profession itself exercise power, defining the process and outcome of work. There is an image of internal unity to those outside the profession. Examples of collegiate professions are those of medicine and law.

• The patronage profession has power exercised between the occupation and the clients, who pay for the service. The practitioners have a degree of power, but set the boundaries of the occupation, the contractual obligations with the clients, the recipients of the service, and the provider of the resources that the practice requires. Examples of patronage professions are accountancy and architecture.

• Mediated profession, where power is exercised through a mediator between the occupation and the clients who use the service. The mediator may be another profession, or, as is often the case, an agency of the State. Examples given are nursing and social work.

Professions may not fit exactly into one of these three categories. For example, pharmacy may be considered to be a mediated profession, with the State acting as the mediator, but it also has elements of a collegiate profession, as shown by the restriction of entry onto the Register of Pharmaceutical Chemists.

Power may be exercised between members of the profession, by the clients who use the services, by social institutions, such as the State, or interprofessionally. Individuals who exercise power may not be aware that they are doing so, because of the lack of conflict in the interaction. Power is not an isolated element of social life, but interweaves occupational and organizational structures with the actions of professionals, both individually and collectively. The profession of medicine has acquired a pre-eminent status in our society with a great deal of prestige and power.

## Hierarchy in professions

The concept of hierarchy in professions relates to the power and structure of the organization. Hierarchy is power and authority in an organization or between occupations. Doctors are regarded as 'higher' than pharmacists in the hierarchical organization of the primary health care team (PHCT), because of their prestige, status and power in society. The more senior the profession, the more secure the power.

Power, and therefore hierarchy, between occupations may be evident in many cases, for example physicians exerting power over nurses. However, this power may be exerted 'both ways': occupations can exercise power by excluding others, or those excluded may challenge the position of the occupation. This is the concept of social closure, where professions define and maintain boundaries of the occupation. The attainment of professional autonomy may be achieved in this way.

There are two concepts involved in exercising power within a hierarchical system: control and resistance. They are occupational concepts because they are based on the nature and scope of the work undertaken by the occupations, rather than on gender, race or any other aspects. Subordinate professions, for example nursing in relation to medicine, exercise power through resistance, whilst a superordinate profession, for example medicine in relation to nursing, exercises power through control of the subordinate profession.

Power of occupations may also be considered by examining the relationship between the members of the occupation and those who are serviced by them. Patients are the clients in both the medical and pharmaceutical professions. It may be said that they are controlled by the professions, although the State gives patients some element of resistance to that power, for example through the Patients' Charter, in the Citizens' Charter.

Gender and race also influence power issues in professions. Medicine is currently a predominantly white, male profession and, based on research evidence, it can be predicted that it is likely to exert power over a predominantly female profession, such as pharmacy. However, female students are now forming the majority of student intake to medical schools. It is likely that 50% of GP principals will be women in the foreseeable future, compared to the situation in 1990, when 24% of GP principals were women and in 1950, when only 10% of GP principals were women.

Qualifications may be used as a device to construct hierarchical levels between professions. Thus doctors spend a longer time gaining their qualification (6 years, with an additional 3 years' vocational training for GPs), compared to pharmacists (5 years).

## Role boundaries and conflict

The potential exists for extension of the pharmacist's occupational role to cause role conflict and tension between the professionals involved. A role can be defined as the pattern of behaviour shared by most occupants of a position, and which becomes expected of them. Roles are generally interlocking, so that if professionals are playing their roles, others have no choice but to play theirs. Role conflict occurs when there are antagonizing pressures from different groups of people, within organizations or between occupations.

One of the most important activities of an occupation is to build and maintain boundaries around its operating activities or tasks. Physicians have been more successful than pharmacists in protecting their task territories. Pharmacists are legally prevented from prescribing restricted drugs, and ethically from diagnosing illness, whilst physicians can, in certain circumstances, dispense drugs.

Research has shown that, in a hospital setting, the expanded boundaries of the pharmacist's clinical role have been accepted by nurses and doctors. Both have welcomed the expertise in medication therapy that the pharmacists had to offer. Other research has, however, indicated that there is role boundary encroachment when pharmacists attempt to expand their occupational role. It has been suggested that all of the pharmacist's new roles were requested and supervised by physicians, and it is concluded that pharmacists have benefited from technological change, but that they have not gained in autonomy, status and power.

The pharmacist's expanding role is defended by stating that pharmacists have responded to technological changes in health care, and have gradually expanded their task boundaries, to influence the activities and roles of the physicians and nurses. All of the professional members of the team have power within the social structure of the hospital. They use various resources through which to exercise this power, including being able to influence others. Therefore those who are subordinate can influence the activities of their superiors by exercising power through resources. Pharmacists in hospital gradually became new members of the 'team', gaining acceptance from the other team members, and actively contributing to patient care.

## Teamwork

Teamwork means operating a system of shared decision making, overlapping roles, shifting leadership focus, and attention to team group processes. A team is a device to coordinate a set of individual activities. Effective teamwork requires the flow of information between team members, emphasizing the need for interprofessional communication. The extent of teamwork is not easy to measure, and teams are not always the most effective means of completing a task.

## Collaboration

Collaboration involves perceptions, values, expectations, assumptions, behaviours and structures. Armitage (1983) provided the following definition of interprofessional collaboration: 'The exchange of information between individuals involved in the delivery of primary health care, which has the potential for action or joint working in the interests of a common purpose'. Collaboration is an ideal of sharing power and authority. The power is based on knowledge and expertise, as opposed to role or role function. Kraus (1980) saw collaboration as having at its core non-competitive, cooperative behaviour and non-hierarchical structures and processes. Interprofessional collaboration will only be successful, therefore, if the primary health care professionals involved are given equal status, prestige or power – this needs to be given by them to each other.

## THE PHARMACEUTICAL AND MEDICAL INTERFACE

The relationship between the general medical practitioner (GP) and community pharmacist has been recognized to be important because of the shared role of providing primary health care. The approximately 9750 community pharmacies in England dispense about 360 million prescriptions a year. These prescriptions are issued by medical and dental practitioners, with the majority originating from GPs. Traditionally, the main role of the community pharmacist has been to dispense prescribed medicines and advise on their safe and effective use. This process consists of reviewing and confirming the product, the dosage and the instructions on each prescription; preparing the items listed on the prescription and supplying the items to the patient with the appropriate advice (see Ch. 9). More recently, other roles performed by the community pharmacist have gained increased recognition, including provision of advice on symptoms, treatment of minor ailments, and the dissemination of health education and health promotion material to the public.

The fulfilment of these roles of the community pharmacist often leads to contact with the prescriber, for example clarification of prescription details. Interprofessional communication between the pharmacists working in community pharmacies and GPs is therefore necessary in the fulfilment of the day-to-day duties of the pharmacist. The contribution of the community pharmacist to other areas of primary care, such as health promotion activities and responding to symptoms, within the primary health care team, also provides opportunity for interprofessional communication and collaboration.

The government White Paper, 'Promoting Better Health' (DoH 1988), promoted the concept of closer liaison between pharmacists and GPs in the community and supported the concept of discussions between pharmacists and doctors about cost-effective prescribing. The White Paper, 'Working for Patients' (DoH 1989), promoted the involvement of hospital and community pharmacists with prescribers in the development and use of local formularies for use in hospitals and the community. Discussions between the Royal College of General Practitioners and the Royal Pharmaceutical Society of Great Britain encouraged the formation of 'local liaison groups', comprising general medical practitioners and community pharmacists serving the same patient cohort.

## The medical and pharmaceutical professions

Historically, owing to the overlap in skill and service of the two professions, pharmacists and the medical profession have had a competitive relationship, associated with many conflicts. At one time the role boundaries between pharmacists and physicians were rather ambiguous, but around the turn of the century, the role of the pharmacist began to undergo significant change. The utilization of pharmacists' compounding and manufacturing skills was gradually reduced, and taken over by large-scale manufacturing. Prepackaged (original pack) medicines became increasingly available, therefore leading to the view that pharmacists are overeducated distributors, with pharmacists describing their role as 'counters and pourers' or 'lickers and stickers'. It has also been suggested that original pack dispensing and computer technology in pharmacy have reduced the need for a highly trained pharmacist and may continue to do so. Research has also indicated that the perceived occupational role of the pharmacist, assessed by attitudes of consumers, physicians and pharmacists themselves, has placed the pharmacist

closer to the concept of technician than that of professional.

The loss of traditional pharmacy functions and role ambiguity led to what has been recognized as a reprofessionalization, beginning in the 1960s. Pharmacy became a profession in transition, and has been described as being uncertain about its status as a health care profession. The direction of the pharmacy profession has become more patient orientated and a clinical role for pharmacists has developed. This move was emphasized by the Pharmaceutical Care document (Report of the Joint Working Party 1992), which presented the results of a Joint Working Party of the Health Department and the pharmaceutical profession (through the RPSGB), to consider ways in which community pharmacy services might be developed to increase their contribution to health care, in areas such as health promotion, effective prescribing and specialist services, such as provision of services for drug misusers. Pharmaceutical care, as a philosophy of pharmacy practice, was defined by Hepler (Hepler & Strand 1990). It is the responsible provision of drug therapy for the purpose of achieving definite outcomes that improve a patient's quality of life. The outcomes are cure of disease, elimination or reduction of patient's symptomatology, arrest or slowing of a disease process or prevention of a disease or symptoms. Hepler also states that pharmaceutical care should be carried out in cooperation with physicians and patients, and recognizes pharmaceutical care as part of the reprofessionalization of pharmacy.

## The primary health care team

A number of health care professions work within the framework of primary health care organizations, including general practitioners, district nurses and health visitors. The importance of teamwork among these professionals within primary health care has been emphasized by different reports. Primary health care includes both the management of illness and the promotion of health. In primary care, a team is generally accepted as an association of different types of professionals who aim to provide the patient with comprehensive care. PHCTs have been described as interdisciplinary or multidisciplinary where two or more professions or occupations are committed to providing care jointly for the same population.

Community pharmacists should, in theory, be members of the PHCT. However, the extent of their involvement is variable. Pharmacies in residential areas have been reported as being more likely to have involvement in the PHCT compared to pharmacies in town or city centres. The extent of interprofessional cooperation was greater in health centres which have a pharmacy on the premises.

## Interprofessional relations within the primary health care team

Interprofessional relations within the PHCT have been investigated but this research has concentrated on members of the primary health care team other than the community pharmacist. Comprehensive research into the extent of collaboration between general practitioners and district nurses and between general practitioners and health visitors has been carried out in England. A measure of professional collaboration between primary health care workers was developed and the taxonomy of collaboration used is illustrated in Table 2.4.

Collaboration was found to exist between general medical practitioners and district nurses, and between general medical practitioners and health visitors, but the level of collaboration was lower than expected. Doctor–nurse collaboration was found to be higher than doctor–health visitor collaboration. Most pairs of professionals did no more than communicate with each other. Structural arrangements, such as working in the same building, were found to be important in contributing to the level of collaboration.

**Table 2.4   A taxonomy of interprofessional collaboration (Gregson et al 1992, after Armitage 1983)**

| Stages of collaboration | Definitions |
|---|---|
| 1. No direct communication | Members who never meet, talk or write to one another |
| 2. Formal, brief communication | Members who encounter or correspond with others but do not interact others meaningfully |
| 3. Regular communication | Members whose encounters, correspondence or consultation includes the transfer of information |
| 4. High level of joint working | Members who act on that information sympathetically; participate in pattern of joint working; subscribe to the same general objectives as others on a one-to-one basis in the same organization |
| 5. Multidisciplinary working | Involvement of all workers in a primary health care setting |

## GP–pharmacist interprofessional relationship

An editorial in the *Journal of the Royal College of General Practitioners* (Taylor 1986) following the publication of the Nuffield Inquiry into Pharmacy stated that: 'Issues of status and inter-professional rivalry must not be allowed to obscure the benefits to patients that would result from more efficient deployment of the expertise of pharmacists in certain aspects of patient care'. The aspects of patient care referred to included responding to symptoms and provision of advice to patients. It was also recognized that increased collaboration between GPs and community pharmacists would reduce misunderstandings between the professions.

The nature of contacts between community pharmacists and other primary health care personnel, and the implications for the primary health care team, has been investigated to a limited extent in the UK. The role of the pharmacist is generally described as being regarded by many as little more than a 'supplier of medication'. Closer liaison with other health care personnel is often suggested for the efficient and effective carriage of many of the primary care functions that the pharmacist wishes to pursue. The most frequent professional contacts that a community pharmacist has are with GPs, usually made by pharmacists to clarify prescription information. Teamwork between the GP and pharmacist could therefore be interpreted as currently serving only to promote efficient prescribing and dispensing. This may be interpreted as stage two in Armitage's (1983) taxonomy of collaboration.

When physicians' perceptions of pharmacists' professional roles have been investigated, they have been more supportive of the pharmacist's role in giving non-prescription drug-related advice than prescription-related advice. It is suggested that pharmacists and physicians actively working together, rather than competing with each other, may offer great benefits. When community pharmacists' perceptions of their professional role have been investigated, they think that provision of medication-related advice should be shared with the physician. This would, therefore, require some degree of communication and collaboration between the professions.

Reasons for misunderstandings between the two groups may be related to different perceptions of roles. Physicians often believe that the most important function of the pharmacist is filling prescriptions, therefore taking on a role of 'supplier of medicines'. Pharmacists, in one survey, believed that their most important function was in advising patients on general health matters. Physicians seem to be more content than pharmacists with the state of the relationship between the two professions. Doctors can have a narrow and somewhat limited image of the pharmacist's role in the health care triangle of pharmacist, physician and patient.

Factors affecting interprofessional consultation have been examined, along with the content and form of the cooperation. Both groups have agreed that cooperation is necessary between the professions. However, there is a difference in opinion between the two professions on the form of the cooperation. The general practitioner wishes to have a reliable and effective information source, and the pharmacist expects to have the opportunity to influence the GP's prescribing habits.

Various methods have been employed to facilitate communication and cooperation between GPs and pharmacists. These include joint educational meetings and liaison groups between GPs and pharmacists serving the same patient cohort. Joint meetings have been shown to bring about a greater mutual understanding and trust between the two professions. Liaison group meetings lead to the GPs having a greater awareness of pharmaceutical issues and also to cooperation between the two professions. Useful points of initial discussion in joint meetings have been analysis of prescribing data, the development of local formularies, prescribing reviews and disease management programmes (see also Ch. 34). These local initiatives fulfil a future role that has been suggested for community pharmacists, of becoming better integrated with prescribing issues, to ensure optimum pharmaceutical care. The local community pharmacist could supplement patient visits to the GP, as a source of local advice and information supplied by the medical and pharmaceutical advisers of the local health authority or board. Pharmacists could also collaborate with local GPs on patient compliance and establishing joint treatment protocols. Pharmaceutical companies may become involved with encouraging GPs and pharmacists to work together. It has been suggested that those companies engaged in promoting interprofessional collaboration would also improve their relationships with the professions.

From the limited research that has been carried out into the interprofessional relationship between community pharmacists and general medical practitioners, it can be seen that close liaison and teamwork, regular communication, joint working and understanding of each other's functions are all thought to be desirable for improved communication and collaboration. This would be equivalent to the two professionals aiming to achieve level five on Armitage's taxonomy of collaboration.

## Health centre pharmacies

The interprofessional relationship within health centre pharmacies has been investigated in more detail. GPs have positive expectations of the pharmacist within health centres, in terms of utilizing the pharmacist's expertise and 'getting on' at a personal level. Working together in a health centre appears to foster a more collaborative approach by pharmacists and GPs towards the provision of health care. Collaboration between GPs and pharmacists in both health centres and the community would be enhanced if the pharmacists developed the confidence to liaise equitably with GPs on a professional basis.

## Information technology

The Pharmaceutical Care document recognized the need to improve communications between prescribers and pharmacists. The report recommended the alteration of restrictions in the conveyance of prescriptions by the doctor to the pharmacist over the telephone. It was felt that a major benefit of telephone prescribing would be that the pharmacist and prescriber would be in contact with each other at the point when a therapeutic decision is made, giving the pharmacist the opportunity to intervene where necessary. Pilot experiments were also recommended to investigate the possibility of faxing or electronically transmitting prescriptions to the pharmacy.

Computers are extensively used in pharmacy already. Extension of the use of information technology may lead to improved interprofessional communication. Electronic links with prescribers may become possible in the future, providing new and exciting opportunities for communication between the professionals. Investigations have been carried out in the use of an electronic document, for example a magnetic card that would contain information from the prescriber and the pharmacist.

## Training and education

The training of pharmacists in the future will have to equip graduates with many skills in order to cope with the changing face of pharmacy and the many challenges and demands that a career in pharmacy will place on practitioners. A greater emphasis on interpersonal skills has become evident in both medicine and pharmacy, in order to be able to deliver effective care to patients and to work in collaboration with members of the primary health care team.

## Undergraduate education

Pharmacists undergo a 4-year degree at one of the 15 schools of pharmacy in the UK, followed by a 1-year pre-registration experience (except for Bradford and John Moore's universities, which run 'sandwich' courses, incorporating the 12 months of pre-registration experience). Six months of the pre-registration year has to be in either community or hospital pharmacy practice. A pre-registration examination was introduced for the first time in 1993, which candidates must pass before they are admitted to the Register of Pharmaceutical Chemists, and become a Member of the Royal Pharmaceutical Society of Great Britain.

Doctors must register with the General Medical Council to practise. Qualifications that are recognized for registration include the degrees of Bachelor of Medicine and Bachelor of Surgery, Doctor of Medicine and Master of Surgery or Licentiate of the Royal College of Physicians of London and Member of the Royal College of Surgeons of England. All general practitioners must undergo a period as a trainee in an approved general practice before they can be employed by the NHS as a 'principal'.

There are few recorded examples of joint educational initiatives on undergraduate courses for medical and pharmacy students. Pharmacists and doctors would probably benefit greatly if there were more integration at undergraduate level, with some subjects being taught to both groups of students. Approximately 10–15% of the pharmacy and medicine undergraduate courses could be common material; however, only two schools of pharmacy in the UK share the same campus as a medical school. It may therefore be difficult to make practical arrangements for joint undergraduate teaching. In one New Zealand university, there is a common first year clinical course for medicine, pharmacy, dentistry and other subjects. Students decide which course to follow after the first year.

Some pharmacists have an input into undergraduate courses in medicine, and physicians also have input into pharmacy undergraduate courses, such as giving lectures on their particular specialities. Pharmacy students from some universities observe a session of GP consultations in practice during their undergraduate degree course. This therefore gives the pharmacy students an insight into the role of the GP.

## Postgraduate education

Continuing education is increasingly important in both the medical and pharmaceutical professions. There are DoH (Department of Health) funded Centres for Postgraduate or Postqualification Pharmaceutical Education (CPPE) in England, Wales, Scotland, and Northern Ireland which provide continuing education for pharmacists. The Royal Pharmaceutical Society of Great Britain provides the guideline of a minimum annual level of 30 hours of continuing education activity for a practising pharmacist. A core syllabus has also been recommended for pharmacists by the RPSGB. General medical practitioners are entitled to claim a postgraduate education allowance (PGEA), providing they have attended 5 days of accredited postgraduate education per year. The three subject areas that must be covered are health promotion and prevention of disease, disease management and service management.

The two professions have a poor understanding of each other's training. Participants in joint educational initiatives have been shown to gain an improved understanding of each other's training and their respective roles in the community. This may be seen as a way of promoting better working relationships between GPs and pharmacists in the community. Bringing the two professions together at a training stage may be beneficial, as attitudes are easier to influence at that stage. The NPA produce a package for community pharmacists to assist them in educating and advising trainee GPs. The training package involves inviting the trainee GP from the local medical practice into the pharmacy, to help him or her understand the role of the community pharmacist.

---

### Key Points

- An individual's attitude to health is derived from the society in which he or she lives.
- The WHO defines health as a 'state of complete physical, mental and social well-being'.
- Many people tolerate major symptoms – the so-called 'symptom iceberg'.
- According to the illness behaviour concept, people assess symptoms using five social triggers.
- The 'sick role' is the way in which society and the individual make illness acceptable. It gives the patient both benefits and obligations.
- Social environment influences the frequency of seeking help from a health professional.

- The 'health belief model' attempts to draw together the many factors which influence a person's decision whether or not to seek professional help.
- Pharmacists have a role in helping individuals decide on a course of action in response to a symptom.
- Patient–pharmacist relationships are most likely to be 'mutual participation'.
- Disease can be described by the 'medical', or 'socioenvironmental' models.
- It is very difficult to establish a causal relationship in disease.
- There is a correlation between social class and health as shown by the standardized mortality rate (SMR) and morbidity.
- Relationships exist between unemployment and health, poverty and health, gender and health, ethnicity and health and age and health.
- Establishing why health is affected by social class has not been achieved because of the many factors involved.
- Patients with chronic conditions have to make many adjustments to life.
- Some diagnoses stigmatize the patient.
- People react to stress with physiological and psychological responses, the exact way being a balance of many factors.
- Personality and motivation will influence the reaction of an individual to any situation, including illness.
- Compliance is the term used to indicate that a patient follows all the intentions of the doctor, including medicine taking and lifestyle changes.
- When changing behaviour, there are five stages – precontemplation, contemplation, preparation, action, maintenance.
- Failure to sustain change is normal, especially with addictive behaviour.
- Placebos produce an effect due to patient expectation.
- Professions may be explained as 'function', 'attribute', 'service' or 'power' in origin.
- Pharmacy has many of the characteristics of a profession, but it has been described as a marginal profession because of the business element in community pharmacy and the reliance on medical authority.
- In a hierarchical system, power is exerted by control or resistance in order to create subordinate and superordinate roles.

- Role boundaries can cause conflict or generate teamworking and collaboration between professions.
- Collaboration is the sharing of power and authority.
- Contact between GPs and pharmacists is necessary in the normal course of dispensing but other opportunities need to be pursued.
- Improved collaboration between GPs and pharmacists will result from improved communication and a clarification of roles.
- Increasing cooperation between pharmacists and GPs is occurring as a result of joint educational meetings and liaison groups.
- The changing role of pharmacists has led to the concept of 'pharmaceutical care' which achieves defined outcomes and improves quality of life.

## REFERENCES

Armitage P 1983 Joint working in primary health care. (Occasional paper) Nursing Times 79: 75–78

Committee of Inquiry into Pharmacy 1986 Pharmacy. A report to the Nuffield Foundation. Nuffield Foundation, London

Department of Health (DoH) 1988 Promoting better health. Cmd 249. HMSO, London

Department of Health (DoH) 1989 Working for patients. Cmd 555. HMSO, London

Donovan J 1984 Ethnicity and Health: a Research Review. Social Science and Medicine 19: 663–670

Dubos R 1959 Mirage of Health. Harper and Row, New York

Gregson B A, Cartlidge A M, Bond J 1992 Development of a measure of professional collaboration in primary health care. Journal of Epidemiology and Community Health 46: 48–53

Harding G, Nettleton S, Taylor K 1990 Sociology for pharmacists. Macmillan, London

Helman C H 1981 Disease versus illness in general practice. Journal of the Royal College of General Practice 31: 548–552

Hepler C D, Strand L M 1990 Opportunities and responsibilities in pharmaceutical care. American Journal of Hospital Pharmacy 47: 533–543

Hugman R 1991 Power in caring Professions. Macmillan Press, London

Johnson T J 1972 Professions and Power. Macmillan Press, London

Kraus W A 1980 Collaboration in organizations. Alternative to hierarchy. Human Sciences Press, New York

Larkin 1983 Occupational Monopoly and Modern Medicine. Tavistock, London

Medicines, Ethics and Practice – a guide for pharmacists, current edn. Royal Pharmaceutical Society of Great Britain, London (Updated twice yearly)

Parsons, T 1951 The Social System. Free Press, London

Prochaska J O, DiClemente C C D 1982 Transtheoretical therapy: towards a more integrative model of change. Psychotherapy: Theory, Research and Practice 19: 276–288

Report of the Joint Working Party on the Future Role of the Community Pharmaceutical Services 1992 Pharmaceutical care: the future for community pharmacy. Royal Pharmaceutical Society of Great Britain, London

Szasz T S, Hollender M H 1956 A contribution to the Philosophy of Medicine: the Basic Models of the Doctor-Patient Relationship. Archives of International Medicine 97: 585–592

Taylor R J 1986 Pharmacists and primary care. Journal of the Royal College of General Practitioners 36: 348

Turner B S 1987 Medical Power and Social Knowledge. Sage Publications, London

Zola I K 1973 Pathways to the Doctor: from Person to Patient. Social Science and Medicine 7: 677–689

## FURTHER READING

Armstrong D 1989 An outline of sociology as applied to medicine, 3rd edn. University Press, Cambridge

Harding G, Nettleton S, Taylor K 1990 Sociology for pharmacists. Macmillan, London

Hart N 1992 The sociology of health and medicine. Causeway Press, Lancashire

Oliver R 1993 Psychology and health care. Baillière Tindall, London

Weinman J 1987 An outline of psychology as applied to medicine, 2nd edn. The Bath Press, Bath

# 3

# Communication skills for the pharmacist

*M. M. Moody, S. L. Hutchinson and E. J. Kennedy*

---

After studying this chapter you will know about:

**Meaning and types of communication**
**Assumptions and expectations in communication**
**Questioning and listening skills**
**Communicating with those with special needs**
**Empathy**
**Non-verbal communication**
**Assertiveness**
**Transactional analysis**
**Barriers to communication.**

## Introduction

When communicating, the purpose is not just to deliver a message to the recipient, but to bring about a change in that person's knowledge, attitude and even behaviour. Effective communication must be a two-way process and the success of it depends on the participants' awareness of this.

## Definition of communication

The dictionary definition of communication is: to announce, correspond, declare, divulge, give, impart, inform, make known, report, reveal, unfold.

This definition illustrates that communication involves more than just words. We use words, both written and spoken, facial and vocal expressions, body posture and even our appearance and the clothing that we wear.

Good communication is difficult to achieve and an awareness of this fact is of utmost importance.

## A requirement for pharmacists?

Communication is important as a life skill, as well as

being particularly important for pharmacists – in dealing with patients, other health care professionals and in business. The pharmacist spends a large proportion of each working day communicating with other people, either verbally or in writing. The extended role for pharmacists requires a greater time to be spent talking to people. Advertising campaigns over recent years have alerted the public to the availability of advice from the community pharmacy. The role of pharmacists in hospitals has an increasing emphasis on talking to patients and medical staff. Poor communication has the potential to cause a range of problems – difficult staff or personal relationships, we may not achieve what we want, life may be frustrating. If there is incomplete communication with health care professionals on correct drug dosage or inappropriate or incomplete advice on the use of medication, potential harm to a patient may occur.

Having identified the need for effective communication skills for pharmacists, it is important to consider how effective our own communication is. We may all be able to talk at length, but do our listeners benefit from our words?

Although we will often embark on a communication process automatically, good communication demands effort, thought, time and a willingness for the process to be effective.

This chapter will cover aspects which are vital for successful communication. It is important to remember that our personality influences our effectiveness as a communicator. It will help you to identify your strengths and weaknesses and enable you to develop the appropriate skills required for your personal and professional fulfilment.

## FACTORS WHICH INFLUENCE COMMUNICATION

Different factors affect people in different ways and

this will have an influence on how they communicate. These can be described as 'drives', which will motivate people towards achieving certain goals. These drives are:

1. Biological needs: for example eating, drinking, feeling healthy or ill
2. Dependency: help, support and guidance from people in positions of power or authority, for example parents or doctors
3. Affiliation: warm and friendly responses, social acceptance by others
4. Dominance: acceptance by others as a leader, gaining a position of power, for example, politicians
5. Gender: physical proximity, bodily contact
6. Aggression: to harm people physically, verbally or in other ways
7. Self-esteem and ego-identity: for other people to make approving responses and to accept the self-image as valid
8. Other motivations which affect social behaviour: needs for achievement, money, interests, medical treatment, for example medicines.

As communicators, both in our personal and professional lives, we need to appreciate how these drives may affect both our own behaviour and attitudes and those of the people with whom we are communicating.

## ASSUMPTIONS AND EXPECTATIONS

It is said that 'You never get a second chance to make a first impression'. When we meet somebody for the first time it is human nature to make assumptions about them. We often put people into categories and these assumptions about people lead to expectations of their behaviour, jobs and character.

No two people experience the same thing in the same way – we are all unique. On the surface we may all be involved in similar activities but we have very different feelings about them.

Our initial judgement of a person is often based purely on what we see and what we hear. This includes the person's appearance, how he or she dresses, age, gender, race, physical disabilities. It is important that we are aware of assumptions that we make in order to avoid stereotyping groups of people.

The impression we have of a person wearing a denim jacket may be very different from that of a person wearing a suit. Conversely, people will make

assumptions about us based on initial impressions; for example, a pharmacist wearing a white coat in a clean, clinical environment may inspire more confidence in a patient than a pharmacist wearing a scruffy jumper and working in a cluttered, untidy environment.

It is well documented that age and gender affect our communication because of assumptions and expectations. We should not assume that people in wheelchairs cannot communicate effectively. We must ensure that we direct our communication at an appropriate physical level and to the appropriate person.

## Demeanour

The way in which people present themselves will lead to certain judgements being made. For example, a person who strides aggressively towards you may make you feel defensive because the assumption may be made that he or she has come to make a complaint. However, a person who approaches hesitantly may lead to the assumption that this person needs help and advice on a potentially embarrassing matter. This will affect our behaviour and attitude in subsequent communication with this person.

## Tone of speech, accents, colloquialisms

All of these have an impact on communication. Our response to a person speaking with a whining, complaining tone will differ from our response to someone who greets us in a friendly welcoming manner. Similarly, a cultured, 'BBC' English accent may invoke a different response from that to someone with a strong local accent.

So remember, no-one experiences the same situation in the same way. We may appear to be doing similar things but have different feelings about them. Do not assume that you know what a person thinks or feels. You need to check with the person – do not make assumptions. We can only guess what people are thinking or feeling from how they look and from their behaviour. For example, we may think that someone is nervous if he or she is moving restlessly or twitching, but that may not be the case. It is useful for us to consider how aware we are of our own behaviour and appearance and what message this may give to other people. We are used to controlling our words but are less skilled at controlling our bodies.

*Exercise 3.1*

To test your awareness of communication and

assumptions spend 5 minutes talking to a person who you do not know very well. After this time, each ask yourselves the following questions:

1. What did you notice about your partner? What type of facial expression did he/she have? What was his/her posture (or gestures) like? How did he/she speak – tone, speed, volume? What does this tell you about him/her?

2. How aware were you of your own non-verbal communication? What was your facial expression? How were you sitting – posture, position in relation to your partner, gestures, way of speaking?

3. What assumptions did you make about your partner? For example, taste in food, political persuasion, favourite TV programmes, family background.

4. How accurate were the assumptions that you made? Ask your partner.

5. Do these assumptions say anything about you and the initial judgements you make of people based on sex, age, class, dress, etc.?

## LISTENING AND QUESTIONING SKILLS

It is said that 'questioning' is one of the most widely used social skills. In the world of pharmacy, good questioning skills are an asset to any pharmacist. However, questioning in itself is not enough. Reinforcement, together with questioning, is required to build up interaction between two people.

We have to ask what the function of a question is. In a pharmacy setting questions are normally asked to encourage the listener to provide information. The type of question asked and the way in which it is asked will dictate the level of response given. Questioning skills can be used to allow communication between the pharmacist and the patient both in the community and hospital sectors and between the pharmacist and other health care professionals. Pharmacists need to be able to respond to patients' enquiries and to try to resolve problems or difficulties they may have in taking prescribed medicines. Pharmacists also need to give advice on over-the-counter (OTC) medicines. Communication between two individuals will only be effective if it succeeds in fulfilling an objective, e.g. establishing what particular medical condition a person is suffering from and being able to recommend appropriate treatment.

## Use of open and closed questions

There are two main types of questions: open and closed.

By definition a closed question is one which is direct and close-ended. It requires the respondent to give a single word reply such as 'yes' or 'no'. Such questions do not include a 'feeling' component, but do provide specific information on a subject area. Examples of closed questions used in a pharmacy setting include:

- Are you taking any medication at present?
- Have you ever taken this medication before?
- Do you understand how to take it?
- Do you have any questions about the medicine?
- Did the medicine work for you?
- Will you work in the dispensary for me next Sunday?

Pharmacists can be inclined to use too many closed questions, but in many pharmacy situations a balanced combination of both open and closed questions is more beneficial.

Open questions are open-ended and often allow people to respond in their own way with a particular reply. They do not set any 'limits' and generally allow the person to provide more detailed information. Open questions encourage elaboration and help people expand on what they have started to say. Examples of open questions include:

- Describe your symptoms to me.
- Tell me about any over-the-counter medicines you are taking just now.
- How do you relieve the symptoms of headache?
- What do you do when that sensation occurs?

The above examples show that open questions are often built around words like 'what' and 'how' and generally allow an element of 'feeling' to be introduced by the patient in the reply.

Pharmacists can also encourage patients to explain more about their symptoms or condition by using open questions which require elaboration, e.g. What can you tell me about the symptoms you have after taking the medicine?

## The funnelling technique

A funnelling technique can be used to allow direction and focusing of ideas on a specific topic. The idea behind this technique is to direct the questions to a particular subject area. This involves initially asking background open questions to provide basic information, then asking specific closed questions to provide more detailed information and clarify points. In these circumstances, it can be useful to paraphrase comments made, to ensure that the understanding of the information being obtained from the patient is accurate. Without this checking procedure the listener may misinterpret something and a misunderstanding can occur. It is possible during any one conversation to use more than one 'funnelling' technique, e.g. establishing a patient's current medical condition, then going on to suggest appropriate action or medication available. In a pharmacy setting, where time can be a limiting factor, using the funnelling technique can be useful for directing and focusing a conversation to enable an end point to be achieved more quickly.

---

**EXAMPLE 3.1**

Hospital clinical pharmacist, on ward round, questioning skills with other health care professionals or when speaking to a patient. A conversation with a patient could be as follows:

'Please tell me about the insulin products you have used in the past.' (background open question)
'What type of insulin do you currently use?' (specific closed question)
'How long have you been using this?' (specific closed question)
'Now that we have established a little about your medication, can we discuss what action we will take in the future to prevent problems with your medication?' (this starts another funnelling technique)

---

**EXAMPLE 3.2**

An industrial pharmacist dealing with other staff in a small working group, responsible for a particular part of product development, e.g. research and development (R & D), quality assurance (QA) or production:

'Please explain about the sampling techniques used.' (background open question)
'Who sampled the sterile water batch yesterday?' (specific closed question)
'Where were the quality control samples taken from?' (specific closed question)
'How many samples were taken?' (specific closed question)

'Now I would like to discuss ways of validating the sampling techniques.' (start of a new funnelling technique)

---

## The use of open and closed questions in a pharmacy setting

If we consider the situation of a pharmacist responding to symptoms, the pharmacist has a number of options available to allow him or her to obtain information from the patient. Choosing the correct type of question can prove to be a difficult decision, particularly bearing in mind the circumstances under which the conversation may be taking place, such as in a busy pharmacy where other customers are waiting for prescriptions or OTC advice. It is tempting to ask a number of closed questions which do provide information, albeit limited to one word answers. However, this could result in the patient being 'bombarded' with a host of questions which takes a great deal of time to establish the patient's condition and makes patients feel as if they have been through an 'interrogation'. Pharmacists must learn to develop good questioning skills to enable them to build up an accurate picture of the patient's condition. This is achieved by using a combination of open and closed questions which can ensure that accurate information is obtained. At the same time, allowing patients adequate time to elaborate on certain points builds their confidence in the pharmacist.

Time pressures may make us reluctant to use open questions. However, although interviews using open-ended questions take longer than interviews based upon protocols of closed questions, they typically elicit more information.

## Skills used for listening

Asking questions is only part of the skill. Listening is of equal importance. This requires good attention to patients' responses, body language, facial expressions, gestures. Good eye contact between the patient and the pharmacist is vital for good one-to-one communication. It is also important to be aware of patients' emotional state when they are communicating with you. Patients are often anxious or embarrassed and find it difficult to communicate in a busy pharmacy where other people can hear their conversations. It is important to be discreet, and be aware of the person's feelings and if necessary, move a little closer to the patient. This situation can, however, create further problems of invading a person's personal space. This is discussed later in this chapter. In the ideal situation, the pharmacist would position himself near the person so that questions can be asked in relative privacy.

The language used by the pharmacist in response to questions which the patient may ask must be appropriate for the patient. Often in a hospital setting, particularly in a ward round, patients can feel very isolated as their condition is discussed using medical jargon which is difficult for them to understand. If pharmacists are involved in this role, it is important to use opportunities to reassure patients about the medication they are being prescribed and to use appropriate language when doing so.

In the community pharmacy, the pharmacist may have the responsibility of staff training. This will involve training in communication skills. A much greater emphasis is now placed upon the requirement for counter staff to adopt certain procedures when responding to a request from a customer for an OTC product or advice. Clearly defined protocols indicate the necessary questions to be asked before OTC prescribing can occur or referral to the pharmacist is required. Counter staff are now required to undertake distance learning packages, e.g. NPA Pharmacy Interaction Scheme, to ensure that they have the relevant knowledge to ask appropriate questions and provide accurate information on OTC medicines for patients.

## Application of questioning skills

Questioning skills do not only apply to the communication between pharmacists and patients, although a large part of their work will be in this area. Good questioning skills are required in staff training and implementation of procedures, dealing with other health care professionals and in ordering and supplying goods.

Questioning skills are not only required for face-to-face communication. Often in a pharmacy setting, the pharmacist may have to communicate by telephone with, for example, a GP, a dentist, a district nurse, nursing home staff, hospital staff or patients' relatives. The major drawback of this type of communication is that reliance is put solely on good verbal communication skills and not on the non-verbal aspect of communication. In these circumstances, it is vital to obtain the information as quickly and efficiently as possible. At the same time, the pharmacist must remain professional, give out accurate advice and offer reassurance if necessary. Examples: a GP phones to order a pre-

scription for a patient, the pharmacist is required to ask specific questions to ensure that all information is accurate; a patient phones to ask about a prescription item that may have been incorrectly dispensed. Using good questioning skills, the pharmacist would check the prescription information, identify the patient's concerns and take appropriate action.

## Special needs

Patients with special needs must be considered carefully when adopting questioning skills. We need to be non-patronizing, avoid the use of jargon and adopt a procedure for obtaining information which is acceptable to the patient.

Many customers who come into pharmacies will suffer from a degree of hearing impairment. Studies have shown that one in six of the adult population in the UK has clinically significant hearing loss. By retirement age (61–70 years old), around 34% of people have significant hearing loss; this increases to 74% in people aged over 70. Considering that the highest number of prescriptions are presented by people in these age groups, it is evident that pharmacists must implement appropriate communication skills.

Recognizing the profoundly deaf is usually simpler than recognizing those who have hearing impairment. The following guidelines may be useful to identify these customers.

### How to recognize the hearing impaired

A person with hearing difficulty is likely to do one or more of the following:

- speak in an unusually loud or soft voice
- turn head to one side or cup hand to ear whilst listening
- concentrate on lips whilst being spoken to
- give inappropriate responses to questions
- have a blank or confused expression during conversation
- frequently ask speakers to slow down or repeat information
- be unable to hear a conversation when back is turned
- be unable to carry on a conversation in a noisy environment.

Having recognized a customer with hearing impairment, you may find the following guidelines helpful.

*Guidelines when speaking to the hearing impaired*

- Ask them how they wish to communicate.
- Make sure that background noise is at a minimum.
- Look directly at the person and do not turn away.
- Make sure sufficient light is on your face.
- Do not hide your face or mouth behind hands, pens, etc.
- Do not shout.
- Keep the normal rhythm of speech but slow down slightly.
- Articulate each word carefully and exactly, particularly emphasizing consonants.
- If a sentence is not heard, rephrase it or write it down.
- Do not change the subject in mid-sentence.

Listening, and being able to demonstrate that you are listening, is very important. Verbal responses are particularly important for telephone calls and the blind; likewise, non-verbal responses for the deaf.

## EMPATHY

Empathetic listening involves more than allowing a stream of consciousness from the patient. It involves the ability to understand accurately what someone is really saying, and then give it back to the person so as to communicate that understanding.

This is where the term 'active listening' comes from. It underlines the fact that effective listening is far from a passive process. It involves grasping what the patient means, then reflecting back this meaning through the skills of paraphrasing, reflective responding, summarizing and focusing.

Active listening is important in all phases of the counselling process. However, it is in the first phase of establishing an empathetic relationship that it is crucial.

Different words can be used to describe an emotion or feeling. However, the strength of the emotion being described will vary depending on which word is selected. Use of these words may be particularly helpful when reflecting back feeling and content to the patient in an empathetic response. Examples of these words are found in Table 3.1.

## DIFFICULT SITUATIONS IN PHARMACY

There are times in all our lives when we have to deal

| Table 3.1 | Feeling vocabulary | | | |
|---|---|---|---|---|
| Feeling | Very strong | Strong | Moderate | Mild |
| Anxiety | Panic-stricken | Tense | Nervous | Worried |
| Fear | Terrified | Frightened | Fearful | Uneasy |
| Happiness | Elated | Joyful | Happy | Pleased |
| Depression | Suicidal | Depressed | Unhappy | Low |
| Sadness | Grief-stricken | Distressed | Sad | Sorry |
| Desire | Craving | Longing | Desirous | Wishful |
| Confusion | Chaotic | Disorganized | Bewildered | Uncertain |
| Confidence | Bold | Self-assured | Secure | Adequate |

with 'difficult situations'. Good communication skills may not always produce the perfect result but can help prevent making a situation worse.

### Exercise 3.2

Read through the following scenarios and think carefully how you would react and deal with such a situation in 'real life'. Consider how the other person would be feeling. Remember, there will no one perfect answer. Discuss the scenarios with a friend or group of friends. This will allow you to identify the different ways people react to the same situation.

1. A young girl returns to your pharmacy to purchase laxatives. You notice that she has been buying them fairly regularly, and decide to tackle the situation. How would you approach this as the pharmacist? How do you think the young girl will react?

2. A drug addict asks to purchase some 1 ml 'insulin' needles. You know that there is a needle exchange scheme at a pharmacy on the other side of town. How do you give this advice to the addict, or advise him on the safe disposal of the needles? How do you think the addict would react?

3. A hospital prescription for morphine, written for pain relief in a terminally ill patient, has been written incorrectly by the houseman. He has already been on duty for 40 hours. How do you approach him? How do you think he will react?

4. You are working on the production of a batch of drug in industry. Your boss is pressing you to release the drug onto the market; however, you feel that it has not fully met all of the quality assurance requirements. How would you present your case to a board of managers?

5. Worried parents ask for your advice as a phar-

macist. They have found some tablets in their son's bedroom. You identify them, and they are drugs that have the potential for misuse and abuse. How do you handle this situation? How do you think the parents will react? Consider the feelings/reaction of the son.

6. A middle-aged man comes storming into your pharmacy. You have given him the wrong strength of tablets and he is very angry. How do you deal with this situation? How do you think the man will react?

7. An older lady wishes to purchase some codeine linctus 'for someone else'. After much soul searching and questioning, you decide to sell her a 100 ml bottle. She returns 10 minutes later with a broken bottle (and not much evidence of codeine linctus). She claims she has dropped it, and wants a replacement. What do you do?

Further examples of difficult situations in pharmacy can be found in Table 3.2.

## NON-VERBAL COMMUNICATION

The meaning of what a person says is made up of several component parts. These comprise the words which are spoken, the tone of voice used, the speed and volume of speech, the intonation and a whole range of body postures and movements. It is generally agreed that in any communication the actual words convey about 10% of the message. This is called verbal communication. The other 90% is transmitted by non-verbal communication which consists of how it is said (40%) and body language (50%).

### Body language

It is well documented that our impression of another person is very often created at first glance. As you get to know a person better, initial impressions are either reinforced or discarded. In many situations in life the opportunity does not present itself to get to know someone better and the first impression is the one which remains. This will not necessarily detract from communication, if the impression which was first given is a favourable one. However, if a poor image was created at first glance, it may cause problems at future meetings or even prevent future encounters taking place. If we consider this in a pharmaceutical context, the pharmacist who creates a friendly approachable impression is more likely to find cus-

**Table 3.2  Types of patients' problems and the communication difficulties which they present**

| Problem type | Examples | Communication difficulties |
|---|---|---|
| Embarrassing problems | Contraception, disorders of the reproductive system, hyperhydrosis, skin conditions | Obtaining privacy in the pharmacy Establishing a common language of understanding Demonstrating empathy and understanding Establishing trust and confidentiality Not exhibiting negative nonverbal behaviour |
| Emotional/ psychological problems | Anxiety, depression, marital problems, drug abuse and dependence, stress | Demonstrating empathy and understanding Insufficient time for counselling Evaluating patient's immediate needs Establishing the nature and amount of advice to be given Establishing two-way listening |
| Problems of handicap | | Making inaccurate judgements regarding personality, intellect, etc. |
| Sensory | Blindness, deafness | |
| Physical | Paralysis, congenital deformity | Providing effective explanations |
| Communicative | Speech impairment | Listening, taking sufficient time with patient |
| Mental | Educationally subnormal | Overcoming social barriers |
| Psychological | Personality disorders | |
| Social | Introversion | |
| Terminal illness | | Knowing what to say and how to say it Establishing patient's feelings |
| Financial problems | | Interpreting cues given off by patient regarding cost of medicines Not embarrassing the patient |

tomers and patients receptive to what he or she has to say. The pharmacist who makes a negative impression will have to work considerably harder to gain the customer's confidence. In the long term, rapport may be established, but the chance may not be given to develop it. If customers perceive the pharmacist as being unfriendly and unhelpful they will probably go elsewhere for advice or will be unreceptive to any information or advice the pharmacist offers.

Body language can be broken down into several component parts which include gestures, facial expression, eye contact, physical contact, body posture, body space and proximity. It is the combination of all these components which gives the overall impression. It is important to ensure that they are all compatible. If you portray a mixture of messages this will cause confusion to observers and they will probably avoid you altogether.

## Gestures

Hand gestures in particular are used in communication. They are useful when emphasizing a point or to help to describe something. Used appropriately, they can greatly enhance communication and improve the listener's understanding. However, it is important not to overuse them, as this can detract from the spoken word and become a distraction to the listener. Pharmacists should use gestures, where appropriate, to emphasize a point or describe a particular procedure. Observing other people's gestures can give useful information on how concerned, agitated or confused they may be. Do a spot of 'people watching'! It is amazing how much information about a person you can pick up just by quietly observing his gestures.

## Facial expression

This is of vital importance in any communication. In fact, it has been suggested that, after the spoken word, facial expression is the most important part of communication. Many of the communication situations in which pharmacists are involved deal with listening and offering advice. In these types of situations the success of the event will be very dependent on how relaxed and comfortable the patient or customer feels. The facial expression of the pharmacist at the start of the conversation may very well determine how receptive the patient will be to any advice or information offered. Facial expression says a lot about mood and emotion, with the eyes and the mouth giving the dominant signs. As

well as ensuring that facial expression is encouraging and welcoming, it is important for pharmacists to be able to read the meaning of facial expressions. In this way important points regarding a patient's level of comprehension or receptiveness can be judged.

## Eye contact

Avoiding eye contact is a very successful way of avoiding communication. This can be very well illustrated by observing a class of students who have just been asked a question by a lecturer!

The maintenance of eye contact during a conversation is vital to ensure the continuation of the process. Eye contact can indicate interest in the subject and is also useful as a means of determining whose turn it is to speak. However, care must be taken. Whilst eye contact is important, an uninterrupted stare can be rather off-putting and may detract from the success of the communication.

## Physical contact

This is an important aspect of any communication process. It can be used to greatly enhance verbal communication. A sympathetic touch on an arm can often say far more than any number of words. However, physical contact is governed by broad social rules and inappropriate use may cause problems. The levels of physical contact vary greatly between cultures, with the British being identified as one of the least 'touching' nations in the world. An awareness of this is important. Pharmacists, in their professional role, come into contact with people from a wide variety of social and cultural backgrounds. What is considered acceptable behaviour in one culture could be unacceptable in another.

## Body posture

We can usually control the words we say, but we are not so good at controlling our body language. Although we may be giving a positive verbal message, our body posture may be giving a negative message. This may be easily picked up by the listener and the verbal message lost.

Body posture can have a major influence on how well a communication progresses, or even if it gets started at all. There are several classic body postures which have been identified as having significant meanings.

- *The closed position.* This would be illustrated by a person standing with his arms folded. This is seen as a rather negative posture and not one likely to encourage initiation of communication.

• *Feet position.* It is often found that a person's feet will be pointing in the direction in which he wants to go. This can be used to check whether the listener is giving you his full attention or would rather be elsewhere.

• *Positive body posture.* Leaning towards the person who is talking, or sitting in a relaxed fashion, are both examples of non-verbal language which can encourage good communication.

As pharmacists, we are constantly trying to build up a complete picture of a patient's problems. In many instances, one of the most important information sources at our disposal is the patient. Good communication will provide much useful information which can then be used to the benefit of the patient.

## Personal space

We all have our own space in which we feel comfortable. Personal space varies between cultures and its extent depends on the situation. The different space zones are generally divided into four main areas. There are different stress levels that are experienced when a simple question or statement is made in each of the four areas of space.

### General space

This is approximately 3 m or more. This is the space we would normally prefer to have round us if we are addressing a group of people or are working alone.

### Sociable area

This is approximately 1–3 m and is the type of distance used when communicating with people we do not know very well.

### Personal area

This is approximately 0.5–1 m. This is the space we would normally feel comfortable with, when at a business or social meeting with people we know reasonably well. It is sufficiently close to allow friendly and meaningful communication without any individuals feeling threatened by having their personal space invaded.

### Intimate area

This is usually 15–50 cm. This space is reserved for people we know very well. Husbands, wives, children, close friends and family are examples of the kind of people with whom we would be comfortable at these distances. If anybody else enters this so-called 'intimate zone' we feel threatened and will generally withdraw into ourselves. There are occasions when we find ourselves in these sorts of situations. Next time you are in a crowded lift watch the behaviour of the people around you. They are all having their personal space invaded. It is unlikely that anyone will talk and eye contact will be avoided.

An awareness of personal space is important for pharmacists as it can play an important role in the success or otherwise of communication. If you carry on a conversation with someone at too great a distance it may be difficult to build up any rapport. However, if you are so close to people that they feel uncomfortable and threatened, they will be so aware of this that it is unlikely that any meaningful dialogue will occur. A simple enquiry, when asked in the general area, can feel like an accusation when asked in the personal area.

## ASSERTIVENESS

Assertiveness is a positive way of relating to other people – a means of communicating as effectively as possible, particularly in potentially awkward situations. Assertive behaviour is useful when dealing with conflict, in negotiation, leadership and motivation, giving and receiving feedback, in cooperative working and in meetings. Assertive communication can give the user confidence, a clearer self-image and leads to a feeling of more control over situations, especially those of conflict. Fundamental assertiveness skills should be useful both in your working life as a pharmacist, and in your personal life.

## Defining behaviour and communication

A number of terms are used in connection with assertiveness:

• Assertiveness may be defined as standing up for personal rights and expressing thoughts, feelings and beliefs in direct, honest and appropriate ways, which do not violate another person's rights. Being assertive involves listening to others and understanding their feelings. An assertive communicator will find a mutually acceptable solution. An important part of being assertive therefore is to formulate your aims and objectives clearly. People who behave assertively deal with other people as equals.

• Aggressive behaviour violates others' rights as the aggressive person seeks to achieve goals at the expense of others. Aggressive behaviour is often frightening, threatening and unpredictable. It will bring out negative feelings in the receiver and communication will be difficult.

• Passive–aggressive behaviour is not as obvious and usually involves a person giving a mixed message; that is, he may agree with what you are saying but then raise his eyebrows and pull a face at you behind your back.

• Submissive behaviour is portrayed by people who behave submissively, have very little confidence in themselves and poor self-esteem. They often allow others to violate their personal rights, in other words, take advantage of them.

People who behave assertively often achieve what they have set out to do in the long term, as do those who have dealt with assertive people (usually). This is in comparison to those who act aggressively, who think that they have achieved their goal, but this is usually at the cost of respect and loyalty from those around them. Submissive people rarely achieve what they want.

## Personal rights and those of others

The following list includes examples of personal rights:

• To state my own needs and priorities
• To be respected as an intelligent and capable equal
• To express my feelings
• To express my own opinions and values
• To say 'Yes' or 'No'
• To make mistakes
• To change my mind
• To say 'I don't understand'
• To ask for what I want (realizing that the other person has the right to say 'No')
• To decline responsibility for others' problems
• To deal with others without being dependent on them for their approval.

## Techniques in assertive communication

### Use of 'I' and 'You' statements

Using 'I' rather than 'You' in a statement places the responsibility of the affect, desire or opinion with the asserter rather than attempting to place the responsibility for personal feelings on the other person. Use of 'I' statements can minimize negative reactions such as anger in communication. For example, compare the following two statements which are effectively saying the same thing. 'You appear to have been arriving rather late for work, recently.' 'I have noticed that you have been arriving rather late for work, recently.' The first statement gives an impression of accusation while the second is more observational and less threatening.

### Repeating the message

If a request for information is not being answered directly by the receiver, a useful assertive technique would be to repeat your request. If this is done firmly and without aggression, the message can be repeated until a reply is obtained. However, there are situations when this technique would not be appropriate, for example when an answer to the request has been given, even though it may not be the desired response. An example of this would be where children repeatedly ask for sweets and the parent has already said 'No!'. Obviously, repeating this request will not be helpful and will aggravate the situation.

### Clear communication

To communicate we use both verbal and non-verbal language; they are both important and it is essential that they match or we will send mixed or confusing messages. An example of a mixed message may arise when asking a patient in a community pharmacy if he understands how to take his dispensed medication. An affirmative reply may be given verbally by the patient but non-verbal signs such as close examination of the label on the dispensed medication and a creased forehead may indicate some confusion which would need to be clarified.

### Extracting the truth

Strong emotions can get in the way of clear communication. Communicators who are angry or upset may cloud the message they are trying to convey with other issues. They may exaggerate or become emotional. It is important, as the receiver, to accept this in an assertive manner. Acknowledge true criticisms but do not be distracted by side issues.

### Self talk

In a situation of conflict we can often 'work ourselves up' to an angry or emotional state which can then lead to unclear and unsuccessful communication. If we use self talk and clarify the issues in a situation, considering the points of view and rights of all those involved, we can often defuse the situation inside ourselves. We can then be ready to undertake clear, unconfused communication which will hopefully lead to a more successful outcome. Self talk does not have to involve 'giving way' to the other person. Rather it is a way of controlling naturally felt emotions and then, instead of 'letting fly', expressing yourself in a manner which is more likely to produce the result you need.

There are a number of steps which you could follow to increase your assertiveness.

- *Choose the right situation.* Choose situations where you believe you have a reasonably good chance of maintaining your assertion, and achieving a mutually acceptable outcome. Changes in behaviour come in small steps, e.g. making requests or giving praise.
- *Prepare for situations.* Spend a short time before an important situation working through the following steps:
  - Get your own objectives clear.
  - Clarify your own and other people's rights.
  - Turn 'faulty' dialogues into sound ones.
  - 'Self talk' the assertive statements with which you want to start the interaction.
  - Consider your response to anticipated hassles.
- *Behave assertively during the situation.* To overcome unexpected hassles, buy brief thinking time, e.g. 'Have I got this right? What you're saying is ...', or 'I'd like to think about that for a moment'.
- *Review the situation afterwards.* Analyse what happened and learn from it. Be honest. Do not play down or exaggerate your success. Never berate yourself. Remember that some people may have a vested interest in your not becoming more assertive.

## TRANSACTIONAL ANALYSIS IN COMMUNICATION

Although communication can be improved using the previously mentioned methods, the way people react and respond in communication is clearly linked to personality. Transactional analysis is a way of looking at the psychological aspects of communication. It suggests that there are three 'ego' states: adult, parent and child. Different situations trigger a particular response out of one main ego state. The par-

ent state, which is powerful, responsible, always right without explanation, may be divided into two: a 'controlling' parent, who is condescending, angry, disapproving and hostile or a 'nurturing' parent, who is loving, encouraging and concerned. The child state can be divided into two states: an 'adapted' child, who is sulky, defiant, aggressive, dejected and hurt or angry if things do not go his way, or a 'natural' child, who is uninhibited, loud, energetic and impulsive. Within the natural child state is the 'little professor' who is creative, curious and intuitive. The adult state is calm, thoughtful, thinks things through clearly, negotiates and uses assertive behaviour. It is generally accepted that the most appropriate response in business or within an inter-professional relationship is an adult–adult consultation, demonstrating objective thinking and confidence. Communication between the prescriber (GP) and the dispenser (pharmacist) would, therefore, generally be conducted on an adult-to-adult basis. Both practitioners must respect each other for having a unique set of knowledge, and the information exchange must reflect this respect. There are occasions, however, where different ego states within the communication process may be more appropriate.

## BARRIERS TO COMMUNICATION

In a pharmacy setting there are a number of factors which can be of benefit to, or can detract from, the quality of any communication. Common barriers which exist can be identified under four main headings:

- environment
- patient factors
- the pharmacist
- time.

## Environment

Community pharmacies, hospital outpatient pharmacies and hospital wards are all areas where pharmacists use their communication skills in a professional capacity. None of these areas is ideal, but an awareness of the limitations of the environment goes part the way to resolving some of the problems. Some examples of potential problem areas are listed below:

- *A busy pharmacy.* This may create the impression that there appears to be little time to discuss personal matters with patients. The pharmacist is supervising a number of different activities at the same time and is unable to devote his or her full attention to an individual matter. It is important that pharmacists organize their work patterns in such a way as to minimize this impression.

- *Lack of privacy*. Some pharmacies, both community and hospital outpatient departments, have counselling rooms or areas but many have not. Many hospital wards could be likened to a busy thoroughfare. For good communication to occur and rapport to be developed it is often necessary for the consultation to take place in a quiet environment, free of interruptions. The aforementioned conditions, in which pharmacists frequently work, require additional skills to overcome the lack of ideal facilities.

- *Noise*. Noise levels within the working environment are an obvious barrier to good communication. People strain to hear what is said, comprehension is made more difficult and, as mentioned previously, particular problems exist for the hearing impaired.

- *Physical barriers*. As already mentioned in the section on personal space, the distance between people when communication occurs is significant. Pharmacy counters and outpatient dispensing hatches are physical barriers which may dictate what this distance is. This in turn can create problems in developing effective communication.

## Patient factors

One of the main barriers to good communication in a pharmacy can be patients' expectations. In today's world people have busy and hectic lifestyles. In many cases they have become used to seeing a 'good' pharmacy as one where their prescription is dispensed quickly. They are not expecting time to be spent with them checking understanding of medication or other health-related matters. Once the purpose of the communication is explained, most patients realize its importance and are quite happy to enter into a dialogue.

- *Physical disabilities*. Dealing with patients who have sight or hearing impairment will require the pharmacist to use additional communication skills. Practical suggestions on help which can be given to patients with sight impairment can be found in the chapter on counselling (Ch. 37). Dealing with the hearing impaired has been discussed in this chapter (p. 40).

- *Comprehension difficulties*. Not all people come from the same educational background and care must be taken to assess a patient's level of understanding and choose appropriate language. In many cases the lack of ability to comprehend may be because English is not the patient's first language. Pharmacists working in areas where there is a high proportion of non-English speakers may find it useful to stock or develop their own information leaflets in appropriate languages.

- *Illiteracy*. An amazingly high proportion of the population of the UK is illiterate. Obviously for these patients any written material will be meaningless. It is not always easy to identify illiterate patients as many feel ashamed and are unlikely to admit to it. However, if a pharmacist identifies any patients who have reading difficulties, pictorial labels can be used and additional verbal advice can be given.

## The pharmacist

It is very easy to talk in theoretical terms about good communication but, as was stated at the start of this chapter, it is not always easy and needs to be worked at. Not all of us are natural, good communicators, but identifying our strengths and weaknesses will assist in improving our communication skills. Some of the weaknesses which can be barriers to good communication are:

- lack of confidence
- lack of interest
- laziness
- a pharmacist who is prone to delegate responsibilities to untrained staff.

If any of these characteristics is present the reason for it should be identified and resolved, if possible.

## Time

In many instances time, or the lack of it, can be a major constraint on good communication. Try developing a meaningful conversation with someone who constantly looks at his watch! Similarly, if the person who has initiated the conversation is short of time, the wrong kind of questions may be used and little opportunity for discussion allowed. It is always worthwhile checking what time people have available before trying to embark on any communication. That way you will make the best use of what time is available.

Not all barriers to good communication can be

removed, but an awareness that they exist and taking account of them will go a long way towards diminishing their negative impact.

As stated at the beginning of this chapter, good communication is not easy and needs to be worked at. We all have different personalities and skills which means we have strengths in some areas and weaknesses in others. If we can become aware of, and maximize, our strengths and minimize our weaknesses, we should become better communicators. Being articulate and able to explain things clearly is of vital importance. However, listening with understanding and empathy is of equal, and in certain situations, of greater importance. We may all hear the words being said but are we really listening to the complete message?

This chapter has emphasized communication skills for pharmacists, particularly in the workplace but remember, good communication is a life skill to be used at all times.

- Assertive behaviour treats other people as equals, and is not to be confused with aggressive behaviour which violates other people's rights.
- Assertive communication will tend to use 'I' rather than 'You', repeat messages, employ clear verbal and nonverbal communication and clarify issues without emotion.
- There are three ego states – adult, parent, child – used in transactional analysis.
- In the working environment there are many potential barriers to effective communication which need to be minimized wherever possible.
- Pharmacists need to maximize their strengths and minimize their weaknesses of communication.

## FURTHER READING

Burnard P 1992 Effective communication skills for health professionals. Chapman & Hall, London
Ley P 1988 Communicating with patients. Croom Helm, London
Pease A 1989 Body language. Sheldon Press, London

## Key Points

- Communication is a two-way process involving words, facial and vocal expression, body posture and appearance.
- A failure to communicate effectively is likely to cause problems.
- 'You never get a second chance to make a first impression.'
- Questions may be open or closed and in most situations a balanced combination is required.
- Questioning skills also involve listening to answers.
- Hearing loss is common in the elderly and will present a barrier to effective communication.
- A number of signs help identify those with hearing loss and many steps can be taken to help the situation.
- Empathy (active listening) involves understanding other people's feelings and reflecting this back to them.
- Body language includes gestures, expression, eye and physical contact, body posture, space and proximity.
- After the spoken word, facial expression is probably the most important part of communication.
- Eye contact must be maintained, but must not become a stare.
- An awareness of personal space is needed to allow effective communication.

# PART 2

# DISPENSING

# 4

# Dispensing techniques (compounding and good practice)

*M. M. Moody*

---

After studying this chapter, the reader will know about:

**Good dispensing practice**
**The working environment and procedures**
**Dispensing equipment and its correct use**
    Balances
    Liquid measuring
    Mortar and pestle
    Tared containers
    Mixing and grinding
**Identification and use of materials**
**Problem solving**
**Methods of counting tablets and capsules.**

---

## Introduction

This chapter deals with aspects of good pharmacy practice. It will concentrate on the small-scale manufacture of medicines from basic ingredients. This process is called compounding or extemporaneous dispensing. In addition, good practice which applies to all aspects of dispensing will be considered and current methods for counting solid dosage forms evaluated.

It is important to remember in any dispensing process that the end product is going to be used or taken by a person or an animal who is ill. It is therefore of the utmost importance that the medicine is of the highest achievable quality. This, in turn, means that the preparation process must be undertaken with the highest standards applied. Quality assurance procedures are of paramount importance in the pharmaceutical manufacturing industry (see Ch. 29) and the same scrupulous attention to detail must be applied to small-scale production.

## ORGANIZATION

The environment in which you work will have considerable influence on your efficiency and therefore it is important to develop a tidy and organized method of working. The pharmacist who works with a dispensing bench cluttered with several containers all containing different ingredients is more likely to select the incorrect one. Always return ingredients to their appropriate shelf when you have measured out the required quantity.

## Cleanliness

The bench that you work at, the equipment and utensils you use and the container which is to hold the final product must all be scrupulously clean. Many medicines provide ideal growth environments for bacteria. Care must be taken to minimize their introduction at the production stage.

Lack of cleanliness is also likely to cause contamination of the preparation with other ingredients. A spatula, which has been used to remove a certain ingredient from a container, if not washed before being used again, will adulterate any subsequent containers.

## Appearance

A clean white overall should be worn. This should be kept buttoned up. Flapping lab coats in laboratory environments are a potential hazard. An overall will also help to prevent outdoor clothes becoming stained if any spillages occur.

Hair should be tied back and any skin lesions covered with a dressing.

## Documenting procedures and results

Keeping comprehensive records is an essential part

of the dispensing process. This may be details of ingredients used, procedures carried out or the calculation of quantities. This should be carried out in a methodical way. An untidy, disorganized approach at this stage can easily lead to errors. In an attempt to produce neat and tidy lab books many students are inclined to do calculations and write details of ingredients on scraps of paper intending to copy the information into the lab book at a later time. This practice should be discouraged. Information may get lost and errors made when transferring details. Good habits learned as an undergraduate should be continued into professional practice.

## EQUIPMENT

The selection of the correct equipment or 'tools' for the job is essential. In addition, this equipment must be used in the correct way.

## Weighing

### Balances

Three types of balance have traditionally been used in dispensing, Class A, Class B (Fig. 4.1) and Class C.

New legislation is now in force and balances are categorized as Class I, Class II, Class III and Class IV. The balance most commonly used in dispensing is a Class B balance. The Class II balance is its nearest equivalent. The main change in the legislation is a stricter control on the maximum and minimum weights which can be weighed. All balances in use which were manufactured after November 1988 must now be marked with both a maximum and minimum weight. The weights previously allowable are shown in Table 4.1.

The minimum weight which can be weighed on the new balances is calculated from the maximum weighable quantity, i.e.

$$\frac{\text{Maximum weight}}{2000} \times 10$$

This means that a balance marked with a maximum of 100 g can weigh a minimum of 500 milligrams or one marked with a maximum of 60 g can weigh a minimum of 300 milligrams. These weights are too high for normal dispensing procedures. Some balances marked with a minimum of 500 milligrams have been given dispensation to weigh down to 250 milligrams. However, manufacturers are cur-

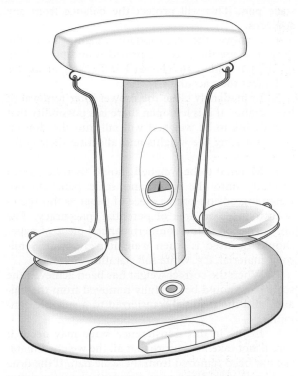

**Fig. 4.1** Dispensing balance.

| Table 4.1 Classes of balances with their weighing capabilities | | | |
|---|---|---|---|
| Type | Minimum weight | Increment | Normal maximum weight |
| Class A | 50 mg | 1 mg | 1 g |
| Class B | 100 mg | 10 mg | 50 g |
| Class C | 1 g | 100 mg | 2 kg |

rently developing balances with a weighing range of 25 g to 125 milligrams. Dispensation has been given to Class B balances and they do not need to be stamped with a maximum or minimum weight. They remain legal and usable until January 2000. At the time of writing it is uncertain what will happen after that date.

Rules for the use of dispensing scales:

1. Ensure that the balance and the scale pans are clean.

2. Check that your instrument is sited in a draught-free area and the pointer is swinging freely.

3. Place a piece of paper under the right-hand

scale pan. This will protect the balance from any spillages.

4. Remove the appropriate weights from the drawer, using the tweezers provided and place them on the left-hand pan. (Never handle weights as this will affect their accuracy.)

5. Immediately close the drawer after removal of the weights. If it is left open there is a possibility that ingredients to be weighed will fall into the drawer, contaminating the weights and affecting their accuracy.

6. Material to be weighed should then be placed carefully onto the right-hand scale pan. Do not weigh ingredients onto a piece of paper as this merely introduces an area of potential inaccuracy. The only occasion that a counterbalanced piece of paper should be used is when weighing greasy or semisolid material, e.g. white soft paraffin.

7. When the correct weight has been achieved the scale pan should be carefully removed from the balance and the material transferred to a suitable container.

8. Errors in this transference stage may occur if care is not taken to ensure that all the weighed material has been removed from the scale pan. If the drug is to be dissolved or incorporated into a suspension it can be washed from the scale pan using some of the appropriate liquid vehicle.

9. It is important, however, not to become overzealous when removing material from a scale pan. There is a temptation to tap the glass scale pan against the side of the container. If the scale pan becomes chipped, this will affect the accuracy of the balance and silvers of glass will not improve the health of the patient!

10. The scale pan should then be washed and dried thoroughly, before any other substance is weighed. A second substance must never be weighed on the remains of the first.

11. The weights should be returned to the drawer. Drawers are normally organized in four sections. The weights should be kept together with those of a similar size, e.g. a 10 milligram weight should not be placed in the same section as a 10 g weight.

In addition to using the balance correctly there are one or two other rules which should be observed, when weighing, to ensure good dispensing practice. These are:

● If using a solid material which requires to be ground or sieved, always ensure that this is done before weighing the required quantity. If a quantity of powder is weighed and then size reduced by grinding in a mortar or sieving, there is a strong possibility that some of the material will be lost in the process and the final preparation will not contain the correct proportions of ingredients. The best approach is to roughly weigh an excess quantity, grind or sieve it as required, then accurately weigh off the required quantity.

● As far as possible never split quantities and do two weighings, as this will increase the inaccuracies.

● If a quantity less than the legal minimum is needed, it is necessary to weigh at least the minimum weight allowable and make an excess of the product or prepare it by trituration (see Ch. 5).

## Measuring liquids

### Liquid measures

Measures for liquids must all comply with current Weights and Measures Regulations and should be stamped accordingly. Traditionally, conical measures (Fig. 4.2) have been used in dispensing, although it could be argued that if not used carefully they can be less accurate than cylindrical measures.

Whichever type of measure is chosen always ensure that:

1. The measure is vertical when reading the meniscus. If this is not done considerable errors in quantities can occur, especially with conical measures, where the error increases with height, because of the slope of the sides.

2. The measure is thoroughly drained. Even if the ingredient is only slightly viscous it is amazing how much can be left in the measure.

3. As far as possible never use more than one measure. Splitting the volume between two measures will increase the potential for error.

4. Always select the smallest measure which will hold the desired volume.

5. If the substance being measured is viscous and it would be virtually impossible to drain the measure effectively then the volume should be measured by difference. This is done by pouring an excess into the measure and then pouring off the liquid until only the excess volume remains.

---

**EXAMPLE 4.1**

25 ml of glycerol is required.
    Because of the viscosity it is difficult to remove it completely from the measure.

It is therefore advisable to measure, say, 35 ml and pour off the 25 ml required, ensuring that 10 ml is left in the measure.

When pouring out liquids to be measured it is important to observe one or two simple rules which ensure good dispensing practice.

- Always hold the liquid container with the label uppermost so that you pour away from the label. This ensures that any liquid which runs down the side of the bottle will not affect the label. There is nothing worse than bottles where the ingredient name has been obscured because large quantities of the liquid have been allowed to run down the side of the bottle. Examine containers of highly coloured substances such as amaranth solution or corrosive substances like acids to see what effect there has been on the label and replace it if necessary.

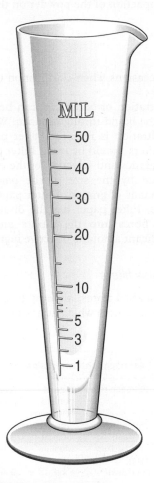

**Fig. 4.2**  Conical dispensing measure.

- If possible, when pouring liquids, hold the cap of the container in your hand, preferably between the fourth finger and the palm of your hand. It is possible you may be measuring more than one liquid and if caps are left lying on the dispensing bench it is all too easy to mix them up and place the wrong one back on the container.

## Measuring small volumes

It is important to select the correct equipment when measuring. The minimum measurable volume for a 10 ml conical measure is 1 ml. Graduated pipettes can be used for volumes from 5 ml down to 0.1 ml. For volumes smaller than this a trituration should be made. The viscosity of the substance being measured should also be considered.

### Correct use of pipettes

Pipettes can be either the 'drainage' or 'blow out' variety. A rubber bulb or teat should be used. On no account should mouth suction be used.

1. A bulb or teat should be placed over the mouth of the pipette, taking care not to push it down too far.
2. The container of the substance to be measured should be ready on the bench.
3. The top of the container should be removed and held in the hand, between the fourth finger and the palm of the hand.
4. The pipette should be put into the container, taking care that only a short length of the pipette is immersed. If a quantity of liquid is allowed to collect on the outside of the pipette the accuracy of the measuring will be affected.
5. The correct amount of liquid should then be drawn up the pipette. Take care at this stage as the liquid may shoot up the pipette into the bulb.
6. If a pipette bulb is being used the appropriate valve is pressed to prevent the liquid running out of the pipette, the pipette removed from the container and the liquid then released.
7. If using a simple teat this should now be flicked off with the thumb and a finger placed firmly over the top of the pipette, taking care not to allow any liquid to be lost. The pipette can then be withdrawn from the container and the liquid measured out by removing the finger from the top of the pipette.

## Tared containers

Liquid preparations should as far as possible be

made up to volume in a measure. There are, however, instances when accurate transfer of the preparation to the final container is difficult. With certain suspensions it can be almost impossible to remove all the insoluble ingredients when pouring from one container to another. Emulsions and viscous preparations can also be difficult to transfer accurately. In these cases it is sometimes considered useful to use a tared container.

### To tare a bottle

A volume of water identical to the volume of the product being dispensed is accurately measured. This is then poured into the chosen medicine container and the meniscus marked with the upper edge of a small adhesive label. The container is then emptied and allowed to drain thoroughly. The preparation is then poured into the container and made up to volume, using the tare mark as a guide.

This procedure should be used with discretion and only in situations when major inaccuracies would occur in the transfer of liquids. It should also only be used when water is present as one of the ingredients. Putting medicines into a wet bottle is generally considered bad practice.

## MIXING AND GRINDING

### Mortar and pestle

The mortar (bowl) and pestle (pounding device) are used to reduce the size of powders, mix powders, mix powders and liquids, and make emulsions. Two types, each in varying sizes, are used.

### Glass mortar and pestle

These are generally small and therefore cannot be used for large quantities of material. The smooth surface of the glass reduces the friction which can be generated. They are therefore not suitable for size reduction, except for friable materials such as crystals. They are useful for dissolving small quantities of ingredients, for mixing small quantities of fine powders and for the mixing of substances such as dyes which are absorbed by and stain composition or porcelain mortars.

### Porcelain or composition mortars and pestles

These are normally larger than the glass variety and have a rougher surface. They are ideal for size reduc-

tion of solids and for mixing solids and liquids, as in the preparation of suspensions and emulsions.

## Correct use of a mortar and pestle

### Size reduction using a mortar and pestle

Selection of the correct type of mortar and pestle is vital for this operation. A flat-bottomed mortar and a pestle with a flat end should be chosen. A flat-ended pestle in a mortar with a round bottom, or vice versa, will mean a lot of wasted effort.

### Using a mortar and pestle for mixing powders

Adequate mixing will only be achieved if there is sufficient space. Overfilling of the mortar should therefore be avoided. The pestle should be rotated in both right and left directions to ensure thorough mixing. Undue pressure should not be used as this will cause impaction of the powder on the bottom of the mortar.

## Filters

There are occasions when clarification of a liquid is required.

Coarse filtration or 'straining' can be carried out by pouring the liquid through muslin. Where a finer degree of filtration is required, filter paper or sintered glass filters should be used. Filter paper comes in different grades and selection of the correct grade is determined by the size of the particles to be removed. Details of grades of filter paper are found in Table 4.2. Filter paper has the disadvantages of introducing fibres into the filtrate and may also absorb significant amounts of active ingredient.

### Sintered glass filters

These do not shed fibres, are easy to clean and can be used for substances which attack filter paper such

| Table 4.2 | Filter paper characteristics | | |
|---|---|---|---|
| Number (Whatman series) | Filtration rate | Size of particle removed | Average pore size (μm) |
| 54 | 1 (fast) | Coarse | 3.4–5.0 |
| 1 | 4 (medium fast) | Medium | 2.1–2.8 |
| 50 | 23 (slow) | Fine | 0.4–1.1 |

as potassium permanganate and zinc chloride. A filter with a pore size 15–40 μm (grade 3) is suitable for most solutions. They will pass through by gravity, although large volumes may be slow and need the assistance of a vacuum. A grade 4 filter (pore size 5–15 μm) requires a vacuum.

## Bunsen burners

Bunsen burners should always be placed on a heat-resistant mat on the dispensing bench. When heating with a Bunsen burner, the flame control should be rotated to produce a blue flame. In most dispensing exercises only gentle heat is required, so only use a fierce blue flame if excessive heat is called for. When not in use the Bunsen burner should be turned to a yellow flame or turned off.

## Water-baths

These are used when melting ointment bases or preparing suppositories. Normally the materials to be heated are placed in a porcelain evaporating basin and placed over the hot water in the water-bath. In most melting exercises the materials should be melted gently. There is no necessity to have the water boiling vigorously, this does not increase the heat, but does increase the risk of scalding.

## MANIPULATIVE TECHNIQUES

Selection of the correct equipment and using it appropriately is fundamental to good compounding. There are, in addition, several basic manipulative techniques which must be practised.

## Mixing

The goal of any mixing operation should be to ensure that even distribution of all the ingredients has occurred. If a sample is removed from any part of the final preparation it should be identical to a sample taken from any other part of the container.

### Mixing of liquids

Simple stirring or shaking is usually all that is required to mix two or more liquids. The degree of stirring or shaking will be dependent on the viscosities of the liquids. Thus mixing liquids of low viscosities will require only minimal stirring, while mixing two liquids, both with a high viscosity, will need more vigorous agitation.

### Mixing solids with liquids

A knowledge of the solubility of the solid should be used. Particle size reduction is also of paramount importance. This will either speed up the dissolution process or improve the uniform distribution of the solid throughout the liquid.

### Mixing solids with solids

As well as the correct use of a mortar and pestle the amounts of material being mixed together must be considered.

Where the quantity of material to be mixed is small and the proportions are approximately the same, the materials can be added to an appropriately sized mortar and effectively mixed.

Where a small quantity of powder has to be mixed with a large quantity, to achieve effective mixing, it must be done in stages.

1. The ingredient with the smallest bulk is placed in the mortar.
2. A quantity of the second ingredient, approximately equal in volume to the first is added and carefully mixed, using the pestle.
3. A further quantity of the second ingredient, approximately equal in volume to the mixture in the mortar, is now added.
4. This process, known as 'doubling-up', is continued until all the powder has been added.

### Mixing semi-solids

This usually occurs in the preparation of ointments where two or more ointment bases may be mixed together. The bases can be mixed together by rubbing them down on an ointment slab, using a spatula. If there is a significant difference in the quantities of bases being mixed the 'doubling-up' process should be used. An alternative method is the fusion method.

*The fusion method:*

1. Place the bases in a porcelain evaporating basin and gently heat them over a water-bath until they have just melted. Excess heat should not be used as overheating may cause physical or chemical changes in some materials.
2. The basin is then removed from the heat and the contents are stirred continuously until the mixture has cooled and set. Stirring at this stage is of

vital importance as otherwise the components may segregate on cooling.

When using the fusion method do not be tempted to add any solid active ingredients to the basin before the bases have set. Addition of any further ingredients is best done by rubbing down on an ointment slab. Further details of methods used in the preparation of ointments can be found in Chapter 14.

## SELECTION OF INGREDIENTS

When dispensing, selection of the correct product is of paramount importance. Dispensary shelves are filled with an increasing number of products and the label on each container must be read carefully and checked to ensure that it contains the product required. Details of manufactured preparations where difficulties may occur are found in Chapter 9. Problems and errors can also occur in extemporaneous dispensing. Some preparations which are dispensed extemporaneously contain several ingredients, so the potential for error is increased.

Pharmacy undergraduates may encounter difficulties when an ingredient occurs in a variety of forms or a synonym is used.

### Variety of forms

The following item has to be prepared: Coal Tar Paste BP.

This paste consists of 7.5% strong coal tar solution in compound zinc paste. Coal tar is available as:

Coal tar solution
Strong coal tar solution
Coal tar.

If all three containers are sitting together on a shelf the wrong item may be selected by accident. Some other materials where confusion can occur are listed in Table 4.3. This list is not meant to be comprehensive. The only foolproof method of avoiding errors is to read the container label carefully.

### Synonyms

Certain substances used in dispensing may be known by more than one name. An awareness of this is useful when selecting ingredients. Some examples of commonly used preparations are found in Table 4.4. It should be noted that this table illustrates a few examples and is not comprehensive.

**Table 4.3  Some substances which occur in a variety of forms**

| Light magnesium carbonate | Because of its lightness and diffusible properties, it is used in suspensions |
| Heavy magnesium carbonate | Normally used in bulk or individual powders |
| Light kaolin | Used in suspensions |
| Heavy kaolin | Used in the preparation of kaolin poultice |
| Precipitated sulphur | This has a smaller particle size than sublimed sulphur and is preferred in preparations for external use, e.g. suspensions, creams and ointments |
| Sublimed sulphur | Slightly gritty powder which does not produce such elegant preparations as precipitated sulphur |
| Yellow soft paraffin | Used as an ointment base |
| White soft paraffin | Bleached yellow soft paraffin normally used when the other ingredients are not strongly coloured |

**Table 4.4  Example of substances with synonyms**

| Substance | Synonym |
| --- | --- |
| Wool fat | Anhydrous lanolin |
| Hydrous wool fat | Lanolin |
| Hard paraffin | Paraffin wax |
| Compound benzoic acid ointment | Whitfield's ointment |
| Macrogol 2000 | Polyethylene glycol 2000 PEG 2000 |
| Theobroma oil | Cocoa butter |

### Concentrated waters

Liquid preparations for oral use are often flavoured to make them more palatable for the patient. In extemporaneously prepared products the flavouring is frequently a flavoured water, e.g. peppermint water, aniseed water. These flavoured waters are available in a concentrated form and are either used as such, or are diluted to provide the vehicle for the preparation. All concentrated waters have the same dilution factor, i.e. 1 part of concentrate plus 39 parts of water yields 40 parts of flavoured water.

---

### EXAMPLE 4.2

In 200 ml of a particular suspension there is 100 ml of peppermint water. The peppermint water is only available as the concentrate. The dilution factor 1 + 39 is used.

1 ml concentrate + 39 ml water = 40 ml peppermint water

If 40 ml of peppermint water contains 1 ml of the concentrate then:

100 ml of peppermint water will contain 2.5 ml of concentrate.

Therefore to 2.5 ml of concentrate is added 97.5 ml of water to produce the 100 ml of flavoured water required.

---

## PROBLEM SOLVING IN EXTEMPORANEOUS DISPENSING

When extemporaneously dispensing, it is always helpful if a method detailing how to prepare the product is available. Methods for 'official' preparations can sometimes be found in reference sources such as the *Pharmaceutical Codex*. However, on many occasions no method is available and one has to be developed. When faced with an extemporaneous preparation and no method, students are often perplexed and unsure of where to start. The application of simple scientific knowledge is often all that is needed.

## Putting theory into practice

### Solubility

Always check the physical properties of the ingredients being used. This provides some very useful information. Always check the solubility of any solid materials. If they are soluble in any of the other ingredients of the product then this will be of considerable benefit in achieving uniform dose distribution. Solution is achieved more quickly if the particle size is small and so size reduction should be considered for any soluble ingredients which are presented in a lumpy or granular form. If the substance is not soluble, or if not already in a finely divided form, it should always be size reduced.

### Volatile ingredients

If an ingredient is volatile then it should be added near the end of the dispensing process. If added too early much may be lost owing to its volatile nature.

### Viscosity

The viscosity of a liquid will have a bearing on how it is measured, i.e. is a pipette suitable, or should it be measured by difference?

The following example illustrates how some very simple facts can be applied to develop an accurate method of preparation.

---

### EXAMPLE 4.3

The following prescription is received:

Sodium Bicarbonate Ear Drops BP
Send 10 ml

*Formula*
Sodium bicarbonate                      500 mg
Glycerol                                        3 ml
Freshly boiled and cooled water    to  10 ml

Points to note:

- Solubility of sodium bicarbonate is 1 in 11 of water.
- Glycerol is a viscous liquid.
- The quantity of water in the ear drops is approximately 6.5 ml.

**Method**

1. The sodium bicarbonate should be size reduced in a mortar and pestle, if necessary.
2. 500 milligrams of sodium bicarbonate is then weighed on a Class B balance and put into a 10 ml conical measuring cylinder.
3. The sodium bicarbonate is soluble, requiring a minimum of 5.5 ml in which to dissolve. Add about 6 ml of water, ensuring that the volume of ingredients does not go beyond the 7 ml mark.
4. Stir the contents of the measure until the sodium bicarbonate is dissolved.
5. Make the volume up to 7 ml with water.
6. The glycerol is viscous and trying to pour 3 ml from a measure is inaccurate. The 3 ml of glycerol can now be added by pouring it into the 7 ml of sodium bicarbonate solution and carefully making the volume in the measure up to 10 ml.

---

The application of a few simple facts and using some problem-solving skills means that a simple accurate method can be developed.

### Expiry date

All extemporaneously prepared products should be awarded an expiry date. Ideally stability studies should be undertaken in order to predict an accurate shelf life for products. This is not usually possible for 'one off' preparations and most hospital pharmacies have guidelines based on previous stability studies. Further information on stability and appropriate expiry dates is found in Chapter 7.

## COUNTING DEVICES

Tablets and capsules form a large proportion of the

medicines which are dispensed today. Many are now presented in patient packs or original packs, but in many instances drugs are supplied in bulk packs and the prescribed amount is counted from them.

Various methods can be used:

- the manual method
- a counting triangle or capsule counter
- a counting tray
- an electronic counter.

These methods all have their advantages and disadvantages and again it is up to each pharmacist to select the most appropriate for the task. Whichever method is selected it must be noted that at no point must the medicines be handled. The equipment should also be carefully cleaned before use, as powder left from one product could cause contamination.

## The manual method

This consists of pouring the product onto a piece of

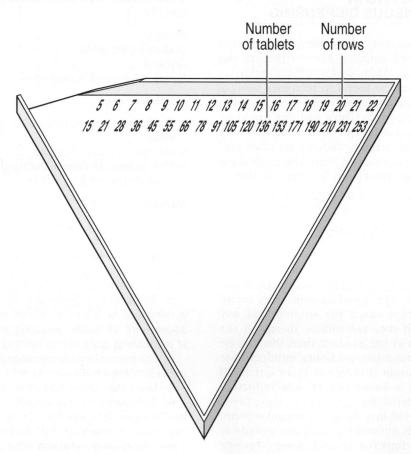

**Fig. 4.3** Counting triangle.

clean white demy paper which overlaps another piece. The products are then counted off in 10s, using a spatula, onto the second piece of paper. This is formed into a small funnel and the tablets or capsules poured into the appropriate container.

Initially this can be a rather slow method but an experienced pharmacist or dispenser can count amazingly quickly. However, concentration must be maintained or the wrong quantity may be counted. The other problem is that white demy paper is becoming increasingly expensive and difficult to obtain.

## Counting triangles and capsule counters

### Counting triangles

This is a fast, accurate and simple way to count tablets. The triangles are made either of metal or plastic. Two rows of figures are printed or etched along the edge. The top row of figures refers to the number of rows and the numbers below refer to the number of tablets contained in that number of rows. This is illustrated in Figure 4.3.

### Capsule counters

Because of their shape, capsules cannot be counted on triangles. A capsule counter, illustrated in Figure 4.4, is a metal tray which consists of 10 rows of grooves. The capsules are poured onto the tray and using a spatula, lined up in the grooves. Each complete row will contain 10 capsules so the number of complete rows multiplied by 10 gives the number of capsules.

Capsule counters are not as easy to manipulate as triangles but are an efficient method for counting capsules. Studies testing the accuracy of the various counting methods have shown these two devices to be the best.

## Perforated counting trays

These are normally made of clear perspex. They consist of a rectangular box with a sliding lid, on top of which is placed a perforated tray. Each box is supplied with several trays with different-sized perforations to accommodate different sizes and types of products (see Fig. 4.5). These trays can be used to count tablets or capsules.

An experienced operator can count quickly and accurately using this type of device. The main disadvantage is the necessity to change the trays for different products.

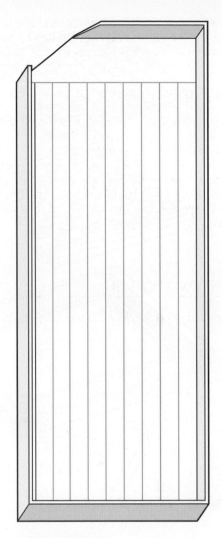

**Fig. 4.4** Capsule counter.

## Electronic counters

There are two types of electronic counter, those which use the weight of the product to count and those which count using a photoelectric cell.

### Electronic balances

Between 5 and 20 of the required dosage form is put on a balance pan or scoop. From the weight of this reference sample, a microprocessor within the device calculates the total number of dosage forms, as they are added. The main problem with this type of device is that for accurate counting, it requires consistent uniformity of the weight of the tablets or capsules.

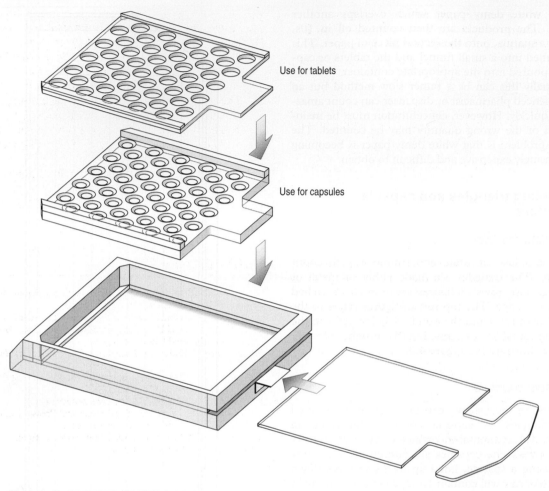

Use for tablets

Use for capsules

**Fig. 4.5** Perforated counting tray.

There can be problems with accuracy when counting sugar-coated or very small tablets.

## Photoelectric cell counters

The product to be counted is poured through a hopper on the top of the machine. The tablets or capsules are then channelled into a straight line and counted as they interrupt the beam of light to the photoelectric cell. This is an efficient method of counting and these devices are widely used. They are not without their problems, however.

- They do not discriminate between whole or broken tablets.
- As the beam of light from the photoelectric cell must be interrupted for counting to occur, these devices cannot count clear capsules, e.g. Zarontin or Atromid S.

- The speed at which the dosage forms are poured through the hopper must be controlled. If pouring becomes too fast the system will not cope.
- They are difficult to clean.

Because of this last point the Council of the Royal Pharmaceutical Society of Great Britain issued the following advice concerning the use of electronic counters:

*Severe allergic reactions can be initiated in previously sensitized persons by very small amounts of certain drugs and of excipients and other materials used in the manufacture of tablets and capsules. In order to minimize that risk, counting devices should be carefully cleaned after each dispensing operation involving any uncoated tablet, or any coated tablet or capsule from a bulk container holding damaged contents.*

*As cross-contamination with the penicillins is particularly serious, special care should be taken when dispensing products containing those drugs.*

This type of device should therefore be reserved for counting only coated tablets or capsules or for prepacking operations.

Because accuracy of counting may not be 100% (99.5% has been claimed by one manufacturer), care should be taken when counting controlled drugs. It is preferable to count these on a triangle and have the quantity checked by a second person.

## CONCLUSION

Developing good practice takes time and requires attention to detail. During the undergraduate course, students should develop the habit of working on their own. If assistance is needed it should be sought from a member of staff. A colleague working nearby may be helpful but may not always know the correct answer. Other examples of good practice are found in Chapter 9.

### Key Points

- Accurate dispensing requires clean, neat methodical work.
- Class B balances are being replaced by Class II balances.
- Ensure that the balance is swinging freely before using it.
- Do not use a Class B balance to weigh less than 100 milligrams.
- Ensure that liquid measures comply with the Weights and Measures Regulations.
- Viscous liquids should be measured 'by difference'.
- Pipettes are used to measure volumes between 0.1 ml and 5 ml.
- Select the smallest measure for the volume of liquid to be measured.
- A glass mortar and pestle can be used for size reduction of friable materials and mixing small quantities of fine powder.
- A porcelain mortar and pestle is used for larger quantities, for mixing solids and liquids, making emulsions and for size reduction.
- 'Doubling-up' is used for mixing a small quantity of powder with a larger quantity.

- Confusion can arise with different forms of the same material and the use of synonyms.
- Concentrated waters are diluted 1 part with 39 parts of water for use as single strength.
- Simple problem-solving techniques can produce a satisfactory method of dispensing a product.
- Tablets and capsules can be counted manually, or by using a triangle, capsule counter, counting tray or an electronic counter.
- Tablets and capsules should not be counted in the hand.

## FURTHER READING

Aulton M E 1988 Pharmaceutics: the science of dosage form design. Churchill Livingstone, Edinburgh

Medicines, Ethics and Practice – a guide for pharmacists, current edn. Royal Pharmaceutical Society of Great Britain, London (Updated twice yearly)

Pharmaceutical Codex 1979 11th edn. Pharmaceutical Press, London

Pharmaceutical Codex 1994 12th edn. Pharmaceutical Press, London

Reynolds J E F (ed) 1996 Martindale: the extra pharmacopoeia, 31st edn. Pharmaceutical Press, London (Updated every 3 years – use current edn)

Wade E (ed) 1980 Pharmaceutical handbook, 19th edn. Pharmaceutical Press, London.

# 5
# Pharmaceutical calculations

*M. M. Moody*

---

After studying this chapter the reader will be able to undertake pharmaceutical calculations dealing with:

**Master formulae to working quantities**
**Solubility**
**Dilutions, additions and mixing**
**Small quantities (trituration)**
**Doses.**

There are some tutorial examples and answers provided to help you assess your progress.

## Introduction

Many pharmacy students approach the calculations involved in dispensing and manufacturing somewhat fearfully. There is no need. Virtually all the calculations which are required are simple arithmetic. Always try to relate the calculation to practice, visualize what you are doing and double check everything. There are many steps in the dispensing process where things can go wrong and calculating quantities is certainly one of them. Careful methodical working will minimize the risk of errors.

## HOW TO MINIMIZE ERRORS

As in all dispensing procedures an organized, methodical approach is essential.

### Write out the calculation clearly

• If you are transferring data from a reference source double check what you have written down. It is all too easy to end up reading from the wrong line.
• Do not take short cuts; you are more likely to produce an error.

• Try not to be totally dependent on your calculator. Have an approximate idea of what the answer should be and then if you happen to hit the wrong button on the calculator you are more likely to be aware that an error has been made.
• Finally, always double check your calculation. There is frequently more than one way of doing a calculation, so if you get the same answer by two different methods the chances are that your answer will be correct.

## CALCULATING QUANTITIES FROM A MASTER FORMULA

In extemporaneous dispensing a product is prepared and usually includes several ingredients. A list of the ingredients is provided on the prescription or is obtained from a recognized reference source where the quantities of each ingredient are indicated. It may be that this 'formula' is for the quantity requested, but more often the quantities provided by the master formula have to be scaled up or down, depending on the quantity of the product you wish to prepare. The following examples illustrate this process.

---

**EXAMPLE 5.1**

You are requested to dispense 200 ml of Ammonium Chloride Mixture BPC. The formula can be found in a variety of reference books such as 'Martindale' (Reynolds 1996). In this example the master formula gives quantities sufficient for 10 ml. As the prescription is for 200 ml, the quantity of each ingredient in the master formula has to be multiplied by 20 to provide the required amount.

---

| Ingredient | Master formula | Scaled quantity |
|---|---|---|
| Ammonium chloride | 1 g | 20 g |
| Aromatic solution of ammonia | 0.5 ml | 10 ml |
| Liquorice liquid extract | 1 ml | 20 ml |
| Water | to 10 ml | to 200 ml |

Because this formula contains a mixture of volumes and weights it is not possible to calculate the exact quantity of water which is required. However, it is always good practice to have an idea of what the approximate quantity will be. The liquid ingredients of the preparation, other than the water, add up to 30 ml and there is 20 g of ammonium chloride. The volume of water required will therefore be in the region of 150 ml.

---

**EXAMPLE 5.2**

Calculate the quantities to prepare the following prescription:

50 g Benzoic Acid Compound Ointment BPC

The formula for this preparation differs from the previous one in that the quantity of each ingredient is specified, so the exact quantities of each ingredient can be calculated and this can be used to check the accuracy of the calculation.

| Ingredient | Master formula | Scaled quantity |
|---|---|---|
| Benzoic acid | 6 g | 3 g |
| Salicylic acid | 3 g | 1.5 g |
| Emulsifying ointment | 91 g | 45.5 g |

*Double check*: the quantities for the master formula add up to 100 g and the scaled quantities add up to 50 g.

---

In most formulae where a combination of weights and volumes is required the formula will indicate that the preparation is to be made up to the required weight or volume with the designated vehicle.

However, occasionally, as can be seen in the next example, a combination of weights and volumes is used and it is not possible to indicate what the exact final weight or volume of the preparation will be. In these instances an excess quantity is normally calculated for and the required amount measured.

**EXAMPLE 5.3**

Calculate the quantities required to produce 300 ml Turpentine Liniment BP 1988.

| Ingredient | Master formula |
|---|---|
| Soft soap | 75 g |
| Camphor | 50 g |
| Turpentine oil | 650 ml |
| Water | 225 ml |

When the total number of units is added up for this formula it comes to 1000; however, this will not produce 1000 ml. The prescription is for 300 ml so calculate for 320 units and this will provide slightly more than 300 ml. The required amount can then be measured.

| Ingredient | Master formula | Quantity for 320 units |
|---|---|---|
| Soft soap | 75 g | 24 g |
| Camphor | 50 g | 16 g |
| Turpentine oil | 650 ml | 208 ml |
| Water | 225 ml | 72 ml |

## SOME VARIATIONS

Not all formulae specify the units of each ingredient, i.e. grams or millilitres. Some specify parts and some will indicate a particular concentration of an ingredient expressed as a percentage.

### Calculations involving parts

In the following example the quantities are expressed as parts of the whole. The number of parts is added up and the quantity of each ingredient calculated, to provide the correct proportion.

**EXAMPLE 5.4**

The quantity which is to be prepared of the following formula is 30 g.

| Ingredient | Master formula | Quantity for 30 g |
|---|---|---|
| Zinc oxide | 12.5 parts | 3.75 g |
| Calamine | 15 parts | 4.5 g |
| Hydrous wool fat | 25 parts | 7.5 g |
| White soft paraffin | 47.5 parts | 14.25 g |

The total number of parts adds up to 100 so the

proportions of each ingredient will be 12.5/100 of zinc oxide, 15/100 of calamine and so on. The required quantity of each ingredient can then be calculated. Zinc oxide 12.5/100 of 30 g, calamine 15/100 of 30 g as indicated above.

There are one or two occasions when extra care in reading the prescription is necessary. Examine the next example.

---

**EXAMPLE 5.5**

Two prescriptions are to be dispensed:

| Betnovate cream | 1 part |
| Aqueous cream | to 4 parts |
| Send 50 g | |

| Haelan ointment | 1 part |
| White soft paraffin | 4 parts |
| Send 50 g | |

Although at first glance these calculations look rather similar the quantities for each are different.

In the Betnovate prescription the total number of parts is 4, i.e. 1 part of Betnovate and 3 parts of aqueous cream to produce a total of 4 parts. However, in the Haelan prescription the total number of parts is 5, i.e. 1 part of Haelan ointment and 4 parts of white soft paraffin.

The quantities required for the prescriptions are as follows:

| Betnovate cream | 12.5 g |
| Aqueous cream | 37.5 g |
| | |
| Haelan ointment | 10 g |
| White soft paraffin | 40 g |

---

## Calculations involving percentages

There are certain conventions which apply when dealing with ingredients indicated as a percentage in a formula.

A solid in a formula where the final quantity is stated as a weight is calculated as weight in weight (w/w).

A solid in a formula where the final quantity is stated as a volume is calculated as weight in volume (w/v).

A liquid in a formula where the final quantity is stated as a volume is calculated as volume in volume (v/v).

A liquid in a formula where the final quantity is stated as a weight is calculated as weight in weight (w/w).

These conventions apply unless an alternative is specified. The definitions are as follows:

1% w/w = 1 g in 100 g
1% w/v = 1 g in 100 ml
1% v/v = 1 ml in 100 ml

If you know this then you can calculate any other percentage concentrations.

---

**EXAMPLE 5.6**

Prepare 250 g of the following ointment.

| Ingredient | Master formula | Master formula | Quantity for 250 g |
|---|---|---|---|
| Sulphur | 2% | 0.2 g | 5 g |
| Salicylic acid | 1% | 0.1 g | 2.5 g |
| White soft paraffin | to 10 g | to 10 g | 242.5 g |

The master formula is for a total of 10 g. To calculate the quantities required for 250 g multiply the amount of each ingredient required to prepare 10 g by 25. Remember, do not multiply the percentage, it remains the same whether you are preparing 250 g, 5 kg or 10 g.

---

In the following example a liquid ingredient, the coal tar solution, is stated as a percentage and a weight in grams of final product is requested. The convention of w/w is applied.

---

**EXAMPLE 5.7**

The quantity requested is 60 g.

| Ingredient | Master formula | Master formula | Quantity for 60 g |
|---|---|---|---|
| Coal tar solution | 3% | 3 g | 1.8 g |
| Zinc oxide | 5 g | 5 g | 3 g |
| Yellow soft paraffin | to 100 g | 92 g | 55.2 g |

---

When dealing with preparations where ingredients are expressed as a percentage concentration it is important to check whether the standard conventions are applied or not.

Some that you should be aware of are:

• Syrup BP is a liquid – a solution of sucrose and water. If the normal convention applied it would be w/v, i.e. a certain weight of sucrose in a final volume of syrup. However, on checking the formula the concentration of sucrose is quoted as w/w. The formula for Syrup BP is:

Sucrose 66.7% w/w
Water to 100%

This means that when preparing Syrup BP the appropriate weight of sucrose is weighed out and water is added to the required weight, not volume.

• Another variation from the convention is a mixture of a gas in a solution. These are always calculated as w/w, unless specified otherwise. The example which is usually used to illustrate this is Formaldehyde Solution BP. This is a solution of 34–38% w/w formaldehyde in water.

## SOLUBILITIES

When preparing pharmaceutical products the solubility of any solid ingredients should be checked. This will give useful information on how the product should be prepared. This is discussed further in Chapters 4, 11 and 12. The objective of this section is to clarify the terminology used when solubilities are stated.

The solubility of a drug will be found in a variety of reference sources, e.g. in individual monographs in 'Martindale' (Reynolds 1996) it will be found in the section dealing with physical properties. The method of stating solubilities is as follows:

Sodium chloride is soluble 1 in 3 of water, 1 in 250 of alcohol and 1 in 10 of glycerol.

This means that 3 ml of water are required to dissolve 1 g of sodium chloride, 250 ml of alcohol will be required to dissolve 1 g of sodium chloride and 10 ml of glycerol are required to dissolve 1 g of sodium chloride. An example of how knowledge of a substance's solubility can help when extemporaneously dispensing can be found in Chapter 4. Some examples of calculating quantities of liquids required to dissolve solids are found in the tutorial section at the end of this chapter (p. 70).

## ALTERING CONCENTRATIONS

### Dilutions

There are situations in pharmacy when the concentration of a preparation has to be altered, e.g. the dilution of a stock concentrate to a suitable strength for use by medical staff or a patient.

---

**EXAMPLE 5.8**

A hospital ward uses a particular disinfectant for two different purposes. A 0.2% w/v solution is used for disinfecting instruments and a 0.05% w/v solution is used for skin disinfection and cleansing. The disinfectant is available as a 10% w/v concentrate. The two strengths, 0.2% and 0.05%, are supplied to the ward in volumes of 500 ml. What quantities of the 10% concentrate are required to prepare 500 ml of each strength?

For this type of calculation always go back to first principles.

100 ml of a 1% w/v solution contains 1 g of solid.
Therefore 100 ml of a 0.2% w/v solution contains 0.2 g of solid (i.e. one-fifth).
Therefore 500 ml of a 0.2% w/v solution contains $5 \times 0.2$ g of solid = 1 g.

To find out the volume of the 10% concentrate needed to produce 500 ml of the 0.2% solution calculate the volume of 10% concentrate which contains 1 g.

10 g of solid is contained in 100 ml of a 10% w/v solution.
Therefore 1 g of solid will be contained in 10 ml of a 10% w/v solution.

10 ml of 10% solution will therefore provide the amount of solid needed to prepare 500 ml of 0.2% w/v solution. Therefore add 490 ml of suitable diluent, e.g. water, to 10 ml of concentrate and 500 ml of 0.2% w/v solution will be produced.

Calculation of the quantities required to prepare 500 ml of 0.05% w/v is done in exactly the same way.

The amount of solid in 500 ml of 0.05% = $0.05 \times 5 = 0.25$ g.
The volume of 10% w/v solution which contains 0.25 g = $100/10 \times 0.25 = 2.5$ ml.
Therefore to prepare 500 ml of 0.05% w/v solution 497.5 ml of a suitable diluent would be added to 2.5 ml of the 10% concentrate.

When doing this type of calculation always try to relate it to practice and visualize what you are doing. Try not to get into the habit of using a formula without understanding the basic concepts.

Terminology used in some dilution calculations can be somewhat confusing and it is important to understand what is meant. The strength of a solution may sometimes be expressed as 'a 1 in 300 solution' or 'a 1 in 2000 solution'.

A 1 in 300 solution is a solution which contains 1 g of solid in 300 ml of the solution and a 1 in 2000 solution contains 1 g of solid in 2000 ml of solution. Do not confuse this with the terminology used to describe solubilities.

---

### EXAMPLE 5.9

What volume of a 3% w/v solution is required to prepare 200 ml of a 1 in 5000 solution?

A 1 in 5000 solution contains 1 g of solid in 5000 ml.
Therefore 200 ml of this solution will contain $1/5000 \times 200 = 0.04$ g, i.e. 40 milligrams.
A 4% w/v solution contains 4 g in 100 ml.
Therefore 40 milligrams or 0.04 g will be contained in $100/4 \times 0.04 = 1$ ml of 4% solution.
To prepare 200 ml of the 1 in 5000 solution 1 ml of 4% solution would be mixed with 199 ml of the appropriate diluent.

---

There are occasions when dilution of a preparation must be carried out, for example when a paediatric strength is requested and only the adult strength is available.

---

### EXAMPLE 5.10

Send 100 ml Linctus Codeine Paediatric BP. Only Linctus Codeine BP is available.

Linctus Codeine BP contains codeine phosphate 15 milligrams/5 ml.
Linctus Codeine Paediatric BP contains codeine phosphate 3 milligrams/5 ml.

100 ml of the paediatric linctus contains 60 milligrams of codeine phosphate. This will be provided by 20 ml of the adult strength.
Therefore to dispense the prescription, 20 ml of the adult linctus will be diluted with 80 ml of the recommended diluent to produce 100 ml of Linctus Codeine Paediatric.

---

Occasionally a product of a particular concentration is produced by mixing two preparations of different strengths of the same drug.

---

### EXAMPLE 5.11

500 ml of a suspension containing 60 milligrams/ 5 ml thioridazine hydrochloride is requested.

Thioridazine hydrochloride suspension is available in two strengths, 100 milligrams/5 ml and 25 milligrams/5 ml. These suspensions cannot be diluted but may be mixed together to provide intermediate doses.
This calculation involves using some very simple algebra.

The total volume requested is 500 ml, therefore the sum of the volumes of the two concentrations of the suspension will equal 500 ml.
Let the volume of the 100 milligrams/5 ml suspension = n.
Therefore the volume of the 25 milligrams/5 ml suspension = 500 − n.
A simple equation can then be written balancing the quantities of drug required on one side and the quantities of drug added on the other.

| | |
|---|---|
| Thus: | $100n + 25(500 − n) = 60 \times 500$ |
| Therefore: | $100n + 12\,500 − 25n = 30\,000$ |
| Rearranging: | $100n − 25n = 30\,000 − 12\,500$ |
| Therefore: | $75n = 17\,500$ |
| So: | $n = 233.33$ ml. |

Therefore the volume of 100 milligrams/5 ml suspension required = 233.33 ml and the volume of the 25 milligrams/5 ml suspension required will = 500 − 233.33 = 266.67 ml. The answer can be checked by calculating the amount of drug in each volume of suspension and ensuring that it totals the total amount required.
The same principles are applied when mixing two ointments of different strengths to produce one of an intervening strength.

---

Some dilution calculations must be read carefully because of the terminology used and the use of synonyms. An example which frequently causes problems is calculations involving dilutions of formaldehyde.

Formaldehyde is available as Formaldehyde Solution BP which contains 34–38% w/w formaldehyde gas. The synonym for Formaldehyde Solution BP is formalin.

### EXAMPLE 5.12

Given Formaldehyde Solution BP, prepare 200 ml of a solution containing 12% formalin.

The standard convention applies of v/v.

100 ml of the required solution will contain 12 ml of formalin.

Therefore 200 ml of the requested solution will consist of 24 ml of Formaldehyde Solution BP (formalin) and 176 ml of water.

In the next example a solution containing a particular concentration of formaldehyde is requested

### EXAMPLE 5.13

Given Formaldehyde Solution BP, prepare 200 ml of a solution containing 12% formaldehyde.

Because solutions of gases are always calculated as w/w a certain weight of solution will have to be prepared and the required volume measured.

The weight per ml of Formaldehyde Solution BP is 1.08 g. The weight of 200 ml of a solution containing 12% w/w formaldehyde gas will therefore be approximately $200 \times 1.08 = 216$ g. If this weight of solution is prepared it will provide slightly more than the volume required.

216 g of a 12% w/w solution of formaldehyde contains 25.92 g of formaldehyde.

100 g of Formaldehyde Solution BP contains 36 g of formaldehyde.

Therefore 25.92 g will be contained in $100/36 \times 25.92 = 72$ g of Formaldehyde Solution BP.

To 72 g of Formaldehyde Solution BP is added 144 g of water to give the required weight of 216 g of solution. The 200 ml requested can then be measured.

## Calculations where the concentration of the active ingredient is increased

### EXAMPLE 5.14

What weight of salicylic acid must be added to

100 g of an ointment containing 2% salicylic acid to increase the concentration to 3% salicylic acid?

There is a temptation to think that the answer is 1 g. This is incorrect. 3 g of salicylic acid would then be contained in 101 g of ointment, which is not 3%.

The quantity of ointment base is the constant.

100 g of 2% ointment contains 98 g of base and 2 g of salicylic acid.

If 98 g of base $= 97\%$ of 3% ointment
then 3% $\quad = 98/97 \times 3$
$\qquad = 3.03$ g.

Therefore the amount of salicylic acid to be added will be $3.03 - 2 = 1.03$ g.

Always be careful with terminology. The following example is worded slightly differently.

### EXAMPLE 5.15

What weight of salicylic acid must be added to an ointment containing 2% salicylic acid to produce 100 g of an ointment containing 3% salicylic acid?

Here, a particular weight has been specified.

100 g of 3% ointment contains 97 g of base and 3 g of salicylic acid.

Find the weight of 2% ointment which contains 97 g of base.

97 g $= 98\%$
Therefore 100% $= 97/98 \times 100$
$\qquad = 98.98$ g
Weight of salicylic acid in this $= 1.98$ g.

Therefore add 1.02 g of salicylic acid to 98.98 g of 2% ointment to produce 100 g of ointment which contains 3 g salicylic acid.

## CALCULATIONS WHERE QUANTITY OF INGREDIENTS IS TOO SMALL TO WEIGH OR MEASURE ACCURATELY

On occasions the quantities of active ingredients required are too small to weigh or measure, using the available equipment. In these instances a triturate should be made. The term 'trituration' describes when an active substance is diluted with an inert diluent.

## Small quantities in powders

---

**EXAMPLE 5.16**

---

Calculate the quantities required to make eight powders each containing 200 micrograms digoxin.

Calculate for an excess to allow for losses during preparation. Calculate for 10 powders. The minimum weight of a divided powder is 120 milligrams, so an inert diluent, such as lactose needs to be used.

The total weight of powder mixture required will be $10 \times 120 = 1200$ milligrams = 1.2 g.

Quantities for 10 powders:

| | |
|---|---|
| Digoxin | 2 mg |
| Lactose | 1198 mg |
| Total | 1200 mg |

The weight of digoxin is too small to weigh (see Ch. 4). The minimum weighable quantity of 100 milligrams is weighed and a triturate is made. A 1 in 10 dilution is produced.

**Trituration 1**

| | |
|---|---|
| Digoxin | 100 mg |
| Lactose | 900 mg |
| Total | 1000 mg |

Each 100 milligrams of this mixture (A) contains 10 milligrams of digoxin.

**Trituration 2**

| | | |
|---|---|---|
| Mixture A | 100 mg | (= 10 mg digoxin) |
| Lactose | 900 mg | |
| Total | 1000 mg | |

Each 100 milligrams of this mixture (B) contains 1 milligram of digoxin.

200 milligrams of mixture B provides the 2 milligrams digoxin required.

**Trituration 3**

| | | |
|---|---|---|
| Mixture B | 200 mg | (= 2 mg digoxin) |
| Lactose | 1000 mg | |
| Total | 1200 mg | |

Each 120 milligrams of this mixture (C) will contain 200 micrograms of digoxin.

The method for preparing divided powders is described in Chapter 16.

## Small quantities in liquids

If the quantity of a solid to be incorporated into a solution is too small to weigh, again dilutions are used. The solubility of the substance needs to be considered, but normally 1 in 10 or 1 in 100 dilutions are used.

---

**EXAMPLE 5.17**

---

Calculate the quantities required to prepare 100 ml of a solution containing 2.5 milligrams morphine hydrochloride/5 ml.

*Quantities for 100 ml*

| | |
|---|---|
| Morphine hydrochloride | 50 mg |
| Chloroform water | to 100 ml |

The solubility of morphine hydrochloride is 1 in 24 of water.

The minimum quantity of 100 milligrams of morphine hydrochloride is weighed and made up to 10 ml with chloroform water.

5 ml of this solution (A) provides the 50 milligrams of morphine hydrochloride required.

Take 5 ml of solution A and make up to 100 ml with chloroform water.

## DOSES OF ORAL LIQUIDS

The practice of diluting oral liquids to provide a dose volume of 5 ml or a multiple of 5 ml is now only carried out if specifically requested by the prescriber. Doses which are fractions of 5 ml are given using an oral syringe. Various calculations are required when dealing with oral liquids.

## Calculation of volume to be dispensed and dosage instructions

---

**EXAMPLE 5.18**

---

The following prescription is received:

Sodium valproate oral solution
100 milligrams given twice daily for 2 weeks.

Sodium valproate oral solution contains sodium valproate 200 milligrams/5 ml.

This prescription is therefore translated as: 2.5 ml to be given twice daily for 2 weeks.

The quantity to be dispensed will be:

$$2.5 \times 2 \times 14 = 70 \text{ ml}$$

## Calculating doses

An overdose of a drug given to a patient can have very serious consequences and may be fatal. It is the responsibility of everyone involved in supplying or administering drugs to ensure that the accuracy and suitability of the dose are checked. The following are some examples of areas where errors can occur.

The standard way to check whether a drug dose is appropriate is to consult a recognized reference book. One of the commonest used for this purpose is the *British National Formulary* (BNF). When first using any reference source be aware of the terminology used. A standard error which many students make is misinterpreting the entries, in particular where doses are quoted as 'x milligrams daily, in divided doses'. An explanation of the terminology will usually be given in the introduction to the book.

---

**EXAMPLE 5.19**

The following prescription is received:

Verapamil tablets 160 milligrams
Send 56
Take two tablets twice daily

There are a variety of doses quoted for verapamil in the BNF depending on the condition being treated. They are as follows:

*By mouth*
Supraventricular arrhythmias 40–120 milligrams three times daily
Angina 80–120 milligrams three times daily
Hypertension 240–480 milligrams daily in two to three divided doses.

The dose given for hypertension is stated in a significantly different way. Whereas the other doses can be given three times daily, indicating a maximum of 360 milligrams in any one day, the hypertension dose is the total to be given in any one day and is divided up and given at a particular frequency, i.e. a maximum of 240 milligrams, given twice daily or a maximum of 160 milligrams, given three times daily.

The prescription presented is for a higher than

---

recommended dose and consultation with the prescriber would be required. Be alert, variation in terminology and a lack of awareness could have very serious consequences.

---

Many doses, in particular those for children, are quoted as 'mg/kg', i.e. the dose for a child of known weight.

---

**EXAMPLE 5.20**

The dose of fentanyl, by intravenous injection, for a child, is 3–5 micrograms/kg. What volume of injection is required for a 4 micrograms/kg dose for a child weighing 20 kg?

Fentanyl intravenous injection contains fentanyl (as the citrate) 50 micrograms/ml.

The dose of fentanyl required is 4 micrograms × 20, i.e. the dose multiplied by the weight of the child, = 80 micrograms.

Since 50 micrograms is contained in 1 ml then the volume of injection required = $1/50 \times 80 = 1.6$ ml.

---

## Key Points

- Always write calculations down clearly and work methodically.
- Check calculations, using a different method where possible.
- Estimate the answer before you start.
- Try to visualize the quantities you are using in the calculation.
- Look carefully to see if a formula gives the quantities of all ingredients or uses 'to' for the vehicle.
- Dilution calculations should be made from first principles, that is by calculating actual weights of material required and then how to obtain them.
- Be very careful to read the wording; small changes in terminology can alter the calculation.
- Triturates with solids and liquids normally use a 1 in 10 dilution per step.
- Be very careful in checking doses, particularly with 'in divided doses' and 'mg/kg' statements in the reference books.

## SELF-ASSESSMENT QUESTIONS

Reminder:

1 g       = 1000 mg
1 mg      = 1000 μg (micrograms)
1 litre   = 1000 ml

% concentration
1% w/v   = 1 g in 100 ml
1% v/v   = 1 ml in 100 ml
1% w/w   = 1 g in 100 g

1.  Express the following as percentages:
    a.  1 milligram of drug in 200 ml of solution
    b.  2 g of drug in 50 ml of solution
    c.  3 ml of drug in 4 litre of solution
    d.  10 g of drug in 250 g of solution
    e.  6 micrograms of drug in 10 ml of solution
    f.  2 litre of drug in 5000 ml of solution
    g.  25 000 p.p.m. (parts per million)
    h.  a 1 in 4000 solution
    i.  a 3 in 10 000 solution.

2.  The following are examples of concentrations expressed as percentages. Indicate the amount of drug present in:
    a.  500 ml of 6% w/v solution
    b.  30 ml of a 15% w/v preparation
    c.  2 litres of a 0.05% v/v preparation
    d.  0.5 ml of a 2% w/v preparation
    e.  20 g of a 0.1% w/w preparation
    f.  150 ml of a 0.002% w/v preparation.

3.  a.  Calculate the concentration of a solution of potassium permanganate, which, when 1 ml is diluted to 100 ml, produces a solution with a concentration of 100 p.p.m.
    b.  Calculate the volume of copper sulphate solution 15% w/v which, when diluted to 100 ml, will produce a 1 in 100 solution.

4.  A drug has a solubility 1 in 50 of water and 1 in 14 of alcohol.
    a.  Will 250 milligrams dissolve in 4 ml of water?
    b.  Will 4 g dissolve in 60 ml of alcohol?
    c.  Will 10 micrograms dissolve in 0.002 ml of water?
    d.  Will 1 kg dissolve in 3 litre of alcohol?
    e.  Will 0.05 g dissolve in 0.2 ml of alcohol?

5.  Calculate the quantity of each ingredient required to prepare the following formulae:
    a.  Coal tar solution          2%
        Zinc oxide                 5 g
        Yellow soft paraffin       to 100 g
        Send 30 g

    b.  Sulphur                    3%
        Salicylic acid             2%
        White soft paraffin        to 10 g
        Send 60 g

    c.  Sodium bicarbonate         0.5%
        Magnesium trisilicate      6%
        Concentrated peppermint emulsion 2.5%
        Water                      to 100 ml
        Send 300 ml

    d.  Zinc oxide                 10 parts
        Calamine                   17.5 parts
        Hydrous wool fat           25 parts
        White soft paraffin        47.5 parts
        Send 500 g

    e.  Concentrated anise water   10 parts
        Amaranth solution          15 parts
        Citric acid monohydrate    25 parts
        Chloroform spirit          60 parts
        Syrup                      to 1000 parts
        Send 150 ml

    f.  Benzoic acid               12 g
        Sulphur                    20 g
        Coal tar                   15 g
        Zinc oxide                 45 g
        Yellow soft paraffin       135 g
        Send 1 kg

    g.  Liquid paraffin            50 ml
        Acacia                     12.5 g
        Water                      to 120 ml
        Send 90 ml

    h.  Aromatic cascara           1 part
        Liquid paraffin            3 parts
        Milk of magnesia           4 parts
        Send 1 litre

    i.  Camphor                    0.8 parts
        Calamine powder            8 parts
        Starch                     9.2 parts
        Talc                       30 parts
        Send 60 g

6. How many grams of ichthammol must be added to 500 g of ointment base to produce an ointment containing 10% w/w ichthammol? Answer to two decimal places.

7. Given 1 litre of a 17% w/v solution (density 1.2 g/ml) calculate what weight of drug must be added to the litre of 17% w/v solution to make a 20% w/w solution.

8. What volume of normal saline (0.9% w/v NaCl) can be made from 1.5 g NaCl?

9. Paregoric is 4% v/v tincture of opium which is 10% w/v opium. If opium contains 10% w/w morphine what weight of morphine is contained in a 30 ml bottle of Paregoric?

10. For the following prescriptions calculate the dose of active ingredient which the patient will be taking on each occasion.
    a. Sudafed elixir
       Mitte 150 ml
       Sig. 3 ml t.i.d.
       (Sudafed elixir contains pseudoephedrine 30 milligrams/5 ml.)
    b. Codeine linctus half strength
       Mitte 200 ml
       Sig. 2.5 ml t.i.d.
       (Codeine linctus contains codeine phosphate 15 milligrams/5 ml.)
    c. Ketotifen elixir
       Mitte 300 ml
       Sig. 7.5 ml b.i.d.
       (Ketotifen elixir contains ketotifen 1 milligram/5 ml.)
    d. Terfenadine suspension
       Mitte 150 ml
       Sig. 10 ml b.i.d.
       (Terfenadine suspension contains terfenadine 30 milligrams/5 ml.)

11. For the following prescriptions calculate the volume of liquid which the patient will take on each occasion.
    a. Hismanal suspension
       Mitte 500 ml
       Sig. 8 milligrams daily
       (Hismanal suspension contains astemizole 5 milligrams/5 ml.)
    b. Dimotane elixir
       Mitte 100 ml
       Sig. 1.5 milligrams q.i.d.
       (Dimotane elixir contains brompheniramine maleate 2 milligrams/5 ml.)
    c. Promethazine elixir
       Mitte 100 ml
       Sig. 12 milligrams daily
       (Promethazine elixir contains promethazine hydrochloride 5 milligrams/5 ml.)

## ANSWERS

1. a. 0.0005% w/v
   b. 4% w/v
   c. 0.075% v/v
   d. 4% w/w
   e. 0.00006% w/v
   f. 40% v/v
   g. 2.5%
   h. 0.025%
   i. 0.03%

2. a. 30 g
   b. 4.5 g
   c. 1 ml
   d. 10 milligrams
   e. 20 milligrams
   f. 3 milligrams

3. a. The concentration required is 1% w/v.
   b. The volume of the 15% w/v solution required is 6.66 ml.

4. a. 250 milligrams of drug requires 12.5 ml of water in which to dissolve, therefore the answer is No.
   b. 4 g of drug requires 56 ml of alcohol in which to dissolve, therefore the answer is Yes.
   c. 10 micrograms of drug requires 0.0005 ml of water in which to dissolve, therefore the answer is Yes.
   d. 1 kg of drug requires 14 litres of alcohol in which to dissolve, therefore the answer is No.
   e. 50 milligrams of drug requires 0.7 ml of alcohol in which to dissolve therefore the answer is No.

5. a. Coal tar solution   0.6 g
      Zinc oxide   1.5 g
      Yellow soft paraffin   27.5 g
   b. Sulphur   1.8 g
      Salicylic acid   1.2 g
      White soft paraffin   57 g
   c. Sodium bicarbonate   1.5 g
      Magnesium trisilicate   18.0 g

Concentrated peppermint
emulsion                              7.5 ml
Water (to 300 ml)          approx. 273 ml

It is not possible to calculate the exact amount of water required because of the mixture of weights and volumes. It is, however, good practice to have an idea of the approximate volume of water required. If it is assumed that the sodium bicarbonate and the magnesium trisilicate occupy in the region of 1.5 ml and 18 ml, respectively, the volume of water required will be approximately 273 ml.

d.  Zinc oxide                        50 g
    Calamine                        87.5 g
    Hydrous wool fat                 125 g
    White soft paraffin            237.5 g

e.  Concentrated anise water         1.5 ml
    Amaranth solution               2.25 ml
    Citric acid monohydrate         3.75 g
    Chloroform spirit                  9 ml
    Syrup (to 150 ml)        approx. 133.5 ml

    Again in this calculation it is not possible to calculate the exact quantity of syrup but it will be in the region of 133.5 ml.

f.  Benzoic acid                    52.9 g
    Sulphur                         88.1 g
    Coal tar                        66.1 g
    Zinc oxide                     198.2 g
    Yellow soft paraffin           594.7 g

g.  Liquid paraffin                 37.5 ml
    Acacia                         9.375 g
    Water (to 120 ml)        approx. 43.0 ml

h.  Aromatic cascara                 125 ml
    Liquid paraffin                  375 ml
    Milk of magnesia                 500 ml

i.  Camphor                            1 g
    Calamine                          10 g
    Starch                          11.5 g
    Talc                            37.5 g

6.  Weight of ichthammol = 55.56 g.
    The 500 g of ointment base will be 90% of the final preparation.
    If 90% = 500 g then:
        10% = 55.56 g, i.e. the required weight of ichthammol.

7.  The weight of drug to be added = 87.5 g.
    Weight of drug in 1 litre of 17% w/v solution is 170 g.

Weight of 1 litre of 17% w/v solution is 1200 g.
The weight of solvent in this is 1200 – 170 = 1030 g.
The weight of the solvent is constant.
In the 20% w/w solution the solvent is 80% of the total.
Therefore 80% = 1030 g.
Then:       20% = 257.5 g.
There is already 170 g of drug present, so amount to be added will be 257.5 – 170 = 87.5 g.

8.  166.66 ml.

9.  30 ml of paregoric contains 12 milligrams of morphine.

10. a.  The patient will take 18 milligrams of pseudoephedrine as a single dose.
    b.  The patient will take 3.75 milligrams of codeine phosphate as a single dose.
    c.  The patient will take 1.5 milligrams of ketotifen as a single dose.
    d.  The patient will take 60 milligrams of terfenadine as a single dose.

11. a.  8 ml of the suspension.
    b.  3.75 ml of the elixir.
    c.  12 ml of the elixir.

## FURTHER READING

British National Formulary, current edn. British Medical Association and Royal Pharmaceutical Society of Great Britain, London (Updated twice yearly)

Diluent Directories (Internal and External), current edn. National Pharmaceutical Association, St Albans

Pharmaceutical Codex 1979 11th edn. Pharmaceutical Press, London

Pharmaceutical Codex 1994 12th edn. Pharmaceutical Press, London

Reynolds J E F (ed) 1996 Martindale: the extra pharmacopoeia, 31st edn. Pharmaceutical Press, London

Rouse S T, Webber M G 1968 Calculations in pharmacy, 2nd edn. Pitman Medical Publishing, London

Stoklosa M J, Ansel H C 1991 Pharmaceutical calculations, 9th edn. Lea & Febiger, London

Wade A (ed) 1980 Pharmaceutical handbook, 19th edn. Pharmaceutical Press, London

# 6

# Packaging

*D. G. Chapman*

After studying this chapter you will know about:

**Definition of a container**
**Considerations made in selecting a container**
**The difference between primary and secondary packaging**
**The materials used for packaging, including glass, plastics, metal and paper**
**Types of container in common use**
**Child-resistant closures and tamper-evident seals**
**Patient pack dispensing**.

## Introduction

Pharmaceutical formulations must be suitably contained, protected and labelled from the time of manufacture until they are used by the patient. Throughout this period the container must maintain the quality, safety and stability of the medicine and protect the product against physical, climatic, chemical and biological hazards. The *British Pharmacopoeia* (BP 1993) identifies the closure as part of the container.

To promote good patient compliance the container must be user-friendly. This is particularly significant for the elderly who have to take more medicines than the general population and have a greater need for improved compliance (see Ch. 42). Thus containers should be easy to open and reclose, most notably for elderly or arthritic patients. However, other factors must also be considered in the selection of the container used to package a pharmaceutical formulation, including the cost and the need for both child-resistant closures and tamper-evident seals.

Manufacturers are responsible for presenting their products in unit packages that will protect the products for their specified shelf life. Repackaging a pharmaceutical product from its original container to another one may alter the level of protection that was given to the product in its original container. The responsibility for determining the shelf life of the repackaged product remains with the person who performs the repackaging procedure. There are, however, some situations where the repackaging is limited, such as with glyceryl trinitrate tablets, owing to the potential loss of the volatile drug.

Sterile products cannot be easily repackaged. These products require effective closure systems to minimize the risk of microbial contamination of the contents within the container. In addition, the pack itself must withstand sterilization procedures. Consequently, care must be applied to the selection of the container and its closure for the packaging of sterile products (see also Chs 22 and 23).

## PRIMARY AND SECONDARY PACKAGING

Primary packaging materials are in direct contact with the container contents. The container must not interact with its contents. By contrast, secondary packages are additional packaging materials that are elegant in appearance such as outer wrappers or labels, but do not directly contact the product (Table 6.1).

The following terms are used to describe containers:

*Singledose containers* hold the product which is intended for single use. An example of such a container is the glass ampoule.

*Multidose containers* hold a quantity of the material that will be used as two or more doses. An example of this system is the multiple dose vial or the plastic tablet bottle.

**Table 6.1 Types of primary and secondary packaging materials and their use**

| Material | Type | Examples of use |
|----------|------|-----------------|
| Glass | Primary | Metric medical bottle, ampoule, vial |
| Plastic | Primary | Ampoule, vial, infusion fluid container, dropper bottle |
| | Secondary | Wrapper to contain primary pack |
| Board | Secondary | Box to contain primary pack |
| Paper | Secondary | Labels, patient information leaflet |

*Well-closed containers* protect the product from contamination with unwanted foreign materials and from loss of contents during use.

*Airtight containers* are impermeable to solids, liquids and gases during normal storage and use. If the container is to be opened on more than one occasion it must remain airtight after reclosure.

*Sealed containers* such as glass ampoules are closed by fusion of the container material.

*Tamper-evident containers* are closed containers fitted with a device that irreversibly indicates if the container has been opened.

*Light-resistant containers* protect the contents from the effect of radiation at a wavelength between 290 nm and 450 nm.

*Child-resistant containers*, commonly referred to as CRCs, are designed to prevent the child accessing the potentially hazardous product.

*Strip packs* have at least one sealed pocket of material with each pocket containing a single dose of the product. The pack is made of two layers of film or laminate material. The nature and the level of protection which is required by the contained product will affect the composition of these layers.

*Blister packs* are composed of a base layer, with cavities which contain the pharmaceutical product, and a lid. This lid is sealed to the base layer by heat, pressure or both. They are more rigid than strip packs and are not used for powders or semi-solids. Blister packs can be printed with day and week identifiers to produce calendar packs. These identifiers will support patient compliance.

*Tropicalized packs* are blister packs with an additional aluminium membrane to provide greater protection against high humidity.

*Pressurized packs* expel the product through a valve. The pressure for the expulsion of the product is provided by the positive pressure of the propellant which is often a compressed or liquefied gas (see Ch. 18).

*Original packs* are pharmaceutical packs that are commercially produced and intended for finite treatment periods. These packs are dispensed directly to the patient in their original form. Manufacturer's information is contained on the pack but the pharmacist must attach a dispensary label.

An important consideration when selecting the packaging for any product is that its main objective is that the package must contribute to delivering a drug to a specific site of effective activity in the patient.

The selection of packaging for a pharmaceutical product is dependent on the following factors:

1. the nature of the product itself: its chemical activity, sensitivity to moisture and oxygen, compatibility with packaging materials
2. the type of patient: is it to be used by an elderly or arthritic patient or by a child?
3. the dosage form
4. method of administering the medication
5. required shelf life
6. use, such as for dispensing or for an over-the-counter product.

## PACKAGING MATERIALS

### Glass

Historically, glass has been the most widely used drug packaging material. It continues to be the preferred packaging material for many pharmaceutical products.

Glass does have several advantages:

1. It is inert to most medicinal products.
2. It is impervious to air and moisture.
3. It allows easy inspection of the container contents.
4. It can be coloured to protect contents from harmful wavelengths of light.
5. It is easy to clean and sterilize by heat.
6. It is available in variously shaped containers.

The disadvantages of glass:

1. It is fragile. Glass fragments can be released into the product during transport or contaminants can penetrate the product by way of cracks in the container.
2. Certain types of glass release alkali into the container contents.

3. It is expensive when compared to the price of plastic.
4. It is heavy resulting in increased transport costs.

The chemical stability of glass for pharmaceutical use is given by the resistance of the glass to the release of soluble minerals into water contacting the glass. This is known as the hydrolytic resistance. Details are given in the BP (1993) for four types of glass.

### Type I glass

This is also known as neutral glass or borosilicate glass. It possesses a high hydrolytic resistance due to the chemical composition of the glass. It is the most inert type of pharmaceutical glass with the lowest coefficient of thermal expansion. As a result, it is unlikely to crack on exposure to rapid temperature changes. Type I glass is suitable for packing all pharmaceutical preparations. However, it is expensive and this restricts its applications. It is widely used as glass ampoules and vials to package fluids for injection. In addition, it is used to package solutions which could dissolve basic oxides in the glass. This would increase the pH of the formulation and could affect the drug potency.

### Type II glass

This is made of soda-lime-silica glass with a high hydrolytic resistance due to surface treatment of the glass. Type II glass is used to package aqueous preparations. In general, it is not used to package parenteral formulations with a pH less than 7. This glass has a lower melting point than Type I glass. It is thus easier to produce and consequently cheaper. It is used as containers for eye treatments and other dropper bottles.

### Type III glass

This is made of a soda-lime-silica glass. It has a similar composition to Type II glass but contains more leachable oxides. Type III glass offers only moderate resistance to leaching and is commonly used as dispensary metric medical bottles. It is also suitable for packaging non-aqueous parenteral products and powders for injection.

### Type IV glass

This is made of a soda-lime-silica glass with a low hydrolytic resistance. This glass must not be used to package parenteral products but it is suitable for packaging solid, liquid and semi-solid formulations.

### Types of glass containers

*Bottles.* These are commonly used in the dispensary as either amber metric medical bottles or ribbed (fluted) oval bottles. Both types of bottle are available in sizes from 50 ml to 500 ml and are supplied with a screw closure.

Amber metric medical bottles have a smooth curved side and a flat side (Fig. 6.1). The bottle was designed to permit the curved side of the bottle to fit into the palm of the hand when pouring from the bottle. The flat side was intended to permit the attachment of a label. In practice, however, the label is commonly attached to the curved surface of the bottle. Amber metric medical bottles are used for packaging a wide range of oral medicines.

Ribbed oval bottles have flutes down one side of the container (Fig. 6.2). The characteristic feel of the flutes warns the user that the contents are not to be taken. A label is attached to the plain front of the bottle. Ribbed oval bottles are used to package various products which are not be taken orally. This includes liniments, lotions, inhalations and antiseptic solutions.

*Dropper bottles.* Eye drop and dropper bottles for ear and nasal use (Fig. 6.3) are hexagonal-shaped

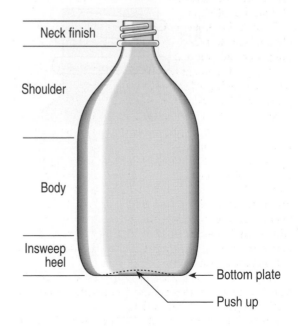

**Fig. 6.1** Metric medicine bottle.

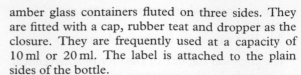

amber glass containers fluted on three sides. They are fitted with a cap, rubber teat and dropper as the closure. They are frequently used at a capacity of 10 ml or 20 ml. The label is attached to the plain sides of the bottle.

*Jars.* Powders and semi-solid preparations are generally packed in wide-mouthed cylindrical jars made of clear or amber glass. The capacity of these jars varies from 15 ml to 500 ml. Ointment jars are used for packing extemporaneously prepared ointments and pastes. They are also used to repackage commercial products where microbial contamination by the patient's fingers is not detrimental to the product.

*Containers for parenteral products.* Small volume parenteral products, such as subcutaneous injections are typically packaged in various containers made of Type I glass. Glass ampoules (Fig. 6.4) are used to package parenteral solutions intended for single use.

Multiple dose vials (Fig. 6.5) are used to package parenteral formulations which will be used on more than one occasion. Large volume parenteral fluids have been packaged in 500 ml glass containers but these have been largely superseded by plastic bags.

## Plastics

Plastics have been widely used for several years as primary packages as containers for the product and

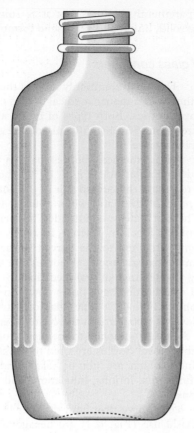

**Fig. 6.2** Ribbed oval bottle.

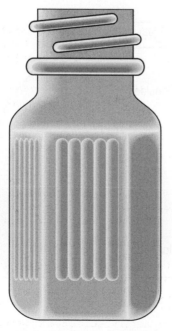

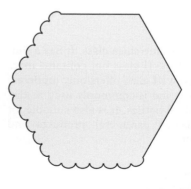

**Fig. 6.3** Hexagonal, ribbed dropper bottle.

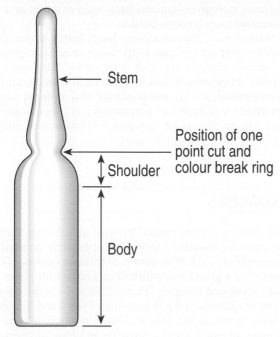

Fig. 6.4 Glass ampoule.

Stem

Position of one
point cut and
colour break ring

Shoulder

Body

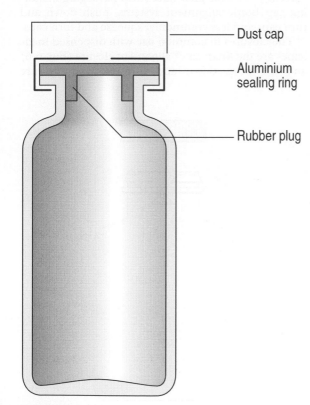

Dust cap

Aluminium
sealing ring

Rubber plug

Fig. 6.5 Glass vial.

**Table 6.2 The application of thermoplastic polymers for the packaging of pharmaceutical products**

| Polymer | Examples of application |
| --- | --- |
| High density polyethylene | Solid dosage form containers |
| Low density polyethylene | Flexible eye drop bottles |
| Linear low density polyethylene | Heat-sealable containers |
| Polypropylene | Container closures i.v. solution bottles |
| Polyvinyl chloride | Laminate for blister packs, i.v. bags |
| Polystyrene | Containers for oils and creams and solid dosage forms |

as secondary packaging in the form of a carton. In more recent times, plastic has evolved for the packaging of parenteral products including infusion fluids and small volume injections.

There are two classes of plastics which are used in the packaging of pharmaceutical products. These are known as thermosets and thermoplastics. The thermosets are used for making screw caps for glass and metal containers. Thermoplastic polymers are used in the manufacture of a wide variety of pharmaceutical packages as detailed in Table 6.2.

The advantages of plastic for packaging are that they:

1. release few particles into the product
2. are flexible and not easily broken
3. are of low density and thus light in weight
4. can be heat sealed
5. are easily moulded into various shapes
6. are suitable for use as container, closure and as secondary packaging
7. are cheap.

The disadvantages of plastic are that:

1. they are not as chemically inert as Type I glass
2. some plastics undergo stress cracking and distortion on contacting some chemicals
3. some plastics are very heat sensitive
4. they are not as impermeable to gas and vapour as glass
5. they may possess an electrostatic charge which will attract particles
6. additives in the plastic are easily leached into the product
7. substances such as the drug and preservatives may be taken up from the product.

Plastic pharmaceutical containers are made of at least one polymer together with additives. The additives used will depend on the composition of the polymer and the production methods used.

Additives used in plastic containers include:

- plasticizers
- resins
- stabilizers
- lubricants
- antistatic agents
- mould-release agents.

### Plastic containers

These are used for many types of pack including rigid bottles for tablets and capsules, squeezable bottles for eye drops and nasal sprays, jars, flexible tubes, strip and blister packs. The composition and the physical shape of the containers vary widely to suit the application.

### The principal plastic materials used in pharmaceutical packaging

*Polyethylene.* This is used as high and low density polyethylene both of which are compatible with a wide range of drugs and are extensively used for the packaging of various pharmacy products. Of these two forms of polyethylene, low density polyethylene (LDPE) is softer, more flexible and more easily stretched than high density polyethylene (HDPE). Consequently, LDPE is usually the preferred plastic for squeeze bottles. By contrast, HDPE is stronger, stiffer, less clear, less permeable to gases and more resistant to oils, chemicals and solvents. It is commonly pigmented or printed white to block light transmission and improve label clarity. HDPE is widely used in bottles for solid dosage forms.

Disadvantages of LDPE and HDPE for packaging are that they:

- are softened by flavouring and aromatic oils
- are unsuitable for packing oxygen-sensitive products owing to high gas permeability
- adsorb antimicrobial preservative agents
- crack on contact with organic solvents.

*Polyvinyl chloride* (PVC). This is extensively used as rigid packaging material and as the main component of intravenous bags.

*Polypropylene.* This is a strong, stiff plastic polymer with good resistance to cracking when flexed. As a result it is particularly suitable for use in closures with hinges which must resist repeated flexing. In addition, polypropylene has been used as tablet containers and intravenous bottles.

*Polystyrene.* This is a clear, hard, brittle material with low impact resistance. Its use in drug packaging is limited due to its high permeability to water vapour. However, it has been used for tubes and amber-tinted bottles where clarity and stiffness are important and high gas permeability is not a drawback. It is also used for jars for ointments and creams with low water content.

## CLOSURES

Any closure system should provide an effective seal to retain the container contents and exclude external contaminants. Child-resistant containers commonly consist of a glass or plastic vial or bottle with a specially designed closure. These CRCs are a professional requirement for dispensing of solid and liquid dosage forms in the UK and are ultimately a compromise between child resistance and ease of opening. Several designs of child-resistant closures are currently used for pharmaceutical packaging including cap–bottle alignment systems, push down and turn caps and less commonly, squeeze and turn caps.

The closures in common use with dispensed medicines are the Snap-safe® alignment closure (Fig. 6.6) and the push down and turn Clic-loc® closure

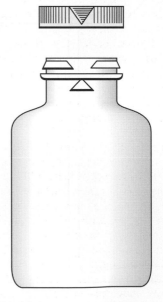

**Fig. 6.6** Snap-safe® closure.

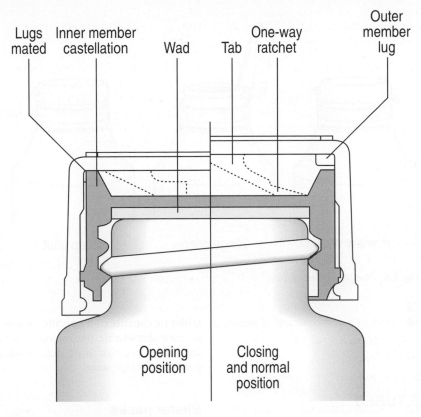

Lugs mated · Inner member castellation · Wad · Tab · One-way ratchet · Outer member lug

Opening position

Closing and normal position

**Fig. 6.7** Clic-loc® closure.

(Fig. 6.7). The Clic-loc® child-resistant closures are based on the assumption that young children are unable to coordinate two separate and dissimilar actions, that is applying pressure and rotating the closure top. The Clic-loc® closure has a two-piece mechanism with springs between the inner and the outer parts. As a result of this design, the closure produces an audible clicking noise when the cap is turned without first being depressed. The inner cap is composed of polypropylene while the outer over-cap is made of HDPE.

Contamination of the screw thread with crystallized sugar arising from syrups can increase the torque necessary to open these Clic-loc® closures. This type of problem can restrict their suitability for use. Owing to opening difficulties experienced by some adults, these closures should not be used on containers supplied to elderly or handicapped patients with poor manual dexterity. They should not be used when a request is made that the product is not dispensed with a child-resistant closure fitted. An individual child-resistant closure must only be dispensed on one occasion as continued use increases the penetration of moisture vapour into the container and decreases the child-resistant properties of the closure.

In recent years greater awareness of the vulnerability of products has led to the development of tamper-evident closures. These closures indicate if unlawful access to the container contents has occurred and are currently available in various designs suitable for different containers and closures. Dispensary stock containers are frequently fitted with a Jaycap® type of tamper-evident closure. These closures are made of either white polypropylene or LDPE. With this closure design the tamper-evident closures snap over a security bead on the neck of the container. The closures cannot be opened until the band connecting the skirt to the tamper-evident ring is torn away (Fig. 6.8). Clic-loc® closures are available with this design whereby an external tamper-evident coloured band must be removed before the closure can be turned. Inner seals are positioned within the closure and isolate the container contents. The seal must be torn or removed from the container to gain access to the packaged product within the container. These

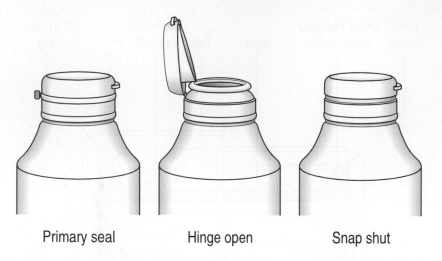

Primary seal    Hinge open    Snap shut

**Fig. 6.8**  Tamper-evident closure.

seals are commonly made of a combination of paper, plastic and foil.

## COLLAPSIBLE TUBES

These are flexible containers for the storage and dispensing of creams and ointments. Tubes made of tin are used to package certain sterile formulations. Typically the formulation is aseptically filled into the pre-sterilized tubes. However, the most common metal tubes in current use are made of aluminium with an internal lacquered surface. With this package the tube remains collapsed as the product is removed. These tubes are frequently sealed at both ends and the nozzle must be punctured to access the product. An alternative seal which can be used with these packages is a heat seal band between the primary closure and the container. This band must be torn to gain access to the container contents.

Metal tubes are being superseded by plastic tubes made from a variety of materials. For example, the tube sleeve may be made of LDPE with either a LDPE or HDPE head or the entire tube may be made of polypropylene.

## UNIT DOSE PACKAGING

This term usually means that a single item such as a tablet or capsule or a specific dose is enclosed within its own disposable packaging. The most commonly used methods for unit dose packaging are blister packs and strip packs.

## Blister packs

These are used for packaging unit doses of tablets and capsules and can act as an aid for patient compliance. The medication is placed in a compartment in a base material made of paper, board, plastic or metal foil or a combination of these. The blister is generally composed of a thermoformed plastic sheet such as PVC. The protection given by the plastic blister depends on its composition, design and the method used to form it. Perforations in the base material allow individual sections of the package to be broken off. Blister packages are rigid, unlike strip packs which are flexible.

## Strip packaging

With strip packaging, two webs of material sandwich various types of medicine such as tablets, capsules, suppositories or pessaries. Each of these dosage forms is contained within its own compartment. The composition of the two webs can be selected to meet the necessary protective requirements for the medicine. Aluminium foil is commonly used to manufacture strip packs and provides a good barrier against moisture penetration. The foil is used as a laminate in which the other components add strength to the fragile aluminium foil. They also block small holes which can occur in the thinner foil layer.

## PAPER

Paper is used more than any other material in packaging. Although it has an insignificant role in primary packaging it remains the predominant secondary and tertiary packaging material. In this role it is used as the carton which contains the primary package and, in the form of board, is the corrugated shipping container which contains both.

## PATIENT PACK DISPENSING

A patient pack consists of a course of medication together with a patient information leaflet in a ready to dispense pack. Liquid formulations are supplied in a standard pack. Solid dose forms are supplied as a strip or blister pack. The size of the sealed patient pack is based on a 28-dose unit. It is supplied in this form unless a doctor prescribes that a different quantity of medicine is to be dispensed. The patient pack contains an information leaflet as an aid to improving patient compliance and to supply information to patients about their medication. Pharmacists should be prepared to respond to enquiries after the patient has read the leaflet. The pack itself is designed as a balance between the need for child resistance and the need for ease of opening by the elderly. If requested by the patient the pack contents can be repackaged in a more suitable container.

### Advantages of patient packs

1. They contain product information such as product and manufacturer identification and the batch number.
2. More efficient dispensing results in greater opportunity for patient counselling.
3. More information is supplied to the patient about the product.

### Disadvantages of patient packs

1. Increased storage space is required.
2. The elderly and debilitated patients may experience difficulty in opening the pack.

## Key Points

- Containers should preserve the quality of a medicine for its stated shelf life.
- Glass has both advantages and disadvantages in use, but remains the preferred material in many situations.
- The types of glass have different uses:
  - Type I for ampoules and vials
  - Type II for eye treatments and dropper bottles
  - Type III for metric medical bottles
  - Type IV for solid, liquid and semi-solid preparations.
- Fluted bottles are used for preparations not intended to be swallowed.
- Plastics may be thermosets or thermoplastics.
- A variety of additives to plastics may enter medicines with which they are in contact.
- Child-resistant closures (CRCs) may be alignment closures (Snap-safe) or push and turn (Clic-loc®).
- Use of CRCs is a professional requirement for dispensed medicines unless requested otherwise.
- Tamper-evident closures indicate that there has been no unlawful access to the medicine.
- Aluminium is being replaced by plastics for collapsible tubes.
- Unit dosage packaging may be either blister or strip packaging.
- The main use for paper is for cartons and boxes.
- A patient pack consists of the medicine and patient information leaflet in a ready to dispense outer pack.

## FURTHER READING

Bellamy K A, Thomas S, Barnett M I 1981 Evaluation of plastic containers for solid dosage forms. Pharmaceutical Journal 226: 466–468
British Pharmacopoeia 1993 Appendix XIX. HMSO, London
Dhalla M 1994 If the cap fits … child resistant closures for liquid medicines. Pharmaceutical Journal 253: 836–837
Hughes D 1994 Child resistant containers for liquid medicines. Pharmaceutical Journal 253: 838–839
Jenkins W A, Osborn K R 1993 Packaging drugs and

pharmaceuticals. Technomatic Publishing Company, Lancaster, Pennsylvania

John E G 1994 Pharmaceutical packaging. In: Lund W (ed) The pharmaceutical codex, 12th edn. The Pharmaceutical Press, London, pp 322–330

Lockhart H, Paine F A 1996 Packaging of pharmaceuticals and healthcare products. Blackie Academic & Professional, Glasgow

Ogden B 1993 Child resistant closures for liquids. Manufacturing Chemist 64: 24–28

# 7

# Storage and stability of medicines

*A. J. Winfield*

---

After studying this chapter, the reader will understand about:

**The reasons for limited life of medicines**
**Nature of storage conditions**
**Expiry dates**
**Estimating shelf life**.

## Introduction

Medicines do not keep indefinitely. Some can be kept for only a short time. There are many reasons why this is the case. In 1984, Rhodes listed six causes for the limited time for which medicines can be kept. These are:

1. loss of drug (such as hydrolysis or oxidation)
2. loss of vehicle (such as evaporation of water or other volatile ingredient)
3. loss of uniformity (such as caking of a suspension or creaming of an emulsion)
4. change in bioavailability (particularly with tablets where ageing can reduce availability)
5. change of appearance (such as colour changes)
6. appearance of toxic or irritant products (as a result of chemical change).

To this list may be added changes which arise from microbiological activity.

The underlying physical and chemical processes, together with the formulation steps that can be taken to improve stability, are discussed in *Pharmaceutics: the Science of Dosage Form Design* (Aulton 1988).

It is important to recognize and be aware of the potential for instability in both manufactured and extemporaneous products. There is a need to specify storage conditions and a shelf life, to ensure effective stock control and pay attention to the packaging used in dispensing. It is also useful to be able to offer advice to a patient where a medicine has been kept at an incorrect temperature. This chapter will consider these practical implications of product instability in pharmacy practice.

## STORAGE CONDITIONS

The *British Pharmacopoeia* (BP) includes storage as a heading in some drug monographs and preparations. These include phrases such as 'protected from moisture' and 'protected from light' which are described as being non-mandatory. Thus they are recommended rather than being required. With commercial products, the manufacturer will specify any special storage requirements on the packaging.

Some products require storage at low temperature. The RPSGB publication *Medicine, Ethics and Practice – a guide for pharmacists* defines the two common requirements. A refrigerator should be between 2 and 8°C and be equipped with a maximum and minimum thermometer. A 'cool place' is between 8 and 15°C. Many pharmacies will not have a room at this temperature, so a refrigerator may be used. It is important that any special storage conditions are complied with, not only in the pharmacy, but also by patients after the medicine has been dispensed. Patients must be given adequate information about the storage of their medicines. The label should state what storage condition is required, and be backed up by a verbal reminder, especially where it is out of the normal. Giving this sort of advice will also be part of the service provided to a residential home (see Ch. 40). It should also be remembered that there are legal requirements, such as a lockable cabinet for the storage of controlled drugs in the pharmacy (see Appendix 1).

## EXPIRY DATE

The expiry date of a medicine is the date after which

it should not be used. Before a shelf life can be given to a medicine, storage conditions must be specified, and a range of chemical, physical or microbiological tests performed. These 'accelerated stability tests' (see Aulton 1988) involve using more extreme conditions to predict behaviour under normal conditions. The results are then confirmed by a series of long-term tests. It is normal to allow the potency of a medicine to fall to 90% of its original. This figure may be varied where toxicity is increased or where an excess is added (such as the addition of a 5% overage above the amount stated on the label). Accelerated testing is time-consuming and costly, but is an important part of the development of a medicine in the pharmaceutical industry.

With extemporaneously dispensed products, a more arbitrary method of arriving at a shelf life is used. The BP (and other pharmacopoeia) uses the terms 'freshly prepared' or 'recently prepared' where preparations have a short keeping time. 'Freshly prepared' is defined as having been made no more than 24 hours before issue for use, but there is no indication of when it should be discarded. 'Recently prepared' is used for products which must be discarded 4 weeks after issue when stored at 15–25°C. Whilst the BP does not give a shelf life for 'freshly prepared' medicines an arbitrary 1-week shelf life is often given. Thus there is no indication of a desirable shelf life for an extemporaneous preparation if the monograph does not mention stability. Some aspects of deciding shelf life for extemporaneous mixtures and diluted creams are discussed later in the chapter.

Special storage requirements apply to eye drops (see Ch. 28).

## Stock control

For economic reasons, pharmacists do not like to have stock on their shelves for long periods of time. The aim is to keep stock at a level which will just meet demand. Most manufactured medicines have a long storage time so stability is not normally an issue. However, it is essential that there is efficient stock rotation, so that the older stock is used first. It is also good practice to check the expiry date as part of the dispensing process. When short shelf life products are involved, stock levels may have to be modified to prevent items regularly expiring on the shelves.

## Packaging

The properties of different types of packaging and containers are discussed in Chapter 6. Containers

**Table 7.1** Some of the stability issues which may arise when redispensing medicines and may cause changes to the expiry date

| Change occurring | Effect produced |
| --- | --- |
| Access of light | Increased oxidation or photochemical degradation |
| Access of oxygen | Increased oxidation |
| Loss of vapour | Loss of water or volatile solvents |
| Access of microorganisms | Increased contamination, growth, spoilage and possible toxicity |
| Access of moisture | Hydrolysis, damage to powders, tablets and capsules |

are designed to afford protection to the medicine which they contain. Part of this may be to protect from light, exclude air and moisture, prevent access of microorganisms or have other more specialized functions.

The official compendia direct to particular containers for some extemporaneous preparations. Manufacturers will have selected the packaging after extensive testing. Any repackaging which takes place during dispensing may reduce the shelf life of the product. Original pack dispensing of manufactured medicines is being introduced. However, progress is slow. Until it is fully implemented, pharmacists have to repackage dispensed medicines. A number of problems may arise, some of which are summarized in Table 7.1.

The pharmacist should include storage conditions on the label. The expiry date may also require to be changed. The decision about this will be based on a consideration of many factors, including the original expiry date, the specified storage condition, a knowledge of the nature of the instability, the properties of the original container and that to be used for the dispensed product, the duration of the treatment and the likely storage conditions at home or on the hospital ward. Particular care will be required if the medicine is being placed in a compliance aid or monitored dosage system where the level of protection will be much reduced (see Ch. 41). A shelf life of a few weeks only may be given to products which have a particular susceptibility to chemical, physical or microbiological change. As with any such decision, the safety of the patient is of the greatest importance. The revised shelf life should be clearly indicated on the label and the patient counselled.

## EXAMPLES OF STABILITY PROBLEMS

Whilst there are many examples of stability problems, three will be considered in more detail.

### Glyceryl trinitrate tablets

The drug glyceryl trinitrate is volatile and soluble in some plastics. The vapour pressure of the drug is relatively low at room temperature. This produces a saturated atmosphere within the container. If it remains tightly closed, further loss of drug would be minimal. If the vapour is in contact with a material which will dissolve or adsorb the drug, this process is likely to occur. Plastic bottles will do this, but so too will some screw-cap liners (such as cork or paperboard) and inserts used to reduce movement of the tablets on transport (such as cotton wool or synthetic fibres). In these situations, the loss of drug will be extensive. However, there are three further complications. One is that, if temperature fluctuates, vaporized drug can condense into other tablets. This has been shown to cause poor content uniformity. This is most likely to happen shortly after packing and can be minimized by the addition of stabilizers to the tablets. Some of these stabilizers reduce drug stability. Secondly, because patients suffering from angina require to carry the tablets around, many transfer a few tablets to a smaller, more convenient container. These are unlikely to have an effective seal and may contain plastics and other adsorbents. Thirdly, the greatest level of loss occurs at elevated temperatures, such as are encountered when the tablets are carried close to the body.

The recommendation is to avoid repackaging on dispensing. The tablets must be in glass containers, fitted with a screw-cap with an aluminium or tin foil lining and with no other packing materials. They should be protected from light and kept below 25°C. A maximum of 100 tablets per container is specified. The recommended shelf life for dispensed tablets is 8 weeks.

### Extemporaneous mixtures

The BP directions on freshly and recently prepared products have been discussed already. However, the actual expiry date will have to be arrived at with an awareness of all the other factors involved. This will include chemical stability (such as hydrolysis or oxidation) and physical stability (such as caking of suspensions or precipitation where tinctures are included). Perhaps the main factor is the possibility of microbiological growth which can occur in aqueous medicines. Whilst many contain chloroform water, the chloroform is volatile and growth has been observed to occur in such systems when it has been lost. Well-filled, well-closed containers appear not to lose much chloroform. However, regular opening of containers can cause the loss of a third or more of the chloroform over 4 weeks. A loss of about one-fifth would probably allow vegetative organisms to grow. The recommendation for mixtures which are preserved with chloroform is that they should be discarded 2 weeks after dispensing (Lynch et al 1977).

### Diluted creams

Creams, being aqueous are prone to microbial growth. Protecting creams is difficult because of the partitioning of preservatives between the aqueous and oily phases and micelles (see Ch. 13). Dilution of a cream, apart from possibly introducing organisms, can also inactivate the preservative system present. This may be through incompatibility, dilution or changes in partition coefficient. The *British National Formulary* recommends that dilution be avoided. Where it is necessary, only the diluent recommended by the manufacturer should be used. The dilution should be freshly prepared and a 2-week expiry date should be applied.

## ESTIMATING SHELF LIFE

Occasionally a product which should have been stored in a refrigerator will have been left at room temperature for a time. It is useful for the pharmacist to be able to advise the patient of a revised expiry date. An accurate calculation is not normally possible, but an estimate is possible using the $Q_{10}$ value (Longland & Rowbotham 1989). The $Q_{10}$ value is defined as the factor by which the rate constant of the decomposition reaction increases for each 10°C rise in temperature. The values are derived from the activation energy and are likely to be between 2 and 4. The equation is:

$$T(T_2) = \frac{T(T_1)}{Q_{10}^{\frac{(T_1 - T_2)}{10}}}$$

where $T(T_1)$ and $T(T_2)$ are the shelf lives at temperatures $T_1$ (accidental storage conditions) and $T_2$ (expected storage conditions).

This equation may be used to estimate the detrimental effect of poor storage on shelf life and the beneficial effects of storage in a refrigerator. The following example illustrates the use of the method.

## EXAMPLE 7.1

A medicine should be stored in the refrigerator (nominal temperature 5°C) and has a shelf life remaining of 12 months. It has been left out of the refrigerator for 2 weeks (nominal temperature 25°C). What is the revised expiry date?

First calculate the time in the refrigerator which is equivalent to the 2 weeks at room temperature.

$$T_5 = \frac{0.5}{Q_{10}^{\frac{-20}{10}}}$$

For the values of $Q_{10} = 2, 3, 4$ the time is 2, 4 or 8 months respectively.

Thus the remaining time is $12 - 2$ months (or $12 - 4$ or $12 - 8$).

Therefore 10, 8 or 4 months remain.

For safety reasons, the 'worst case' is always taken, therefore a 4-month expiry date is used. It must be emphasized that the answer is only an estimate.

## Key Points

- Storing in a cool place means 8–15°C and storing in a refrigerator means at 2–8°C.
- Shelf life is normally the time that a medicine can be kept before the potency has fallen to 90% of the original.
- Expiry date is calculated from the shelf life at the time of preparation.
- Extemporaneous preparations often have to be given arbitrary shelf lives.
- 'Freshly prepared' is defined in the BP as prepared no more than 24 hours before issue.
- 'Recently prepared' is defined in the BP as discarded after 4 weeks.
- Dispensing may inadvertently involve shortening the shelf life of a product in view of its susceptibility to chemical, physical or microbiological challenge.
- Glyceryl trinitrate tablets must be dispensed in glass containers with a metal foil cap liner, protected from light, and stored below 25°C with fewer than 100 per container. The shelf life is 8 weeks.

- Preparations made with chloroform water as preservative should normally have a shelf life of 2 weeks.
- Cream dilutions should be avoided, but if prepared a 2-week shelf life is used.
- The $Q_{10}$ value is a method for estimating shelf life following inappropriate storage.

## FURTHER READING

Aulton M E 1988 Pharmaceutics: the science of dosage form design. Churchill Livingstone, Edinburgh

British Pharmacopoeia, current edn. HMSO, London

British National Formulary, current edn. British Medical Association and Royal Pharmaceutical Society of Great Britain, London (Updated twice yearly)

Longland P W, Rowbotham P C 1989 Room temperature stability of medicines recommended for cold storage. Pharmaceutical Journal 243: 589–595

Lynch M, Lund W, Wilson D A 1977 Chloroform as a preservative in aqueous systems. Pharmaceutical Journal 219: 501–510

Medicines, Ethics and Practice – a guide for pharmacists, current edn. Royal Pharmaceutical Society of Great Britain, London (Updated twice yearly)

Pharmaceutical Codex 1994 12th edn. The Pharmaceutical Press, London

Rhodes C T 1984 An overview of kinetics for the evaluation of the stability of pharmaceutical systems. Drug Development and Pharmaceutical Industry 10: 1163–1174

# 8
# Labelling of dispensed medicines

*M. M. Moody*

---

After studying this chapter you will know about:

**The reasons for having labels**
**Requirements for labels**:
    Producing labels
    Standard details on labels
    Additional information on some labels
**Specific legal requirements**.

## Introduction

The label on a dispensed medicine has two main functions. One is to uniquely identify the contents of the container. The other is to ensure that patients have clear and concise information which will enable them to take or use their medication in the most effective and appropriate way.

There are several legal and professional requirements which must be complied with when labelling a dispensed medicine and it is the pharmacist's responsibility to ensure that these requirements are satisfied and all labelling is accurate and comprehensible. The regulations indicate standard details which must appear on every label and in certain circumstances additional details are also required.

## STANDARD REQUIREMENTS FOR LABELLING DISPENSED MEDICINES

All labels must be typewritten or computer generated. This means that the information on the label should be legible; however, there have been reports of labels which were unreadable because the printing was too faint. Check printer ribbons regularly and make sure that the print is clear. It is easier to read what is on a faintly printed label when you know what is supposed to be there. The patient may not be so lucky!

Details which must appear on the label of a dispensed medicine:

- the name of the preparation
- the quantity
- instructions for the patient
- the patient's name
- the date of dispensing
- the name and address of the pharmacy
- 'Keep out of reach of children'.

## Additional labelling requirements

- Where appropriate, warning or advisory labels should be either attached to the container, or indicated.
- A batch number should be indicated if the preparation has been prepared extemporaneously.
- An expiry date should be indicated if the preparation has been prepared extemporaneously or the shelf life has been shortened, e.g. a diluted preparation.
- Additional legal requirements, e.g. 'For animal treatment only' on veterinary prescriptions.

## The name of the preparation and the quantity

The name which appears on the label must be the same as the one which appears on the prescription. The preparation may be prescribed generically but only be available as a proprietary or branded product; however, the prescribed name must be used. The reason for this is to avoid the patient becoming confused with a variety of names.

Occasionally a prescriber may not wish the name of the preparation to appear on the container. To do this they will delete the NP instruction on the prescription (see p. 98). In these cases the name of the product should be replaced by the form, i.e. 'the tablets', 'the mixture'.

Another occasion when the name may be omitted is when the product contains several active ingredients and has no official or proprietary name. It would be extremely difficult to list all the ingredients on the label. In these instances the pharmaceutical form name is used, e.g. 'the ointment', 'the mixture'.

If the preparation occurs as more than one strength, in order to uniquely identify the product, the strength must be included on the label.

Normally the quantity which appears on the label will be the quantity which has been prescribed. However, in some cases multiple packs are required to complete a prescription. In these instances, when more than one container of the same medicine is dispensed, the quantity on the label should be the amount in each container.

## The instructions

No patient should leave a pharmacy without knowing, how much, how often and how to use his or her medication. Although the label should be seen as a back-up to the verbal counselling and advice given by the pharmacist, it is still essential to ensure that the wording on the label is clear, concise and comprehensible to the patient. The prescriber's instructions should therefore be translated into an appropriate form. If instructions are missing or incomplete it is the pharmacist's professional duty to obtain instructions from the prescriber or use professional discretion to interpret *British National Formulary* (BNF) statements on dosage.

The way in which instructions are worded is of paramount importance and will greatly influence how easily a patient understands the message. Pharmacists should therefore give serious consideration to the wording on medicine labels.

The Royal Pharmaceutical Society Working Party Report (1990) on 'The labelling of dispensed medicines' made several recommendations. The use of active verbs is preferred, i.e. 'take' instead of 'to be taken', 'apply' instead of 'to be applied'. The reason for this is that research has shown that active verbs are more easily understood and remembered than passive verbs. The use of active verbs may cause slight problems in that it is bad practice to have two numbers appearing together in instructions, e.g. 'take two three times daily'. It is all too easy for a patient to mentally transpose the position of the numbers and the previous instruction is changed, in the patient's mind, to 'three twice daily'. This could seriously compromise the effect of the medication. In these situations the numbers should *always* be

**Table 8.1 Recommended wording for directions**

| Recommended wording | Wording to be replaced |
|---|---|
| Do not swallow | Not to be taken |
| Take 'x' times a day, spaced evenly through the day. This wording was considered preferable for antibiotics. For analgesics it remains desirable to use the previous wording | Take every 'y' hours |
| Put two drops in the affected eye | Instil two drops in the affected eye |
| For creams or ointments: Spread thinly | Use sparingly |
| For pessaries or suppositories: Gently put one into the vagina/rectum | Insert one into the vagina/rectum |
| Patient information leaflets: Where appropriate, reference should be made to the patient information leaflet for instructions on how the product should be used | |

separated by using the formulation name, e.g. 'take two tablets', 'two capsules', 'two powders three times daily'.

Other Working Party recommendations can be seen in Table 8.1.

Numbers which are part of an instruction must always be written as words except in the case of 5 ml, when referring to a 5 ml spoonful, or oral syringe quantities, e.g. a 2.5 ml dose using the oral syringe provided.

## The patient's name

It is a legal requirement that on all dispensed medicines the name of the patient for whom the medication has been prescribed must appear on the label. If possible, the status of the patient, i.e. Mr, Mrs, Miss, Master, Child or Baby should be included in order to clearly differentiate from other members of a household, where there may be persons with the same name. A full first name should also be included, if possible, rather than an initial e.g. Mr James Burnett instead of J. Burnett.

## The date and name and address of the pharmacy

The majority of pharmacies use computer systems for prescription labelling and this information will normally appear automatically, with the date being re-set daily.

## 'Keep out of reach of children'

Virtually all labels which are to be used with typewriters or computer systems, for dispensing purposes, come preprinted with 'Keep out of reach of children' but it is always worth checking that this is the case. Any pharmacist who issues a dispensed medicine without this warning on the label is guilty of contravening the Medicines Act.

## ADDITIONAL LABELLING REQUIREMENTS

In addition to the standard details required on all dispensed medicines there are several extra details which are required in certain circumstances.

### Additional information specific to a particular type of formulation

#### Storage

Certain formulations may require special storage and this information should be attached to the label, e.g. transdermal patches should be stored in a cool place. Any specific pharmaceutical precautions relating to storage should always be indicated. Information for individual preparations can be found in the relevant chapters in this book. Information on proprietary medicines can be accessed in the Association of British Pharmaceutical Industries (ABPI) *Compendium of Data Sheets*.

#### Warnings for patients

Ideally, any liquid preparation should state 'Shake the bottle'.

Preparations for external use should state 'Do not swallow' or similar instruction, alerting the patient.

Many drugs cause side effects about which the patient should be informed. Information on these can be found in Appendix 9 of the BNF. It is a professional requirement, subject to the pharmacist's discretion, that if indicated, these special warnings should be affixed to the container. Nowadays many computer systems will automatically print these warnings when a label for a particular drug is being

produced. However, there are instances when use of this information is inappropriate and, again, professional discretion should be used. For example, the antihistamine chlorpheniramine requires the warning: 'Warning. May cause drowsiness. If affected do not drive or operate machinery. Avoid alcoholic drink'. Young children may be prescribed a drug such as this and clearly this warning would be inappropriate. It is obviously important to draw attention to the problem of sedation and in this case the more suitable warning 'Warning. May cause drowsiness' could be used.

Other BNF warning labels which have been known to cause confusion are numbers 5, 6, 7, 11 and 14. All of these may require additional explanation to be given to the patient.

- Label number 5: 'Do not take indigestion remedies at the same time of day as this medicine'.
- Label number 6: 'Do not take iron preparations or indigestion remedies at the same time of day as this medicine'.
- Label number 7: 'Do not take milk, iron preparations or indigestion remedies at the same time of day as this medicine'.

Some patients misunderstand the information on these three labels and think that milk, iron preparations and indigestion remedies must not be taken at all. It should be explained to the patient that as long as there is an interval of approximately 2 hours between taking the medication and any of the substances mentioned there is not a problem.

- Label number 11: 'Avoid exposure of skin to direct sunlight or sunlamps'.

There have been reports of patients who were frightened to venture outside when taking medication which carried this warning. Again an explanation that as long as exposed areas of skin are adequately covered, e.g. a long-sleeved shirt, a sunhat to shade the face, the patient should not suffer any ill effects.

- Label number 14: 'This medicine may colour the urine'.

In this instance it is useful to give the patient an indication of what the colour might be.

#### A batch number

When a product has been prepared extemporaneously it is always good practice to award it a batch number and incorporate this onto the label. This is standard practice in hospital pharmacy. When preparing an extemporaneous product, details of the ingredients used should be recorded. The batch number allows referral back to this information and assists pharmacists in complying with the Consumer Protection Act (see Appendix 1).

### Expiry date

It is not normally necessary to put an expiry date on the label of a dispensed medicine although with the increasing dispensing of manufacturers' original packs this information will be part of the pack labelling. Manufacturers' expiry dates relate to ideal storage conditions but, unfortunately, when a product has been dispensed and given to the patient there is no longer any control over how it is stored. For this reason, under current legislation, when a product is repackaged for dispensing no expiry date is stated. Patients should be encouraged to complete the course of medication or, if for any reason, a supply is not finished and is no longer required, to bring any remainder back to the pharmacy.

There are, however, specific occasions when an expiry date must be added to the label.

- An expiry date should always be put onto any extemporaneously prepared item.
- An expiry date should always be used when a product has been diluted, thereby affecting the stability and shelf life.
- An expiry date should always be indicated when the preparation is sterile, e.g. eye drops. Once opened the product is no longer sterile and if used beyond a certain timescale there is a serious risk of infection. It is therefore recommended that eye drops and eye ointment, unless otherwise specified by the manufacturer, should be discarded 4 weeks after opening. This instruction should be indicated on the label.
- Glyceryl trinitrate tablets lose their efficacy owing to the volatility of the active ingredient and an expiry date must be attached to the container (see Ch. 7). The tablets must be disposed of 8 weeks after the container is first opened.

Although the majority of patients will understand what 'expiry date' means it is important to express the information in a clear and unambiguous way. 'Any unused to be discarded on...(date)' or 'Do not use after...(date)' are preferred methods of expressing expiry dates.

## LEGAL REQUIREMENTS IN CERTAIN CIRCUMSTANCES

### Veterinary dispensed products

The words 'For animal use only' or similar must always be added to the label of a dispensed veterinary product.

Instead of the patient's name the name of the animal's owner should appear, along with the owner's address or address where the animal lives.

### Emergency supply

When a preparation is dispensed using the emergency supply procedures (see Appendix 1) the words 'Emergency supply' must appear on the label.

### Private prescriptions

A label for a medicine dispensed from a private prescription must bear a reference number. This reference number will relate to the entry in the private prescription register and will also be endorsed on the private prescription.

## ERRORS

The potential for making errors when producing a label is considerable and it is important that constant checking is carried out. Practice procedures should be such that the chances of errors occurring are minimized. One of the commonest ways that errors occur is reading what we think is on a label not what is actually there. Dispensing is usually carried out in a busy environment with many distractions and it takes considerable effort to maintain the 100% concentration required to ensure that errors do not occur.

Apart from errors in interpreting prescribers' instructions or missing off any of the details already mentioned the advent of computerized labelling has brought its own problems, two of which will be mentioned.

### Patient's name

When using a computer system, if a patient presents a prescription for several items, the patient's name is typed in once and the number of items to be dispensed bearing that patient's name is entered. Occasionally an item may not be dispensed or the number of items is entered incorrectly. This means that when the next prescription is to be dispensed, if care is not taken, the drug details will be entered and the label produced with the correct drug information but bearing the wrong patient name.

## Transposition of labels

Commonly two labels have been produced on the pharmacy computer and two medicines have been prepared. At this point the labels are applied but to the incorrect container.

An awareness of how easily these errors can occur is at least one step to ensuring that they do not happen.

---

### Key Points

- A label is used to identify and instruct on use of a medicine, so simple language should be used.
- All labels must be typewritten or computer generated.
- All labels must state the name and quantity of the preparation, patient's name and instructions, name and address of pharmacy, date of dispensing and 'Keep out of reach of children'.
- Warning labels may also be required.
- Active verbs should be used on the label.
- Adjacent numbers should be separated by the formulation name, e.g. 'take two tablets three …' on a label.
- As full a name of the patient as possible should be included on the label.
- The BNF contains details of side effect warnings which should be used unless there is a good reason not to do so.
- Some warning labels may require verbal explanation.
- It is good practice to give an extemporaneous preparation a batch number.
- Expiry dates are required on the label when dispensing diluted, sterile and extemporaneous preparations and for glyceryl trinitrate tablets.
- Computer labelling systems can increase the risk of some types of error.

---

## SELF-ASSESSMENT QUESTIONS

1. The following NHS prescription was received:

   Tabs Ibuprofen 400 mg
   Mitte 60
   one t.i.d.

   The name of the patient was Mrs Marjory Nicol. Comment on the accuracy of the following labels produced for this prescription. (Assume that the name and address of the pharmacy and 'Keep out of the reach of children' are included.)

   a. 60 Tabs Ibuprofen
      Take one tablet three times daily
      with or after food
      Mrs Marjory Nicol                    [12/5/96]

   b. 60 Tabs Ibuprofen 400 mg
      Take one three times daily
      with or after food
      Mrs Marjory Nicol                    [12/5/96]

   c. 60 Tabs Ibuprofen 400 mg
      Take one tablet three times daily
      with or after food
      M Nicol                              [12/5/96]

   d. 60 Tabs Ibuprofen 400 mg
      One to be taken three times daily
      with or after food
      Mrs Marjory Nicol                    [12/5/96]

   e. 60 Tabs Ibuprofen 400 mg
      Take three tablets daily with
      or after food
      Mrs Marjory Nicol                    [12/5/96]

2. The following NHS prescription is received:

   Betnovate Ointment Half Strength
   Mitte 50 g
   Sig. apply to affected area m. et n.
   Mr James Hill                          [12/5/96]

   Comment on the following label:

   50 g Betnovate ointment Half strength
   Apply to affected area morning and night
   Mr James Hill                          [12/5/96]

3. You will need to consult Appendix 9 in the *British National Formulary* to complete this exercise.

   Using the BNF, indicate the cautionary and advisory labels which should appear on the following products. Are there any where you consider additional information may need to be given?

a. Tildiem Retard tablets
b. Ledermycin capsules
c. Solpadol caplets
d. Madopar capsules.

## ANSWERS

1. a. The strength of the drug has been omitted from the label. This will cause problems of identification.
   b. The instructions have been written with the number of tablets and the dose frequency together, i.e. 'Take one three times...'. This is bad practice and may lead to errors in dosing.
   c. The status of the patient and first name have not been included, i.e. M Nicol instead of Mrs Marjory Nicol.
   d. The passive form of the verb has been used, i.e. 'to be taken'. The active form 'take' is the preferred form.
   e. The instructions are not clear. Although the patient has been told the correct number of tablets to take in a 24-hour period, information about frequency is missing. This will lead to loss of efficacy and a possible increase in the incidence of adverse effects.

2. This preparation has been diluted, i.e. Betnovate ointment, 25 g and 25 g of recommended diluent. This has affected the stability and consequently the shelf life so an expiry date should have been indicated on the label. The manufacturer's recommendation is a shelf life of 14 days. This preparation is for external use and the label should have indicated this.

3. a. Tildiem Retard tablets require:

   Label 25: 'Swallowed whole, not chewed'.

   This is a reasonably simple instruction but the patient's attention should be drawn to it and an explanation of why it is necessary given. The modified release of the preparation will be destroyed if the tablets are crushed or chewed.

   b. Ledermycin capsules require:

   Label 7: 'Do not take milk, iron preparations or indigestion remedies at the same time of day as this medicine'.
   Label 9: 'Take at regular intervals. Complete the prescribed course unless otherwise directed'.

Label 11: 'Avoid exposure of skin to direct sunlight or sun lamps'.
Label 23: 'Take an hour before food or on an empty stomach'.

The main problem here is the considerable amount of information. The patient's understanding of the information should be checked and further explanation given if necessary.

c. Solpadol caplets require:

Label 2: 'Warning. May cause drowsiness. If affected do not drive or operate machinery'.
Label 29: 'Do not take more than 2 at any one time. Do not take more than 8 in 24 hours'.
Label 30: 'Contains paracetamol'.

Again there is a considerable amount of information given, all of which is important. The pharmacist should alert the patient to the paracetamol warning and explain that other paracetamol-containing preparations should not be taken.

d. Madopar capsules require:

Label 14: 'This medicine may colour the urine'.
Label 21: 'Take with or after food'.

Reinforcement of dosing in relation to food intake should be given if the pharmacist considers it necessary. If the patient has not received the medication before, an indication that the urine colour will be reddish, should be given.

## FURTHER READING

ABPI Compendium of data sheets and summaries of product characteristics, current edn. Datapharm Publications, London (Updated annually)
British National Formulary, current edn. British Medical Association and Royal Pharmaceutical Society of Great Britain, London (Updated twice yearly)
Medicines, Ethics and Practice – a guide for pharmacists, current edn. Royal Pharmaceutical Society of Great Britain, London (Updated twice yearly)
Royal Pharmaceutical Society Working Party Report 1990 Labelling of dispensed medicines. Pharmaceutical Journal 245: 128–129

# 9
# The prescription

*M. M. Moody*

After studying this chapter you will know about:

**Differences between NHS and private prescriptions**
**'Repeat' prescribing and dispensing**
**Steps to be taken in responding to a prescription**
**Procedures for checking a prescription**
**The structure of and abbreviations used on a prescription**
**Generic prescribing**
**Endorsing NHS and private prescriptions**
**Record keeping**
**Steps needed to reduce errors being made during dispensing a prescription.**

## Introduction

The majority of prescriptions dispensed in the UK are National Health Service (NHS) prescriptions. These can be issued by general medical practitioners (GPs), dental practitioners, hospital doctors and certain qualified nurses. The Government pays the cost of these prescriptions with some patients paying a tax on receipt of the dispensed item to defray the cost to the Government. The NHS prescription form is illustrated in Figure 9.1.

Some prescribers will provide patients with private prescriptions where the patient pays the full cost of the medication. Medical practitioners, dental practitioners and veterinary surgeons may prescribe, using private prescriptions. An example of a private prescription is seen in Figure 9.2A.

## Repeatable prescriptions

One of the main areas where private prescriptions differ from NHS forms is that the prescriber can indicate that the item can be repeated (see Fig. 9.2B), unless

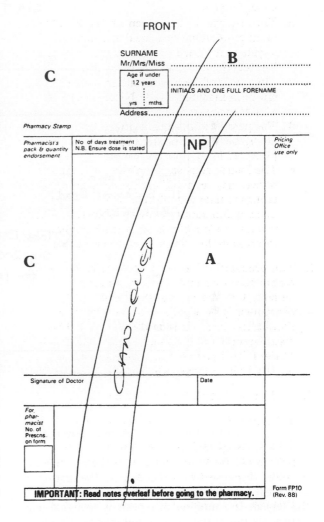

**Fig. 9.1** NHS prescription form (reproduced by permission of the Family Practitioner Committee).

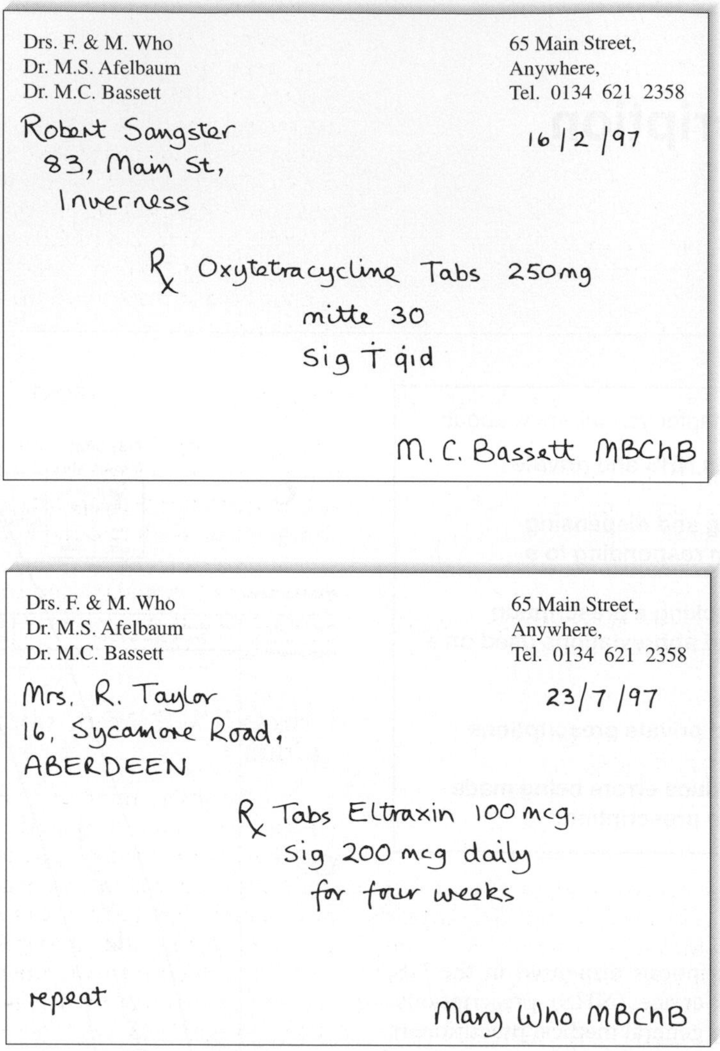

Drs. F. & M. Who
Dr. M.S. Afelbaum
Dr. M.C. Bassett

65 Main Street,
Anywhere,
Tel. 0134 621 2358

Robert Sangster
83, Main St,
Inverness

16/2/97

℞ Oxytetracycline Tabs 250mg
mitte 30
Sig Ṫ qid

M. C. Bassett MBChB

A

Drs. F. & M. Who
Dr. M.S. Afelbaum
Dr. M.C. Bassett

65 Main Street,
Anywhere,
Tel. 0134 621 2358

Mrs. R. Taylor
16, Sycamore Road,
ABERDEEN

23/7/97

℞ Tabs Eltraxin 100 mcg.
Sig 200 mcg daily
for four weeks

repeat

Mary Who MBChB

B

**Fig. 9.2** Private prescriptions.

the drug prescribed belongs to Schedule 2 or 3 of the Misuse of Drugs Act (see Appendix 1).

If the prescriber writes 'repeat' on the prescription it can be dispensed on two occasions; the first occasion is the first dispensing and the second occasion is the repeat. If a number of repeats is specified, e.g. 'repeat six times' the prescription may be dispensed seven times in total. The exception is where the prescription is for an oral contraceptive. If the prescription states 'repeat' the item can be dispensed six times, i.e. five repeats.

As well as the repeat facility there are differences in the endorsing and administrative procedures for NHS and private prescriptions. These will be dealt with later in the chapter. However, the checking procedures, which should be undertaken by the pharmacist, when dispensing either type of prescription are fundamentally the same.

As in all pharmacy practice procedures an organized, structured approach will reduce the likelihood of errors and ensure good practice. When presented with a prescription the following method should be adopted:

## 1. Read the prescription

- Is the prescription legal?

- Who is it for? Adult, child, elderly, animal?
- What is the name of the preparation?
- What are the instructions for the patient?
- What quantity is to be dispensed?

### 2. Find out information

- What is it?
- How does it act and how is it used?
- Are the prescriber's instructions correct?
- How is it prepared?
- What advice does the patient require?

### 3. Carry out procedures (i.e. put knowledge into practice)

- Make or assemble the preparation.
- Pack into appropriate container.
- Label the container.
- Endorse the prescription.
- Make appropriate records.
- Hand over to the patient with appropriate advice.
- Correctly dispose of the prescription.

## READ THE PRESCRIPTION

### Legality

It is every pharmacist's responsibility to check that the prescription to be dispensed is legal. The details required for a legally written prescription are found in the RPSGB publication *Medicines, Ethics and Practice – a Guide for Pharmacists*. The current edition should be consulted in conjunction with this chapter. There are, however, one or two areas worthy of mention.

### Date

An area where errors may occur is the date of the prescription. In order to be legal a prescription must be appropriately dated. Occasionally the date may be omitted when the prescription is written. An undated prescription is illegal and must be returned to the prescriber to be amended. In addition, prescriptions for prescription-only medicines (POM) are only valid for limited times. These are 6 months for a POM and 13 weeks for a POM which is also a Schedule 2 or 3 drug in the Misuse of Drugs Act. If the prescription is a private, repeatable prescription, the first dispensing must take place within 6 months of the date on the prescription. Subsequent dispens-

ing can occur at any time interval. There is, however, a professional issue to be considered. If considerable time has elapsed between repeats it is good practice to check whether the medication is still appropriate for the patient. The patient may have developed a condition which means that the drug is contraindicated or he may now be taking other drugs for the condition or drugs which could interact.

There are occasions when a prescriber may postdate a prescription. In these cases the prescription cannot be dispensed until the date indicated on the prescription.

### Signature

Many prescriptions are computer generated. The appropriate prescription details are printed out by the computer and the prescription is then signed by the prescriber. Occasionally a prescription may be overlooked by the prescriber and is presented for dispensing with the signature missing. It is therefore important that all details are carefully checked on every prescription.

## Who is it for? Adult, child, elderly, animal?

It is obviously important to know whether the patient is an adult or a child in order that the dose can be checked. Any prescription where this is unclear should not be dispensed until the necessary information has been obtained. Where a child is under 12 years old it is a legal requirement to indicate the child's age on the prescription. Do not assume just because the age is not indicated that the child is over 12 years old.

Some drugs should be given in smaller doses when the patient is elderly. Although not checked as frequently as it should be, this type of information can help in reducing the level of side effects or other drug-induced problems from which the elderly may suffer.

If the prescription is for an animal, information on the type and possibly the weight of the animal is needed, in order to check that the drug and dose are appropriate.

## What is the name of the preparation?

There are several abbreviations which are still commonly used in prescription writing. The symbol 'R' appears on the prescription. This is an abbreviation for the Latin word 'recipe' which means 'take'. This is an instruction from the prescriber. The name of

| Table 9.1 Some names which may cause confusion | |
|---|---|
| Aldactide | Aldactone |
| Alrheumat | Aldomet |
| Betaloc | Berotec |
| Betnesol | Betnelan |
| Carbamazepine | Carbimazole |
| Cardene | Codeine |
| Daonil | Danol |
| Ergotamine | Ergometrine |
| Eugynon | Euglucon |
| Fucidin | Fulcin |
| Gliclazide | Glipizide |
| Ketotifen | Ketoprofen |
| Mebendazole | Metronidazole |
| Migril | Mictral |
| Nicardipine | Nifedipine |
| Promazine | Promethazine |
| Quinine | Quinidine |
| Ranitidine | Famotidine |
| Selegiline | Stelazine |
| Zocor | Zoton |

the preparation to be dispensed is written after this abbreviation. Many prescriptions are computer generated and the typescript means that they are often easier to read than hand-written prescriptions. However, whichever way a prescription has been produced, great care must be taken when reading details of the product to be dispensed. There are many product and drug names which can be confused if checking is not thorough and careful. Some examples are given in Table 9.1.

A more comprehensive list of confusing names can be obtained from the National Pharmaceutical Association (NPA).

## What are the instructions for the patient?

Certain conventions and abbreviations are used when instructions are written on a prescription.

'Signetur', or more commonly the abbreviation 'sig.', means 'let it be labelled' and indicates the instructions which have to be attached to the dispensed medicine. The instructions are often written in Latin abbreviations, e.g. 't.i.d.', which means 'three times daily'. Further information on common terms and abbreviations used is given in Appendix 4.

## What quantity is to be dispensed?

The word 'mitte', or its abbreviation 'M', is used. This translates as 'send' and is an indication of the quantity of the drug which is to be dispensed.

Typical prescription details are as follows:

R. Tabs Paracetamol
Mitte 50
Sig. 1 t.i.d.

Some prescribers indicate the quantity to be dispensed by writing the length of treatment, e.g. 30 days or 2 weeks. Again some abbreviations are used. A fraction of 7 may be used to signify the number of days and a fraction of 52 signifies the number of weeks. This is illustrated in Examples 9.1 and 9.2.

---

### EXAMPLE 9.1

Tablets atenolol 50 mg
Sig. 1 twice daily for 4/52

Although no quantity appears on the prescription it is implicit in the instructions. The length of treatment is 4 weeks, i.e. 28 days and two tablets have to be taken each day. The total to be dispensed is 56 tablets.

---

### EXAMPLE 9.2

Tablets penicillin 250 mg
Sig. 2 four times daily for 5/7

The quantity to be dispensed is 40, i.e. eight tablets daily for 5 days.

---

Another variation used is when the dose of the drug to be taken is given as the instruction. This involves a small calculation.

---

### EXAMPLE 9.3

Tablets penicillin 250 mg
Sig. 500 mg four times daily for 5 days

This translates to two tablets four times daily for 5 days. The total to be dispensed is therefore 40 tablets.

---

In the following example the strength of the preparation is not stated but is implicit in the instructions.

---

### EXAMPLE 9.4

Tablets diazepam
Sig. 4 mg t.i.d.
Mitte 30 days supply

Diazepam tablets are made in three strengths:
2 mg, 5 mg and 10 mg. For this prescription the
2 mg strength will be dispensed. Two tablets will be
taken three times daily for a total of 30 days. The
quantity to be dispensed will be 180 tablets.

---

Important information should be being noted at this time for use in patient counselling, e.g. are there potential compliance problems if the therapy is long term or the dosage instructions are complicated? Is it a drug where additional advice needs to be given? Is there potential for interaction?

## FIND OUT INFORMATION

Through education and work experience pharmacists gain considerable knowledge about drug therapy and its implications for the patient. However, new drugs are continually being marketed and theories on optimum therapy and doses of drugs for particular disease states change. It is essential that pharmacists keep up to date with these changes. Reference sources should be consulted frequently. Important reference works which should be available in every pharmacy include:

- *Martindale: the Extra Pharmacopoeia*
- *The British National Formulary* (always use the most recent edition)
- *The Pharmaceutical Codex*
- The ABPI *Compendium of Data Sheets*.

Further details of useful information sources can be found in Chapter 37 and Appendix 7.

Information about the drug being dispensed should be checked. Is the prescribed dose appropriate? On occasions a higher than recommended dose will be prescribed. In some instances the prescriber will circle and initial a higher than normal dose to indicate that it is appropriate. However, even if this has been done, if the pharmacist has misgivings about the prescribed dose the prescriber's intentions should be verified. In any case of doubt it is the pharmacist's responsibility to check the prescriber's intentions. If this is not done and an overdose is dispensed the pharmacist is held responsible.

If a drug has been prescribed which will interact with the patient's existing medication this should be investigated. It may be that the situation has already been recognized and dealt with, e.g. the doses of the interacting drugs have been modified appropriately or the patient is being monitored. However, if the pharmacist is uncertain that the therapy is appropriate, the prescriber should be contacted. The pharmacist should be in a position to explain his or her concerns and offer suggestions to resolve the problem. Clinical practice must be applied throughout the dispensing process.

## CARRY OUT PROCEDURES

If all the details on the prescription are appropriate the items can then be dispensed.

### Make or assemble the preparation

Details of extemporaneous dispensing are found in Chapter 4 and the chapters dealing with particular formulations. Nowadays for the majority of prescriptions the items to be dispensed will be manufactured preparations such as tablets or capsules. Selecting the correct item must be done carefully and with 100% concentration. There are many products with similar names which can cause confusion, e.g. prednisolone and prednisone, chlorpromazine and chlorpropamide. A list of some names which can cause confusion can be found in Table 9.1.

### Generic prescribing

In the UK prescribers are encouraged to prescribe drugs by the generic name. Pharmacists may then dispense any suitable product. Some drugs are produced by several generic manufacturers and are also available in several brands. Although all are the same drug and the same dosage form, the appearance of these products may differ. Different manufacturers' products should not be dispensed together as the variation in appearance and the possibility of differences in bioavailability may affect the patient. Certain drugs such as lithium and theophylline from different manufacturers have significant differences in bioavailability. In these instances the patient must be maintained on the same brand.

If a branded product is prescribed that brand must be dispensed. At present, generic substitution is not allowed.

## Liquids for oral use

It is a requirement that any liquid for oral use should be dispensed with a 5 ml spoon or if the prescribed dose is a fraction of 5 ml an oral syringe should be supplied.

## Labelling the dispensed medicine

Details of labelling are found in Chapter 8. Details of advice for specific dose forms will be found in the relevant chapters. Care should also be taken when labelling, to check the NP instruction on the prescription. The abbreviation 'NP' is printed on all NHS prescriptions. This stands for 'nomen propium' meaning 'proper name'. It is a legal requirement that all medicines dispensed in the UK are labelled with their name. On some occasions the prescriber may not wish the name of the product to appear on the label. In these instances the NP instruction will be deleted by the prescriber. If this is deleted the preparation must be labelled with the formulation name only, e.g. the tablets, the capsules.

## Endorsing requirements

### NHS prescriptions

NHS prescriptions are submitted to the Pricing Division for pricing. It is important that the prescription should be appropriately endorsed before being submitted. Clear information on what was dispensed and in what quantity, should be indicated. The prescription must be stamped with the name and address of the pharmacy from which it was dispensed. Prescriptions for Schedule 2 and 3 drugs must be endorsed with the date of dispensing and the letters 'CD' (controlled drugs).

### Incomplete prescriptions

If certain details are missing from a prescription, such as the prescriber's signature or the date, the prescription must be returned to the prescriber to be corrected. However, unless the prescription is for a Schedule 2 or 3 drug and governed by the Misuse of Drugs Act handwriting requirements, certain drug details may be added by the pharmacist. The prescriber is contacted over the telephone and missing details such as strength, quantity and dosage can be added. The prescription is endorsed 'p c' (prescriber contacted) and dated and initialled by the pharmacist.

If the prescriber cannot be contacted and the pharmacist has sufficient information to make a professional judgement, the missing details may be obtained from the patient, computer-held medication records or other reliable source. The prescription is then endorsed 'p n c' (prescriber not contacted). If, however, there is any doubt as to the accuracy of the information, the prescription must not be dispensed and the patient must be referred back to the prescriber. For NHS prescriptions where the quantity is omitted, a quantity sufficient for 5 days' treatment or the smallest original pack may be supplied and the prescription endorsed 'p n c'.

Further details of NHS endorsing can be found in Appendix 2.

### Endorsing of private prescriptions

Because the patient pays the pharmacist the full cost of the drugs, including a dispensing fee, there is no necessity to endorse private prescriptions with price details. However, they must be stamped with the pharmacy name and address. The date of dispensing and the reference number which relates to the entry in the private prescription book should be indicated on the prescription. If the prescription is a repeatable one, the number of the repeat should be indicated. An illustration of private prescription endorsing is shown in Figure 9.3.

## Record keeping

Apart from ensuring that all prescriptions dispensed satisfy the legal and clinical requirements, pharmacists must also comply with certain record-keeping requirements.

### NHS prescriptions

Unless the drug dispensed belongs to Schedule 2 of the Misuse of Drugs Act no records need to be kept for NHS prescriptions. Details of Schedule 2 records are found in *Medicines, Ethics and Practice – a Guide for Pharmacists*.

### Private prescriptions

For private prescriptions full details of the prescription must be kept. The law states that only records of prescriptions for POM drugs need to be kept but for ethical and professional reasons it is good practice to keep records of all private prescriptions dispensed. The details should be entered into a private prescription register which should be a hard-backed, bound book. A loose-leaf format is not considered suitable.

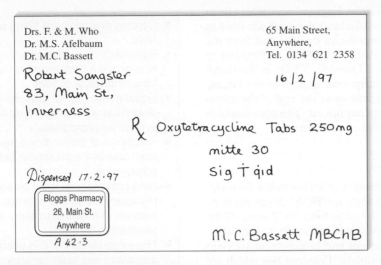

Drs. F. & M. Who
Dr. M.S. Afelbaum
Dr. M.C. Bassett

65 Main Street,
Anywhere,
Tel. 0134 621 2358

Robert Sangster
83, Main St,
Inverness

16/2/97

℞ Oxytetracycline Tabs 250mg

mitte 30

Sig T qid

Dispensed 17.2.97

Bloggs Pharmacy
26, Main St.
Anywhere

A 42.3

M. C. Bassett MBChB

**Fig. 9.3** Private prescription endorsing.

The book must be retained for 2 years from the date of the last entry. Details which should be recorded are:

- the name and address of the patient; for a veterinary prescription the name and address of the animal's owner should be recorded
- full details of the drug dispensed, i.e. name, form, strength, quantity, instructions to the patient
- the name and address of the prescriber
- the date on which the drug was prescribed
- the date of dispensing; these two dates may be the same but two entries indicating the dates must be recorded
- details of any repeat indications.

The entry should then be awarded a reference number which should be endorsed on the prescription and should also appear on the label of the dispensed medicine.

*Records for repeat prescriptions.* Where a prescription is being repeated and a full record of the initial dispensing is already documented in the private prescription book, there is no need to made a further full record. The following details are all that are required:

- the date of dispensing
- an indication of what number of repeat is being dispensed
- the reference number of the original entry
- the charge made to the patient
- the date of the repeat dispensing should be indicated in the original entry.

If the prescription is being repeated but has not previously been dispensed in the pharmacy there will be no record of it in the private prescription book. A full entry must be therefore be made.

## Hand over to the patient with appropriate advice

When the medicine has been dispensed it should be checked by the pharmacist. Any information which needs to be given to the patient should be noted. It is then ready for collection by the patient. Ideally, prescriptions should always be handed to patients by the pharmacist. It is always wise to ask for the patient's address and use this as a double check that the medicine is being handed to the correct person. It is possible for people of the same name to be collecting prescriptions from the same pharmacy. Having verified the identity of the person collecting the prescription, appropriate advice about the medication can be given. In many instances the prescription is not collected by the patient, but by a relative, friend or carer. Where an oral syringe is being supplied with the medicine, a check should be made that the patient or carer knows how to use it. Chapter 37 on counselling gives details of the type of advice which should be offered to patients. No one should leave a pharmacy without knowing how to use medication or appliances correctly.

## Disposal

### NHS prescriptions

The prescriptions are sorted into groups. Because of

differences in the NHS in England and Wales from Scotland and Northern Ireland the methods used in each country vary. Details can be obtained from the Prescription Pricing Authority (PPA) in England or the Pharmacy Practice Division (PPD) in Scotland. Once sorted, the prescriptions are sent to the Pricing Division either fortnightly or at the end of the calendar month, where they are priced. The pharmacist is then reimbursed for the costs incurred.

### Private prescriptions

When completed, unless it is a repeatable prescription, private prescriptions for POM drugs must be filed and retained in the pharmacy for 2 years. If the prescription has a repeat indication on it, it must be offered back to the patient and is only retained when all the repeats are complete. Prescriptions which are for pharmacy category (P) or general sales list (GSL) medicines are also returned to the patient unless the prescriber has indicated 'not to be repeated'.

## PRESCRIBING IN HOSPITALS

Drug therapy is prescribed for hospital inpatients by the doctors and consultants caring for the patients. Different hospitals use different systems for recording prescribing details. However, pharmacists must carry out the same rigorous checking system to ensure that the drug details are correct, an appropriate dose is prescribed and the request for the drugs has been initiated and signed by an appropriately qualified medical practitioner.

### Key Points

- Prescriptions may be written by a GP, dentist, veterinary surgeon, hospital doctor or some nurses (NHS only).
- Only private prescriptions may be endorsed 'repeat'.
- The legality of a prescription must be checked.
- A prescription must state the age of a child under 12 years.
- Great care is required to avoid errors arising through confusing names.
- A series of conventions and abbreviations are used on prescriptions.
- It is the pharmacist's responsibility to verify the dose to be dispensed.

- Generic prescribing is being encouraged in the NHS.
- Bioavailability variations with drugs such as lithium make it important to use the same brand for an individual patient.
- Liquid medicines for oral use must be dispensed with either a 5 ml spoon or an oral syringe as appropriate.
- The name of the medicine must appear on the label unless the prescriber deletes 'NP' on the prescription.
- NHS prescriptions must be endorsed with the pharmacy name and address stamp and other relevant information to allow appropriate payment to be made.
- The endorsement 'p c' is used when the prescriber has been contacted to allow the pharmacist to add missing details to a prescription. The endorsement 'p n c' is used when the information was obtained from another reliable source, such as a patient medical record (PMR).
- Private prescriptions are endorsed with the pharmacy stamp and a reference number relating to the entry in the private prescription book, and the number of the repeat if relevant.
- The only requirement to record an NHS prescription is for a drug in Schedule 2 of the Misuse of Drugs Act.
- Whilst the law only requires a record of POM drugs dispensed on private prescription, it is good professional practice to record all private prescriptions.
- The private prescription register must be a hard-backed, bound book, which must be retained for 2 years after the last entry.
- There are differences in the bundling requirements in different parts of the UK when submitting NHS prescriptions to the Pricing Division.
- POM private prescriptions must be retained for 2 years when dispensing is complete.
- Different hospitals may have their own form of writing prescriptions, but the same procedures apply to their dispensing.

## FURTHER READING

ABPI Compendium of data sheets and summaries of product characteristics, current edn. Datapharm Publications, London (Updated annually)

British National Formulary, current edn. British Medical
    Association and Royal Pharmaceutical Society of Great
    Britain, London (Updated twice yearly)
Drug Tariff, current edn. HMSO, London (Published
    monthly)
Drug Tariff, current edn. SOHD, Edinburgh (Published
    quarterly)
Medicines, Ethics and Practice – a guide for pharmacists,
    current edn. Royal Pharmaceutical Society of Great Britain,
    London (Updated twice yearly)
Pharmaceutical Codex 1994 12th edn. Pharmaceutical Press,
    London
Reynolds J E F (ed) 1996 Martindale: the extra
    pharmacopoeia, 31st edn. Pharmaceutical Press, London
    (Updated every 3 years – use current edn)

# 10
# Routes of administration and dosage forms

*M. M. Moody*

After studying this chapter the reader will know about:

**The different routes of administration of drugs**
**The advantages and disadvantages of each route**
**The types and uses of dosage forms**.

## Introduction

After administration of a drug, a successful therapeutic response will only be achieved if the drug reaches the appropriate site of action or 'receptor' site in sufficient concentration to exert its pharmacological action. This is achieved by the drug being absorbed into the body tissues from the site of administration. The choice of administration site will be dependent on a variety of factors, such as whether a local or systemic action is required, or how quickly a response to the drug is needed. This chapter deals with the various routes of administration used for drug delivery and discusses some of their advantages and disadvantages. Brief details of a variety of dosage forms are also given.

## THE ORAL ROUTE

The oral route is used to obtain either systemic or local effects. The drug, formulated in either a solid or a liquid form, is absorbed from the gastrointestinal tract (GIT). This is the most commonly used route for drug administration. There are a variety of reasons for this.

- From a patient's point of view it is the simplest.
- Self-administration of drugs can be carried out.
- If used properly, it is also the safest route.

However, there are certain disadvantages which should be borne in mind:

- The onset of action is relatively slow.
- Absorption from the GIT may be irregular.
- Certain drugs are destroyed by enzymes and other secretions found in the GIT and by first pass metabolism.
- Drug solubility can be altered by the presence of other substances in the GIT, e.g. calcium.
- Slow gastric emptying may cause a drug to be inactivated by gastric juices, owing to prolonged contact. This can be a particular problem in the elderly.
- It is an unsuitable route of administration in unconscious or vomiting patients and for immediate pre- or postoperative use.

## THE BUCCAL ROUTE

A drug is administered by this route by being formulated as a tablet and absorbed from the buccal cavity. The highly vascular nature of the tongue and buccal cavity, and the presence of saliva which facilitates the dissolution of the drug, make this a highly effective and useful route for drug administration. It can be used for both systemic and local actions.

Two sites are used for absorption from the buccal cavity.

- For sublingual absorption, the area under the tongue is used. This gives a very fast onset of action of the drug but duration is usually short.

- For buccal absorption, the buccal sulcus is used. This is the area between the lip and the gum. Tablets formulated for absorption from the buccal sulcus give a quick onset of action but will also give a reasonably long duration of action.

It is important that patients are made aware of the

different sites and they should be given full instructions on how to administer their tablets, otherwise the full benefit of using this route of administration may not ensue. For details of suitable patient instructions see Chapter 17.

The advantages of the buccal route are:

- a relatively quick onset of action
- drugs are absorbed into the systemic circulation, thereby avoiding the 'first pass' effect
- drugs can be administered to unconscious patients
- because the tablet is not swallowed, anti-emetic drugs can be given by this route.

## THE RECTAL ROUTE

For administration by this route drugs are formulated as liquids; solid dosage forms, e.g. suppositories; and semi-solids such as creams, ointments and foams (see Ch. 15). The chosen preparation is inserted into the rectum from where the drug may be absorbed. This route is used for both systemic and local effects.

The rectum is supplied by three veins, namely the middle and inferior rectal veins which drain directly into the general circulation and the upper rectal vein which drains into the portal vein. The latter flows into the liver. This means that some of the drug absorbed from the rectum can be subject to the 'first pass' effect. Bioavailability therefore, may be less than 100%. It is often better than absorption from the GIT.

The amount of fluid present in the rectum is small, estimated at approximately 3 ml. This affects the rate of dissolution of the drug released from the suppository. However, this is counterbalanced by the muscular movement in the rectum which spreads the drug over a large area and promotes absorption.

The advantages and disadvantages of this route of administration are as follows.

### Advantages

- Can be used when the oral route is unsuitable, e.g. severe vomiting, unconscious patient, patient is uncooperative such as children, elderly or mentally disturbed, patients with dysphagia.
- Useful when the drug causes GIT irritation.
- Can be used for local action.

### Disadvantages

- Absorption can be irregular and unpredictable, giving rise to a variable effect.

- Less convenient than the oral route.
- There is low patient acceptability of this route in the UK. A wider acceptance is found in Europe.

## THE VAGINAL ROUTE

For administration by this route, drugs are formulated as pessaries, which are solid dosage forms, or as semi-solids such as creams, ointments and foams. These are inserted into the vagina. Again, this route can be used for both local and systemic effects. Drugs absorbed from the vagina are not subject to the 'first pass' effect and because of the higher fluid content in the vagina, drug dissolution is more efficient than by the rectal route.

## THE INHALATION ROUTE

In this route drugs are inhaled through the nose or mouth to produce either local or systemic effects. This route is used predominantly to treat respiratory conditions. For this, drugs are delivered directly to the site of action, namely the lungs. Because of the high blood flow to the lungs and their large surface area, drug absorption by this route is extremely rapid. A variety of dosage forms are used, from simple inhalations consisting of volatile ingredients such as menthol to sophisticated inhaler devices (see Ch. 18). A major benefit of the inhaled route is that the drug dose required to produce a systemic effect is much smaller than for the oral route, with a consequent reduction in side effects.

## THE TOPICAL ROUTE

In the topical route the skin is used as the site of administration. This route is most commonly used for local effects. The formulations used include ointments, creams and pastes (see Ch. 14). In recent years specialized dosage forms have been developed which, when applied to the skin, allow the drug to pass through the skin layers to produce a systemic effect. These are known as transdermal therapeutic systems. The skin is the largest and one of the most complex organs of the body. A more detailed discussion of this route of administration can be found in Chapters 14 and 18.

## THE PARENTERAL ROUTE

This is the term used to describe when drugs are given by injection. Within this general term there are a variety of specialized routes. The main ones are:

• *Intravenous route*, where drugs are injected directly into the systemic circulation. This produces a very fast onset of action.

• *Subcutaneous route*, where drugs are injected into the subcutaneous layer of the skin. This is the easiest and least painful type of injection to administer.

• *Intramuscular route*, where drugs are injected into muscle layers. This method can be used to produce a fairly fast onset of action when the drug is formulated as an aqueous solution. A slower and more prolonged action will occur when the drug is presented as a suspension or in an oily vehicle.

These and other specialized types of injections are discussed more fully in the chapter on parenteral products (see Ch. 25).

## DOSAGE FORMS

Drugs are presented in a wide variety of dosage forms. How a drug is formulated is dependent on a variety of factors and the same drugs may be presented in several different dosage forms. It is important for pharmacists to appreciate the different properties of the varying dosage forms in order that the most appropriate or most acceptable formulation is given to the patient. This section gives brief information on the different types of dosage forms. Additional, more detailed, information is found in the chapters dealing with specific formulations and in *Pharmaceutics: the Science of Dosage Form Design* (Aulton 1988).

### Aerosols

These consist of pressurized packs which contain the drug in solution or suspension and a suitable propellant. They are most commonly used for their systemic effect in the treatment of asthma. These devices are fitted with a metering valve which allows a known dose of drug to be delivered each time the device is fired. Some aerosols are for topical use, particularly in the treatment of muscle sprains and injuries. These may contain substances such as non-steroidal anti-inflammatory drugs or counter-irritants.

### Applications

This is the name given to solutions, suspensions or emulsions which are for topical use. They contain substances such as ascaricides or antiseptics.

### Capsules

These are solid dosage forms, generally for oral use. Some drugs formulated as capsules are intended to be inhaled. It is therefore important to inform the patient on appropriate use. For both types of capsule the drug is contained in a gelatin shell, usually as a powder or a liquid. Modified-release preparations are available where the drug is presented in the gelatin container as small pellets with different coatings.

### Collodions

These are liquid preparations for external use. The liquid is painted on the skin, where it forms a flexible film. They contain substances such as salicylic acid which is useful in the treatment of warts.

### Creams

These are semi-solid emulsions for external use. Because of the water content they are susceptible to microbial contamination and either include a preservative or are given a short shelf life. Creams are easier to apply and are less greasy than ointments, so they are often preferred by patients.

### Dusting powders

These are finely divided powders for external use. Their main uses are as lubricants to prevent friction between skin surfaces and for disinfection and antisepsis in minor wounds.

### Ear drops

These are used topically to treat a variety of ear problems. The drug, or mixture of drugs, is presented as a solution or suspension in a suitable vehicle such as water, glycerol, propylene glycol or alcohol. The drops are inserted into the ear, using a dropper. Some vehicles, such as alcohol, may cause a degree of stinging when applied to the ear. Ensure that the patient is aware of this and is assured that it is a normal sensation. If patients find the degree of stinging unacceptable they may have to be given ear drops with an aqueous vehicle. Oils such as almond or olive are often recommended for the alleviation of impacted ear wax. It is usually suggested that such oils, before being dropped into the ear, should be warmed. This must be done very carefully and only minimal heat applied, i.e. the oil placed on a warm spoon. Excessive heat will have very serious consequences for the integrity of the ear.

## Elixirs

An elixir is for oral use and is a solution of one or more drugs. The vehicle generally contains a high proportion of sucrose or, increasingly nowadays, a 'sugar-free' vehicle such as sorbitol solution, which is less likely to cause dental caries. The therapeutic action of drugs presented as elixirs varies widely and includes antihistamines, antibiotics and decongestants.

## Emulsions

These are mixtures of two immiscible liquids, usually oil and water. When the term 'emulsion' is used this refers to a preparation for oral use. Emulsions are dealt with in detail in Chapter 13.

## Enemas

An enema is an oily or aqueous solution which is administered rectally. A variety of drugs are formulated as enemas and are used to treat conditions such as constipation or ulcerative colitis. They are also used in X-ray examination of the lower bowel.

## Eye drops

These are used to administer drugs to the eye and are dealt with in detail in Chapter 28, along with other eye preparations.

## Gargles

Gargles are aqueous solutions used to treat infections of the throat. They are often presented in a concentrated form with instructions to the patient for dilution. Gargles should not be swallowed but held in the throat while exhaling through the liquid. After a suitable time period, usually a minute or so, the patient should spit out the gargle.

## Gels

Gels are semi-solid dosage forms for topical use. They are usually transparent or translucent and have a variety of uses. Spermicides and lubricants are often presented in a gel form. Preparations containing coal tar or other drugs used in the treatment of psoriasis and eczema are also presented in this form. Many patients prefer this formulation.

The term 'gel' is also used to describe colloidal suspensions of drugs such as aluminium and magnesium hydroxides.

## Granules

This term is used to describe a drug which is presented in small irregularly shaped particles. Granules may be packed in individual sachets containing a unit dose of medicament or may be provided in a bulk format where the dose is measured using a 5 ml spoon. Certain laxatives are examples of drugs currently presented as granules. Other uses of granules are found in Chapter 16.

## Implants

This term refers to solid dosage forms which are inserted under the skin by a small surgical incision. They are most commonly used for hormone replacement therapy and more recently an implant containing a progestogen has been developed for use as a contraceptive. Release of the drug from implants is generally slow and long-term therapy is achieved. In the case of the contraceptive implant the effect continues for up to 5 years. A testosterone implant used in the treatment of male hypogonadism will maintain adequate hormone levels in the patient for 4–5 months. Implants must be sterile.

## Inhalations

These are preparations which contain volatile medicaments which may have a beneficial effect in upper respiratory tract disorders such as nasal congestion. Some inhalations contain substances which are volatile at room temperature and the patient can obtain a degree of relief by adding a few drops to a handkerchief or a pillowcase and breathing in the vapour. Other inhalations are added to hot water and the impregnated steam is then inhaled. Many users of this latter type of inhalation use boiling water. Pharmacists should advise against this as the steam produced is too hot and can damage the delicate mucous membranes of the upper respiratory tract. Overuse of this type of preparation should also be avoided as it may cause a chronic condition to develop. The use of these strong aromatic decongestants is contraindicated in children under 3 months owing to the risk of apnoea.

## Injections

These are used parenterally and are sterile. They are discussed in detail in Chapter 25.

## Insufflations

This term is used to describe drugs presented in a dry powder form, usually in a capsule, which is inserted into a specially designed device where the capsule is broken, the contents released and the patient inhales the powder. Today, the most common use being made of insufflations is in the treatment of asthma. Some patients find these 'breath-actuated' devices easier to use than aerosol devices.

## Irrigations

These are sterile solutions most commonly used in the treatment of infected bladders. Sterile solutions of sodium chloride 0.9% (physiological saline) are used to treat a wide range of common urinary tract pathogens. Antifungal drugs such as amphotericin and locally acting cytotoxics, e.g. doxorubicin and epirubicin, are introduced into the bladder, as irrigations, to treat mycotic infections and bladder tumours, respectively.

## Linctuses

A linctus is a viscous liquid for oral use. The majority of products formulated as linctuses are for the relief of cough. The viscous nature of the preparation coats the throat and helps to alleviate the irritation which is causing the problem. Previously, many linctuses contained a high level of sucrose; however, many have been reformulated as 'sugar-free' products to reduce the risk of dental caries. Because the viscous nature of linctuses is beneficial they should not be diluted prior to administration.

## Liniments

These are liquids for external use. They are used to alleviate the discomfort of muscle strains and injuries. Because of the rubefacient nature of some of the ingredients some sportsmen will use them prior to starting a sporting activity in an attempt to avoid any muscle damage. Examples of active ingredients found in liniments are turpentine oil and methyl salicylate.

## Lotions

These are liquids for external use and may be solutions, suspensions or emulsions. They have a variety of uses which include antiseptic, parasiticidal and soothing. Care should be taken when recommending lotions for the treatment of head lice. Those which have an alcohol base should be avoided in asthmatics and young children, as the alcoholic fumes may cause breathing difficulties. Aqueous-based products should be advised.

## Lozenges

These are large tablets designed to be sucked and remain in the mouth for up to 15 minutes. They do not contain a disintegrant and the active ingredient is normally incorporated into a sugar base, such as sucrose or glucose. The main use of lozenges is in the treatment of mouth and throat infections.

## Mixtures

This is a generic term which is used for many liquid preparations for oral use.

## Mouthwashes

These are similar to gargles but are used specifically to treat conditions of the mouth. The active ingredients are usually antiseptics or bactericidal agents.

## Nasal drops

These are isotonic solutions used to treat conditions of the nose. Locally acting decongestants are commonly presented as nose drops. The container includes a dropper device to allow the patient to deliver the appropriate dose into the affected nostril(s). Overuse of nose drops is common as patients find it difficult to judge the number of drops being delivered. Some nose drop preparations are presented as sprays which may improve ease of use.

## Ointments

Ointments are semi-solids for topical use. Full details are found in Chapter 14.

## Paints

Paints are solutions for application to the skin or mucous membranes. Those used on the skin are often formulated with a volatile vehicle. This evaporates on application and leaves a film of active ingredient on the skin surface. Paints to be used on the throat and mucous surfaces normally include a viscous vehicle such as glycerol, which enables the preparation to remain in contact with the affected area. Paints are used for their antiseptic, analgesic, caustic or astringent properties and should be supplied with a brush to assist application.

## Pastes

These are semi-solids for external use. They differ from creams and ointments in that they contain a high proportion of fine powder, such as starch. This makes them very stiff and means they do not spread readily over the skin's surface. Corrosive drugs such as dithranol are often formulated as pastes. The paste is applied to the lesions but will not spread onto healthy skin and compromise its integrity.

## Pastilles

Pastilles are for oral use and like lozenges, are designed to be sucked. They contain locally acting antiseptics, astringents or anaesthetics and are used to treat, or give symptomatic relief of, conditions affecting the mouth and throat. They are jelly like in consistency due to their basis of gelatin or acacia.

## Pessaries

Pessaries are solid dosage forms for insertion into the vagina. They are used for both local and systemic action. Full details of pessaries are found in Chapter 15.

## Pills

Pills are oral dosage forms which have been superseded by tablets and capsules. The term is still used, incorrectly, to describe any solid oral dose form.

## Powders (oral)

These occur as both bulk and divided powders. Bulk powders usually contain non-potent active ingredients such as antacids. The dose is measured using a 5 ml spoon.

Individual powders consist of more potent drugs where accuracy of dosage is more important. An individual dose is packaged separately, either in a sheet of paper or in a sachet.

Details of powders for oral use are found in Chapter 16.

## Suppositories

These are solid dosage forms for insertion into the rectum. They are used for both local and systemic actions. Details of suppositories are given in Chapter 15.

## Suspensions

Suspensions are liquid dose forms where the active ingredient is insoluble. Suspensions are available for both oral and external use. Details of suspensions are given in Chapter 12.

## Syrups

These are concentrated aqueous solutions of sugars such as sucrose. The term 'syrup' is frequently, but incorrectly, applied to certain sweetened liquids intended for oral use. The term 'syrup' should nowadays only be used to refer to flavouring vehicles. Sucrose is being replaced by sorbitol as the sweetening agent in many preparations to reduce the risk of dental caries.

## Tablets

This is the term used to describe solid dosage forms generally intended for oral use, although some pessaries may be referred to as vaginal tablets. As well as the standard tablet made by compression, there are many different types of tablet designed for specific uses, e.g. dispersible, enteric coated, modified release or buccal. Details of these and other tablet types are given in Chapter 17.

## Transdermal delivery systems

This term is used to describe the adhesive patches which, when applied to the skin, deliver a controlled dose of drug over a specified time period. They are used for a systemic effect. Additional information on these dosage forms is given in Chapter 18.

## Key Points

- The route can be chosen to give local or systemic effects, fast or slow onset.
- The oral route is the most commonly used route.
- Availability of drug from the oral route may be limited by gastric emptying, stability and other materials present.
- Sublingual absorption gives a short, fast-onset activity.
- Buccal absorption takes place between the gum and lip.
- Buccal administration can be used with unconscious patients.
- Rectal absorption partially avoids first pass metabolism.
- Rectal administration is useful for nil-by-mouth patients and in cases of gastric irritation. However, it is poorly accepted in the UK.
- Vaginal administration can give systemic effects avoiding first pass metabolism.
- Inhalation requires a much lower dose than the oral route, with a rapid onset.
- Administration to the skin may be used for local or systemic effects.
- Injections can give the fastest onset of action but prolonged action is possible with oily intramuscular injections.
- The same drug may usefully be used in different formulations to assist different types of patients.

## FURTHER READING

ABPI Compendium of data sheets and summaries of product characteristics, current edn. Datapharm Publications, London (Updated annually)

Aulton M E (ed) 1988 Pharmaceutics: the science of dosage form design. Churchill Livingstone, Edinburgh

British National Formulary, current edn. British Medical Association and Royal Pharmaceutical Society of Great Britain, London (Updated twice yearly)

Pharmaceutical Codex 1979 11th edn. Pharmaceutical Press, London

Pharmaceutical Codex 1994 12th edn. Pharmaceutical Press, London

Reynolds J E F (ed) 1996 Martindale: the extra pharmacopoeia, 31st edn. Pharmaceutical Press, London (Updated every 3 years – use current edn)

Wade A (ed) 1980 Pharmaceutical handbook, 19th edn. Pharmaceutical Press, London

# 11
# Solutions

*E. J. Kennedy*

After studying this chapter, the reader will know about:

**Definitions of solutions and expressions of solubility**
**Methods of controlling solubility**
**Advantages and disadvantages of using solutions**
**Selection of vehicles**
**Use of preservatives in solutions**
**Principles of dispensing**:
   Solutions for oral use
   Mouthwashes
   Nasal, oral and aural solutions
   Enemas.

## Introduction

Solutions are stable homogeneous mixtures of two or more components. They contain one or more solutes dissolved in one or more solvents. The solvent is often aqueous but can be oily or alcoholic. In medicines, solid-in-liquid systems are the most widely used, having the most applications in practice.

There are many classifications of pharmaceutical solutions, based on their composition or medical use. Solutions may be used as oral dosage forms, mouthwashes, gargles, nasal drops, ear drops and externally, for example as lotions or paints. Solutions may also be used in ophthalmic preparations and injections, which are discussed in Chapters 28 and 25 respectively.

## FORMULATION OF SOLUTIONS

Solutions will comprise the medicinal agent in a solvent as well as any additional agents. These addi-

tional agents are usually included to provide colour, flavour, sweetness or stability to the formulation. Most solutions are now manufactured on a large scale although it may be occasionally required to make up a solution extemporaneously. When compounding a solution, information on solubility and stability of each of the solutes must be taken into account.

Chemical and physical interactions that may take place between constituents must also be taken into account, as these will affect the preparation's stability or potency. For example, esters of *p*-hydroxybenzoic acid, which can be used as preservatives in oral solutions, have a tendency to partition into certain flavouring oils. This could reduce the effective concentration of the preservative agent in the aqueous vehicle of the preparation to a level lower than that required for preservative action.

## Solubility

The solubility of an agent in a particular solvent indicates the maximum concentration to which a solution may be prepared with that agent in that solvent. When a solvent, at a given temperature, has dissolved all of the solute it can, it is said to be saturated. Solubilities for medicinal agents in a given solvent are stated in the *British Pharmacopoeia* (BP) and 'Martindale' (Reynolds 1996) as well as in other reference sources. Solubilities are usually stated as the number of parts (by volume) that will dissolve one part (by weight or volume of a liquid) of the substance. Most solutions for pharmaceutical use are not saturated with solute.

---

**EXAMPLE 11.1**

Potassium chloride is soluble in 2.8 to 3 parts of water.

---

This means that 1 g of potassium chloride will dissolve in 2.8 to 3 ml of water at a temperature of 20°C (taken as normal room temperature).

---

**EXAMPLE 11.2**

Diazepam is described as being very slightly soluble in water (1 in 1000 to 1 in 10 000), soluble in alcohol (1 in 10 to 1 in 30) and freely soluble in chloroform (1 in 1 to 1 in 10).

This means that 1 g of diazepam will dissolve in between 10 and 30 ml of alcohol, but would need 1000–10 000 ml of water to dissolve, at a temperature of 20°C.

---

### Factors affecting solubility

Compounds that are predominantly non-polar tend to be more soluble in non-polar solvents, such as chloroform. Polar compounds tend to be more soluble in polar solvents, such as water and ethanol. The pH will also affect solubility, as many drugs are weak acids or bases. The ionized form of a compound will be the most water soluble, therefore a weakly basic drug will be most soluble in an aqueous solution that is acidic. Acid or alkali may therefore be added to form salts and improve solubility. Most compounds are more soluble at higher temperatures. Particle size reduction will increase the rate of solution.

## Increasing the solution of compounds with low solubility

### Cosolvency

The addition of cosolvents, such as ethanol, glycerol, propylene glycol or sorbitol can increase the solubility of weak electrolytes and non-polar molecules in water. They work by decreasing the interfacial tension between the hydrophobic solute and the aqueous environment.

### Solubilization

Surfactants may be used as solubilizing agents. At the critical micelle concentration (CMC) dispersed surfactant molecules in a liquid aggregate to form micelles of colloidal dimensions. In aqueous solution, the hydrophobic areas of the solubilizing agent will point towards the centre of the micelle with the hydrophilic areas orientating themselves towards the solvent. The reverse is true for a non-polar solvent.

Micelles are used to help dissolve poorly soluble compounds. The dissolved compound may be in the centre of the micelle, adsorbed onto the micelle surface or sit at some intermediate point depending on the polarity of the compound. Examples of surfactants used in oral solutions are polysorbates, and soaps are used to solubilize phenolic disinfectants.

## Expression of concentration

Strengths of pharmaceutical solutions can be expressed in a number of ways. The two most commonly used are in terms of percentage strengths or amount of drug contained in 5 ml of vehicle. For example a 100 mg/5 ml solution contains 100 mg of drug in each 5 ml dose. A percent weight in volume (% w/v) describes the number of grams of a constituent in 100 ml of preparation. For example, a 2% w/v preparation contains 2 g of a constituent in 100 ml of preparation. A percent volume in volume (% v/v) describes the number of millilitres of a constituent in 100 ml of preparation. For example, a 1% v/v preparation contains 1 ml of a constituent in 100 ml of preparation.

## Vehicles

In pharmacy the medium which contains the ingredients of a medicine is called the vehicle. This may be a solvent. The choice of a vehicle depends on the intended use of the preparation and on the nature and physicochemical properties of the active ingredients.

### Water as a vehicle

Water is the vehicle used for most pharmaceutical preparations. It is widely available, relatively inexpensive, palatable and non-toxic for oral use and non-irritant for external use. There are different types of water available.

*Potable water.* Potable water is drinking water, usually drawn freshly from a mains supply. It should be palatable and safe for drinking. Its chemical composition may include mineral impurities which could react with medicaments, for example, calcium carbonate in hard water.

*Purified water.* This is prepared from suitable potable water by distillation, by treatment with ion-exchange materials or by any other suitable treatment method. Distilled water is purified water that has been prepared by distillation.

*Water for preparations.* This is potable or freshly boiled and cooled purified water, used in oral liquid or external preparations which are not intended to be sterile. Any stored water, for example drawn from a local storage tank, should not be used because of the risk of contamination with microorganisms. Boiling removes dissolved oxygen and carbon dioxide from solution in the water.

*Water for injections.* This is pyrogen-free distilled water, sterilized immediately after collection and used for parenteral products (for further details see Ch. 25).

*Aromatic waters.* Aromatic waters are saturated aqueous solutions of volatile oils or other aromatic or volatile substances, and are often used as a vehicle in oral solutions. Some have a mild carminative action, for example dill. Aromatic waters are usually prepared from a concentrated ethanolic solution, in a dilution of 1 part to 39 parts with water. Chloroform water is used as an antimicrobial preservative and also adds a sweetness to preparations.

### Other vehicles used in pharmaceutical solutions

*Syrup* is a solution of sucrose in water. It will promote dental decay and is unsuitable for diabetic patients.

*Alcohol (ethyl alcohol, ethanol).* This is rarely used for internal preparations but is a useful solvent for external preparations.

*Glycerol (Glycerin)* may be used as a vehicle in some external preparations. It is miscible both with water and alcohol. It is used as a stabilizer and sweetener in internal preparations. In concentrations above 20% v/v it acts as a preservative.

*Propylene glycol* is a less viscous liquid and a better solvent than glycerol.

*Oils.* Bland oils such as fractionated coconut oil and arachis oil may be used for fat-soluble compounds, for example Calciferol Oral Solution BP.

*Acetone* is used as a cosolvent in external preparations.

*Solvent ether* can be used as a cosolvent in external preparations for preoperative skin preparation. The extreme volatility of ether and risk of fire and explosion limit its usefulness.

### Preservation of solutions

Most pharmaceutical solutions will support microbial growth, particularly aqueous solutions. Raw materials may introduce microbial contamination; therefore care is needed when selecting these.

Preservatives may be added to the formulation. Chloroform is the most widely used in oral prepara-

tions although there are disadvantages to its use, including its high volatility and reported carcinogenicity in animals. Use in the UK is limited to a chloroform content of 0.5% (w/w or w/v). For oral solutions, chloroform at a strength of 0.25% v/v will usually be incorporated as Chloroform Water BP. Double strength chloroform water is usually included in pharmaceutical formulae as half the total volume of the solution, to effectively give single strength chloroform water as the vehicle. Benzoic acid at a strength of 0.1% w/v is also suitable for oral administration, as are ethanol, sorbic acid, the hydroxybenzoate esters and syrup. Few of these are active in alkaline pH.

Syrups can be preserved by the maintenance of a high concentration of sucrose as part of the formulation. High sucrose concentrations, greater than 65% w/w, will usually protect an oral liquid from growth of most microorganisms owing to osmotic effects. A problem in formulation occurs when other ingredients are added to syrups, as this would lead to a decrease in the sucrose concentration. Consequently, this may cause a loss in the preservative action of the sucrose.

Preservatives used in external solutions include chlorocresol (0.1% w/v), chlorbutol (0.5% w/v) and the parahydroxybenzoates (parabens).

## SHELF LIFE OF SOLUTIONS

There may be individual variations, but most solutions which are prepared extemporaneously should be freshly or recently prepared. The data sheets should be consulted for information about particular manufactured solutions and for storage conditions.

## SOLUTIONS FOR ORAL DOSAGE

Oral solutions are usually formulated so that the patient receives the usual dose of the medicament in a conveniently administered volume, usually a multiple of 5 ml, given to the patient using a 5 ml medicine spoon. A teaspoon should not be used as an expression of a dose for an oral liquid as this is not an accurate measure.

Advantages of solutions for oral use over a solid dosage form are that the medicament is readily absorbed into the gastrointestinal tract and liquids are much easier to swallow than tablets or capsules. This is especially so for children, elderly patients or those with chronic conditions such as Parkinson's disease, who may have difficulty swallowing a solid oral dosage form. An advantage of solutions over suspensions is that the medicament is dispersed homogeneously throughout the preparation, without the need to shake the bottle. This makes the preparation easier for the patient to use. Substances with a low aqueous solubility may be made into solution by the addition of another solvent to give complete dissolution rather than formulate the medicament as a suspension.

Disadvantages of solutions are that they are bulky and not as convenient to carry around as a solid dosage form. They are also less microbiologically and chemically stable than their solid counterparts, for example drugs that are susceptible to hydrolysis. Drugs that have an unpleasant taste may not be suitable for administration as an oral solution.

The different forms of oral solutions may be described as:

• *Syrups*, which are aqueous solutions that contain sugar. An example is Epilim syrup (sodium valproate).

• *Elixirs*, which are clear, flavoured liquids containing a high proportion of sucrose or a suitable polyhydric alcohol and sometimes ethanol. An example is phenobarbitone elixir.

• *Linctuses*, which are viscous liquids used in the treatment of cough. They should be sipped and swallowed slowly and usually contain a high proportion of sucrose, other sugars or a suitable polyhydric alcohol or alcohols. Examples are Simple Linctus BP and pholcodine linctus.

• *Mixtures* is a term often used to describe pharmaceutical oral solutions and suspensions. Examples are chloral hydrate mixture and ammonium chloride and morphine mixture.

• *Oral drops* are oral solutions or suspensions which are administered in small volumes, using a suitable measuring device. A proprietary example is Abidec vitamin drops.

## Additional ingredients

Solutions that are intended for oral use may contain excipients such as flavouring agents, sweetening agents and sometimes colouring agents. These are added to improve the palatability and appearance of a solution for the patient. The solubility of sparingly soluble drugs can be enhanced by the addition of cosolvents such as ethanol, glycerol or propylene glycol. These are all suitable for oral use, although the amount of ethanol in oral medicines is kept to a minimum because of pharmacological effect, cost and burning taste in high concentration. Stabilizing agents may also be used.

### Flavouring agents

Flavours added to solutions can make a medicine more acceptable to take, especially if the drug has an unpleasant taste. Certain flavours should be chosen to disguise certain tastes, for example a fruit flavour helps to disguise an acid taste. The age of the patient should be taken into account when selecting a flavour, as children will tend to enjoy fruit or sweet flavours. Some flavours are associated with particular uses, for example peppermint is associated with antacid preparations. Flavours may be incorporated using juices (raspberry), extracts (liquorice), spirits (lemon and orange), syrups (blackcurrant), tinctures (ginger) and aromatic waters (anise and cinnamon). Some synthetic flavours are used commercially.

### Sweetening agents

Many oral solutions are sweetened with different sugars, including glucose and sucrose. Sucrose enhances the viscosity of liquids and also gives a pleasant texture in the mouth. Prolonged use of liquid medicines containing sugar will lead to an increased incidence of dental caries, particularly in children. Attempts should be made to formulate oral solutions without sugar as a sweetening agent, using sorbitol, mannitol, xylitol, saccharin and aspartame as alternatives. Oral liquid preparations that do not contain fructose, glucose or sucrose are labelled 'sugar free' in the *British National Formulary* (BNF). These alternatives should be used where possible.

### Colouring agents

Colouring agents are added to pharmaceutical preparations to enhance the appearance of a preparation or to increase the acceptability of a preparation to the patient. Colours are often matched to the flavour of a preparation, for example a yellow colour for a banana-flavoured preparation. Colour is also useful to give a consistent appearance where there is natural batch variation between materials.

Colours can give distinctive appearances to some medicines, for example the green colour of the Drug Tariff formula of methadone mixture. Colouring agents should be non-toxic and free of any therapeutic activity themselves.

Natural colourants include materials derived from

plants and animals, for example carotenoids, chlorophylls, saffron, red beetroot extract, caramel and cochineal. As with all natural agents, the disadvantage is that batches may vary in quality. Mineral pigments such as iron oxides are not often used in solutions because of their low solubility in water. Synthetic organic dyes such as the azo compounds are alternatives for colouring pharmaceutical solutions as they give a wide range of bright, stable colours. Colours appear in pharmaceutical formulae less often now, especially in children's medicines. Their use is seen as unnecessary by some consumers and some colouring agents were recently implicated in hyperactivity of children and rare allergic reactions, for example tartrazine. Additionally, coloured dyes in medicines can lead to confusion when diagnosing diseases, for example a red dye appearing in vomit could be wrongly assumed to be blood. In the European Union, colours are selected from a list permitted for medicinal products, with designated E numbers between 100 and 180.

### Stabilizers

Antioxidants may be used where ingredients are liable to degradation by oxidation, for example in oils. Those which are added to oral preparations include ascorbic acid, citric acid, sodium metabisulphite and sodium sulphite. These are odourless, tasteless and non-toxic.

### Viscosity-enhancing agents

Syrups may be added to increase the viscosity of an oral liquid. They also improve palatability and ease pourability. Other thickening agents may also be used (see Ch. 12).

## Oral syringes

If fractional doses are prescribed for oral liquids, they should not be diluted, but an oral syringe should be given with the dispensed oral liquid. An oral syringe is marked in 0.5 ml divisions from 1 to 5 ml to measure doses of less than 5 ml. An adapter to fit the neck of the medicine bottle and full instructions should be supplied with the oral syringe. An example of a patient information leaflet that accompanies an oral syringe is given in Figure 11.1. Pharmacists should ensure that parents understand how to use and care for the oral syringe, for example to clean the syringe after use and allow it to dry out fully.

## Diluents

If a prescriber insists that a manufactured solution is diluted, then a suitable diluent must be selected. Information sources to obtain this information are the ABPI *Data Sheet Compendium* or the National Pharmaceutical Association (NPA) *Diluent Directory*. An indication of the expiry date for the diluted preparation is also given in these references. The dilution should be freshly prepared.

A short shelf life for a diluted solution may require patients to return to the pharmacy to collect the balance of their medication. This may happen, for instance, where an oral sodium chloride solution has been prescribed for 1 month. The solution has a 2-week expiry, and must therefore be supplied in two instalments. The patient, or the patient's representative, should be issued with an owing slip, or some similar documentation. This should state the name of the patient, the pharmacy, the item and quantity of medicine owed and the date of issue. A record should also be kept in the pharmacy.

## Containers for dispensed solutions for oral use

Plain, amber medicine bottles should be used, with a reclosable child-resistant closure. Exceptions to this are if the medicine is in an original pack or patient pack or if there are no suitable child-resistant containers for a particular liquid preparation. Advice to store away from children should then be given. A 5 ml measuring spoon or an appropriate oral syringe should be supplied to the patient.

## Special labels and advice for dispensed oral solutions

An expiry date should appear on the label for extemporaneously prepared solutions. Most 'official' mixtures and some oral solutions are freshly or recently prepared. 'Official' elixirs and linctuses and manufactured products are generally more stable, unless diluted. Diluted products generally have a shorter shelf life than the undiluted preparation. Linctuses should be sipped and swallowed slowly, without the addition of water.

## SOLUTIONS FOR OTHER PHARMACEUTICAL USES

Topical solutions for external use are considered in

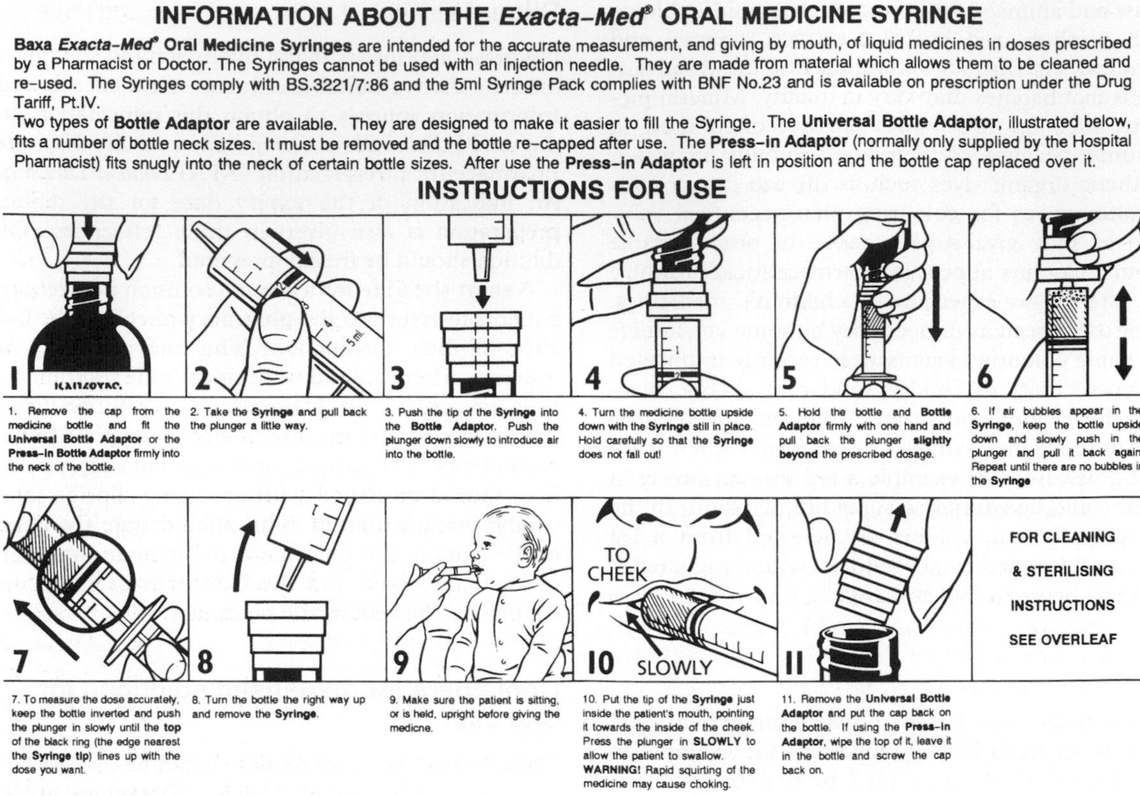

## INFORMATION ABOUT THE *Exacta-Med®* ORAL MEDICINE SYRINGE

Baxa *Exacta-Med®* **Oral Medicine Syringes** are intended for the accurate measurement, and giving by mouth, of liquid medicines in doses prescribed by a Pharmacist or Doctor. The Syringes cannot be used with an injection needle. They are made from material which allows them to be cleaned and re-used. The Syringes comply with BS.3221/7:86 and the 5ml Syringe Pack complies with BNF No.23 and is available on prescription under the Drug Tariff, Pt.IV.

Two types of **Bottle Adaptor** are available. They are designed to make it easier to fill the Syringe. The **Universal Bottle Adaptor**, illustrated below, fits a number of bottle neck sizes. It must be removed and the bottle re-capped after use. The **Press-in Adaptor** (normally only supplied by the Hospital Pharmacist) fits snugly into the neck of certain bottle sizes. After use the **Press-in Adaptor** is left in position and the bottle cap replaced over it.

### INSTRUCTIONS FOR USE

1. Remove the cap from the medicine bottle and fit the **Universal Bottle Adaptor** or the **Press-in Bottle Adaptor** firmly into the neck of the bottle.

2. Take the **Syringe** and pull back the plunger a little way.

3. Push the tip of the **Syringe** into the **Bottle Adaptor**. Push the plunger down slowly to introduce air into the bottle.

4. Turn the medicine bottle upside down with the **Syringe** still in place. Hold carefully so that the **Syringe** does not fall out!

5. Hold the bottle and **Bottle Adaptor** firmly with one hand and pull back the plunger **slightly beyond** the prescribed dosage.

6. If air bubbles appear in the **Syringe**, keep the bottle upside down and slowly push in the plunger and pull it back again. Repeat until there are no bubbles in the **Syringe**.

7. To measure the dose accurately, keep the bottle inverted and push the plunger in slowly until the **top** of the black ring (the edge nearest the **Syringe** tip) lines up with the dose you want.

8. Turn the bottle the right way up and remove the **Syringe**.

9. Make sure the patient is sitting, or is held, upright before giving the medicine.

10. Put the tip of the **Syringe** just inside the patient's mouth, pointing it towards the inside of the cheek. Press the plunger in **SLOWLY** to allow the patient to swallow. **WARNING!** Rapid squirting of the medicine may cause choking.

11. Remove the **Universal Bottle Adaptor** and put the cap back on the bottle. If using the **Press-in Adaptor**, wipe the top of it, leave it in the bottle and screw the cap back on.

FOR CLEANING & STERILISING INSTRUCTIONS SEE OVERLEAF

**Fig. 11.1** Patient information leaflet with instructions for the use of an oral syringe (reproduced by permission of Baxa Corporation).

Chapter 14. Some topical solutions are designed for instillation into body cavities, such as the nose, mouth and ear.

## Mouthwashes and gargles

Gargles are used to relieve or treat sore throats and mouthwashes are used on the mucous membranes of the oral cavity, rather than the throat, to refresh and mechanically clean the mouth. Both are concentrated solutions but gargles tend to contain higher concentrations of active ingredients than are present in mouthwashes. Both are usually diluted with warm water before use. They may contain antiseptics, analgesics or weak astringents. The liquid is usually not intended for swallowing. Examples are Phenol Gargle BPC and Compound Sodium Chloride Mouthwash BP. Proprietary examples are chlorhexidine (Corsodyl) mouthwash and povidone-iodine (Betadine) mouthwash.

### Containers for mouthwashes and gargles

An amber, ribbed bottle should be used for extemporaneously prepared solutions. Medicine bottles may be used for products which are intended to be swallowed. Manufactured mouthwashes and gargles are usually packed in plain bottles.

### Special labels and advice for mouthwashes and gargles

Directions for diluting the preparations should be given to the patient. If the preparation is not intended for swallowing, the following label is appropriate: 'Not to be swallowed in large amounts'.

### Nasal solutions

Most nasal preparations are solutions, administered as nose drops or sprays. They are isotonic to nasal secretions (equivalent to 0.9% normal saline) and buffered to the normal pH range of nasal fluids (pH 5.5–6.5) to prevent damage to ciliary transport in the nose. The most frequent use of nose drops is as a decongestant for the common cold or to administer local steroids for the treatment of allergic rhinitis. Examples are normal saline nose drops and ephedrine nose drops, 0.5% or 1%. Overuse of topical decongestants can lead to oedema of the nasal mucosa and they should only be used for short periods of time (about 5 days) to avoid rebound congestion, called rhinitis medicamentosa. The nasal route may also be useful for new biologically active peptides and polypeptides which need to avoid the first pass metabolism and destruction by the gastrointestinal fluids. The nasal mucosa rapidly absorbs medicaments applied there to give a systemic effect. There are some products utilizing nasal delivery currently available on the market, for example desmopressin (Desmospray, DDAVP) used in the treatment of pituitary diabetes insipidus.

## Ear drops

Ear drops are solutions of one or more active ingredients which exert a local effect in the ear, for example by softening ear wax or treating infection or inflammation. They may also be referred to as otic or aural preparations. Propylene glycol, glycerol and water may be used as vehicles. Examples are aluminium acetate ear drops, almond oil ear drops and Sodium Bicarbonate Ear Drops BP.

### Containers for nasal and aural preparations

Nose and ear drops that are prepared extemporaneously should be packed in an amber, ribbed hexagonal glass bottle which is fitted with a rubber teat and dropper. Manufactured nasal solutions may be packed in flexible plastic bottles which deliver a fine spray to the nose when squeezed, or in a plain glass bottle with a pump spray or dropper. Manufactured ear drops are usually packed in small glass or plastic containers with a dropper.

### Special labels and advice for nasal and aural preparations

Patients should be advised not to share nasal sprays or nose and ear drops in order to minimize contamination and infection. Manufactured nasal sprays and nose and ear drops will usually contain instructions for administration. Patients should be given advice on how to administer extemporaneously prepared nose and ear drops, accompanied by written information if possible (see Fig. 11.2). For nose drops it may be easier if the patient is lying flat with the head tilted back as far as comfortable, preferably over the edge of a bed. The patient should remain in this position for a few minutes after the drops have been administered to allow the medication to spread in the nose.

For ear drops, it may be easier for someone other than the patient to administer the drops. The drops can be warmed by holding the bottle in the hands before putting them in. The ear lobe should be held up and back in adults, down and back in children, to allow the medication to run in deeper. They may cause some transient stinging. If the drops are intended to soften ear wax, then the ears should be syringed after use.

Extemporaneous preparations should be labelled with the appropriate expiry date following the official monographs. 'For external use' would not be an appropriate label and 'Not to be taken' is advisable.

## Enemas

Enemas are oily or aqueous solutions that are administered rectally. They are usually anti-inflammatory, purgative or sedative or given to allow X-ray exami

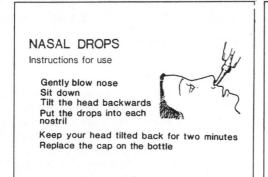

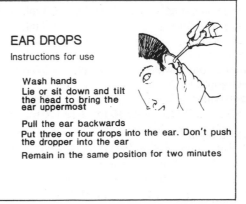

**Fig. 11.2**  Patient instruction leaflets for use of nose and ear drops.

nation of the lower bowel. Examples are arachis oil enema and magnesium sulphate enemas. Retention enemas are administered to give either a local action of the drug, for example prednisolone, or for systemic absorption, for example diazepam. They are used after defecation. The patient lies on one side during administration and remains there for 30 minutes to allow distribution of the medicament. Microenemas are single dose, small volume solutions. Examples are solutions of sodium phosphate, sodium citrate or docusate sodium. They are packaged in plastic containers with a nozzle for insertion into the rectum. Large volume (0.5–1 litre) enemas should be warmed to body temperature before administration.

## Containers for enemas

If extemporaneously produced, enemas are packed in amber, fluted glass bottles. Manufactured enemas will usually be packed in disposable polythene or polyvinyl chloride bags sealed to a rectal nozzle.

## Special labels and advice for enemas

Patients should be advised on how to use the enema if they are self-administering and the time that the product will take to work. The label 'For rectal use only' should be used.

---

### EXAMPLE 11.3

℞ Ammonium and Ipecacuanha Mixture BP. Mitte 100 ml.

|  | Master formula | For 100 ml |
|---|---|---|
| Ammonium bicarbonate | 200 mg | 2 g |
| Liquorice liquid extract | 0.5 ml | 5 ml |
| Ipecacuanha tincture | 0.3 ml | 3 ml |
| Concentrated camphor water | 0.1 ml | 1 ml |
| Concentrated anise water | 0.05 ml | 0.5 ml |
| Double strength chloroform water | 5 ml | 50 ml |
| Water | to 10 ml | to 100 ml |

#### Action and uses
Expectorant cough preparation. The benefit of expectorant mixtures is doubtful, but they may be a useful placebo and they are inexpensive.

#### Formulation notes
Ammonium bicarbonate, ipecacuanha and

camphor water are mild expectorants. Anise water acts as a mild expectorant and a flavouring agent. Liquid liquorice extract is used as a mild expectorant, flavouring and sweetening agent. Chloroform water acts as a sweetener and a preservative. Ammonium bicarbonate is soluble 1 in 5 of water.

#### Method of preparation
The ammonium bicarbonate should be weighed on a Class B balance and dissolved in approximately 15 ml water, in a 100 ml conical measure. The double strength chloroform water should be added to this solution. The other liquid ingredients should be measured and added to the solution. The mixture should then be made up to volume in the conical measure. It should be packed into an amber medicine bottle with a child-resistant closure. The bottle should be polished and labelled, and a 5 ml spoon should be given with the medicine.

#### Shelf life and storage
Store in a cool, dry place. It is recently prepared, therefore a shelf life of 2–4 weeks is applicable.

#### Advice and labelling
Shake well before use.

---

### EXAMPLE 11.4

℞ 200 ml of Diamorphine linctus.

|  | Master formula | For 200 ml |
|---|---|---|
| Diamorphine hydrochloride | 3 mg | 120 mg |
| Oxymel | 1.25 ml | 50 ml |
| Glycerol | 1.25 ml | 50 ml |
| Compound tartrazine solution | 0.06 ml | 2.4 ml |
| Syrup | to 5 ml | to 200 ml |

#### Action and uses
A cough suppressant in terminal care.

#### Formulation notes
Oxymel is a solution of acetic acid, water and purified honey, used as a demulcent and sweetening agent in linctuses. Glycerol is also a demulcent and sweetener. Compound tartrazine solution is a colouring agent and syrup is a demulcent vehicle. Diamorphine is soluble 1 in 1.6 of water and 1 in 12 of alcohol.

#### Method of preparation
Weigh 120 mg diamorphine on a Class B balance.

Transfer to a 200 ml measuring cylinder. Dissolve the diamorphine in the oxymel and glycerol. Add about 50 ml of syrup, then add the compound tartrazine solution. Transfer to a previously tared amber medicine bottle. Make up to volume with the syrup in the tared bottle in order to overcome difficulties in draining all the viscous mixture from a measure. Close with a child-resistant closure, polish and label the bottle and give a 5 ml medicine spoon or oral syringe with the medicine (depending on the dosage prescribed).

### Shelf life and storage
Store in a cool, dry place. It is recently prepared, therefore a shelf life of 2–4 weeks is applicable.

### Advice and labelling
Shake well before use. The linctus should be sipped and swallowed slowly, undiluted. The medicine may cause drowsiness. This patient is unlikely to be driving or operating machinery (terminally ill). Alcohol should be avoided as this will increase the sedative effect (BNF Label 2).

---

### EXAMPLE 11.5

℞ 50 ml Chloral elixir, paediatric. For an 8-month-old baby.

|  | Master formula | For 50 ml |
|---|---|---|
| Chloral hydrate | 200 mg | 2 g |
| Water | 0.1 ml | 1 ml |
| Blackcurrant syrup | 1 ml | 10 ml |
| Syrup | to 5 ml | to 50 ml |

### Action and uses
For short-term use in insomnia.

### Formulation notes
Chloral hydrate is soluble 1 in 0.3 of water and has an unpleasant taste. Blackcurrant syrup is used as a flavouring agent to mask this.

### Method of preparation
Weigh 2 g chloral hydrate on a Class B balance. Transfer to a 50 ml measuring cylinder and dissolve in water. Add the blackcurrant syrup. Add some of the syrup (rinsing the measure used for the blackcurrant syrup). Transfer the mixture to a tared, 50 ml amber medicine bottle and make up to volume, to avoid loss of the viscous product in the measures. Polish and label the bottle and give a 5 ml medicine spoon with the medicine.

### Shelf life and storage
Store in a cool, dry place. Chloral hydrate is volatile and sensitive to light. It is recently prepared and a shelf life of 2 weeks is appropriate.

### Advice and labelling
Shake well before use. An appropriate dose for a child up to 1 year is one 5 ml spoonful to be given, well diluted with water, at bedtime. The parent should be advised that this may make the child drowsy (BNF Labels 1 and 27).

---

### EXAMPLE 11.6

℞ 200 ml Potassium Citrate Mixture BP.

|  | Master formula | For 200 ml |
|---|---|---|
| Potassium citrate | 3 g | 60 g |
| Citric acid monohydrate | 500 mg | 10 g |
| Syrup | 2.5 ml | 50 ml |
| Quillaia tincture | 0.1 ml | 2 ml |
| Lemon spirit | 0.05 ml | 1 ml |
| Double strength chloroform water | 3 ml | 60 ml |
| Water | to 10 ml | to 200 ml |

### Action and uses
Alkalinization of urine to relieve discomfort in mild urinary tract infections or cystitis.

### Formulation notes
Citric acid and potassium citrate are the active ingredients, both are soluble 1 in 1 of water. Lemon spirit is a flavouring agent and consists of lemon oil in alcoholic solution. The oil tends to be displaced from solution in an aqueous medium, especially in the presence of a high concentration of salts. The quillaia tincture is a surfactant used to emulsify any displaced lemon oil. Syrup is a sweetening agent.

### Method of preparation
The solids should be size reduced, weighed and dissolved in the double strength chloroform water and syrup. The quillaia tincture should be added before the lemon spirit is added with stirring, so that emulsification of the oil will be achieved. Make up to volume with water. Pack in an amber medicine bottle with a child-resistant closure. Polish and label the bottle and give a 5 ml medicine spoon with the medicine.

### Shelf life and storage
Store in a cool, dry place. It is recently prepared, therefore a shelf life of 2–4 weeks is applicable.

**Advice and labelling**

Shake well before use. The medicine should be well diluted with water (BNF Label 27).

---

## EXAMPLE 11.7

℞ Compound Sodium Chloride Mouthwash BP. Mitte 500 ml.

|  | Master formula | For 200 ml |
|---|---|---|
| Sodium chloride | 1.5 g | 7.5 g |
| Sodium bicarbonate | 1 g | 5 g |
| Concentrated peppermint emulsion | 2.5 ml | 12.5 ml |
| Double strength chloroform water | 50 ml | 250 ml |
| Water | to 100 ml | to 500 ml |

**Action and uses**

Mechanically cleans and freshens the mouth.

**Formulation notes**

Concentrated peppermint emulsion is used as a flavouring and the chloroform water is a sweetener and preservative. Sodium chloride is soluble 1 in 3 of water and sodium bicarbonate is soluble 1 in 11–12 of water.

**Method of preparation**

The solids are weighed on a Class B balance and dissolved in a 500 ml conical measure in approximately 100 ml of water. Add the double strength chloroform water and the concentrated peppermint emulsion. Make up to volume with water. Pack in an amber fluted bottle with a child-resistant closure. Polish and label the bottle.

**Shelf life and storage**

Store in a cool, dry place. It is recently prepared, therefore a shelf life of 2–4 weeks is applicable.

**Advice and labelling**

Shake well before use. The patient should be directed to use about 15 ml diluted in an equal volume of warm water, usually morning and night, unless otherwise directed. The solution should be used as a mouthwash and should not be swallowed, although reassure the patient that it is not harmful to swallow small amounts of the mouthwash.

---

## EXAMPLE 11.8

℞ 10 ml Sodium Bicarbonate Ear Drops BP.

|  | Master formula | For 10 ml |
|---|---|---|
| Sodium bicarbonate | 5 g | 500 g |
| Glycerol | 30 ml | 3 ml |
| Water | to 100 ml | to 10 ml |

**Action and uses**

For the softening and removal of ear wax (usually prior to syringing with warm water).

**Formulation notes**

Sodium bicarbonate is soluble 1 in 11–12 of water. Glycerol is a viscous liquid, which may present problems in measuring accurately.

**Method of preparation**

Weigh 500 mg sodium bicarbonate and dissolve in 6 ml of water, using a 10 ml conical measure. Carefully make up to 7 ml using water. Carefully add glycerol up to the 10 ml mark (this will result in 3 ml of glycerol being added to the solution). Pack in a 10 ml hexagonal, amber, ribbed bottle with a dropper. Polish and label the bottle on the three smooth sides.

**Shelf life and storage**

Store in a cool, dry place. The drops are recently prepared, therefore a shelf life of 2–4 weeks is applicable.

**Advice and labelling**

Shake well before use and Not to be taken. The bottle may be warmed in the hands before placing drops in the ears. A patient information leaflet should be used to describe how to use the drops (see Fig. 11.2).

---

## Key Points

- Pharmaceutical solutions are given different names depending on their nature and use.
- Saturation solubility of a drug in a solvent is affected by polarity of both drug and solvent.
- Saturation solubility can be increased by techniques such as cosolvency and solubilization.
- Many different vehicles may be used in pharmaceutical solutions.
- Water is available in different forms for different uses.

- Antimicrobial preservation is required for most aqueous solutions.
- There are both advantages and disadvantages in the use of oral solutions.
- Various additives such as flavours, sweeteners and colours may be added to improve the palatability of oral solutions.
- Oral syringes will be required for doses of less than 5 ml.
- Most oral solutions would be freshly or recently prepared.
- Solutions may also be used for mouthwashes, gargles, nasal drops and sprays, ear drops and enemas.

## FURTHER READING

ABPI Compendium of data sheets and summaries of product characteristics, current edn. Datapharm Publications, London (Updated annually)

Ansel H C, Popovich N G, Allen L V 1995 Pharmaceutical dosage forms and drug delivery systems, 6th edn. Williams & Wilkins, Malvern, USA

British National Formulary, current edn. British Medical Association and Royal Pharmaceutical Society of Great Britain, London (Updated twice yearly)

British Pharmacopeia, current edn. HMSO, London

British Pharmaceutical Codex 1973 Pharmaceutical Press, London

Diluent Directories (Internal and External), current edn. National Pharmaceutical Association, St Albans

Pharmaceutical Codex 1979 11th edn. Pharmaceutical Press, London

Pharmaceutical Codex: Principles and practice of pharmaceutics 1994 12th edn. Pharmaceutical Press, London

Reynolds J E F (ed) 1996 Martindale: the extra pharmacopoeia, 31st edn. Pharmaceutical Press, London (Updated every 3 years – use current edn)

Wade A (ed) 1980 Pharmaceutical handbook, 19th edn. Pharmaceutical Press, London

# 12
# Suspensions

*E. J. Kennedy*

---

After studying this chapter, the reader will know about:

**The nature of suspensions**
**The pharmaceutical uses of suspensions**
**The properties of an ideal suspension**
**Matters which need to be considered in formulating a suspension**
**Ingredients which may be added to suspensions**
**The dispensing of suspensions for internal and external use**.

## Introduction

Suspensions contain one or more insoluble medicaments in a vehicle, with other additives such as preservatives, flavours, colours, buffers and stabilizers. Most pharmaceutical suspensions are aqueous, but an oily vehicle is sometimes used. Suspensions may be used for oral administration, inhalation, topical application, as ophthalmic preparations, for parenteral administration and as aerosols.

A definition of a pharmaceutical suspension is a disperse system in which one substance (the disperse phase) is distributed in particulate form throughout another (the continuous phase). A coarse suspension is a dispersion of particles with a mean diameter greater than 1 mm and a colloidal suspension is a dispersion of particles with a mean diameter less than 1 mm. Suspended solids may slowly separate on standing, but may be redispersed.

## PHARMACEUTICAL APPLICATIONS OF SUSPENSIONS

Suspensions may be used pharmaceutically for a number of reasons. Some are given below.

- Drugs that have very low solubility are usefully formulated as suspensions.
- If people have difficulty swallowing solid dosage forms, the drug may need to be dispersed into a liquid form.
- Drugs that have an unpleasant taste in their soluble form can be made into insoluble derivatives, and formulated as a suspension, which will be more palatable. For example chloramphenicol (soluble) → chloramphenicol palmitate (insoluble).
- In oral suspensions the drug is delivered in finely divided form, therefore dissolution occurs immediately in the gastrointestinal (GI) fluids. The rate of absorption of a drug from a suspension is usually faster than when delivered as a solid oral dosage form, but slower than the rate from solution. The rate of availability of drug from a suspension is dependent on the viscosity; the more viscous the product, the slower the release of drug.
- Insoluble forms of drugs may prolong the action of a drug by preventing rapid degradation of the drug in the presence of water.

Oxytetracycline
in aqueous solution

Hydrochloride (soluble, tablet form): hydrolyses rapidly

Calcium salt (insoluble): stable

- When the drug is unstable in contact with the vehicle, suspensions are prepared immediately prior to handing out to the patient in order to reduce the amount of time that the drug particles are in contact with the dispersion medium. For example with ampicillin suspension, water is added to powder or granules prior to giving out to the patient. A 14-day expiry date is given, if kept in the fridge.
- Drugs which degrade in aqueous solution may be suspended in a non-aqueous phase, for example

tetracycline hydrochloride suspended in a fractionated coconut oil for ophthalmic use.

- Bulky, insoluble powders can be formulated as a suspension so that they are easier to take, for example kaolin or chalk (see Example 12.2). Examples of suspensions for oral use are Kaolin Mixture Paediatric BP, kaolin and morphine mixture and antacids such as Magnesium Trisilicate Mixture BP.
- Intramuscular, intra-articular or subcutaneous injections are often formulated as suspensions to prolong the release of the drug.
- Lotions containing insoluble solids are formulated to leave a thin coating of medicament on the skin. As the vehicle evaporates, it gives a cooling effect and leaves the solid behind. Examples are Calamine Lotion BP (see Example 12.5) and Sulphur Lotion Compound BPC.

## PROPERTIES OF A GOOD PHARMACEUTICAL SUSPENSION

In preparing a pharmaceutically elegant product, several desirable properties are sought:

- There is ready redispersion of any sediment produced on storage.
- After gentle shaking, the medicament stays in suspension long enough for a dose to be accurately measured.
- The suspension is pourable.
- Particles in suspension are small and relatively uniform in size, so that the product is free from a gritty texture.

## FORMULATION OF SUSPENSIONS

The three steps that can be taken to ensure formulation of an elegant pharmaceutical suspension are:

1. Control particle size. On a small scale, this can be done using a mortar and pestle, to grind down ingredients to a fine powder.
2. Use a thickening agent to increase viscosity of vehicle, using suspending agents or viscosity-increasing agents.
3. Use a wetting agent.

Some of the theoretical and practical aspects of these will be considered.

The insoluble medicament may be a diffusible solid or an indiffusible solid:

1. *Diffusible solids (dispersible solids)*. These are insoluble solids that are light and easily wetted by water. They mix readily with water, long enough for an adequate dose to be measured. Examples include light kaolin, magnesium trisilicate, light magnesium carbonate, bismuth carbonate.

2. *Indiffusible solids*. Most insoluble solids are not easily wetted, and may form large porous clumps in the liquid. These solids will not remain evenly distributed in the vehicle long enough for an adequate dose to be measured. Examples for internal use include aspirin, chalk, phenobarbitone, sulphadimidine and for external use calamine, hydrocortisone, sulphur, zinc oxide.

## Problems encountered when formulating insoluble solids into a suspension

Various factors need to be considered when formulating insoluble solids into a suspension.

### Sedimentation

The factors affecting the rate of sedimentation of a particle are described in Stokes' equation.

*Stokes' Law:*

$$\upsilon = \frac{2r^2 (\sigma - \rho) \, g}{9\eta}$$

where $\upsilon$ = velocity of a spherical particle of radius $r$, and density $\sigma$, in a liquid of density $\rho$, and viscosity $\eta$, and where $g$ is the acceleration due to gravity.

The basic consequences of this equation are that the velocity of fall of a suspended particle in a vehicle of a given density is greater for larger particles than it is for smaller particles. Also, the greater the density of the particles, the greater the rate of descent. Increasing the viscosity of the dispersion medium within limits, so that the suspension is still pourable, should reduce the rate of sedimentation of a medicament. Thus a decrease in settling rate in a suspension may be achieved by reducing the size of the particles and by increasing the density and the viscosity of the continuous phase.

### Flocculation

The natural tendency towards aggregation of particles will determine the properties of a suspension. In a deflocculated suspension, the dispersed solid particles remain separate and settling is very slow. However, the sediment that eventually forms is hard to redisperse and is described as a 'cake' or clay. In a flocculated suspension, individual small particles aggregate into clumps or floccules. Because these are larger, there is a more rapid rate of sedimentation, but the sediment is loose and easily redispersible. Excess flocculation may prevent 'pourability'.

The ideal is to use either a deflocculated system with a sufficiently high viscosity to prevent sedimentation, or controlled flocculation with a suitable combination of rate of sedimentation, type of sediment and pourability.

### Wetting

Air may be trapped in the solid particles which causes them to float to the surface of the preparation and prevents them from being readily dispersed throughout the vehicle. Wetting of the particles can be encouraged by reducing the interfacial tension between the solid and the liquid, so that adsorbed air is displaced from solid surfaces by liquid. Suitable wetting agents increase the affinity of the particles for the surrounding medium, but decrease interparticular forces.

Hydrophilic colloids such as acacia and tragacanth act as wetting agents. However, care should be taken when using these agents as they can promote deflocculation. Polysorbates and sorbitan esters are surface-active agents used for internal preparations. Solvents such as ethanol, glycerol and the glycols also facilitate wetting. Sodium lauryl sulphate and quillaia tincture are used in external preparations.

## Suspending agents

Suspending agents modify the vehicle viscosity, thereby slowing down sedimentation rates. Most agents can form thixotropic gels which are semisolid on standing, but flow readily after agitation. Care must be taken when selecting a suspending agent for oral preparations, as the acid environment of the stomach may alter the physical characteristics of the suspension, and therefore the rate of release of the drug from suspension. Some suspending agents may also bind to certain medicaments, making them unavailable for their therapeutic use.

Suspending agents can be divided into five broad categories: natural polysaccharides, semi-synthetic polysaccharides, clays, synthetic agents and miscellaneous compounds. Brief information on these classes of suspending agents is given below, with more detailed information available from the

*Pharmaceutical Codex* or the companion volume to this book (Aulton 1988).

### Natural polysaccharides

The main problem with these agents is their natural variability between batches and microbial contamination. Tragacanth is a widely used suspending agent and becomes less viscous at pH 4–7.5. As a rule of thumb, 0.2 g tragacanth powder is added per 100 ml suspension or 2 g compound tragacanth powder per 100 ml suspension. Compound Tragacanth Powder BP 1980 contains tragacanth, acacia, starch and sucrose. Other examples include acacia gum, starch, agar, guar gum, carrageenan, sodium alginate.

### Semi-synthetic polysaccharides

These are derived from the naturally occurring polysaccharide, cellulose. Examples include methylcellulose (Cologel, Celacol), hydroxyethylcellulose (Natrosol 250), sodium carboxymethylcellulose (Carmellose sodium), microcrystalline cellulose (Avicel).

### Clays

These are naturally occurring inorganic materials which are mainly hydrated silicates. Examples include bentonite, aluminium magnesium silicate, magnesium aluminium alginate.

### Synthetic thickeners

These were introduced to overcome the variable quality of natural products. Examples include carbomer (Carboxyvinyl polymer, Carbopol), colloidal silicon dioxide (Aerosil, Cab-o-sil), polyvinyl alcohol.

### Miscellaneous compounds

Gelatin is used as a suspending and viscosity-increasing agent.

## Preservation of suspensions

Water is the most common source of microbial contamination. All pharmaceutical preparations that contain water are therefore susceptible to microbial growth. Also the naturally occurring additives such as acacia and tragacanth may be sources of microbes and spores. Preservative action may be diminished because of adsorption of the preservative onto solid particles of drug, or interaction with suspending agents. Useful preservatives include chloroform water, benzoic acid and hydroxybenzoates.

## THE DISPENSING OF SUSPENSIONS

The method of dispensing of suspensions is the same for most, with some differences for specific ingredients.

1. Crystalline and granular solids are finely powdered in the mortar. The suspending agent should then be added and mixed thoroughly in the mortar. Do not apply too much pressure, otherwise gumming or caking of the suspending agent will occur and heat of friction will make it sticky.

2. Add a little of the liquid vehicle to make a paste and mix well until smooth and free of lumps. Continue with gradual additions until complete.

### Variations

- If syrup and/or glycerol are in the formulation, use this to form the initial paste.
- If wetting agents are included in the formulation, add them at the end of stage one, before forming the paste.
- If soluble solids are being used, dissolve them in the remaining vehicle after making a paste.
- Leave addition of volatile components, colourings or concentrated flavouring tinctures such as chloroform spirit, liquid liquorice extract and compound tartrazine solution until the end.

Most 'official' suspensions will be prepared from the constituent ingredients. There may be some occasions where an oral solid dosage form, such as a tablet or capsule will have to be reformulated by the pharmacist into an oral suspension, for example where the medicine is for a child. It is important to obtain as much information (physical, chemical and microbiological) as possible about the manufactured drug and its excipients. Typically, the tablet will be crushed or capsule contents emptied into the mortar and a suspending agent added. A paste is formed with the vehicle and then diluted to a suitable volume, with the addition of any other suitable ingredients such as preservative or flavourings. A short expiry of no more than 2 weeks (more likely to be 7 days) should be given owing to the lack of knowledge about the stability of the formulation.

## Preparation of suspensions from dry powders and granules for reconstitution

Suspensions may be prepared from previously manufactured dry powders or granules if the liquid preparation has a limited shelf life because of chemical or physical instability. Powders should firstly be loosened from the bottom of the container by lightly tapping against a hard surface. The specified amount of cold, purified water should then be added, sometimes in two or more portions, with shaking, until all the dry powder is suspended. The container is usually over-sized in order to allow adequate shaking for reconstitution. Some suspensions may be prepared by the patient immediately before taking from individually packed sachets of powder or from bulk solids. This is considered in more detail in the chapter on powders (Ch. 16).

## Containers for suspensions

Suspensions should be packed in amber bottles, plain for internal use and ribbed for external use. There should be adequate air space above the liquid to allow shaking and ease of pouring. A 5 ml medicine spoon or oral syringe should be given when the suspension is for oral use.

## Special labels and advice for suspensions

The most important additional label for suspensions is 'Shake well before use', as some sedimentation of medicament would normally be expected. Shaking the bottle will redisperse the medicament and ensure that an accurate or aliquot dose can be measured by the patient.

'Store in a cool place.' Stability of suspensions may be adversely affected by extremes and variations of temperature. Some suspensions, such as those made from reconstituting dry powders, may need to be stored in the refrigerator.

Extemporaneously prepared and reconstituted suspensions will have a relatively short shelf life. They are usually required to be recently or freshly prepared, with a 1–4-week expiry date. Some official formulae state an expiry date, but many do not. The pharmacist may have to make judgements about the expiry date for a particular preparation, based on its constituents and likely storage conditions. The manufacturer's literature for reconstituted products will give recommended storage conditions.

## Inhalations

Suspensions are useful formulations for inhalations. The volatile components are adsorbed on a diffusible solid to ensure uniform dispersion throughout the liquid. When hot water is added the oils vaporize. Where quantities are not stated, 1 g of light magnesium carbonate is used for each 2 ml of oil (such as eucalyptus oil) or 2 g of volatile solid (such as menthol). An example of an inhalation is menthol and eucalyptus inhalation (see Example 12.4).

---

### EXAMPLE 12.1

R. 150 ml Kaolin and Morphine Mixture BP.

|  | Master formula | For 150 ml |
|---|---|---|
| Light kaolin | 2 g | 30 g |
| Sodium bicarbonate | 500 mg | 7.5 g |
| Chloroform and morphine tincture | 0.4 ml | 6 ml |
| Water | to 10 ml | to 150 ml |

#### Action and uses
As an adjunct to fluid replacement in treatment of acute diarrhoea.

#### Formulation notes
Light kaolin is a diffusible solid, therefore no suspending agent is required.

#### Method of preparation
Weigh the light kaolin and place in the mortar. Dissolve the sodium bicarbonate in about 100 ml of water. Gradually add this to the light kaolin in the mortar with mixing to disperse the solid. Add the chloroform and morphine tincture. Wash the mixture into a tared, amber medicine bottle, and make up to volume with water. Seal with a child-resistant closure. Polish and label the bottle and give a 5 ml medicine spoon with the medicine.

#### Shelf life and storage
Store in a cool, dry place. It is recently prepared (unless the kaolin has been sterilized), therefore a shelf life of 2–4 weeks is applicable.

#### Advice and labelling
Shake well before use. The usual dose is 10 ml every 4 hours in water. The importance of rehydration therapy should be stressed to the patient.

---

### EXAMPLE 12.2

R. Chalk Mixture, Paediatric BP. Mitte 100 ml.

|  | Master formula | For 100 ml |
|---|---|---|
| Chalk | 100 mg | 2 g |
| Tragacanth | 10 mg | 200 mg |
| Syrup | 0.5 ml | 10 ml |
| Concentrated cinnamon water | 0.02 ml | 0.4 ml |
| Double strength chloroform water | 2.5 ml | 50 ml |
| Water | to 5 ml | to 100 ml |

#### Action and uses
As an antidiarrhoeal mixture for children, in addition to fluid replacement.

#### Formulation notes
Chalk is an indiffusible solid, practically insoluble in water and requires a suspending agent, tragacanth, in its formulation. The concentrated cinnamon water is a flavouring agent and the syrup increases the viscosity as well as acting as a sweetener. Chloroform water is the preservative.

#### Method of preparation
The chalk and tragacanth should be weighed and lightly mixed in a mortar and pestle. Add the syrup and mix to make a paste. The double strength chloroform water should be gradually added, with mixing, followed by the concentrated cinnamon water. The mixture should be rinsed into a previously tared 100 ml amber medicine bottle and made up to volume with water. Shake the suspension well and seal with a child-resistant closure. Polish and label the bottle and give a 5 ml medicine spoon with the medicine.

#### Shelf life and storage
Store in a cool, dry place. It is freshly prepared, therefore a shelf life of 1–2 weeks is applicable.

#### Advice and labelling
Shake well before use. A dose of 5 ml every 4 hours is normally used. Advise on the importance of fluid replacement, using oral rehydration sachets if necessary.

---

### EXAMPLE 12.3

R. Spironolactone suspension 15 mg/5 ml. Sig. 5 ml t.d.s. Mitte 100 ml. For a 4-year-old child.

| | Master formula | For 100 ml |
|---|---|---|
| Spironolactone | q.s.* | 300 mg |
| Compound orange spirit | 0.2% | 0.2 ml |
| Cologel | 20% | 20 ml |
| Water | to 100% | 100 ml |

*Sufficient

### Action and uses
A potassium-sparing diuretic used in oedema of heart failure and nephrotic syndrome.

### Formulation notes
Spironolactone is practically insoluble in water. Cologel (methylcellulose) acts as the suspending agent. Compound orange spirit is a flavouring agent.

### Method of preparation
Tablets may be used, and sufficient crushed in a mortar and pestle to give 300 mg spironolactone (for example 6 × 50 mg tablets). Alternatively, weigh the powder and transfer to a mortar and pestle. Add the Cologel and mix to a paste. Gradually add some of the water. Add the compound orange spirit. Rinse the suspension into a tared, amber medicine bottle and make up to volume with water. Shake the bottle well and seal with a child-resistant closure. Polish and label the bottle and give a 5 ml medicine spoon with the medicine.

### Shelf life and storage
It is recently prepared with a shelf life of 4 weeks when stored in a refrigerator. Spironolactone should be protected from light.

### Advice and labelling
Shake well before use and give one 5 ml spoonful three times a day.

---

### EXAMPLE 12.4

℞ Menthol and Eucalyptus Inhalation BP 1980. Mitte 100 ml.

| | Master formula |
|---|---|
| Menthol | 2 g |
| Eucalyptus oil | 10 ml |
| Light magnesium carbonate | 7 g |
| Water | to 100 ml |

### Action and uses
For relief of nasal congestion.

### Formulation notes
Light magnesium carbonate is used to adsorb the volatile ingredients which helps to ensure a uniform dispersion. Menthol is freely soluble in fixed and volatile oils.

### Method of preparation
Grind the menthol to a fine powder in a glass mortar and add the eucalyptus oil, which will dissolve the menthol. Gradually add the light magnesium carbonate to the mortar and mix well. Add the water gradually to produce a pourable suspension. Rinse into a tared, amber ribbed bottle and make up to volume. Seal with a child-resistant closure.

### Shelf life and storage
Store in a cool, dry place. It is recently prepared, therefore a shelf life of 2–4 weeks is applicable.

### Advice and labelling
Shake well before use and not to be taken. The patient should be told to add one teaspoonful to 1 pint of hot, not boiling, water. A towel should be placed over the head and the vapour inhaled for 5–10 minutes. Patients should be aware of the potential danger of scalding to themselves and others, particularly small children.

---

### EXAMPLE 12.5

℞ 200 ml Calamine Lotion BP

| | Master formula | For 200 ml |
|---|---|---|
| Calamine | 15 g | 30 g |
| Zinc oxide | 5 g | 10 g |
| Bentonite | 3 g | 6 g |
| Sodium citrate | 500 mg | 1 g |
| Liquefied phenol | 0.5 ml | 1 ml |
| Glycerol | 5 ml | 10 ml |
| Water | to 100 ml | to 200 ml |

### Action and uses
As a cooling lotion for sunburn or skin irritation.

### Formulation notes
Calamine is a coloured zinc carbonate and is practically insoluble in water, as is zinc oxide. Both are indiffusible solids. Sodium citrate is added to control the flocculation of calamine. Bentonite and glycerol are thickening agents and liquefied phenol acts as a preservative and antiseptic.

### Method of preparation
The dry powders should be weighed and mixed in

a mortar so that the bentonite is well distributed. Add the glycerol to the powders and mix. The sodium citrate is dissolved in about 140 ml of water, and gradually added to the mixture in the mortar, so that a smooth paste is produced. Add the liquefied phenol, taking care not to splash as it is caustic. Transfer the mixture to a tared, amber ribbed glass bottle, adding washings from the mortar and make up to volume. Seal with a child-resistant closure.

### Shelf life and storage

Store in a cool, dry place. It is recently prepared, therefore a shelf life of 2–4 weeks is applicable.

### Advice and labelling

For external use only, shake well before use and do not apply to broken skin. The lotion should be applied to the affected areas when required and allowed to dry.

---

### Key Points

- Suspensions can be used to administer an insoluble solid by the oral route.
- Suspensions are used to replace tablets, to improve dissolution rate and to mask some bad tastes.
- Solids may be diffusible or indiffusible.
- Stokes' equation can be applied when formulating a suspension.
- Flocculated particles settle quickly and redisperse easily, whilst deflocculated particles settle slowly but tend to cake.
- Hydrophobic solids may require wetting agents.
- Suspending agents are added to slow down the rate of settling of the solid.
- Suspending agents may be natural polysaccharides, semi-synthetic polysaccharides, clays or synthetic polymers.
- Some suspensions are made by adding water to reconstitute manufactured powders when stability is a problem.
- 'Shake well before use' and 'Store in a cool place' should be part of the labels on a suspension.

---

## FURTHER READING

ABPI Compendium of data sheets and summaries of product characteristics, current edn. Datapharm Publications, London (Updated annually)

Ansel H C, Popovich N G, Allen L V 1995 Pharmaceutical dosage forms and drug delivery systems, 6th edn. Williams & Wilkins, Malvern, USA

Aulton M E 1988 Pharmaceutics: the science of dosage form design. Churchill Livingstone, Edinburgh

British National Formulary, current edn. British Medical Association and Royal Pharmaceutical Society of Great Britain, London (Updated twice yearly)

British Pharmacopeia, current edn. HMSO, London

British Pharmaceutical Codex 1973 Pharmaceutical Press, London

Diluent Directories (Internal and External), current edn. National Pharmaceutical Association, St Albans

Pharmaceutical Codex 1979 11th edn. Pharmaceutical Press, London

Pharmaceutical Codex: Principles and practice of pharmaceutics 1994 12th edn. Pharmaceutical Press, London

Reynolds J E F (ed) 1996 Martindale: the extra pharmacopoeia, 31st edn. Pharmaceutical Press, London (Updated every 3 years – use current edn)

Wade A (ed) 1980 Pharmaceutical handbook, 19th edn. Pharmaceutical Press, London

# 13

# Emulsions

*E. J. Kennedy*

After studying this chapter, the reader will know about:

**The uses of pharmaceutical emulsions**
**The different types of emulsion**
**The methods of identification of the emulsion type**
**Considerations during the formulation of emulsions**
**Selection of emulsifying agents and other ingredients**
**The dispensing processes for emulsions.**

## Introduction

An emulsion consists of two immiscible liquids one of which is uniformly dispersed throughout the other as droplets of diameter greater than 0.1 µm. To prepare a stable emulsion a third phase, an emulsifying agent, is required. Oral emulsions are stabilized oil-in-water dispersions that may contain one or more active ingredients. They are a useful way of presenting oils and fats in a palatable form. Emulsions for external use only are known as lotions, applications or liniments if liquid, or creams if semi-solid in nature. Some parenteral products may also be formulated as emulsions. These are covered in more detail in Chapter 27. Pharmaceutically the term 'emulsion' when no other qualification is used, is taken to mean an oil-in-water preparation for internal use.

## PHARMACEUTICAL APPLICATIONS OF EMULSIONS

Emulsions have a wide range of uses, including:

- Oral, rectal and topical administration of oils and oil-soluble drugs.

- To enhance palatability of oils when given orally by disguising taste and oiliness.
- They can increase absorption of oils and oil-soluble drugs through intestinal walls. An example is griseofulvin suspended in oil in an oil-in-water emulsion.
- Intramuscular injections of some water-soluble vaccines to provide slow release and therefore a greater antibody response and longer-lasting immunity.
- Total parenteral nutrition makes use of an emulsion formulation. Sterile oil-in-water emulsions are used to deliver oily nutrients intravenously to patients, using non-toxic emulsifying agents, such as lecithin (see Ch. 27).

Examples of emulsions for oral use are cod liver oil emulsion, liquid paraffin oral emulsion and castor oil emulsion. Examples of emulsions for external use are Turpentine Liniment BP and Oily Calamine Lotion BP.

## EMULSION TYPES

Emulsions may be oil-in-water emulsions (o/w), where oil is the disperse phase in a continuous phase of water, or water-in-oil emulsions (w/o), where water is the disperse phase in a continuous phase of oil. It is also possible to form a multiple emulsion, for example a water droplet enclosed in an oil droplet, which is itself dispersed in water – a w/o/w emulsion. These may be used for delayed-action drug delivery systems.

If the emulsion is for oral or i.v. administration it will always be oil-in-water. Intramuscular injections may be water-in-oil for a depot therapy. When selecting emulsion type for preparations for external use, the therapeutic use, texture and patient acceptability will be taken into account. Oil-in-water emulsions are less greasy, easily washed off the skin and more cosmetically acceptable than water-in-oil emulsions. They have an occlusive effect, which hydrates upper layers of skin (called an emollient, see Ch. 14). Water-in-oil emulsions rub in more easily.

## Identification of emulsion type

More than one test should be carried out in order to confirm the type of emulsion. Some of the tests that can be used are outlined below.

*Miscibility tests.* An emulsion will mix with a liquid that is miscible with the continuous phase. Therefore an o/w emulsion is miscible with water, a w/o emulsion with an oil.

*Conductivity measurement.* Systems with an aqueous continuous phase will conduct electricity, whilst systems with an oily continuous phase will not.

*Staining tests.* Filter paper soaked in cobalt chloride solution and allowed to dry turns from blue to pink on exposure to stable o/w emulsions.

*Dye tests.* If an oil-soluble dye is used, o/w emulsions are paler in colour than w/o emulsions and vice versa. If examined microscopically, an o/w emulsion will appear as coloured globules on a colourless background whilst a w/o emulsion will appear as colourless globules against a coloured background.

## FORMULATION OF EMULSIONS

An ideal emulsion has globules of disperse phase that retain their initial character, that is the mean size does not change and the globules remain evenly distributed. The formulation of emulsions involves the prevention of coalescence of the disperse phase and reducing creaming.

## Emulsifying agents

Emulsifying agents help the production of a stable dispersion by reducing interfacial tension and then maintaining the separation of the droplets by forming a barrier at the interface. Effective emulsifying agents are surface-active agents. These have hydrophilic polar groups which are orientated towards the water and lipophilic non-polar groups that are orientated towards the oil. Emulsion type is determined by the solubility of the emulsifying agent. If the emulsifying agent is more soluble in water, i.e. hydrophilic, then water will be the contin-

uous phase and an o/w emulsion will be formed. If the emulsifying agent is more soluble in oil, i.e. lipophilic, then oil will be the continuous phase and a w/o emulsion will be formed. If a substance is added which alters the solubility of the emulsifying agent, this balance may be altered and the emulsion may change type. This is called phase inversion. The ideal emulsifying agent is colourless, odourless, tasteless, non-toxic, non-irritant and able to produce stable emulsions at low concentrations.

Emulsifying agents can be classed into three groups: naturally occurring, surfactants and finely divided solids.

### Naturally occurring emulsifying agents

These agents come from animal or vegetable sources. Therefore the quality may vary from batch to batch and they are susceptible to microbial contamination.

*Polysaccharides.* Acacia is the best emulsifying agent for extemporaneously prepared oral emulsions as it forms a thick film at the oil–water interface to act as a barrier to coalescence. It is too sticky for external use. Tragacanth is used to increase the viscosity of an emulsion and prevent creaming. Other polysaccharides, such as starch, pectin and carrageenan, are used to stabilize an emulsion.

*Semi-synthetic polysaccharides.* Low viscosity grades of methylcellulose and carboxymethylcellulose will form o/w emulsions.

*Sterol-containing substances.* These agents act as water-in-oil emulsifying agents. Examples include beeswax, wool fat and wool alcohols.

### Surfactants

These agents contain both hydrophilic and lipophilic regions in the molecule. They are classified according to their ionic characteristics as anionic, cationic, non-ionic and ampholytic. The latter are used in detergents and soaps but are not widely used in pharmacy.

*Anionic surfactants.* These are organic salts which, in water, have a surface-active anion. They are incompatible with some inorganic cations and with large organic cations such as cetrimide. They are widely used in external preparations as o/w emulsifying agents. They must be in their ionized form to be effective and emulsions made with anionic surfactants are generally stable at alkaline pH.

Many different ones are used pharmaceutically. Some examples include:

- alkali metal and ammonium soaps such as sodium stearate (o/w)

- soaps of divalent and trivalent metals such as calcium oleate (w/o)
- amine soaps such as triethanolamine oleate (o/w)
- alkyl sulphates such as sodium lauryl sulphate (o/w).

*Cationic surfactants.* These are usually quaternary ammonium compounds which have a surface-active cation and so are sensitive to anionic surfactants such as the soaps. They are used in the preparation of o/w emulsions for external use and must be in their ionized form to be effective. Emulsions formed by a cationic surfactant are generally stable at acidic pH. The cationic surfactants also have antimicrobial activity. Examples include cetrimide and benzalkonium chloride.

*Non-ionic surfactants.* These are synthetic materials and make up the largest group of surfactants. They are used to produce either o/w or w/o emulsions for both external and internal use. The non-ionic surfactants are compatible with both anionic and cationic substances and are highly resistant to pH change. The type of emulsion formed depends on the balance between hydrophilic and lipophilic groups which is given by the HLB (hydrophilic–lipophilic balance) number (see below). Examples of the main types include glycol and glycerol esters, polysorbates, macrogol ethers and esters, sorbitan esters, higher fatty alcohols, polyvinyl alcohols.

*The HLB (hydrophilic–lipophilic balance) system.* An HLB number, usually between 1 and 20, is allocated to an emulsifying agent and represents the relative proportions of the lipophilic and hydrophilic parts of the molecule. High numbers (8–18) indicate a hydrophilic molecule, and produce an o/w emulsion. Low numbers (3–6) indicate a lipophilic molecule and produce a w/o emulsion. Oils and waxy materials have a 'required HLB number' which helps in the selection of appropriate emulsifying agents when formulating emulsions. Liquid paraffin, for example, has a required HLB value of 5 to obtain a w/o emulsion and 12 for an o/w emulsion. Two or more surfactants can be combined to achieve a suitable HLB value and often give better results than one surfactant alone. (See Aulton (1988) or the *Pharmaceutical Codex* for more details.) HLB values of some commonly used emulsifying agents are given in Table 13.1.

### Finely divided solids

Finely divided solids can be adsorbed at the oil–water interface to form a coherent film that prevents coalescence of the dispersed globules. If the particles

| Table 13.1 HLB values of emulsifying agents | |
|---|---|
| Emulsifying agent | HLB value |
| Acacia | 8.0 |
| Sorbitan monolaurate | 8.6 |
| Sorbitan monostearate | 4.7 |
| Polysorbate 20 | 16.7 |
| Polysorbate 60 | 14.9 |
| Polysorbate 80 | 15.0 |
| Sodium lauryl sulphate | 40.0 |
| Sodium oleate | 18.0 |
| Tragacanth | 13.2 |
| Triethanolamine oleate | 12.0 |

are preferentially wetted by oil, a w/o emulsion is formed. Conversely, if the particles are preferentially wetted by water, an o/w emulsion is formed. They form emulsions with good stability which are less prone to microbial contamination than those formed with other naturally derived agents. Examples are bentonite, aluminium magnesium silicate, hectonite. Colloidal aluminium and magnesium hydroxides are used for internal preparations.

## Choosing an emulsifying agent

The active ingredients that are to be emulsified and the intended use of the product will determine the choice of emulsifying agent. Emulsifying agents for internal preparations should be non-toxic and non-irritant. Thus the non-ionic emulsifying agents and natural polysaccharides will be useful. Quillaia can be used in low concentrations, but soap emulsions irritate the gastrointestinal tract and have a laxative effect. The taste should be bland and palatable, again suggesting the natural polysaccharides. Polysorbates have a disagreeable taste, therefore flavouring ingredients are necessary. Only certain non-ionic emulsifying agents are suitable for parenteral use including lecithin, polysorbate 80, methylcellulose, gelatin and serum albumin. A wider range of emulsifying agents can be used externally, although the polysaccharides are normally considered too sticky.

## Antioxidants

Some oils are liable to degradation by oxidation and therefore antioxidants may be added to the formulation. They should be preferentially soluble in the oily phase. Antioxidants used in oral emulsions which are odourless and tasteless include ascorbic acid, citric acid, sodium metabisulphite and sodium sulphite.

## Antimicrobial preservatives

Emulsions contain water, which will support microbial growth. Microbes produce unpleasant odours, colour changes and gases and may have an effect on the emulsifying agent, possibly causing breakdown of the emulsion. Other ingredients of emulsions can provide a growth medium for microbes. Examples include arachis oil which supports *Aspergillus* species and liquid paraffin which supports *Penicillium* species. Contamination may be introduced from a variety of sources including:

- natural emulsifying agents, for example, starch, acacia gum
- water, if not properly stored
- carelessly cleaned equipment
- poor closures on containers.

Antimicrobial preservative agents should be free from toxic effects, odour, taste and colour. They should be bactericidal rather than bacteriostatic, have a rapid action and wide antibacterial spectrum over a range of temperatures and pH. Additionally their activity should not be affected by emulsion ingredients and they should be resistant to attack by microorganisms. The effect of the partition coefficient in the emulsion is also important. Microbial growth normally occurs in the aqueous phase of an emulsion, therefore it is important that a sufficient concentration of preservative is present in the aqueous phase. A preservative with a low oil/water partition coefficient will have a higher concentration in the aqueous phase. A combination of preservatives may give the best preservative cover for an emulsion system. The ratio of the disperse phase volume to the total volume is known as the phase volume or phase volume ratio. If a preservative is soluble in water and if the proportion of oil is increased, the concentration of preservative in the aqueous phase increases, and vice versa.

Some preservatives in use are listed below:

- Benzoic acid: effective at a concentration of 0.1% at a pH below 5
- Esters of parahydroxybenzoic acid such as methyl paraben (0.01–0.3%)
- Chloroform, as chloroform water (0.25% v/v)
- Chlorocresol (0.05–0.2%)
- Phenoxyethanol (0.5–1.0%)
- Quaternary ammonium compounds, for example cetrimide which can be used as a primary emulsifying agent but at concentrations of 0.002–0.01% can be used as a preservative
- Organic mercurial compounds such as phenyl mercuric nitrate and acetate (0.001–0.002%).

## Colours and flavourings

Colour is rarely needed in an emulsion, as most have an elegant white colour and thick texture. Emulsions for oral use will usually contain some flavouring agent.

## Stability of emulsions

### Phase inversion

This is the process in which an emulsion changes from say o/w to w/o. The most stable range of disperse phase concentration is 30–60%. If the amount of disperse phase approaches or exceeds a theoretical maximum of 74% of the total volume, then phase inversion may occur. Addition of substances which alter the solubility of an emulsifying agent may also cause phase inversion.

### Creaming

The term 'creaming' is used to describe the aggregation of globules of the disperse phase on the top or bottom of the emulsion, similar to cream on milk. It is a reversible process and gentle shaking redistributes the droplets throughout the continuous phase. Creaming is undesirable because it is inelegant in appearance and inaccurate dosing is possible if shaking is not thorough. Additionally, creaming increases the likelihood of coalescence of globules and therefore breakdown of the emulsion due to cracking.

### Cracking

Cracking is the coalescence of dispersed globules and separation of the disperse phase as a separate layer. It is an irreversible process and redispersion cannot be achieved by shaking.

## What causes emulsions to crack or cream?

- Incorporation of excess disperse phase as discussed above.
- Globule size. Stable emulsions require a maximal number of small sized (1–3 μm) globules and as few as possible larger (15–20 μm) diameter globules. A homogenizer will efficiently reduce droplet size and may additionally increase the viscosity if more than 30% of disperse phase is present. Homogenizers force the emulsion through a small aperture to reduce the size of the globules.
- Storage temperature. Extremes of temperature

will sometimes lead to an emulsion cracking. When water freezes, undue pressure is exerted on dispersed globules, which may lead to cracking. Conversely, an increased temperature decreases the viscosity of the continuous phase. An increasing number of collisions between droplets of the disperse phase will occur, leading to creaming and an increased chance of cracking. The integrity of the interfacial film is also reduced.

● Potential for globule coalescence. Increasing the viscosity of the continuous phase will reduce the potential for globule coalescence as this reduces the movement of globules. Emulsion stabilizers which increase the viscosity of the continuous phase may be used in o/w emulsions, for example tragacanth, sodium alginate and methylcellulose.

● Changes which affect the interfacial film formed by the emulsifying agent. These changes may be chemical, physical or biological effects:
– microbiological contamination may destroy the emulsifying agent
– addition of a common solvent
– addition of an emulsifying agent of opposite type, for instance cationic to anionic.

## DISPENSING EMULSIONS

Emulsions can be extemporaneously prepared on a small scale using a mortar and pestle. Electric mixers can also be used, although incorporation of excess air may be a problem. All equipment used must be thoroughly clean and dry. All oil-soluble and water-soluble components of the emulsion are separately dissolved in the appropriate phase. A suitable emulsifying agent must then be chosen.

### Emulsions for oral use

Acacia gum is usually used when making o/w emulsions for oral use, unless otherwise specified. A primary emulsion should be prepared first, which is a thick, stable emulsion.

#### Calculating quantities for primary emulsions

Proportions or 'parts' for preparation of primary emulsions are given in Table 13.2. These refer to parts by volume for the oils and water and weight for the acacia gum (and oleo-resin). If more than one oil is to be incorporated, the quantity of acacia for each is calculated separately and the sum of the quantities used.

| Table 13.2 | Quantities for primary emulsions | | | |
|---|---|---|---|---|
| Type of oil | Examples | Oil | Water | Gum |
| Fixed | Almond, arachis, cod liver, castor | 4 | 2 | 1 |
| Mineral (hydrocarbon) | Liquid paraffin | 3 | 2 | 1 |
| Volatile | Turpentine, cinnamon, peppermint | 2 | 2 | 1 |
| Oleo-resin | Male fern extract | 1 | 2 | 1 |

---

**EXAMPLE 13.1**

Calculate the quantities for a primary emulsion for the following:

| Cod liver oil | 30 ml |
|---|---|
| Water | to 100 ml |

**Primary emulsion quantities**
Cod liver oil is a fixed oil, therefore the primary emulsion proportions are 4:2:1. Hence:

| Cod liver oil | 30 ml | 4 |
|---|---|---|
| Water | 15 ml | 2 |
| Powdered acacia gum | 7.5 g | 1 |

---

#### Variations to primary emulsion calculations

If the proportion of oil is too small, modifications must be made. Acacia emulsions containing less than 20% oil tend to cream readily. A bland, inert oil, such as arachis oil, should be added to increase the amount of oil and so prevent this from happening.

---

**EXAMPLE 13.2**

Calciferol solution, 0.15 ml per 5 ml dose.
The percentage of oil in each dose is 3%. The oil content must be made up to 20% to produce a stable emulsion.
Since 20% of 5 ml = 1 ml
the volume of bland oil required is 1 − 0.15 = 0.85 ml.

**Formula for primary emulsion (for 50 ml)**

| Calciferol solution | 1.5 ml | 4 |
|---|---|---|
| Arachis oil | 8.5 ml | |
| Water | 5 ml | 2 |
| Acacia | 2.5 g | 1 |

## METHODS OF PREPARATION

There are two possible methods, with the dry gum method being the most popular.

### Dry gum method of preparation

1. Measure the oil very accurately in a dry measure.
2. Allow measure to drain into a dry mortar with a large, flat, bottom.
3. Weigh acacia gum.
4. Measure water for the primary emulsion in a clean measure.
5. Add acacia to the oil and mix lightly to disperse lumps. Do not over-mix, and keep the suspension in the bottom of the mortar.
6. Immediately add all of the water and stir continuously and vigorously until the mixture thickens and the primary emulsion is formed. This is characterized by a 'clicking' sound.
7. Continue triturating for a further 2–3 minutes to produce the white stable emulsion. The whiter the product, the smaller the globules.
8. Gradually dilute the primary emulsion with small volumes of the vehicle, ensuring complete mixing between additions.
9. Gradually add any other ingredients, transfer to a measure and make up to final volume with vehicle.

### Wet gum method of preparation

Water is added to the acacia gum and quickly triturated until the gum has dissolved, to make a mucilage. Oil is added to this mucilage in small portions, triturating the mixture thoroughly after each addition, until a thick primary emulsion is obtained. The primary emulsion should be stabilized by mixing for several minutes and then completed in the same way as for the dry gum method.

### Problems when producing the primary emulsion

The primary emulsion may not form and a thin oily liquid is formed instead. Possible causes are:

- the primary emulsion has become oily and translucent owing to phase inversion
- incorrect quantities of oil or water
- cross-contamination of water and oil
- use of a wet mortar

- mortar too small and curved, or pestle head too round, therefore insufficient shear
- excessive mixing of oil and gum (dry gum method)
- diluting primary emulsion too early
- too rapid dilution of primary emulsion
- poor quality acacia.

## EMULSIONS FOR EXTERNAL USE

Liquid or semi-liquid emulsions may be used as applications, liniments and lotions (see Ch. 14). The extemporaneous preparation of emulsions for external use does not require the preparation of a primary emulsion. Soaps are commonly used as the emulsifying agent and some are prepared 'in situ' by mixing the oily phase containing a fatty acid and the aqueous phase containing the alkali. Alternatively the emulsifying agent can be dissolved in the oily or aqueous phase and the disperse phase added to the continuous phase, either gradually or in one portion.

Creams are viscous semi-solid emulsions which may be o/w (for example aqueous cream) or w/o (for example oily cream). These are considered in more detail in Chapter 14.

## SHELF LIFE AND STORAGE

Emulsions should be stored at room temperature and will either be recently or freshly prepared. Some official preparations will have specific expiry dates. They should not be frozen.

## CONTAINERS

An amber medicine bottle is used, plain for internal use and ribbed for external use, with an airtight child-resistant closure. Containers with a wide mouth are useful for very viscous preparations.

## SPECIAL LABELLING AND ADVICE FOR EMULSIONS

- Shake well before use.
- Store in a cool place. This is to protect the

emulsion against extremes of temperature which will adversely affect its stability.

- Expiry date.
- For external use only, for external emulsions.

---

### EXAMPLE 13.3

Prepare 200 ml cod liver oil emulsion to the following formula:

| | |
|---|---|
| Cod liver oil | 60 ml |
| Chloroform | 0.4 ml |
| Cinnamon water | to 200 ml |

#### Action and uses
A rich source of vitamins A and D.

#### Formulation notes
Cod liver oil is a fixed oil that requires the addition of acacia gum as an emulsifying agent. The proportions are 4 oil : 2 water : 1 gum. Therefore 60 ml cod liver oil, 30 ml of cinnamon water and 12.5 g of acacia gum will be used to prepare the primary emulsion. Cinnamon water acts as a flavouring agent and vehicle. It may need to be prepared from concentrated cinnamon water, at a dilution of 1 part to 39 parts of water. Chloroform is dense and only slowly soluble and acts as a preservative.

#### Method of preparation
Use the dry gum method. Weigh 12.5 g of acacia and place in a dry, flat-bottomed mortar. Measure 60 ml of cod liver oil and 30 ml of cinnamon water, which will be used to create the primary emulsion. Add the cod liver oil and mix very lightly and briefly. Immediately add the prepared cinnamon water, mixing vigorously until a clicking sound is heard and a white primary emulsion is formed. Continue mixing for a few minutes to stabilize the primary emulsion. Scrape the mortar and pestle with a spatula to ensure that all the oil is incorporated. Add the chloroform and mix thoroughly. Gradually add most of the remainder of the cinnamon water to the emulsion in the mortar, stirring well between additions. Transfer the emulsion to a 200 ml measure, rinsing the mortar and adding these washings to the measure. Make up to volume with cinnamon water and pack in an amber medicine bottle with a child-resistant closure. Polish and label the bottle and give a 5 ml medicine spoon with the medicine.

#### Shelf life and storage
Store in a cool, dry place. It is recently prepared, therefore a shelf life of 2–4 weeks is applicable.

#### Advice and labelling
This is an unofficial formula, and should be labelled 'Cod liver oil 30% v/v emulsion'. 'Shake well before use.' A normal dose is 10 ml three times a day, with or after food.

---

### EXAMPLE 13.4

100 ml Liquid Paraffin Oral Emulsion BP 1968.

| | |
|---|---|
| Liquid paraffin | 50 ml |
| Vanillin | 50 mg |
| Chloroform | 0.25 ml |
| Benzoic acid solution | 2 ml |
| Methylcellulose 20 | 2 g |
| Saccharin sodium | 5 mg |
| Water | to 100 ml |

#### Action and uses
A lubricant laxative for chronic constipation.

#### Formulation notes
Methylcellulose 20 at a concentration of 2% acts as an emulsifying agent for the mineral oil, liquid paraffin. Benzoic acid and chloroform act as preservatives and vanillin and saccharin sodium act as flavouring and sweetening agents. The amount of saccharin sodium is not weighable and will be obtained by trituration using water as the diluent (since this is the vehicle for the emulsion). Trituration for saccharin sodium:

| | |
|---|---|
| Saccharin sodium | 100 mg |
| Water | to 100 ml |

5 ml of water will contain 5 mg of saccharin sodium.

#### Method of preparation
Firstly, prepare a mucilage by mixing the methylcellulose 20 with about six times its weight of boiling water and allow to stand for 30 minutes to hydrate. Add an equal weight (about 15 g) of ice and stir mechanically until the mucilage is homogeneous. Dissolve the vanillin in the benzoic acid solution and chloroform, as it is more soluble in organic solvents. Add this solution to the mucilage and stir for 5 minutes. Make up the saccharin sodium trituration and stir in the appropriate volume of solution to the mucilage. Make the volume of the mucilage up to 50 ml, taking care to ensure that there is no entrapped air in the mucilage. Make the emulsion by adding together 50 ml of liquid paraffin and 50 ml of prepared mucilage with constant stirring. The

emulsion is more stable if passed through a hand homogenizer. Pack in an amber medicine bottle with a child-resistant closure. Shake well to ensure that the emulsion is thoroughly mixed. Polish and label the bottle and give a 5 ml medicine spoon with the medicine.

### Shelf life and storage
Store in a cool, dry place. This is an official preparation and should remain stable on storage.

### Advice and labelling
Shake well before use. The emulsion should not be taken within 30 minutes of meal times and preferably on an empty stomach. The importance of fibre and fluid intake in the diet should be emphasized.

---

### EXAMPLE 13.5

100 ml Oily Calamine Lotion BP 1980.

| | |
|---|---|
| Calamine | 5 g |
| Wool fat | 1 g |
| Oleic acid | 0.5 ml |
| Arachis oil | 50 ml |
| Calcium hydroxide solution | to 100 ml |

### Action and uses
Soothing lotion for the treatment of eczema, sunburn and other inflammatory conditions.

### Formulation notes
The emulsifying agent for the arachis oil is the soap calcium oleate produced from the calcium hydroxide and oleic acid when they are shaken together. Wool fat is included as an emulsion stabilizer. This is a w/o emulsion.

### Method of preparation
The wool fat, oleic acid and arachis oil should be warmed together in an evaporating basin on a water bath until melted. Mix them together well. The calamine should be sieved and weighed and placed on a warm ointment tile. Add a little of the oily mixture and rub in with a large spatula until smooth. Gradually add more of the oily mixture until it is fluid. Transfer back to the evaporating basin and stir to evenly distribute the calamine powder. Pour into a previously tared, amber ribbed bottle and add the calcium hydroxide solution to the bottle in small amounts, shaking well between additions. Make up to volume and seal with a child-resistant closure. Polish and label the bottle.

### Shelf life and storage
Store in a cool, dry place. It is unpreserved, therefore a shelf life of 2–4 weeks is applicable.

### Advice and labelling
Shake well before use and For external use only.

---

## Key Points

- Emulsions may be oil-in-water (o/w) or water-in-oil (w/o).
- Oral emulsions are always o/w.
- Emulsions may be used orally, externally or by intramuscular and intravenous injection.
- The type of emulsion may be determined by miscibility, conductivity, staining and dye tests.
- Emulsifying agents are required to reduce the interfacial tension and act as a barrier between the oil and water phases.
- Naturally occurring emulsifying agents include polysaccharides (acacia), semi-synthetic polysaccharides (methylcellulose) and sterols (wool fat).
- Synthetic surfactants can be used and are selected using the HLB number.
- Care is required to avoid anion–cation incompatibilities.
- Some finely divided solids will stabilize emulsions.
- Emulsions require antimicrobial preservation.
- Phase inversion, creaming and cracking are physical instabilities of emulsions which must be avoided.
- A primary emulsion is prepared when making an emulsion using acacia as the emulsifying agent.
- The ratio of oil : water : acacia will vary with the type of oil in the formulation.
- Liquid emulsions should have a 'Shake well before use' label and should not be frozen.

---

## FURTHER READING

ABPI Compendium of data sheets and summaries of product characteristics, current edn. Datapharm Publications, London (Updated annually)

Ansel H C, Popovich N G, Allen L V 1995 Pharmaceutical dosage forms and drug delivery systems, 6th edn. Williams & Wilkins, Malvern, USA

Aulton M E 1988 Pharmaceutics: the science of dosage form design. Churchill Livingstone, Edinburgh

British National Formulary, current edn. British Medical Association and Royal Pharmaceutical Society of Great Britain, London (Updated twice yearly)

British Pharmacopeia, current edn. HMSO, London

British Pharmaceutical Codex 1973 Pharmaceutical Press, London

Diluent Directories (Internal and External), current edn. National Pharmaceutical Association, St Albans

Pharmaceutical Codex 1979 11th edn. Pharmaceutical Press, London

Pharmaceutical Codex: principles and practice of pharmaceutics 1994 12th edn. Pharmaceutical Press, London

Reynolds J E F (ed) 1996 Martindale: the extra pharmacopoeia, 31st edn. Pharmaceutical Press, London (Updated every 3 years – use current edn)

Wade A (ed) 1980 Pharmaceutical handbook, 19th edn. Pharmaceutical Press, London

# 14

# External preparations

*A. J. Winfield*

After studying this chapter you will know about:

**Skin structure and sites of action of drugs**
**The types and function of solid, liquid and semi-solid skin preparations**
**The ingredients used in skin preparations**
**Dispensing preparations for use on the skin.**

## Introduction

Skin is the largest organ in the body and has three distinct regions. The hypodermis is the innermost and is often called subcutaneous fat. The dermis is the bulk of the thickness of the skin and contains the blood vessels, the nerve fibres, the sweat glands and the hair follicles. The outermost region is the epidermis, which is made up of several layers. Cells divide in the stratum basale, and as they move towards the surface change appearance and function. The outermost layer is called the stratum corneum, which acts as the skin barrier. It is made up of about 20 layers of dead keratinized cells. The hair follicles and sweat ducts pass through the stratum corneum to reach the surface. A simplified diagram showing the main skin structures is given in Figure 14.1.

There are a large number of diseases which may affect different regions of the skin. Any drug used will require to reach the site of the disease in order to act. Unless it is for a surface effect only, the drug must either pass through the stratum corneum or go

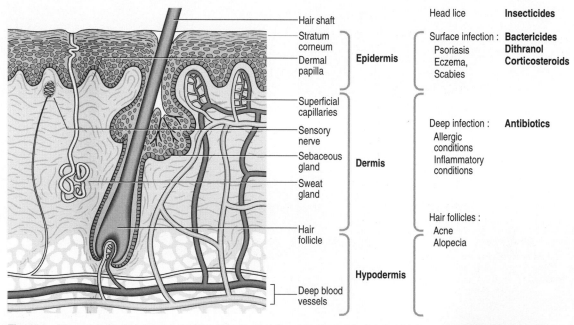

**Fig. 14.1** Diagrammatic representation of the skin showing the main structures, location of diseases and the sites of action of drugs.

through a follicle or sweat gland. Examples of drugs applied to the skin and their sites of action are shown in Figure 14.1. Once in the skin, a lipid-soluble drug will tend to accumulate in lipid regions, whilst more water-soluble drugs will tend to enter the blood capillaries and be removed from the skin. There are also many metabolic enzymes in the skin which can deactivate drugs. Pharmacokinetics is seldom applied to skin administration and dosage is often imprecise.

There are an increasing number of drugs that are effective against skin diseases, but they are not the only way of treating skin conditions. Beneficial changes can be brought about by creating physiological change in the skin. The main one is to control the moisture content of the skin. Normal skin has 10–25% moisture in the stratum corneum. This level may be reduced in, for example, eczema, or increased, as in skin maceration between the toes. By using an occlusive product (that is an oily product), water leaving the body through the skin will be trapped and moisture content will increase. These products are called emollients. An excess of moisture may be removed using an astringent, a hygroscopic material or, to a lesser extent, a dusting powder. Where an oily vehicle is needed but moisture must not increase, adding solid particles to the vehicle will allow water to escape. Lubrication of sensitive skin is achieved by using finely divided solids, applied either as a powder or, more efficient-

ly, as a suspension. Cooling the skin relieves inflammation and eases discomfort. It is achieved by evaporating a solvent, usually water or a water and alcohol mixture. Volatile solvents sprayed on the skin give intense cooling.

## TYPES OF SKIN PREPARATION

There are a large number of different types of external medicine, ranging from dry powders through semi-solids to liquids. The names are often traditional. Figure 14.2 illustrates the formulation of the main types of preparation used on the skin.

### Solids

Dusting powders are applied to the skin for a surface effect such as drying or lubricating, or an antibacterial action. They are made of fine particle size powders together with any medicament.

### Liquids

*Soaks* have an active ingredient dissolved in an aqueous solvent and are often used as astringents, for cooling or to leave a film of solid on the skin. Oily

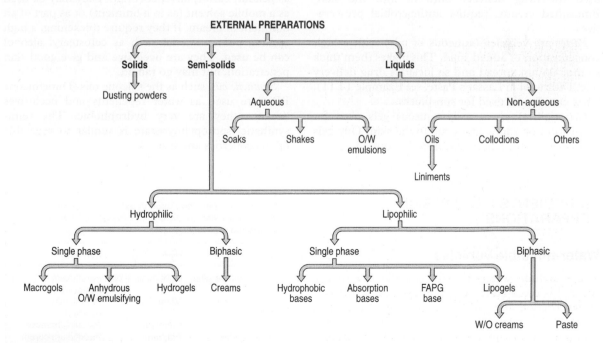

**Fig. 14.2** Schematic representation of types of external medicines.

vehicles can be used in bath additives to leave an emollient film on the skin surface.

*Applications* are solutions or emulsions that frequently contain parasiticides.

*Liniments* are alcoholic or oily solutions or emulsions designed to be rubbed into the skin. The medicament is usually a rubefacient.

*Lotions* are aqueous solutions, suspensions or emulsions that cool inflamed skin and deposit a protective layer of solid.

*Paints* and *tinctures* are concentrated aqueous or alcoholic antimicrobial solutions.

*Collodions* are organic solvents containing a polymer and keratolytic agent for treating corns and calluses.

There are also many other liquid products including shampoos, pomades, foot washes.

## Semi-solids

*Ointments* are usually oily vehicles that may contain a surfactant to allow them to be washed off easily (barrier creams). They are used as emollients, or for drug delivery either to the surface or for deeper penetration.

*Creams* are traditionally o/w emulsions whilst *oily creams* are w/o emulsions. However, there are also 'creams' that are not emulsions. They usually give cooling, are less greasy than ointments and can be used for drug delivery onto or into the skin. Emulsified creams require antimicrobial preservatives.

*Pastes* are vehicles (aqueous or oily) with a high concentration of added solid. This makes them thick so they do not spread and so localizes drug delivery (e.g. Dithranol in Lassar's Paste, see Example 14.11). They can also be used for sun-blocks.

*Gels* (jellies) are usually aqueous gels used for lubrication or applying a drug to the skin. Oily gels are also available where occlusion is required.

## INGREDIENTS USED IN SKIN PREPARATIONS

### Water-miscible vehicles

These include water, alcohol and the Macrogols. Alcohol is often added to water to increase the rate of evaporation and produce a more intense cooling effect. Industrial methylated spirit (IMS) is normally used for external preparations because it is exempt from excise duty. The Macrogols (polyethylene gly-cols), are available with a range of molecular weight. As chain length increases, so the properties change from liquid, through semi-solid to waxy solid. They have good solvent properties for a wide range of drugs and can be blended to produce intermediate consistencies. They do tend to dry the skin, inactivate some antimicrobials, interact with some plastics and can give poor release of drugs.

### Oily vehicles

Oils used in external preparations come from one of three sources.

*Mineral oils* (paraffins) are the most widely used. They are complex mixtures of mainly saturated hydrocarbons which are available in different fractions. Different names are used in different pharmacopoeias (see Table 14.1).

Light liquid paraffin is not normally used in external medicines. Soft paraffin is the main ingredient in many products, with liquid or hard paraffin being used to thin or thicken them respectively. There are two forms of soft paraffin – yellow and white. The latter has been bleached, residues of which may remain. As a rule, white is used in white or pale-coloured products, whilst yellow is used for darker products. The paraffins are occlusive and chemically inert, but do not give good skin penetration.

*Vegetable oils* come from many plant sources such as peanut, castor, olive, coconut. They may be used as a mobile solvent (as in a liniment) or as part of an ointment or cream. If they require thickening, a high melting point material such as cetostearyl alcohol can be used. They are occlusive and give good skin penetration, but may go rancid.

*Synthetic oils*, such as the silicone oils (Dimethicone BP), are used as water repellents and occlusives because they are very hydrophobic. The semi-synthetic isopropylmyristate is similar to vegetable oil in properties and use.

| Table 14.1 Paraffins used in external preparations: the names used are different in the UK, USA and European pharmacopoeias | | |
|---|---|---|
| UK | USA | European |
| Light liquid paraffin | Light mineral oil | Paraffinium perliquidum |
| Liquid paraffin | Mineral oil | Paraffinium liquidum |
| Soft paraffin | Petrolatum | Paraffinium molle |
| Hard paraffin | Paraffin | Paraffinium durum |

## Emulsifying agents

Liquid and semi-solid emulsions, both o/w and w/o, are used externally and require the addition of emulsifying agents. The latter may also be added to an oil without water as in Emulsifying Ointment BP. The presence of a surfactant usually increases the skin penetration of any drug. A wide range of materials can be used as surfactants, either alone or in combinations. Selection is made in view of the type of emulsion required (o/w or w/o) and the charge on the other ingredients (anionic, cationic or non-ionic).

### W/o emulsifiers

Wool fat, obtained from sheep wool, is a pale yellow sticky material. It is a complex mixture of fatty acid esters of cholesterol and other sterols and alcohols. Whilst it is similar to human sebum, it can cause sensitization in some people. Wool alcohols, a solid, is richer in cholesterol and lanesterol and freer of impurities. Both it and wool fat increase the 'water holding' capacity of greasy bases. Hydrous wool fat is 7 parts wool fat and 3 parts water and is a softer material. Different names are used as shown in Table 14.2. Beeswax is a traditional w/o emulsifier which is occasionally used.

### O/w emulsifiers

The main group of materials used extemporaneously are the emulsifying waxes. Each one has two ingredients – cetostearyl alcohol and a surface-active agent as shown in Table 14.3. All three are waxy solids that mix with oily materials. Addition of water produces an o/w emulsion – a cream. Both the non-aqueous blends and the creams are easily washed off the skin. Consistency can be controlled by varying the amount of bodying agent, usually cetostearyl alcohol. The ratio of oil to water will also alter the consistency of a cream.

**Table 14.2  Materials based on wool fat: different names are used in the UK, USA and European pharmacopoeias**

| UK | USA | European |
|---|---|---|
| Wool Fat | Lanolin | Adeps lanae |
| Wool Alcohols | Lanolin alcohols | Alcoholes adipis lanae |
| Hydrous Wool Fat | Hydrous lanolin | Adeps lanae cum aqua |

**Table 14.3  The ingredients used in the emulsifying waxes described in the *British Pharmacopoeia* (BP) and *British Pharmaceutical Codex* (BPC)**

| Charge | Surfactant | CSA/SAA ratio | Name |
|---|---|---|---|
| Anionic | Sodium lauryl sulphate | 9 : 1 | Emulsifying Wax BP |
| Cationic | Cetrimide | 9 : 1 | Cetrimide Emulsifying Wax BPC |
| Non-ionic | Cetomacrogol 1000 | 8 : 2 | Cetomacrogol Emulsifying Wax BPC |

### Other emulsifiers

The gums, used in oral emulsions (see Ch. 13), are too sticky for external use, but a number of other emulsifying agents are used.

Calcium soaps are produced by mixing a fatty acid with lime water (calcium hydroxide solution) to form a soap in situ. They form w/o emulsions. Soft soap is a sticky green material that can be used to make o/w emulsions.

Synthetic surface active agents can also be used. Low HLB materials will produce w/o emulsions, whilst higher HLB surfactants give o/w emulsions.

## Suspending agents

These materials can be used for suspending solids in shake lotions, or to produce gels, depending on the concentration used. Those used in oral suspensions (see Ch. 12) are too sticky for use in external liquid suspensions. The main group of materials used for this purpose are the clays, of which there are many forms including bentonite, attapulgite, montmorrilonite, Veegum (aluminium magnesium silicate). They leave a lubricant layer of powder on the skin. They are unsuitable for use below pH 3.5 and their consistency may be affected by alcohol and electrolytes.

Gelling agents can be used to produce a wide range of consistency from slightly thickened (as in artificial tears), through lubricants and semi-solids for the delivery of drugs to very thick bases used to immobilize the skin. For aqueous gels the materials used include tragacanth, alginates, pectin, gelatin, methylcelluloses, carbomer, polyvinyl alcohol and clays. Oils may be thickened using cetostearyl alcohol, hard paraffin, beeswax, wool alcohols and polyvalent soaps such as magnesium stearate. The latter, when heated with an oil, produces a clear 'lipogel'.

## Other ingredients

Wetting agents are required for hydrophobic solids. Tincture of quillaia is the traditional material, but alcohol alone may be effective. Synthetic materials, such as Manoxol OT, can also be used.

Humectants are materials added to reduce the rate of water loss from creams and gels. They are all hygroscopic materials and include glycerol, propylene glycol, PEG 300 and sorbitol syrup, typically used at a concentration of 5–15%.

Solids may be added to semi-solid occlusive bases. They provide channels for the migration of water from the skin surface and so reduce the occlusiveness. Solids used include zinc oxide, talc, starch, Aerosil. Some, such as talc, must be sterilized to kill bacterial spores (see Ch. 16).

Whenever there is a danger of microbial growth, antimicrobial preservation is required.

## DISPENSING OF EXTERNAL PREPARATIONS

A wide range of dispensing techniques are used in compounding external medicines some of which have been reviewed in other chapters (Chs 11, 12, 13 and 16). In the section which follows, only those types of product which require different dispensing techniques are described in detail.

## Dusting powders

A simple mixing in a mortar and pestle using 'doubling-up' is used (see Ch. 16). Sieving may be necessary to disperse aggregates in cohesive powders. A 180 μm sieve should be used. Powders such as starch, which contains a lot of moisture, may need drying to ensure optimum flow properties. With coloured materials, considerable working with the pestle is required before proceeding to 'doubling-up' otherwise a speckled product may result. A liquid may be added by pipette to a small quantity of the powder and be worked in before further mixing. A worked example of a dusting powder is given in Example 16.3.

## Liquid preparations

These include solutions, suspensions and emulsions. The same basic dispensing techniques employed in making the corresponding oral systems are used (see Chs 11, 12 and 13). Most liquid preparations are used unsterilized, but if they are intended for application to broken skin, eyes or body cavities, they should be sterilized. They should be packed in ribbed bottles, labelled 'For external use only' and carry a 'Shake the bottle' label if they are emulsions or suspensions. Worked examples are given of a lotion in Example 12.5 and of an oily lotion in Example 13.5.

---

**EXAMPLE 14.1**

### Compound Sulphur Lotion BPC
Send 100 ml Compound Sulphur Lotion BPC.

|  | Formula | For 100 ml |
|---|---|---|
| Precipitated sulphur | 40 g | 4 g |
| Quillaia tincture | 5 ml | 0.5 ml |
| Glycerol | 20 ml | 2 ml |
| Industrial methylated spirit | 60 ml | 6 ml |
| Calcium hydroxide solution | to 1000 ml | to 100 ml |

#### Action and uses
This is used as a treatment for acne, scabies and as a mild antiseptic.

#### Formulation notes
This an example of a shake lotion, an aqueous suspension prepared without a suspending agent, but including a wetting agent for the hydrophobic sulphur.

#### Method of preparation
Sieve the precipitated sulphur. Weigh out 4 g and place in a glass mortar. Using a 1 ml pipette add 0.5 ml quillaia tincture and work well into the sulphur using a pestle. Add 6 ml of industrial methylated spirits followed by 2 ml glycerol working in after each addition (thus achieving maximum wetting before water is added). Add 20–30 ml calcium hydroxide solution to produce a pourable suspension. Transfer this to a tared bottle. Rinse the mortar with calcium hydroxide solution, adding it to the bottle, before making up to volume.

#### Shelf life and storage
There are no special requirements for storage. An expiry date of 4 weeks is suitable.

---

**EXAMPLE 14.2**

### Methyl Salicylate Liniment BP
Prepare 100 ml methyl salicylate liniment.

| | Formula | For 100 ml |
|---|---|---|
| Methyl salicylate | 250 ml | 25 ml |
| Arachis oil | to 1000 ml | to 100 ml |

### Action and uses

Methyl salicylate is a rubefacient, used to treat muscular aches and pains.

### Formulation notes

The methyl salicylate requires to enter the skin. The vegetable oil, arachis oil, is used as the solvent to assist in this process. Other suitable fixed oils can be used.

### Method of preparation

Measure 25 ml of methyl salicylate in a 100 ml measure and add arachis oil to make up to volume. Transfer to a dry 100 ml amber ribbed bottle.

### Shelf life and storage

This liniment should be kept in a well-closed container in a cool place. An expiry date of 4 weeks is appropriate.

---

### EXAMPLE 14.3

### Turpentine Liniment BP

Prepare 100 ml of turpentine liniment.

| | Formula | To send 100 ml |
|---|---|---|
| Turpentine oil | 650 ml | 78 ml |
| Racemic camphor | 50 g | 6 g |
| Soft soap | 75 g | 9 g |
| Purified water, freshly boiled and cooled | 225 ml | 27 ml |

### Action and uses

Both turpentine oil and camphor are rubefacients which are rubbed into the skin to relieve muscular aches and pains.

### Formulation notes

The BP formula adds up to 1000. However, these are a mixture of weight and volume so the final volume is not known. It is usual to calculate in the ratio 120 'units' per 100 ml.

This is an emulsion made using an alkali soap. When using soft soap, it is usual to use it at 10% weight of a fixed oil (as in this example), or 20% weight of a fat.

### Method of preparation

Weigh the camphor and place in a porcelain mortar. Grind it to a small particle size. Choose the softer, greener parts of the soap. Weigh (on a piece of paper) and mix thoroughly with the camphor. Measure the turpentine oil and add small aliquots (5–10 ml at first) to the soap and camphor followed by thorough mixing. When an even dispersion is obtained, transfer this to a 250 ml stoppered measuring cylinder. Use the remaining oil to rinse the mortar and add to the cylinder. Measure the water and add it, as quickly as possible, to the measure, stopper and shake it vigorously until a creamy white emulsion is formed. Allow it to stand for a few minutes (for air bubbles to separate) before transferring 100 ml to a tared bottle. Avoid plastic containers because turpentine reacts with some plastics.

### Shelf life and storage

There are no special storage requirements. An expiry date of 4 weeks is appropriate.

---

### EXAMPLE 14.4

### Benzyl Benzoate Application BP

Prepare 100 ml of benzyl benzoate application.

| | Formula | For 100 ml |
|---|---|---|
| Benzyl benzoate | 250 g | 25 g |
| Emulsifying wax | 20 g | 2 g |
| Purified water, freshly boiled and cooled | to 1000 ml | to 100 ml |

### Action and uses

Benzyl benzoate is a liquid insecticide used for treating scabies and lice. It is usually applied with a brush over the whole body below the neck. It should not be applied to broken or inflamed skin.

### Formulation notes

Benzyl benzoate is water immiscible and is being emulsified using the anionic Emulsifying Wax BP. The application is an o/w emulsion.

### Method of preparation

Weigh the emulsifying wax and place it in an evaporating basin on a water-bath to melt. Add the benzyl benzoate and mix and warm. Warm about 75 ml of the water to the same temperature. Add about half of this to the evaporating basin and mix very gently. Transfer the mixture, again very gently to avoid frothing, to a tared bottle. Add warmed water to volume. Close the bottle and shake vigorously. Care is required to avoid frothing when water is present, because it will be very difficult to make up to the tare mark when froth has formed. Shake frequently whilst the application cools.

## Shelf life and storage

The application should be kept in a cool place, but not be allowed to freeze. An expiry date of 4 weeks is appropriate.

# Semi-solid preparations

## Mixing by fusion

The compounding of many semi-solid preparations includes the blending together of oily materials, some of which are solids at room temperature. This is achieved by the process called 'mixing by fusion'. As the name implies, it involves melting the ingredients together (see Example 14.5). The process is carried out in an evaporating basin on a water-bath. It should be noted that a high temperature is not required so 60–70°C is usually adequate. Waxy solids should be grated before weighing and should be added first, so that melting can start whilst other ingredients are being measured. When all the ingredients are melted, remove the basin from the water-bath and gently stir until cold. Mixing, which should be gentle to avoid air bubbles, is necessary to avoid lumps forming. This could happen because the higher melting point ingredients in the eutectic system may precipitate out. A medicament may be added at different stages of preparation depending on its properties. If soluble and stable, it can be added when the base is molten. If it is less stable, or insoluble but easy to disperse, it can be added during cooling. However, if it is unstable or if dispersion is difficult, it should be added when cold using mixing by trituration.

When evaporating basins are being used, recovery of all the product is not possible. Thus, in order to be able to pack the prescribed amount, it is necessary to make an excess of about 10%.

---

**EXAMPLE 14.5**

---

### Simple Ointment BP

Send 50 g simple ointment.

|  | Formula | For 60 g |
|---|---|---|
| Wool fat | 50 g | 3 g |
| Hard paraffin | 50 g | 3 g |
| Cetostearyl alcohol | 50 g | 3 g |
| Yellow or white soft paraffin | 850 g | 51 g |

### Action and uses

Simple ointment is used for making other ointments, or as an emollient.

## Formulation notes

This is a simple blend of solid and semi-solid oily ingredients made by fusion. Yellow or white soft paraffin is chosen according to the colour of the finished product. In this case, since there is nothing else to be added, white soft paraffin should be used.

## Method of preparation

Grate the hard paraffin and cetostearyl alcohol. Weigh 3 g of each and place in an evaporating basin on a water-bath. Weigh the wool fat, using a piece of paper to allow full recovery of the material, and add it to the evaporating basis, followed by the soft paraffin. Stir gently until fully melted. Remove from the heat and continue to stir gently until cold. Weigh 50 g of base into a tared ointment jar or pack into a collapsible tube (see Example 14.10). If an ointment jar is used, a greaseproof paper disc should be placed on the surface of the ointment to protect the liner of the lid.

## Shelf life and storage

Store in a cool place. An expiry date of 4 weeks is appropriate.

---

## Mixing by trituration

Insoluble solid or liquid medicaments are incorporated into bases using the technique called 'mixing by trituration'. Any powders should be passed through a 180 μm sieve before weighing to avoid grittiness. Mixing by trituration is carried out on an ointment slab or tile, which may be made of glass or glazed porcelain. A flexible spatula is used to work the materials together. Powders are placed on the tile and incorporated into the base using 'doubling-up' as it is worked in. However, it is usually necessary to have two to three times the volume of base to powder, otherwise it will 'crumble'. Liquids, if present, are usually small volumes. A portion of the base is placed on the slab and a recess made to hold the liquid which is then worked in gently. Larger quantities of liquid should be added a little at a time using the same method. These processes can be carried out in a mortar with a flat base using a pestle with a flat head. However, because recovery of the product is difficult, this is usually reserved for larger-scale batches.

---

**EXAMPLE 14.6**

---

### Sulphur Ointment BP

Send 50 g sulphur ointment.

|  | Formula | For 50 g |
|---|---|---|
| Precipitated sulphur, finely sifted | 100 g | 5 g |
| Simple ointment | 900 g | 45 g |

## Action and uses

The ointment is used to treat acne and scabies.

## Formulation notes

The BP directs that the simple ointment be prepared with white soft paraffin. If simple ointment is available, the trituration can be carried out on a slab and all the product recovered. However, if simple ointment is also being made, 50 g should be adequate to ensure that 45 g is available. Precipitated sulphur, whilst of smaller particle size than sublimed sulphur, can give a gritty feel unless it is passed through a 180 μm sieve.

## Method of preparation

Sieve and then weigh out 5 g of precipitated sulphur and place it on the slab. Weigh 45 g of simple ointment (using a piece of paper to prevent it sticking to the balance), and place it on a different part of the slab. Take a portion of the base of about three times the volume of the sulphur and work it and the sulphur together vigorously until there is no sign of any particles of sulphur. This can be checked for by spreading a thin layer on the slab. Collect the ointment together on the slab using the spatula and pack 50 g.

## Shelf life and storage

Store in a cool place. An expiry date of 4 weeks is appropriate.

---

### EXAMPLE 14.7

## Methyl Salicylate Ointment BP

Prepare 30 g methyl salicylate ointment.

|  | Formula | For 35 g |
|---|---|---|
| Methyl salicylate | 500 g | 17.5 g |
| White beeswax | 250 g | 8.75 g |
| Hydrous wool fat | 250 g | 8.75 g |

## Action and uses

Methyl salicylate is a volatile material used as a rubefacient.

## Formulation notes

With the high proportion of the liquid methyl salicylate, the product would be runny without the addition of the beeswax as a thickening agent. The base ingredients require to be blended by fusion.

## Method of preparation

Grate and weigh the beeswax. Melt it with the hydrous wool fat (weighed on a piece of paper) in an evaporating basin on a water-bath. Remove from the heat and stir until almost cold before adding the methyl salicylate. Continue stirring until cold. Pack 30 g in a glass ointment jar (plastic should be avoided with methyl salicylate).

## Shelf life and storage

Store in a cool place. An expiry date of 4 weeks is appropriate.

---

Creams are emulsified preparations containing water. They are susceptible to microbial growth which may cause spoilage or disease. Whilst preservatives are included, they are usually inadequate to cope with a heavy microbial contamination and so the possibility of microbial contamination during preparation should be minimized. Ideally aseptic technique should be used, but this is not normally possible and so thorough cleanliness is employed. As a minimum, all apparatus and final containers should be thoroughly cleaned and rinsed with freshly boiled and cooled purified water before drying. Swabbing of working surfaces, spatulas and other equipment with ethanol will also reduce the possibility of microbial contamination.

The basic method of making an emulsified cream is to warm the oily phase and aqueous phase to a temperature of about 60°C, mix the phases and stir until cold. It is important that the temperatures of the two phases are within a few degrees the same and it is advisable to use a thermometer to check this. Rapid cooling will cause the separation of high melting point materials, and excessive aeration as a result of vigorous stirring can also produce a granular product. Medicaments may, if they are stable, be dissolved in the appropriate phase before emulsification, or can be added by trituration when cold.

---

### EXAMPLE 14.8

## Aqueous Cream BP

Send 50 g aqueous cream.

|  | Formula | For 55 g |
|---|---|---|
| Emulsifying ointment | 300 g | 16.5 g |
| Phenoxyethanol | 10 g | 0.55 g |
| Purified water, freshly boiled and cooled | 690 g | 37.95 g |

## Action and uses

Aqueous cream is an emollient and can be used as a base for drugs.

## Formulation notes

This is an o/w cream made using an anionic emulsifying agent. To reduce the risk of microbial contamination all equipment should be washed before use. Phenoxyethanol is present as an antimicrobial preservative. It is a liquid, so has to be weighed, or, if its density is obtained, it could be measured by pipette. If the emulsifying ointment has to made, exactly 16.5 g can be made because the emulsification can be carried out in the same evaporating basin.

## Method of preparation

The phenoxyethanol is dissolved in the water warmed to 60°C. Weigh the emulsifying ointment (using a piece of paper to prevent it sticking) and melt it in an evaporating basin on a water-bath. Ensure that both phases are close to 60°C, then add the aqueous phase to the melted ointment. Remove from the heat and stir continuously until cold, taking care not to incorporate too much air. Weigh 50 g and pack in an ointment jar or collapsible tube.

## Shelf life and storage

The preparation should be stored in a cool place, but not allowed to freeze. A shelf life of 2–4 weeks is appropriate because the preparation has not been made in the cleanest conditions.

---

### EXAMPLE 14.9

## Hydrous Ointment BP (also known as Oily Cream)

Send 50 g oily cream.

|  | Formula | For 60 g |
|---|---|---|
| Wool alcohols ointment | 500 g | 30 g |
| Phenoxyethanol | 10 g | 0.6 g |
| Dried magnesium sulphate | 5 g | 0.3 g |
| Purified water, freshly boiled and cooled | 485 g | 29.1 g |

## Actions and uses

Oily cream is used as an emollient in treating dry skin conditions.

## Formulation notes

This is a w/o cream prepared using wool alcohols as the emulsifying agent. Phenoxyethanol is present as preservative, but all equipment should be washed before use. Phenoxyethanol is a liquid and so must be weighed, or, if its density is obtained, it can be measured by pipette. Quantities

for 55 g produce amounts that cannot be weighed on a dispensing balance, so 60 g is made. If the wool alcohols ointment is also to be made, exactly 30 g is adequate, because it does not have to be removed from the evaporating basin.

## Method of preparation

All equipment should be thoroughly cleaned before use. Dissolve the magnesium sulphate and phenoxyethanol in the water and warm to 60°C on a water-bath. Weigh the wool alcohols ointment, using a piece of paper, and melt it in an evaporating basin at 60°C. Check that the two temperatures are the same. Add the water, little by little, to the ointment, stirring constantly until a smooth cream, whilst maintaining the temperature at 60°C. When all the water is added, stir gently until the cream is at room temperature. Pack 50 g in an ointment jar or collapsible tube.

## Shelf life and storage

Store in a cool place but do not allow to freeze. If liquid separates on storage it may be re-incorporated by stirring. An expiry date of 4 weeks is appropriate.

---

# Dilution of creams

It is sometimes necessary to prepare a dilution of a commercially produced cream, although the practice is undesirable. Choice of diluent is crucial, since the diluent may impair the preservative system in the cream, may affect the bioavailability of the medicament, or be incompatible with other ingredients. The process of dilution also increases the risk of microbial contamination. Thus, dilutions should only be made with the diluent(s) specified in the manufacturer's data sheet. All diluted creams should be freshly prepared and be given a 2-week shelf life.

---

### EXAMPLE 14.10

## A method for filling a collapsible tube extemporaneously

1. Cut a piece of greaseproof paper about 5 cm longer than the tube and of a width that will go round the tube about twice. Place this on a clean slab, and fold up about 1 cm on one long edge (see Fig. 14.3).

2. Place the cream on the paper, parallel to the fold, so that the length is about the same as that of the tube. Then fold the loose edge of the paper into

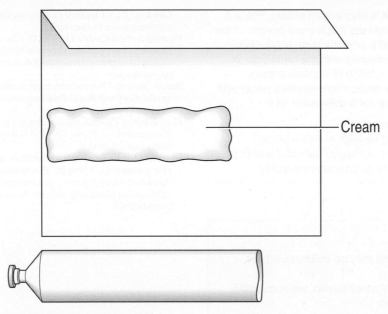

**Fig. 14.3**  Filling a collapsible tube.

the fold, so covering the cream (This stage is rather like wrapping a powder – see Ch. 16.) Roll the paper from the fold, so that the cream is held in a cylinder of paper which will slide inside the tube.

3.  Push the paper and cream right down the tube. Then, using a spatula or fingers, close the paper at the open end and gently pull it out, leaving the cream behind in the tube.

4.  When fully withdrawn hold a spatula blade firmly down on the open end of the tube, about 2.5 mm in from the end and raise the cap end to produce a fold. Use the spatula, or a crimping tool if one is available, to complete the fold. Repeat this to produce a second fold.

## Pastes

Pastes are dispersions of high concentrations of solid in either an aqueous or oily vehicle. They can be used to treat infections by making use of their high osmotic pressure, or as very thick materials to prevent irritant drugs spreading over the skin surface. Incorporation of the solid is by mixing on a slab.

---

### EXAMPLE 14.11

**Dithranol Paste BP**
Send 100 g of weak dithranol paste.

|  | Formula | For 100 g |
|---|---|---|
| Dithranol | 1 g | 0.1 g |
| Lassar's paste | 999 g | 99.9 g |

**Lassar's Paste**

|  | Formula | For 110 g |
|---|---|---|
| Zinc oxide | 240 g | 24 g |
| Salicylic acid | 20 g | 2 g |
| Starch | 240 g | 24 g |
| White soft paraffin | 500 g | 50 g |

#### Action and uses
Dithranol is used to treat psoriasis. There are two strengths of dithranol paste, 'weak' is 0.1% and 'strong' is 1%, although a range of intermediate strengths is prescribed by dermatologists.

#### Formulation notes
The Lassar's paste has to be made first before incorporating the dithranol. Dithranol is prone to oxidation, so contact with metal should be avoided.

#### Method of preparation
Sieve the zinc oxide and salicylic acid through a 180 µm sieve before weighing. Weigh the soft paraffin (on a piece of paper) and melt in an evaporating basin on a water-bath. Take some of the powder and stir into the melted base. Continue until all the powder is added, then stir gently until cold. Weigh out the Lassar's paste (using paper to avoid sticking). Only when the Lassar's paste has been completed, weigh out the dithranol. Care is

required because it is very irritant to skin. Place it on a slab and incorporate it in a small portion of the paste, ensuring that a smooth, even product is produced. Dilute gradually with the remainder of the paste. Pack in a 120 g (4 ounces) brown ointment jar, with a circle of greaseproof paper and a tight-fitting closure, or a collapsible tube.

### Shelf life and storage

The product should be kept in a cool place, protected from light. An expiry date of 2 weeks is appropriate because of chemical instability.

---

## Key Points

- Skin preparations may be solids, liquids or semi-solids.
- Vehicles may be water based, water miscible, oily or emulsified.
- Emulsifying agents may be used to produce either o/w or w/o emulsions.
- Suspending agents used on the skin are usually clays.
- Other ingredients include wetting agents, humectants and finely divided solids.
- Dusting powders are simple mixtures made by 'doubling-up'.
- Lotions are aqueous solutions, suspensions or emulsions.
- Liniments are oily solutions or emulsions.
- Mixing by fusion is the process of melting together the ingredients of ointment bases followed by stirring until cold.
- Mixing by trituration is the incorporation of solids or liquids into semi-solid vehicles on an ointment slab.
- Cleanliness is essential when making creams to avoid excessive microbial contamination.
- Powders should normally be passed through a 180 μm sieve before use.
- Containers for liquid preparations should be brown and ribbed.
- All skin preparations should carry the label 'For external use only'.

---

## FURTHER READING

British Pharmacopoeia, current and earlier edns. HMSO, London

Pharmaceutical Codex 1994 12th edn. Pharmaceutical Press, London (Part 1 includes a very useful chapter on administration to the skin)

Pharmaceutical Codex 1979 11th edn. Pharmaceutical Press, London (This and the previous British Pharmaceutical Codex have many details on formulation of external preparations)

British National Formulary, current edn. British Medical Association and Royal Pharmaceutical Society of Great Britain, London

Handbook of Pharmaceutical Excipients, 1994 2nd edn. Pharmaceutical Press, London (Gives technical details on many ingredients)

Reynolds J E F (ed) 1996 Martindale: the extra pharmacopoeia, 31st edn. Pharmaceutical Press, London (Updated every 3 years – use current edn. Has a lot of information about ingredients, formulae and uses of preparations)

# 15
# Suppositories and pessaries

*M. M. Moody*

---

After studying this chapter, the reader will understand about:

**Ideal suppository bases**
**Types of base**
**Suppository moulds and mould calibration**
**Displacement values**
**Methods of preparation of suppositories and pessaries**
**Containers, labelling and patient advice for suppositories and pessaries.**

## Introduction

Drug administration by the rectal and vaginal routes is achieved using drugs formulated as suppositories and pessaries, respectively. This chapter gives details of how these two dose forms are prepared, the substances and equipment used in their preparation and the calculations involved.

A suppository is a drug delivery system where the drug is incorporated into an inert vehicle. This vehicle, generally referred to as the base, must have certain properties.

## PROPERTIES OF AN IDEAL SUPPOSITORY BASE

An ideal suppository base must:

- melt at, or just below body temperature or dissolve in body fluids
- solidify quickly after melting
- be miscible with many ingredients
- be bland, i.e. non-toxic and non-irritant
- be stable on storage
- be resistant to handling
- be stable to heating above its melting point

- release the active ingredient readily
- be easily moulded and removed from the mould.

The substances which satisfy these properties fall into two groups, the fatty bases and the water-soluble or water-miscible bases.

## The fatty bases

These bases melt at body temperature and consist of the naturally occurring theobroma oil and synthetic hard fats.

Theobroma oil exhibits many of the properties of an ideal suppository base.

- It has a melting point range of 30–36°C and therefore is solid at normal room temperature.
- It readily liquefies on heating but sets rapidly when cooled.
- It is miscible with many ingredients.
- It is bland, therefore no irritation occurs.

However, although it has been used as a suppository base for over 200 years, theobroma oil has now been largely superseded by the newer synthetic bases. The reasons for this are as follows:

- Theobroma oil is polymorphic, i.e. when it is heated and cooled it solidifies in a different crystalline form. If theobroma oil is melted at 36°C and slowly cooled, stable beta crystals (melting point 34.5°C) are formed, but if it is overheated, unstable alpha and gamma crystals are formed, which have a much lower melting point (alpha crystals melt at 23°C and gamma crystals melt at 18°C). These unstable forms do eventually return to the stable form but this may take several days. Meanwhile the preparation is unsuitable for use.
- Theobroma oil shrinks only slightly on cooling and therefore may tend to adhere to the walls of the suppository mould. For this reason the mould must be lubricated before use.

- The relatively low melting point makes it unsuitable for use in hot climates.
- The melting point is reduced if the active ingredients are soluble. This can be counteracted by adding beeswax, but care must be taken not to raise the melting point too high, as the suppository would not melt when inserted into the rectum.
- Theobroma oil deteriorates on storage and is prone to oxidation.
- It does not have a high water-absorbing capacity.
- In common with many naturally occurring substances, the quality of theobroma oil may vary from batch to batch and it can be expensive.

### Synthetic fats

These are prepared by hydrogenating suitable vegetable oils. They have all the advantages but none of the disadvantages of theobroma oil. However, there are one or two points worthy of note.

- The viscosity of the synthetic fats, when melted, is lower than that of theobroma oil. There is, therefore, a greater risk of the active ingredient sedimenting during the preparation process, leading to a lack of uniform drug distribution. This is compensated to a degree in that the synthetic bases set very quickly.
- These bases become brittle if cooled too rapidly, so should not be refrigerated during the preparation period.
- Most manufacturers market a series of grades of synthetic fatty bases, e.g. Witepsol. These have slightly different degrees of hardness and melting point ranges. Release and absorption of the drug in the body may vary depending on the base being used, so any new formulation must be thoroughly investigated prior to marketing.

Further information on these bases can be found in the *Pharmaceutical Codex* (1994).

## Water-soluble and water-miscible bases

### Glycero-gelatin bases

These bases comprise a mixture of glycerol and water, which is stiffened with gelatin. The commonest in use is Mass for Glycerol Suppositories BP which has 14% w/w gelatin and 70% w/w glycerol. In hot climates the gelatin content can be increased to 18% w/w. Gelatin is a purified protein produced by the hydrolysis of the collagenous tissue of animals such as skins and bones. Grades of gelatin for phar-

maceutical use must be heat treated during their preparation to ensure that the product is pathogen free.

Two types of gelatin are used for pharmaceutical purposes, Type A, which is prepared by acid hydrolysis and is cationic and Type B, which is prepared by alkaline hydrolysis and is anionic. Type A is compatible with substances such as boric acid and lactic acid while Type B is compatible with substances like ichthammol and zinc oxide. The 'jelly strength' or 'Bloom rating' of gelatin is important, particularly when it is used in the preparation of suppositories or pessaries.

This type of base is less frequently used than the fatty bases for a variety of reasons.

- Glycero-gelatin bases have a physiological effect. They dissolve in the mucous secretions of the rectum but, because of the small amount of liquid present, osmosis occurs. This is useful if a laxative effect is required but otherwise is undesirable.
- They are much more difficult to prepare and handle.
- The solution time depends on the content and quality of the gelatin and also the age of the suppository.
- They are hygroscopic and therefore require careful storage and may cause rectal irritation.
- Because of the water content, microbial contamination is more likely than with the fatty bases. Preservatives may require to be added to the product, which in turn can lead to problems of incompatibilities.

### Macrogols

These are polyethylene glycols which are blended together to produce suppository bases which vary in melting point, dissolution rates and physical characteristics. High polymers produce preparations which release the drug slowly. They are also brittle. Less brittle products which release the drug more readily can be prepared by mixing high polymers with medium and low polymers. Drug is released as the base dissolves in the rectal contents. Details of combinations which are used are found in the *Pharmaceutical Codex* (1994 p. 172). Macrogols have several properties which make them ideal suppository bases.

*Advantages:*

- They have no physiological effect, e.g. do not produce a laxative effect.
- They are not prone to microbial contamination.
- Some polymers have a high melting point.

These are useful for drugs which lower the melting point of other bases.

- They have a high water-absorbing capacity.
- In solution, viscosity is high, which means there is less likelihood of leakage from the body.

*Disadvantages:*

- They are hygroscopic which means they must be carefully stored. Irritation of the rectal mucosa can also occur. This can be alleviated by dipping the suppository in water prior to insertion.
- They are incompatible with several drugs and materials, e.g. benzocaine, penicillin and plastic. The latter can cause problems when choosing packaging material.
- They become brittle if cooled too quickly and also may become brittle on storage.
- Crystal growth occurs with some active ingredients. This can cause irritation in the rectal mucosa and if the crystals are large, dissolution time may be prolonged.

## PREPARATION OF SUPPOSITORIES

Suppositories are made using a suppository mould (Fig. 15.1). The mould is generally made of metal in two halves which are clamped together with a screw. The internal surface is normally plated. This ensures that the suppositories have a smooth surface.

Before use it is essential to ensure that the mould is completely clean and it should be washed carefully in warm, soapy water and thoroughly dried. Care should be taken not to scratch the internal surface.

The moulds are made in four sizes, 1 g, 2 g, 4 g and 8 g. Unless otherwise stated, the 1 g size is used. The same moulds are used to prepare pessaries, when the two larger sizes are generally used. The capacity of a suppository mould is nominal and each mould will have minor variations. In addition, because they are filled by volume, the weight of material contained in each mould will vary, depending on the base being used. It is therefore essential that each mould is calibrated for each different base.

## Mould calibration

The capacity of the mould is confirmed by filling the mould with the chosen base. The total weight of the perfect products is taken and a mean weight calculated. This value is the calibration value of the mould for that particular base.

---

**EXAMPLE 15.1**

A 1 g suppository mould is to be used to prepare a batch of suppositories. The base to be used is a synthetic fat, Witepsol. Some base is melted in an evaporating basin, over a water-bath. When about two-thirds of the base has melted the basin is removed from the heat. The contents of the basin are stirred and the remaining base melts with the residual heat. Continue stirring the base until it is almost on the point of setting. The base is then poured into the mould cavities, slightly overfilling to allow for shrinkage. After about 5 minutes the domed tops are trimmed off. The unmedicated

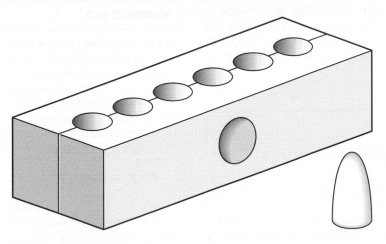

**Fig. 15.1** Dispensing suppository mould.

suppositories are then left to set. Depending on room temperature this may take about a further 10–15 minutes. The mould is then opened and the suppositories removed. Only the perfect products should be weighed. Any which are chipped or damaged should be discarded.

From the above exercise five perfect products were obtained. The total weight was 5.05 g. The mould calibration figure is therefore 5.05/5 = 1.01 g. This is the value which should be used for that particular mould and for that base.

## Displacement values

The volume of a suppository from a particular mould is uniform but its weight will vary because the density of the medicaments usually differs from the density of the base. For example a drug which has twice the density of the base will occupy half the volume which the base occupies, and a drug whose density is a quarter that of the base will occupy four times the volume which the same weight of base occupies. Allowance must be made for this by using displacement values (DVs).

The displacement value of a drug is the number of parts by weight of drug which displaces 1 part by weight of the base.

Displacement values for a variety of medicaments are given in Table 15.1. Other reference sources such as the *Pharmaceutical Handbook* (Wade 1980) and the *Pharmaceutical Codex* also give information on displacement values. Minor variations may occur in the values quoted so it is always advisable to indicate the source of your information.

Displacement values in the literature normally refer to values for theobroma oil. These values can be used for other fatty bases. For glycero-gelatin suppository base approximately 1.2 g occupies the same volume as 1 g of theobroma oil. Using this information the relevant displacement values can be calculated.

**Table 15.1  Displacement values with respect to fatty bases**

| Medicament | Displacement value |
|---|---|
| Aspirin | 1.1 |
| Bismuth subgallate | 2.7 |
| Chloral hydrate | 1.4 |
| Cinchocaine hydrochloride | 1.0 |
| Codeine phosphate | 1.1 |
| Hamamelis dry extract | 1.5 |
| Hydrocortisone | 1.5 |
| Ichthammol | 1.0 |
| Liquids | 1.0 |
| Metronidazole | 1.7 |
| Morphine hydrochloride | 1.6 |
| Paracetamol | 1.5 |
| Pethidine hydrochloride | 1.6 |
| Phenobarbitone | 1.1 |
| Zinc oxide | 4.7 |

A 1 g mould is used with mould calibration = 1.
Weight of bismuth subgallate = 8 × 300 mg = 2.4 g.
DV of bismuth subgallate = 2.7.
2.4 g of bismuth subgallate will displace 1/2.7 × 2.4 g of base = 0.89 g base.
The weight of base required to prepare eight unmedicated suppositories = 8 × 1 = 8 g.
Therefore, weight of base required for medicated suppositories = 8 − 0.89 = 7.21 g.

There may be occasions when information on the DV of a drug is not available. In these situations the DV must be calculated.

---

**EXAMPLE 15.3**

**To calculate the DV of a drug**
A batch of unmedicated suppositories is prepared and the products weighed.

A batch of suppositories containing a known concentration of the required drug is prepared and the products are weighed.
Weight of six unmedicated suppositories = 6 g.
Weight of six suppositories containing 40% drug = 8.8 g.
Weight of base in this  = 60%
= 60/100 × 8.8
= 5.28 g.
Weight of drug in suppositories  = 40%
= 40/100 × 8.8
= 3.52 g.

---

**EXAMPLE 15.2**

Prepare six suppositories each containing 300 mg bismuth subgallate.

To allow for unavoidable wastage calculate for eight suppositories.
DV of bismuth subgallate = 2.7 (*Pharmaceutical Codex*), i.e. 2.7 g of bismuth subgallate displaces 1 g of base.

Weight of base displaced by drug $= 6 - 5.28$
$= 0.72$ g.

If 0.72 g of drug is displaced by 3.52 g of base, then 1 g of base will be displaced by 3.52/0.72 g = 4.88 g.

Therefore displacement value of drug = 4.9 (rounded to one decimal place).

*Calculation of quantities when the active ingredient is stated as a percentage*

A displacement value is not required when calculating quantities stated as percentages.

---

**EXAMPLE 15.4**

Prepare eight suppositories containing 18% zinc oxide.

| | |
|---|---|
| Calculate for 10 suppositories | |
| Mould calibration | $= 1$ |
| Weight of base required to fill mould | $= 10 \times 1$ |
| | $= 10$ g. |
| Zinc oxide is 18% of total | $= 1.8$ g |
| Weight of base required | $= 10 - 1.8$ |
| | $= 8.2$ g. |

---

*Calculation of quantities where more than one active ingredient is present*

In this situation the quantity of each medicament is calculated and the amount of base is calculated using the displacement value for each ingredient.

---

**EXAMPLE 15.5**

Calculate the quantities required to make 15 suppositories each containing 150 mg hamamelis dry extract and 560 mg of zinc oxide. A 2 g mould is to be used.

Calculate for 18 suppositories.
Mould calibration = 2.04.
DV of hamamelis dry extract = 1.5 (PC).
DV of zinc oxide = 4.7 (PC).

| | |
|---|---|
| Weight of hamamelis dry extract | $= 18 \times 0.15$ |
| | $= 2.7$ g. |
| Weight of zinc oxide | $= 18 \times 0.56$ |
| | $= 10.08$ g. |
| Weight of base | $= 18 \times 2.04 - (2.7/1.5 +$ |
| | $10.08/4.7)$ |

$= 36.72 - (1.8 + 2.14)$
$= 32.78$ g.

---

## Preparation of suppositories containing an active ingredient which is insoluble in the base

The bases used most commonly for extemporaneous preparation of suppositories and pessaries are the synthetic fats and glycero-gelatin base.

1. It is always advisable when calculating the quantity of ingredients to calculate for an excess to allow for unavoidable wastage, e.g. if required to prepare 12 suppositories, calculate for 14.
2. The mould should be carefully washed and dried.
3. Ensure that the two halves fit together correctly. This is necessary to ensure that there is no leakage of material.
4. For some bases the mould will need to be lubricated. The lubricants are given in Table 15.2.
5. If lubricant is necessary, apply it carefully to the two halves of the mould using gauze or non-fibrous material. Do not use cotton wool as fibres may be left on the mould surface and become incorporated into the suppositories.
6. Invert the mould to allow any excess lubricant to drain off.
7. Accurately weigh the required amount of base. If large lumps are present the material should be grated.
8. Place in a porcelain basin and put on a water-bath, over gentle heat. Allow approximately two-thirds of the base to melt and remove from the heat. The residual heat will be sufficient for the rest of the base to melt.
9. Reduce the particle size of the active ingredient, if necessary. This will be done by either grinding in a mortar and pestle or sieving.
10. Weigh the correct amount of medicament and place on a glass tile.
11. Add about half of the molten base to the powdered drug and rub together with a spatula.

| Table 15.2 Lubricants for use with suppository bases | |
|---|---|
| Base | Lubricant |
| Theobroma oil | Soap spirit |
| Glycero-gelatin base | Almond or arachis oil |
| Witepsol | No lubricant required |
| Macrogols | No lubricant required |

12. Scrape this mixture off the tile, using the spatula and place back into the porcelain basin.

13. If necessary, put the basin back over the water-bath to re-melt the ingredients.

14. Remove from the heat and stir constantly until almost on the point of setting. If the mixture is not stirred at this stage the active ingredient will sediment and uniform distribution of the drug will not be achieved.

15. Quickly pour into the mould, slightly overfilling each cavity. This is to allow for contraction on cooling. Do not be tempted to start pouring the suppositories while the mixture is still very molten. If this is done, the drug sediments to the bottom of the mould, the base shrinks and the tops become concave.

16. Leave the mould and its contents to cool for about 5 minutes and then, using a spatula, trim the tops of the suppositories. Do not leave the suppositories too long before trimming as they will be too hard and trimming becomes very difficult.

17. Allow to cool for another 10–15 minutes until the suppositories are completely firm and set. Do not be tempted to speed up the cooling process by putting the mould in a refrigerator. Synthetic fats, in particular, are inclined to become brittle and break if cooled too quickly.

18. Unscrew the mould and remove the suppositories

19. Each perfect suppository should then be carefully wrapped in greaseproof paper, packed in an appropriate container and labelled.

When preparing suppositories where the active ingredient is a semi-solid, is soluble in the base or is a liquid which is miscible with the base the melting point of the base is lowered. In these situations a base with a higher than normal melting point needs to be used. The base is melted as normal and the active ingredient is added directly to the base and incorporated by stirring.

## Preparation of suppositories using a glycero-gelatin base

The formula for Glycerol Suppository Base BP is:

| | |
|---|---|
| Gelatin | 14% |
| Glycerol | 70% |
| Water | to 100% |

1. The gelatin strip is cut into small pieces, approximately 1 cm square, trimming off any hard outer edges.

2. The correct amount of gelatin is weighed out and placed in a previously weighed, porcelain evaporating basin.

3. Sufficient water to just cover the gelatin is added and the contents left for about 5 minutes.

4. When the gelatin has softened any excess water is drained off. This step is not necessary if powdered gelatin is being used.

5. The exact amount of glycerol is then weighed into the basin.

6. The basin is placed on a water-bath, over gentle heat and the mixture gently stirred until the gelatin has melted. Do not stir vigorously as this will cause air bubbles to become incorporated. At this stage the base may need to be heat treated as noted below.

7. When the gelatin is melted the basin is removed from the heat and weighed. If the weight is less than the required total, water is added, to the correct weight. If the contents of the basin are too heavy it must be put back on the heat and the excess water evaporated off.

8. When the correct weight is achieved the active ingredient is added, with careful stirring.

9. The mixture is then poured into the prepared mould, lubricated with either arachis or almond oil. It is not necessary to overfill the moulds and this type of product does not require to be trimmed.

10. The preparation is left to set. After unmoulding each should then be smeared with liquid paraffin before being wrapped in greaseproof paper.

*Note:* Gelatin which is of a grade suitable for pharmaceutical use should not contain any pathogens but as a precaution, the base may be heat treated. This is done by heating the base for 1 hour at 100°C in an electric steamer. This should be done before the base is adjusted to weight (at Stage 7 above).

This base is commonly used for the preparation of pessaries, as described in the following example.

---

**EXAMPLE 15.6**

Prepare 10 pessaries containing 10% ichthammol. A 4 g mould is used.

Calculate for 14 pessaries to allow for wastage.
  Mould calibration for glycero-gelatin base is 4.8 (4 × 1.2 g).

  Displacement value is not required as the active ingredient, ichthammol, is expressed as a percentage.

  Formula for the base:

| | |
|---|---|
| Gelatin | 14 g |
| Glycerol | 70 g |
| Water | to 100 g |

Formula for the pessaries:

| | |
|---|---|
| Ichthammol | 10% w/w |
| Glycero-gelatin base | 90% w/w |

The total weight required to prepare the pessaries is $14 \times 4.8$ g = 67.2 g. For ease of calculation prepare 70 g.

Quantities are therefore:

| | |
|---|---|
| Ichthammol | 7 g |
| Base | 63 g |

It is advisable to make a small excess of base, taking care to choose quantities which give easily weighable amounts, i.e. do not try to weigh to several decimal points. In this case 65 g can be prepared.

Using the method described above, prepare the chosen quantity of the base. Take care that the correct type of gelatin is chosen. Because the active ingredient is ichthammol, Type B should be used.

When the 65 g of base has been prepared 2 g should be removed from the basin, leaving the required 63 g. The base is removed from the heat, allowed to cool and 7 g of ichthammol added, with careful stirring. The mixture is then poured into the lubricated mould and left to set.

## CONTAINERS FOR SUPPOSITORIES

Glass or plastic screw-topped jars are possibly the best choice of container for extemporaneously prepared suppositories and pessaries. Cardboard cartons may be used but these offer little protection from moisture or heat. They are therefore not suitable for hygroscopic materials.

## LABELLING FOR SUPPOSITORIES

Adequate information should appear on the label so that the patient knows how to use the product. In addition the following information should appear:

- 'Store in a cool place'
- 'For rectal use only' or 'For vaginal use only', whichever is appropriate.

'Do not swallow' can be put on the label but do not use 'For external use only'. The preparation is being inserted into a body cavity and this instruction is therefore incorrect.

An expiry date should be indicated for all extemporaneously prepared products. As long as they are well packaged and the storage temperature is low, suppositories and pessaries are relatively stable preparations. Unless other information is available, an expiry date of 1 month is appropriate.

## PATIENT ADVICE

In addition to what appears on the label, patients should be told to unwrap the suppository or pessary (this may appear to be unnecessary advice but there is sufficient evidence to show that it is not always done) and insert it as high as possible into the rectum or vagina. It may be helpful to provide the patient with a diagram and instruction leaflet, such as that produced by the National Pharmaceutical Association (see Ch. 37).

---

### Key Points

- Bases may be fatty or water miscible.
- Synthetic bases, made from hydrogenated vegetable oils are easier to use than theobroma oil.
- Glycero-gelatin base produces a laxative effect.
- Type A (anionic) or Type B (cationic) gelatin can be used to avoid incompatibilities.
- Because glycero-gelatin base has a higher density than fatty bases, moulds hold approximately 1.2 times the nominal weight.
- Macrogol bases are blends of high and low molecular weight polymers which dissolve in rectal contents.
- Suppository moulds have nominal capacities of 1, 2, 4 and 8 g and must be calibrated with the base to be used.
- Unless the density of the drug and base are the same, a displacement value is required to calculate the amount of base displaced by the drug.
- When using theobroma oil and glycero-gelatin base the mould has to be lubricated.
- To allow for contraction on cooling, overfilling with oily bases is required.
- Labels should include either 'For rectal use only' or 'For vaginal use only' and 'Store in a cool place'.

## FURTHER READING

Aulton M E 1988 Pharmaceutics: the science of dosage form design. Churchill Livingstone, Edinburgh

British National Formulary, current edn. British Medical Association and Royal Pharmaceutical Society of Great Britain, London (Updated twice yearly)

British Pharmacopoeia 1988 HMSO, London

British Pharmacopoeia 1993 HMSO, London

Pharmaceutical Codex 1979 11th edn. Pharmaceutical Press, London

Pharmaceutical Codex 1994 12th edn. Pharmaceutical Press, London

Pharmaceutical Society 1988 Information leaflets. Pharmaceutical Journal 240: 98

Wade A (ed) 1980 Pharmaceutical handbook, 19th edn. Pharmaceutical Press, London

# 16
# Powders and granules

*E. J. Kennedy*

> After studying this chapter, the reader will know:
>
> **The pharmaceutical uses of powders**
> **Bulk and divided powders**
> **The mixing of powders**
> **Diluents used with powders**
> **Calculations required when preparing powders**
> **How to dispense powders**
> **The folding of powders**.

## Introduction

A powder may be defined as solid material in a finely divided state. Granules are powders agglomerated to produce larger free-flowing particles. Most medicinal products in use today occur in powdered or crystalline form. Powders and granules are used to prepare other formulations, such as solutions, suspensions and tablets. Powders may be used as pharmaceutical preparations for oral administration of a drug, when it is usually mixed with water first, or for external application. A single active ingredient may be presented as powders, called a simple powder or may be blended with different ingredients. These are termed 'compound powders', for example compound tragacanth powder.

## POWDERS FOR INTERNAL USE

Powders for oral administration will comprise the active ingredients with excipients such as diluents, sweeteners and dispersing agents. These may be presented as undivided powders (bulk powders) or divided powders (individually wrapped doses).

Magnesium Trisilicate Powder, Compound BP and Compound Kaolin Powder BP are examples of bulk powders for internal use. Proprietary powders and granules include Dioralyte, Rehidrat (oral rehydration salts), Normacol (sterculia) and Fybogel (ispaghula husk). Individually wrapped powders tend not to be official formulas (see Examples 16.1 and 16.2).

## Bulk powders

Bulk powders can be dispensed to the patient although this is rarely seen nowadays because the dosage form is inconvenient to carry around and there are possible inaccuracies in measuring the dose. Supplying an undivided powder is useful for non-potent, bulky drugs with a large dose, for example antacids, and when the dry powder is more stable than its liquid-containing counterpart. Some liquid mixtures may be prepared in the pharmacy from a bulk powder by the addition of a specific volume of water, for example, Magnesium Trisilicate Mixture BP. This reduces transport and packaging costs.

## Individually wrapped powders

Individually wrapped powders are used to supply some potent drugs, where accuracy of dose is extremely important. Extemporaneously produced powders are wrapped separately in paper. They are convenient dosage forms for children's doses of drugs which are not commercially available at the particular strength, such as aspirin and phenobarbitone (see Example 16.2). Sealed sachets of powders are available commercially, for example Paramax (paracetamol and metoclopramide), Stemetil (prochlorperazine) and oral rehydration sachets. They are mixed with water prior to taking and are useful for patients who have difficulty swallowing or where rapid absorption of the drug is required.

## GRANULES FOR INTERNAL USE

Some preparations are supplied to the pharmacy as granules, for reconstitution immediately before dispensing, for example antibiotic suspensions. This protects drugs which are susceptible to hydrolysis, or other degradation, in the presence of water until absolutely necessary in order to give an adequate shelf life (see Ch. 12).

### Particle size

The particle size of a powder is described using standard descriptions given in the *British Pharmacopoeia* (BP). These refer to the standardized sieve size that they are capable of passing through in a specified time under shaking, or to the particle size determined microscopically. Thus powders for oral use would normally be a 'moderately fine' or a 'fine' powder. The former is able to pass through a sieve of nominal mesh aperture $355\,\mu m$ and the latter of $180\,\mu m$. Comminution is the process of particle size reduction. On a small scale, this can be done using a mortar and pestle when it is often called trituration. This is a common first step in dispensing, after which the powder should be passed through a sieve of appropriate size before weighing.

### Mixing the powder

Ingredients of powders should be mixed thoroughly, using the technique of 'doubling-up' to ensure an even distribution. This process involves starting with the ingredient which has the smallest bulk. In Example 16.1 this would be hyoscine hydrobromide. The other ingredient(s) are added in approximately equal parts by volume. In this way the amount in the mortar is approximately doubled at each addition. Mixing in between additions continues until all the ingredients are incorporated. The powder can then be packed.

### Preparing individually wrapped powders

The minimum weight of an individually wrapped powder is $120\,mg$. Dilution of a drug with a diluent, usually lactose, is often necessary to produce this weight.

Occasionally manufactured tablets or capsules may be used to prepare oral powders. This involves crushing the tablet in a mortar and pestle, or emptying the contents of the capsule and adding a suitable diluent. Lactose is used as a diluent because it is colourless, odourless, soluble and generally harmless. It also has good flow properties. Some patients may be unable to tolerate lactose and a suitable inert alternative diluent, for instance light kaolin, would then be used.

## Powder calculations

Quantities should be calculated to allow for loss of powder during manipulation. It is usual to allow for at least one extra powder. If the total amount of active ingredient required is less than the minimum weighable quantity, dilutions will be necessary. In this process, also called trituration, the minimum quantity of the active ingredient(s) is weighed and diluted, over several steps if necessary, in order to obtain the dose(s) required. Example 16.1 illustrates the process where two dilution steps are required.

---

**EXAMPLE 16.1**

℞ Hyoscine hydrobromide 300 micrograms
Mitte 4 powders
Label 'One to be given 30 minutes before the journey'.

**Action and uses**
Antimuscarinic drug used in the prevention of motion sickness.

**Calculation and method of preparation**
Calculate for five powders. Use lactose as the diluent, each powder to weigh 120 mg.

Hyoscine hydrobromide $(5 \times 300) =$  1.5 mg
(1500 μg)
Lactose $(5 \times 120\ mg)$  to 600 mg

The minimum weighable quantity (Class B balance) is 100 mg.

*Step 1*
Hyoscine hydrobromide  100 mg
Lactose  900 mg

Mix, by doubling-up and remove 100 mg (triturate A). 100 mg of triturate A contains:
$100 \div 1000 \times 100 = 10$ mg hyoscine hydrobromide.

*Step 2*
Triturate A  100 mg
Lactose  900 mg

Mix, by doubling-up and remove 150 mg (triturate B). 150 mg of triturate B contains:
$10 \div 1000 \times 150 = 1.5$ mg hyoscine hydrobromide.

---

*Step 3*

| | |
|---|---|
| Triturate B | 150 mg |
| Lactose (5 × 120 mg − 150 mg) | 450 mg |

Mix, by doubling-up. 120 mg portions of this final powder will contain 300 micrograms of hyoscine hydrobromide. Weigh 120 mg aliquots and wrap in a powder paper.

## Folding papers

White glazed paper, called demy paper, is used for wrapping powders. A suitable size is 120 mm × 100 mm. The wrapping should be carried out on a clean tile or larger sheet of demy to protect the product. The papers should be folded with their long edges parallel to the front of the bench. Follow the steps illustrated in Figure 16.1 in order to fold the paper.

The long edge, furthest away from the dispenser, should be turned over to about one-seventh of the paper width (step A).

The powder should be weighed accurately and placed towards the folded edge of the paper (step B).

The unfolded long edge should then be brought over the powder to meet the crease of the turned edge (step C).

This upturned edge should then be folded over (towards the front of the dispenser) so that it covers about half the powder packet (step D).

The short edges of the powder packet should be folded over, using a powder cradle, if available, so that the flaps are of equal lengths and the folded powder fits neatly into a box or jar (steps E and F).

The creases can be sharpened with a spatula, taking care not to tear the paper or use excessive pressure which would compress the powder inside the pack.

The powders can be packed in pairs, back to back, or in one bundle, with the final powder placed back to back. They should be held together with an elastic band. In a well-wrapped product, there will be no powder in the fold or flaps, so that all the powder is available for easy administration when unwrapped.

Powders are subject to a uniformity of weight test, or uniformity of content test if each dose contains less than 2 mg of active ingredient or the content of active ingredient represents less than 2% of the total weight.

## Shelf life and storage of internal powders

Extemporaneously prepared powders should have an expiry of between 2 and 4 weeks. Proprietary

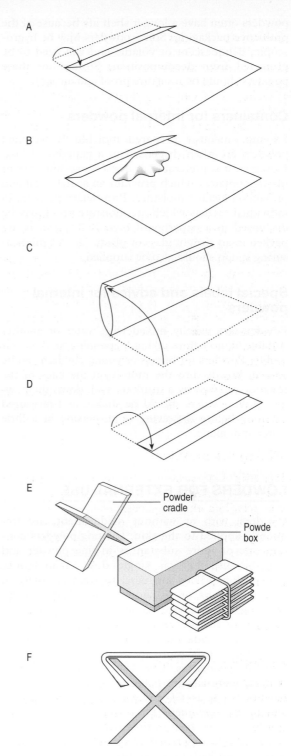

**Fig. 16.1**  Steps for the folding of individually wrapped powders.

powders often have a longer shelf life because of the protective packaging. Some powders may be hygroscopic, deliquescent or volatile and will need to be protected from decomposition. Storage for these powders should be moisture proof and airtight.

## Containers for internal powders

Extemporaneously prepared individually wrapped powders are often dispensed in a paperboard box. However, it is preferable to use a screw-top glass or plastic container which provides an airtight seal and protection against moisture. Proprietary powders in individual sachets which are moisture proof may be dispensed in a paperboard box. Bulk powders are packed in an airtight glass or plastic jar. A 5 ml measuring spoon should also be supplied.

## Special labels and advice for internal powders

Powders are usually mixed with water or another suitable liquid before taking, depending on their solubility. Powders for babies or young children can be placed directly into the mouth on the back of the tongue, followed by a drink to wash down the powder. Bulk powders should be shaken and measured carefully before dissolving or dispersing in a little water and taking.

## POWDERS FOR EXTERNAL USE

Powders, with or without medicament, are frequently applied to the skin. Dusting powders contain one or more substances in fine powder and may be dispensed as single dose or multidose preparations. They are used to treat a variety of skin conditions or to soothe skin. Examples are antifungal powders for athlete's foot or talc dusting powder for the prevention of chafing and skin irritation. Zinc oxide and starch are added to formulations to absorb moisture and talc is used for lubricant properties. Talc, kaolin and other natural mineral materials are liable to contamination with bacteria such as *Clostridium tetani, C. perfringens* and *Bacillus anthracis*. These ingredients should be sterilized by dry heat or the final product should be sterilized. Dusting powders should be sterile if they may be applied to large areas of open skin or wounds. They should not be used where there is a likelihood of large volumes of exudate, as hard crusts will form.

## Preparing powders for external use

A sieve size of 180 μm should be used to obtain the finely divided powder. The constituents should be mixed using the doubling-up method, as described previously.

## Shelf life and storage for powders for external use

Dry powders should remain stable over a long period of time if packaged and protected from the atmosphere. For extemporaneously prepared products, a maximum expiry of 4 weeks is reasonable.

## Containers for powders for external use

Powders for external use may be packed in glass, metal or plastic containers with a sifter-type cap. Some are also available commercially in pressurized containers, containing other excipients such as a propellant and lubricants.

## Special labels and advice for powders for external use

- For external use only
- Store in a cool, dry place

Examples of official powders for external use include Zinc Oxide Dusting Powder Compound BPC, Chlorhexidine Dusting Powder BP, Talc Dusting Powder BP. Proprietary examples of powders for external use include Daktarin (miconazole), Cicatrin (neomycin sulphate, bacitracin zinc, cysteine, glycine and threonine) and Ster-zac powder (hexachlorophene, zinc oxide, talc and starch).

---

**EXAMPLE 16.2**

Send 10 aspirin powders for a child of 3 years (14 kg).

|  | For 1 powder | For 12 powders |
|---|---|---|
| Aspirin | 200 mg | 2.4 g |

**Action and uses**
Non-steroidal anti-inflammatory drug, used to treat juvenile arthritis at a dose of 80 mg/kg, five to six times daily.

**Formulation notes**
Diluent is not required, since the weight of each

powder will be above the minimum 120 mg required. Manufactured 300 mg aspirin tablets can be used to prepare these powders.

## Method of preparation

Take 8 × 300 mg aspirin tablets (contain 2.4 g aspirin) and weigh. Grind to a fine powder in mortar and pestle. Pass the resulting powder through a 250 μm sieve and lightly remix. Divide the original weight of tablets by 12, and weigh aliquots of the resulting amount of powder. Pack into individual powder papers. Fasten the 10 powders together with an elastic band and pack in an amber glass jar or plastic container with a screw cap.

## Shelf life and storage

Store in a cool, dry place. A short shelf life of about 2 weeks is appropriate.

## Advice and special labels

The powders should be given after food, in water (or directly into the child's mouth, followed by a drink of water).

---

## EXAMPLE 16.3

℞ Zinc, Starch and Talc Dusting Powder BPC. Mitte 100 g.

|  | Master formula | For 100 g |
|---|---|---|
| Zinc oxide | 25% | 25 g |
| Starch | 25% | 25 g |
| Sterilized purified talc | 50% | 50 g |

## Action and uses

A soothing preparation to absorb moisture and act as a lubricant, preventing friction in skin folds.

## Method of preparation

Sieve the powders, using a 180 μm sieve, weigh and mix them by doubling-up in a mortar and pestle. Pack in an amber glass jar or plastic container with a screw cap (with a perforated, recloseable lid if possible).

## Shelf life and storage

Store in a dry place.

## Advice and special labels

Lightly dust the powder onto the affected area. The area should not be too wet as the powder will cake and abrade the skin. It should not be applied to broken skin or large raw areas.

---

## EXAMPLE 16.4

℞ Compound Magnesium Trisilicate Oral Powder BP 1988. Mitte 200 g.

|  | Master formula | For 200 g |
|---|---|---|
| Magnesium trisilicate | 250 mg | 50 g |
| Chalk | 250 mg | 50 g |
| Heavy magnesium carbonate | 250 mg | 50 g |
| Sodium bicarbonate | 250 mg | 50 g |

## Action and uses

Antacid preparation for dyspepsia.

## Method of preparation

Sieve the powders, using a 250 μm sieve, weigh and mix them by doubling-up, using a mortar and pestle. Pack in an amber glass jar or plastic container with a screw cap.

## Shelf life and storage

Store in a dry place. A 4-week expiry date is reasonable if kept dry.

## Advice and special labels

A normal dose is 1–5 g of the powder taken in liquid, when required. Antacids are usually taken between meals and at bedtime.

---

## Key Points

- Powders may be prepared as bulk powders, divided powders or granules.
- Powders may be used internally or externally.
- The particle size of a fine powder should be less than 180 μm.
- The minimum weight of a divided powder is 120 mg.
- Lactose is a good diluent for internal powders.
- Trituration is the process used to obtain small doses which are below the minimum weighable quantity.
- Ideally powders should be packed in a glass or plastic container.
- A 5 ml spoon should be provided with bulk powders for oral use.
- When dispensing divided powders, an excess of one or two should be prepared to allow for loss during processing.

# FURTHER READING

ABPI Compendium of data sheets and summaries of product characteristics, current edn. Datapharm Publications, London (Updated annually)

Ansel H C, Popovich N G, Allen L V 1995 Pharmaceutical dosage forms and drug delivery systems, 6th edn. Williams & Wilkins, Malvern, USA

British National Formulary, current edn. British Medical Association and Royal Pharmaceutical Society of Great Britain, London (Updated twice yearly)

British Pharmacopeia, current edn. HMSO, London

British Pharmaceutical Codex 1973 Pharmaceutical Press, London

Diluent Directories (Internal and External) current edn. National Pharmaceutical Association, St Albans

Pharmaceutical Codex 1979 11th edn. Pharmaceutical Press, London

Pharmaceutical Codex: principles and practice of pharmaceutics 1994 12th edn. Pharmaceutical Press, London

Reynolds J E F (ed) 1996 Martindale: the extra pharmacopoeia, 31st edn Pharmaceutical Press, London (Updated every 3 years – use current edn)

Wade A (ed) 1980 Pharmaceutical handbook, 19th edn. Pharmaceutical Press, London

# 17

# Oral unit dosage forms

*E. J. Kennedy*

---

After studying this chapter the reader will know about:

**Different types of tablets**
**Excipients used in tablets and capsules**
**Dispensing commercially produced tablets and capsules**
**Extemporaneous dispensing of capsules**
**Pastilles and cachets**.

## Introduction

Tablets and capsules are the most popular way of delivering a drug for oral use. They are convenient for the patient and are usually easy to handle and identify. A high accuracy of dosage is achievable with oral unit dosage forms and they are free from the problems of stability found in aqueous mixtures and suspensions. Packaging in blister packs can enhance the stability of these dosage forms (see Ch. 6). They are mass produced on a commercial scale at a relatively low manufacturing cost. Their main disadvantage is that some people cannot swallow solid oral dosage forms, for example the very young or very old.

## TABLETS

Tablets are solid preparations each containing a single dose of one or more active ingredients. They are normally prepared by compressing uniform volumes of particles, although some tablets are prepared by moulding. The process of tablet production is not covered here, please refer to Aulton (1988) or the *Pharmaceutical Codex*.

Many different types of tablets are available which may be in a variety of shapes and sizes. The types include dispersible or effervescent, chewable, sublingual and buccal tablets, lozenges, tablets for vaginal administration and solution tablets. Some tablets are designed to release the medication slowly for prolonged drug release and sustained drug action (see Ch. 10).

In addition to the active ingredient, several excipients, or inactive ingredients must be added. These will aid the process of tableting and ensure that the active ingredient will be released in the body as intended. Excipients include:

1. Diluents or fillers. These add bulk to make the tablet easier to handle. Examples include lactose, mannitol, microcrystalline cellulose and calcium carbonate.

2. Binders or adhesives. These enable granules to be prepared which improves flow properties of the mixture and compression. Examples include acacia, mucilage, glucose, povidone and starch mucilage.

3. Disintegrators or disintegrating agents. These ensure that the tablet breaks down into its component particles after ingestion. Examples include sodium alginate, carmellose sodium, microcrystalline cellulose, sodium glycine carbonate and starch.

4. Antiadherents, glidants, lubricants or lubricating agents. These are essential for flow of the tablet material into the tablet dies and preventing sticking of the compressed tablet in the punch and die. Examples of lubricants are magnesium and calcium stearate, sodium lauryl sulphate and sodium stearyl fumarate. Finely divided silica is usually the glidant of choice.

5. Miscellaneous agents may be added, such as colours and flavours in chewable tablets.

Some tablets have coatings, such as sugar coating or film coating. Coatings can protect the tablet from environmental damage, mask an unpleasant flavour, aid identification of the tablet and enhance its appearance. Enteric coatings on tablets resist dissolution or

161

disruption of the tablet in the stomach, but not in the intestine. This is useful when a drug is destroyed by gastric acid, is irritating to the gastric mucosa, or when bypassing the stomach aids drug absorption.

## Dispensing of tablets

The majority of tablets in the UK are packaged by the manufacturer into patient packs suitable for issue to the patient without repacking by the pharmacist. Patient information leaflets are also contained in these patient packs. When dispensing these packs to patients, the pharmacist must ensure that they are labelled correctly, according to the prescriber's instructions (see Ch. 8) and that the patient is counselled on the use of the medication (see Ch. 37). For some controlled-release tablets, variations in bioavailability may occur with different brands. It is important that patients are given the brand that they are stabilized on to maintain therapeutic outcome. This applies in particular to formulations of theophylline, lithium and phenytoin.

Some tablets will still be supplied in a bulk container. The required number of tablets needs to be counted out (see Ch. 4) and placed in a suitable container for dispensing to the patient (see Ch. 6). It is important to minimize errors by ensuring that the correct bulk container has been selected and the correct drug dispensed. This should be verified by the pharmacist by checking the label of the bulk container and by examining the shape, size and markings on the dispensed tablets where appropriate, with the prescription.

## Shelf life and storage

Most tablets should be stored in air-tight packaging, protected from light and extremes of temperature. When stored properly they generally have a long shelf life. The expiry date will be printed on the package or the individual strip packs. Some tablets need to be stored in a cool place, for example, Ketovite (store between 2 and 8°C) and Leukeran (chlorambucil) (store under 15°C). Some tablets contain volatile drugs, for example glyceryl trinitrate, and must be packed in glass containers with tightly fitting metal screw caps. An additional warning must be placed on the tablets, when dispensed to patients, to advise them to throw away the tablets 8 weeks after opening, as they loose potency.

## Containers

Strip or blister packs are dispensed in a paperboard box and tablets counted from bulk containers are placed in amber glass or plastic containers with air-tight, child-resistant closures.

## Special labels and advice on tablets

Most tablets should be swallowed with a glass or 'draught' of water. A draught of water refers to a volume of water, about 50 ml. This prevents the dosage form becoming lodged in the oesophagus, which can cause problems such as ulceration. Some tablets are coated and shaped to aid swallowing.

Some tablets should be dissolved or dispersed in water before taking, for example effervescent analgesic tablets. Some tablets, particularly those with coatings or modified-release properties, should be swallowed whole. Some tablets should be chewed or sucked before swallowing, for example antacid tablets. Appropriate labels should be placed on the container (see Ch. 8).

If there are coatings on tablets, for example enteric coatings, there will be specific advice on avoidance of indigestion remedies at the same time of day, as these will affect the pH of the stomach, and therefore cause premature breakdown of the enteric coating on the tablet.

Buccal and sublingual tablets are not swallowed whole and it is important that patients know how to use them. If these formulations are swallowed then they will not have their intended therapeutic effect. Figure 17.1 illustrates the positioning for buccal tablets. Sublingual tablets are placed under the tongue.

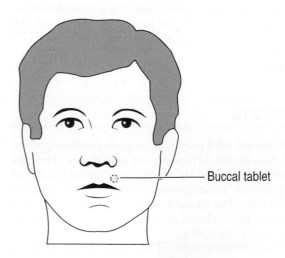

**Fig. 17.1** Positioning of a buccal tablet.

## CAPSULES

Capsules are solid preparations intended for oral administration made with a hard or soft shell. One or more medicaments are enclosed within this gelatin container. Most capsules are swallowed whole, but some contain granules which provide a useful pre-measured dose for administering in a similar way to a powder, for example formulations of pancreatin. Some capsules enclose enteric-coated pellets, for example Erymax (erythromycin). Capsules are elegant, easy to swallow and can be useful in masking unpleasant tastes. Capsules may also be used to hold powder or oils for inhalation, for example Intal capsules (sodium cromoglycate) or Karvol (see Ch. 18) or for rectal and vaginal administration (see Ch. 15).

### Soft shell capsules

A soft gelatin capsule consists of a flexible solid shell containing powders, non-aqueous liquids, solutions, emulsions, suspensions or pastes. Such capsules allow liquids to be given as solid dosage forms, for example cod liver oil. They also offer accurate dosage, improved stability and overcome some of the problems of dealing with powders. They are formed, filled and sealed in one manufacturing process.

### Hard shell capsules

Empty capsule shells are made from a mixture of gelatin, acacia, sugar and water. They are clear, colourless and essentially tasteless. Colourings and markings can be easily added for light protection and easy identification. The shells are used in the preparation of most manufactured capsules and for the extemporaneous compounding of capsules. The shell comprises two sections, the body and the cap, both being cylindrical and sealed at one end. Powder or particulate solid, such as granules and pellets, can be placed in the body and the capsule closed by bringing the body and cap together (see Fig. 17.2). Some capsules have small indentations on the body and cap which 'lock' together. If not, they must be sealed by moistening the outside top of the body before putting the top in place.

### Compounding of capsules

Occasionally hand filling of capsules may be

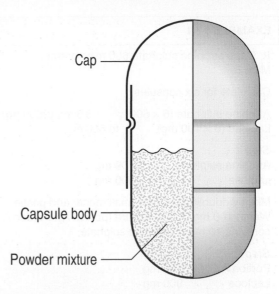

**Fig. 17.2** Hard gelatin capsule shell: body and cap.

**Table 17.1 Sizes of hard gelatin capsules and their approximate capacities**

| Capsule no. | 000 | 00 | 0 | 1 | 2 | 3 | 4 | 5 |
|---|---|---|---|---|---|---|---|---|
| Content (mg) | 950 | 650 | 450 | 300 | 250 | 200 | 150 | 100 |

required, particularly in a hospital pharmacy setting or when preparing materials for clinical trials. A suitable size of capsule shell should be selected so that the finished capsule looks reasonably full. Hard shell capsules are available in eight sizes. These are listed in Table 17.1, with the corresponding approximate capacity (based on lactose). The density of a powder mixture will also affect the choice of capsule size.

### Calculations for compounding capsules

The recommended minimum weight for filling a capsule is 100 mg. If the required weight of the drug is smaller than this a diluent should be added by trituration (see Ch. 16). If the quantity of the drug for a batch of capsules is smaller than the minimum weighable amount, 100 mg, then trituration will also be required. Lactose, magnesium carbonate, starch, kaolin and calcium phosphate are commonly used diluents. To allow for small losses of powder, a small excess should be calculated for, for example an extra capsule. Example 17.1 gives a worked example.

---

**EXAMPLE 17.1**

R. Caps atropine sulphate 600 micrograms.
Mitte 5.

Calculate for six capsules.

Atropine sulphate (6 × 600)    3.6 mg (3600 µg)
Lactose (6 × 100 mg)    to 600 mg

*Step 1*
Atropine sulphate    100 mg
Lactose    900 mg

Mix, by doubling-up, in a small mortar and pestle.
Weigh 100 mg of this mixture (portion A). Portion A
contains 10 mg of atropine sulphate.

*Step 2*
Portion A    100 mg
Lactose    900 mg

Mix, by doubling-up, in a small mortar and pestle.
Weigh 360 mg of this mixture (portion B). Portion B
contains 3.6 mg of atropine sulphate.

*Step 3*
Add sufficient lactose to portion B to make the final
weight up to 600 mg.
   The powder mixture is now ready to be placed
into capsules.

---

## Filling capsules

The number of capsules to be filled should firstly
be taken and set aside. This avoids the danger of
contaminating empty capsules. The powder to be
encapsulated should be prepared and finely sifted
(250 µm sieve). Magnesium stearate (up to 1%
w/w) and silica may be added as a lubricant and glidant respectively, to aid filling of the capsule.
Various methods of filling capsules on a small scale
are possible.

### Filling from a powder mass

The prepared powder can be placed on a clean tile
and powder pushed into the capsule body with the
aid of a spatula, until the required weight has been
enclosed. The empty capsule body could also be
'punched' into a heap of powder until filled.
Alternatively create a small funnel from white
paper and fill the capsule body with the required
weight. Gloves or rubber finger cots should be
worn to protect the capsules from handling with
bare fingers.

### Filling with weighed aliquots

Weighed aliquots of powder may be placed on paper
and channelled into the empty capsule shell.
Alternatively, simple apparatus is useful for small-
scale manufacture of larger numbers of capsules. A
plastic plate with rows of cavities to hold the empty
capsule bodies is used, different rows holding different sizes of capsules. A plastic bridge containing
a row of holes corresponding to the position of the
capsule cavities can then be used to support a long-
stemmed funnel. The end of the funnel passes into
the mouth of the capsule below. The stem of the
funnel should be as wide as possible for the size of
the capsule. A weighed aliquot of powder can then
be poured into the capsule via the funnel. A thin
glass or plastic rod or wire may be used as a 'tamper' to break blockages or to compress the material
inside the capsule. After filling the capsule, the top
can be fitted loosely and the weight checked before
sealing.

Capsules are subject to tests of uniformity of weight
and content of active ingredient and uniformity of
content where the content of active ingredient is less
than 2 mg or less than 2% by weight of the total capsule fill.

## Shelf life and storage

If stability data are not available for extemporaneously filled capsules, then a short expiry date, up to
4 weeks, should be given. Manufactured capsules
will generally be very stable and will be assigned
expiry dates on the container or on the packed
strips or blister packs. Most capsules need to be
stored in a cool, dry place. Some capsules need to
be stored in a cool place, for example Restandol
(testosterone), which needs to be stored in the
refrigerator until it is dispensed to the patient,
when it can be stored at room temperature for
3 months.

## Containers

Containers used are similar to those for tablets.
Some capsules are susceptible to moisture absorption, and desiccants may be included in the packaging, either integrally (for example in the cap of the
container for Losec capsules) or as separate units.
These capsules have a limited shelf life once dispensed to a patient. Desiccants should not be dispensed to patients, in case they are mistaken for a
capsule and ingested.

## Special labels and advice on capsules

Capsules should be swallowed whole with a glass of water or other liquid. Advice may be sought from the pharmacist about whether it is acceptable to empty the contents of a capsule onto food or into water for ease of swallowing. In giving this advice, the release characteristics of the dosage form should be considered; for instance, whether there is an enteric coating or a prolonged-release formulation. Additional labels and advice may be required for capsules, depending on the drug contained.

## OTHER ORAL UNIT DOSAGE FORMS

## Pastilles

These contain a glycerol and gelatin base. They are sweetened, flavoured and medicated and are popular over-the-counter remedies for soothing coughs and sore throats.

## Cachets

These are very rarely used in practice today. They are made from rice flour and each cachet comes in two halves ready to be filled with powder. They are available as dry seal or wet seal. They are swallowed whole with water and prevent the patient from tasting the powder. Filled cachets are packed in cardboard boxes.

---

### EXAMPLE 17.2

R. Droperidol 10 mg capsules, with 1% w/w magnesium stearate. Mitte 8 caps.

|  | For 1 capsule | For 10 capsules |
|---|---|---|
| Droperidol | 10 mg | 10w0 mg |
| Magnesium stearate | 1 mg | 10 mg |
| Lactose | 89 mg | 890 mg |

#### Action and uses
Antipsychotic drug, used for tranquillization and control in mania.

#### Formulation notes
Magnesium stearate is added to act as a lubricant to aid flow of the powder into the capsule. 10 mg is not weighable, so a trituration must be carried out. Lactose acts as a diluent to bring the weight of each capsule fill to 100 mg.

#### Trituration for magnesium stearate

| Magnesium stearate | 100 mg |
|---|---|
| Lactose | 900 mg |

Take a 100 mg portion of this mixture, which will contain 10 mg of magnesium stearate and 90 mg of lactose.

#### Method of preparation
Sieve the powders using a 250 μm sieve. Prepare the magnesium stearate triturate. Weigh 100 mg of droperidol, and mix this with the magnesium stearate triturate in a mortar and pestle. Gradually add 800 mg of lactose to this mixture, by doubling-up. This gives a total powder quantity of 1000 mg (equivalent to 10 × 100 mg capsules). Fill the capsule shells (size 4 or 5) with 100 mg aliquots, checking the weight of each capsule before sealing. Pack eight capsules in an amber glass or plastic tablet container with a child-resistant closure.

#### Storage and shelf life
Store in a cool dry place and protect from light. Expiry date of 2 weeks, since stability in capsule form is unknown.

#### Advice and labelling
The medicine will cause drowsiness. The patient should not drive or operate machinery if he/she is affected. Alcoholic drinks should be avoided.

---

### Key Points

- Tablets and capsules are the most popular way of giving a medicine.
- Excipients are added to improve manufacture, handling and release of the drug.
- Bioavailability of some tablets may vary between manufacturers.
- Checking of labels and contents of bulk containers is essential in minimizing errors.
- Tablets should be swallowed with about 50 ml of water.
- Ensure that the patient knows how to take the tablet – chew, dissolve, swallow whole, buccal or sublingual.
- Indigestion remedies should be avoided with enteric-coated tablets and capsules.
- Tablets cannot be made extemporaneously, but capsules are filled, especially in hospitals and preparing for clinical trials.
- Capsule size is selected so that they look reasonably full.

- The minimum weight of contents in an extemporaneous capsule is 100 mg.
- Capsules may be subject to uniformity of weight and drug content tests.
- Pastilles are popular for coughs and sore throats.
- Cachets are little used today.

## FURTHER READING

ABPI Compendium of data sheets and summaries of product characteristics, (current edn.) Datapharm Publications, London (Updated annually)

Ansel H C, Popovich N G, Allen L V 1995 Pharmaceutical dosage forms and drug delivery systems, 6th edn. Williams & Wilkins, Malvern, USA

Aulton M E 1988 Pharmaceutics: the science of dosage form design. Churchill Livingstone, Edinburgh

British National Formulary, current edn. British Medical Association and Royal Pharmaceutical Society of Great Britain, London (Updated twice yearly)

British Pharmaceutical Codex 1973 Pharmaceutical Press, London

British Pharmacopoeia 1988 HMSO, London

Diluent Directories (Internal and External), current edn. National Pharmaceutical Association, St Albans

Pharmaceutical Codex 1979 11th edn (incorporating the British Pharmaceutical Codex). Pharmaceutical Press, London

Pharmaceutical Codex: principles and practice of pharmaceutics 1994 12th edn. Pharmaceutical Press, London

Reynolds J E F (ed) 1996 Martindale: the extra pharmacopoeia, 31st edn. Pharmaceutical Press, London (Updated every 3 years – use current edn)

Wade A (ed) 1980 Pharmaceutical handbook, 19th edn. Pharmaceutical Press, London

# 18

# Aerosols and other dosage forms

*M. M. Moody*

---

After studying this chapter you will know about:

**The types of pressurized aerosols**
**Dry powder inhaler devices**
**The reasons for the use of the inhalation route, the aids available and how they are used**
**Transdermal drug delivery.**

## Introduction

This chapter deals with three types of drug delivery system: pharmaceutical aerosols, dry powder or 'breath-actuated' inhaler devices and transdermal delivery systems. All three are used to produce systemic effects but use a route other than the oral route. Aerosols are also used to produce local effects, using the topical route.

## PHARMACEUTICAL AEROSOLS

Pharmaceutical aerosols consist of solutions, suspensions or emulsions of drugs mixed with inert propellants. These mixtures are normally contained, under pressure, in metal canisters which are fitted with a valve. On depression of the valve the canister is 'fired' and the medicament expelled. Two types of valve are used in aerosol production, the continuous spray valve and the metered-dose valve. Aerosols fitted with a continuous spray valve will deliver the medicament for as long as the valve is depressed. The metered-dose valve functions similarly to the continuous spray valve but incorporates a reservoir which holds a specific quantity of medicament. When the valve is depressed the aerosol will deliver a spray of precise volume, containing a known dose of drug. If a further dose is required the valve must be

depressed again. A detailed description of the production of pharmaceutical aerosols is found in the *Pharmaceutical Codex* (1994).

Pharmaceutical aerosols are used to deliver drugs to produce both local and systemic effects.

## Local effects

A wide variety of medicaments have been formulated as aerosols for topical use. These include antiseptics, antifungals, anti-inflammatory drugs, local anaesthetics, antibiotics and protective films. Some drugs such as steroids are incorporated into aerosols and are produced as foams. The aerosol is fitted with a metered-dose valve which delivers a known dose of steroid. These foam preparations are useful in the treatment of conditions such as ulcerative colitis and Crohn's disease.

## Systemic effects

The most common use for pharmaceutical aerosols is in the treatment of asthma and other chronic obstructive airways diseases. The drug is delivered using the inhaled route. Firing the device releases a measured dose of the drug in droplets with a diameter of 50 μm or less. The drug is inhaled through the mouth and delivered directly to the site of action, i.e. the lungs. Because the drug is delivered directly to the site of action the dose needed to produce an adequate therapeutic response is much lower than the oral dose. There is therefore a consequent reduction in side effects. The simplest inhaler is an unmodified, pressurized aerosol fitted with a metered-dose valve. An example of an unmodified pressurized aerosol inhaler or metered-dose inhaler (MDI) is illustrated in Figure 18.1.

### Method of use

1. The cap should be removed and the inhaler

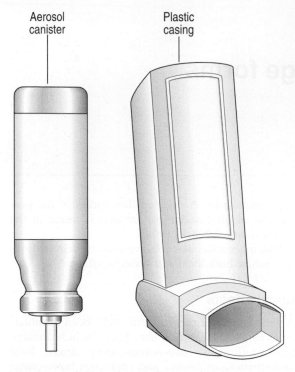

Aerosol
canister

Plastic
casing

**Fig. 18.1** Metered-dose inhaler.

shaken to disperse the drug. Many patients forget, or are unaware of, the need to shake the container. This should be emphasized when counselling patients on inhaler technique.

2. The patient should breathe out normally, but not fully. The inhaler mouthpiece is then put in the mouth and the lips closed round it.

3. The patient then breathes in slowly and at the same time activates the aerosol by pressing down on the canister.

4. The breath should be held for 10 seconds or as long as the patient can comfortably manage.

5. The patient then slowly exhales.

6. If another dose has to be taken at least 1 minute should elapse before repeating the exercise.

Unfortunately, some patients find these devices difficult to use and because of poor technique many patients do not get the expected response. There are several reasons for patients' problems. These include:

• Patients may not be able to synchronize breathing in and firing the aerosol. Some patients have difficulty pressing hard enough to fire the aerosol.

• The inhaled drug does not travel in a straight line and there are many areas en route where drug

particles or droplets can be deposited. The breath in, therefore, must be slow, as this will reduce the impaction of particles in the mouth and pharynx.

• The breath must be held at the end of the inspiration period to allow the particles to deposit on the site of action. If the breath is not held, the particles will merely be exhaled.

• When the propellant hits the back of the throat it causes the 'cold freon effect'. This interrupts breathing in some patients and renders this type of inhaler device useless in these cases.

Even with perfect technique, only 10% of the drug released reaches the bronchi. Of the remainder, 10% remains in the mouthpiece and 80% in the back of the throat. Studies have shown that only 50% of adult patients can use this type of inhaler. They are unsuitable for use by children under 5 years of age.

For these reasons much work has gone into developing devices which will overcome the various problems. Four devices which are currently in common use are described below.

### The Haleraid

This is a simple device illustrated in Figure 18.2 which fits over certain makes of pressurized aerosols. Instead of firing the aerosol by pressing down on the canister with the forefinger, the Haleraid is gently squeezed using the whole hand. This fires the device, making the operation much easier. This is a very simple compliance aid which is useful for certain elderly or arthritic patients who have difficulty pressing the canister.

### The spacer inhaler

This is illustrated in Figure 18.3. It is a standard pressurized inhaler with an elongated mouthpiece. The benefit of this device is that the delivered dose of drug and propellant is more diffuse when it arrives at the mouth and the 'cold freon effect' is considerably reduced. For that reason these devices can be beneficial. However, they are slightly awkward to manipulate for some patients, particularly the elderly and those with arthritic hands.

### Large volume inhaler

This is a spacer attachment for use with a metered-dose inhaler as illustrated in Figure 18.4. It overcomes the problems of coordination, the 'cold freon effect' and generally gives the patient more time.

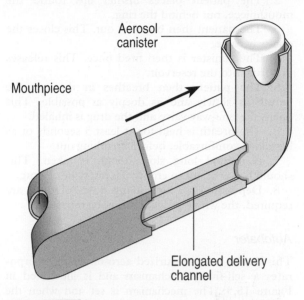

**Fig. 18.3** Spacer inhaler (courtesy of Astra Pharmaceuticals Ltd).

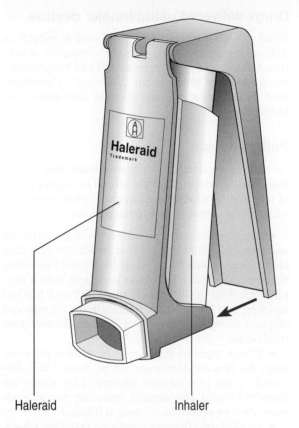

**Fig. 18.2** Haleraid (courtesy of Allen & Hanburys Ltd).

They can be used by children and are also useful where the patient has poor inspiratory flow.

A much larger dose of drug reaches the lungs using this device. Studies have shown that 30–35% of the delivered drug reaches the lungs, which is far more than with an unmodified pressurized aerosol. Because of their size they are less convenient to use, but because of the higher doses of drug being delivered, they are of particular benefit for use with prophylactic drugs.

*Method of use for large volume spacer*

1. The aerosol canister is fitted into the holder and the whole device shaken.

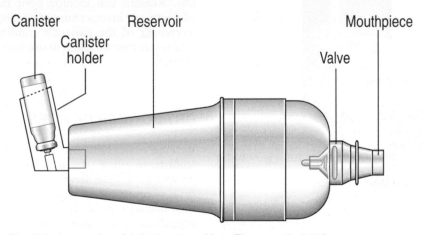

**Fig. 18.4** Large volume inhaler (courtesy of Astra Pharmaceuticals Ltd).

2. The patient places his/her lips round the mouthpiece, but behind the ring.

3. The patient then breathes out. This closes the one-way valve.

4. The canister is then fired once. This releases the drug into the reservoir.

5. The patient then breathes in through the mouth as slowly and as deeply as possible. This opens the one-way valve and the drug is inhaled.

6. The breath is held for at least 5 seconds or as long as is comfortable, before breathing out.

7. A second long slow breath is taken. This should be sufficient to empty the reservoir of drug.

8. Depending on how many doses of drug are required, the whole procedure can be repeated.

### Autohaler

This device is a pressurized aerosol which incorporates a self-firing mechanism and is illustrated in Figure 18.5. The mechanism is set and when the patient inhales, the device fires, delivering the drug dose. These are useful for patients who have difficulty depressing the canister. Studies have shown that approximately 21% of the delivered drug reaches the lungs.

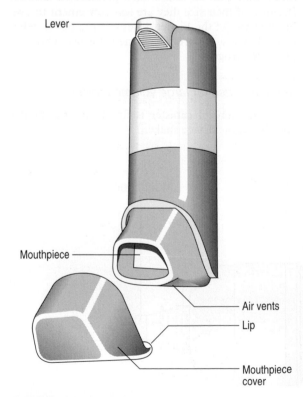

**Fig. 18.5**  Autohaler (courtesy of 3M Health Care Ltd).

## Drugs delivered using inhaler devices

Many patients are prescribed drugs such as steroids or sodium cromoglycate to prevent asthmatic attacks (prophylactic therapy – 'preventers') and bronchodilators for use if an attack occurs ('relievers'). Commonly used bronchodilator drugs include salbutamol and terbutaline.

## Patient advice

As well as checking that patients know how to use their inhaler devices there are several important pieces of information relating to the type of drug being used which the pharmacist should tell patients.

• Many patients are prescribed both prophylactic and bronchodilator drugs. It is important that they know which is which and when they should be taken. Some patients have been confused and used a prophylactic drug to alleviate an attack. When it has had no effect they have lost confidence in the therapy and stopped using it. Overuse of bronchodilators may then occur.

• If both types of drug are to be used at the same time, the bronchodilator should be inhaled first, followed by the prophylactic therapy. This allows the bronchi to relax and expand, ensuring that an optimum dose of prophylactic drug is inhaled.

• Prophylactic therapy should be taken on a regular basis, unlike bronchodilators which may be taken, up to a maximum dose, on an 'as necessary' basis. If prophylactic drugs are delivered using a large volume device the more efficient drug delivery should lead to a better therapeutic response. This in turn should reduce the need for bronchodilator therapy.

• If the patient's use of inhalers increases, the pharmacist should attempt to identify the reason for this. Reasons can include poor inhaler technique, ineffective or incorrect use of prophylactic therapy or worsening of the patient's condition. Appropriate action can then be taken to improve the health of the patient.

## DRY POWDER DEVICES

Because of the problems of synchronization and the 'cold freon effect', dry powder or 'breath-actuated' devices have been developed. In these devices the drug is presented in a finely divided form. Rather than being propelled from the container by an inert propellant it is removed from the device by the action of the patient breathing in.

While these breath-actuated devices overcome the previously mentioned problems, they do have some disadvantages.

• The dry powder may cause reflex coughing in the patient, which may worsen the condition.

• The bioavailability of the drug in dry powder devices appears to be lower than with pressurized aerosols. This means that, in order to achieve the same therapeutic response, drug doses in dry powder devices are normally twice those of pressurized aerosols

• Some devices, such as the Rotahaler, cannot be kept preloaded. This could cause problems for a patient suffering a severe attack, as the drug would not be immediately ready for inhalation.

Two dry powder devices currently available are illustrated in Figures 18.6 and 18.7.

In the Diskhaler (Fig. 18.6) the drug is presented in small blisters in a circular, foil container. The foil circle is loaded into the inhaler device. When required for use, a blister is punctured and the powdered drug is inhaled by the patient.

In the Rotahaler (Fig. 18.7) the drug is presented as a capsule. When required for use the capsule is inserted into the Rotahaler. The device is twisted which splits the capsule in two. The patient then breathes in deeply through the mouthpiece and inhales the powdered drug.

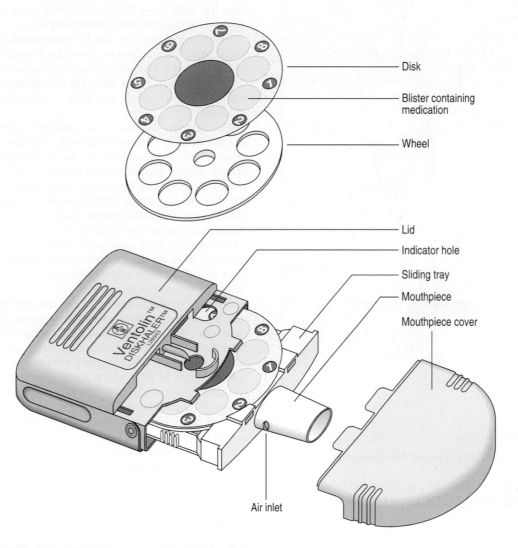

Disk

Blister containing medication

Wheel

Lid

Indicator hole

Sliding tray

Mouthpiece

Mouthpiece cover

Air inlet

**Fig. 18.6** Diskhaler (courtesy of Allen & Hanburys Ltd).

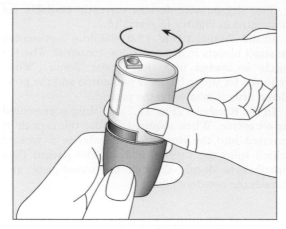

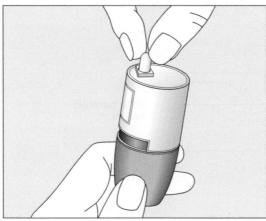

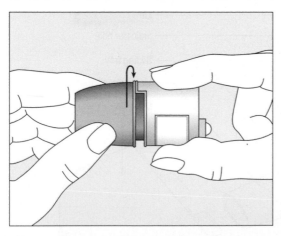

**Fig. 18.7** Rotahaler (courtesy of Allen & Hanburys Ltd).

# TRANSDERMAL DELIVERY SYSTEMS

Traditional oral dosage forms have a number of disadvantages as drug delivery systems. They produce plasma levels which have peaks and troughs. These fluctuations may result in undesirable side effects and lack of efficacy of the drug. If the time interval between drug dosage is short the frequency of dosing may cause problems with compliance. Transdermal drug delivery aims to overcome these problems by providing continuous drug release over a period of time which can be from 1 to 7 days.

The principle of this dosage form is that the drug is absorbed through the skin into the systemic circulation. The drug is incorporated into an adhesive patch which is applied to the surface of the skin. The patch releases a known dose of drug, over a specific time. Because absorption through the skin is variable, the rate of release of the drug must be controlled. To achieve constant absorption at a specific dose the drug must be released from the patch at a slower rate than the skin can absorb it.

Transdermal patches can be categorized into two main types, depending on how the release of drug is controlled. The membrane or reservoir type (Fig. 18.8) uses a rate-limiting membrane to control the rate at which the drug is released from a reservoir.

The matrix type occurs in a variety of forms. In all, the drug is incorporated into a matrix and the release rate is dependent on the properties of the matrix. In one type of matrix patch the rate of drug release is controlled by using a concentration gradient (Fig. 18.9). In this type of patch the drug is present in a multilayered matrix. Each layer contains a different concentration of drug, the least concentrated being in the layer next to the skin. As each layer is depleted of drug the concentration gradient causes drug to diffuse from a level of higher concentration to one of lower concentration.

A recent development has been the incorporation of drug into water-based, pressure-sensitive adhesive. As in the previous two types, drug transport through the skin is by passive diffusion. Initial results show that this system appears to give a constant steady state concentration of drug which is closer to the theoretical ideal than is achieved by the earlier systems.

Steady state plasma levels are usually achieved with all types of patch within 1–4 hours and maintained for at least 24 hours.

Drugs currently available as transdermal therapeutic systems include:

- Glyceryl trinitrate for the treatment of angina. Both membrane and matrix devices are available. These patches are designed to deliver the drug over a 24-hour period.
- Oestradiol for the alleviation of menopausal

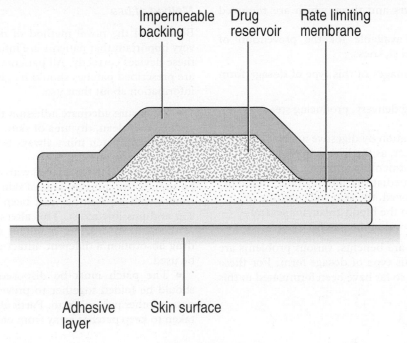

**Fig. 18.8** Membrane or reservoir type of transdermal patch.

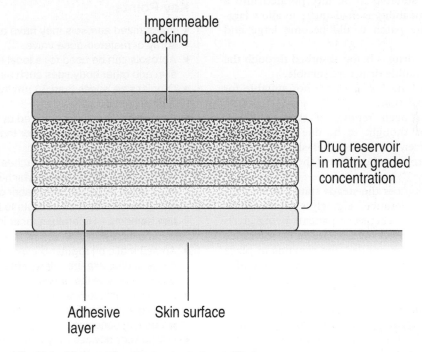

**Fig. 18.9** Matrix patch using a concentration gradient.

symptoms and the prevention of osteoporosis. These patches are designed to deliver a therapeutic dose of drug for 72 hours.

● Nicotine, in the alleviation of withdrawal symptoms in smoking cessation. Two types of patches are available: those which deliver the drug dose over 24 hours and those which are removed after 16 hours.

• Hyoscine is available for the prevention of symptoms of travel sickness.

The main advantages of this type of dosage form are:

• continuous drug delivery, producing steady state plasma levels
• no drug deactivation by digestive juices
• no first pass effect, as the liver is bypassed
• cessation of treatment by removing the patch. (This is not immediate as, although the source of the drug is removed, the skin will continue to deliver drug into the bloodstream for several hours after removal of the patch.)

Although these are benefits, various problems are associated with this type of dosage form. For these reasons few drugs so far have been formulated in this way.

## Disadvantages

• Only potent drugs, i.e. those with a small therapeutic dose are suitable to be incorporated into a patch. Skin permeability is inadequate to allow larger doses and the patch would become large and cumbersome.
• Because the drug is being absorbed through the skin, only lipid-soluble drugs are suitable.
• Drugs with long half-lives are not suitable for this type of formulation.
• There have been reports of skin reactions. Initially this was thought to be due to the patch adhesive. However, further studies showed that it was caused by prolonged contact of the skin with the drug.
• In some instances the steady state blood levels have produced tolerance, e.g. glyceryl trinitrate. This has led to the practice of patients being given a 'nitrate-free' period which prevents tolerance occurring. A patch is applied and remains in place for 16 hours and is then removed. A period of 8 hours is allowed to elapse before a new patch is applied.
• Steady state blood levels of nicotine have caused central nervous system disturbance, in particular, patients have reported suffering nightmares. Normally nicotine levels in a smoker will fall during the hours of sleep as no cigarette smoking occurs. No such fall will occur when 24-hour nicotine patches are used. For this reason one manufacturer has developed a patch which is applied for 16 hours then removed. A new one is applied 8 hours later.

## Method of use

Because of the novel method of drug delivery it is very important that patients are informed how to use these devices correctly. All patients who purchase or are prescribed patches should be given the following information about their use.

• To ensure adequate adhesion the patch must be applied to a clean, dry area of skin.
• The old patch must always be removed before applying a new one.
• When a patch is replaced with a new one it must be applied to a different area of skin. The area of skin from which a patch has just been removed will be soft and possibly moist. This alters the permeability of the skin. In order to maintain the same level of drug absorption a different, intact area of skin must be used.
• The patch must be disposed of carefully. It should be folded together to prevent it being stuck onto another person's skin. Particular care should be taken to keep patches away from children.

## Key Points

• Pressurized aerosols may have a continuous spray or metered-dose valve.
• Aerosols can be used for a local effect on the skin and other body sites such as the colon.
• Droplet size is less than 50 μm from a pressurized inhaler.
• A much lower dose is required by the inhalation route than orally for the same effect on asthma.
• A maximum of 10% drug reaches the alveoli from a pressurized inhaler which is increased to 35% with a large volume spacer device.
• Compliance aids are available to help patients use aerosols – Haleraid, spacer inhaler, large volume inhaler.
• An asthmatic on regular preventer and reliever drugs should use the reliever first to improve dose delivery of the preventer.
• Increasing inhaler use indicates a poor technique, ineffective use of prophylaxis or a worsening condition.
• Dry powder devices may assist patients who have difficulty with aerosols, but can cause cough, have reduced bioavailability and cannot be preloaded.
• Skin patches may be of reservoir or matrix design.

- Patches produce steady state plasma levels and drug administration can be stopped by removing the patch.
- Transdermal delivery is only feasible for lipid-soluble drugs requiring small doses.
- Side effects and tolerance may develop with drugs administered over a 24-hour period.

## FURTHER READING

ABPI Compendium of data sheets and summaries of product characteristics, current edn. Datapharm Publications, London (Updated annually)

ABPI Compendium of patient information leaflets, current edn. Datapharm Publications, London (Updated annually)

Aulton M E 1988 Pharmaceutics: the science of dosage form design. Churchill Livingstone, Edinburgh

British National Formulary, current edn. British Medical Association and Royal Pharmaceutical Society of Great Britain, London (Updated twice yearly)

Jenkins A W 1995 Developing the Fematrix transdermal patch. Pharmaceutical Journal 255: 179–181

Livingstone C, Livingstone D 1988 Transdermal systems. Pharmaceutical Journal 241: 130–131

Pharmaceutical Codex 1994 12th edn. Pharmaceutical Press, London

# 19

# Wound management, stoma and incontinence products

*J. H. Musset and A. J. Winfield*

After studying this chapter you will know about:

**Types of wounds and selection of wound management products**
**The form and use of dressings**
**Elastic support hosiery**
**The types of stoma and problems associated with them**
**Different types of stoma appliances**
**Incidence and causes of incontinence**
**The management of incontinence and the use of incontinence appliances**
**Pharmaceutical advice for stoma and continence patients.**

## WOUNDS

A wound may be defined as any damage to the skin. Wounds are caused by mechanical injuries, burns and underlying medical conditions giving rise to ulcers.

The complex process of wound healing involves the growth of fibrous and vascular tissue within the wound and the migration of epithelial cells from the edges of the wound. Normally a hard scab forms at the wound surface and underlying dehydrated tissue slows down the movement of cells. If the wound is kept moist, epithelial cells can move unimpeded and the epidermis is regenerated within half the time.

### Types of wounds

However a wound has been generated, treatment will depend largely upon the present condition of the wound. The same wound may go through several stages in the healing process, and the most appropriate choice of wound management product will change accordingly.

### Necrotic wounds

Necrotic wounds are covered with a hard, dry, black layer of dead tissue known as eschar (pronounced eskar). It often occurs in pressure sores. The eschar needs to be removed before healing can begin.

### Sloughy wounds

Slough (pronounced sluff) is white, yellow or brown soft material formed from dead cells on the surface of the wound. Again, it needs to be removed for healing to occur.

### Granulating wounds

Granulating wounds are red, granular and moist. This is due to granulation tissue, consisting of blood vessels, collagen and other connective tissue, being laid down in the base of the wound. The ideal dressing here would promote moist wound healing and provide thermal insulation; wounds heal more quickly at body temperature.

### Epithelializing wounds

Epithelializing wounds are pink in colour as a new epidermis is being formed. This occurs within 24 hours with shallow superficial wounds. In others it follows the granulation stage. A suitable dressing is one which provides a moist environment and does not adhere to the wound.

### Exuding wounds

Granulating and epithelializing wounds produce varying amounts of liquid exudate, which usually decreases as healing proceeds. A dressing should be sufficiently absorbent to contain excess exudate while still maintaining a moist wound surface.

## Infected and malodorous wounds

Infected wounds are often surrounded by red, hot inflamed tissue, and pus may be present. As infection delays healing, it should be treated. Minor infections can be treated with dressings containing antimicrobial substances. For more serious infection, a course of appropriate antibiotics given systemically is safer than topical application. Infected burns often respond successfully to Flamazine, a hydrophilic cream containing silver sulphadiazine.

Infection with anaerobic bacteria also causes an unpleasant odour. Metronidazole given orally or topically will eradicate the bacteria. In addition, charcoal dressings will help to remove the offensive odour.

# TRADITIONAL DRESSINGS

Dressings have been used for centuries and some of these are still in use today. Most are passive in that they cover and hide the wound, but have little impact on the healing process.

## Absorbents

Absorbent dressings are used to:

- clean and swab wounds
- absorb excess wound exudate
- apply medicaments to the skin
- protect the wound from future knocks.

The dressings can be used in the original fibrous form, e.g. absorbent cotton and cellulose wadding. Alternatively, the fibres are spun into a yarn and woven into a fabric, to be used as fabric absorbents. These include gauzes made from loosely woven cotton or combined cotton and viscose. They are used extensively in surgery. A combination of fibrous and fabric absorbents is found in Gamgee Tissue, where absorbent cotton is enclosed in gauze.

Absorbent dressings should not be left directly on a moist wound for several reasons:

- dehydration of the wound surface
- adhesion – as the wound exudate dries out it forms a powerful glue between the dressing and the dermis; removal of the dressing destroys new epidermis and causes fresh bleeding
- formation of capillary loops as new blood vessels grow round the threads of the fabric
- shedding of fibres into the wound
- absorption of antibacterial exudate, so removing part of the body's natural defence mechanism

- strike through of exudate to the outer surface of the dressing, providing a pathway for bacteria.

## Bandages

The *British National Formulary* (BNF 1996) classifies bandages as retention, support and compression, and medicated.

## Retention bandages

Retention bandages are used to:

- protect absorbent dressings and keep them in place
- provide light support for minor sprains and strains
- secure splints.

They may be extensible (stretch) or non-extensible. Examples of non-stretch products are Open-wove Bandage and Domette Bandage. The latter contains wool which imparts warmth. Stretch retention bandages include Cotton Conforming Bandage, which is made of cotton crimped mechanically to impart elasticity in both directions. This helps it to retain dressings in difficult positions such as over joints. Tubular bandages are knitted fabrics, some of which include rubber to increase their elasticity.

## Support and compression bandages

Support and compression bandages are one-way stretch products. The support and compression they give increase with the weight of the dressing and its elasticity. Non-adhesive products include crepe bandage, where elasticity is imparted by the inclusion of wool and double twisted cotton threads. This gives light support for strains and sprains. Greater support is given by elastic web bandage which incorporates rubber threads in its structure. A coloured thread running down the centre acts as a guide in its application, to provide even compression.

Adhesive support and compression bandages have the advantage of remaining secure once applied. They are useful in the treatment of fractured ribs and collar bones, leg ulcers and varicose veins especially in patients who are mobile. Unfortunately, their application and particularly their removal may be painful and may damage fragile skin. Another disadvantage is a possible sensitivity to ingredients of the adhesive, e.g. rubber. Bandages may be:

- self-adhesive, e.g. elastic adhesive bandage

- diachylon, e.g. Lestreflex – the bandage is warmed prior to application in order to produce adhesion
- cohesive, e.g. Coban – the bandage adheres to itself but not to the patient's skin.

### Medicated bandages

Medicated bandages consist of a cotton bandage impregnated with a medicament formulated in a moist paste. They are used in the treatment of dermatological conditions, such as eczema and inflammation associated with leg ulcers. They may be left in position for up to 2 weeks. They are usually covered by a support and compression bandage. Most are zinc paste bandages containing zinc oxide. Additional ingredients include calamine, coal tar (a fungicide), clioquinol and ichthammol (antibacterials). Some also contain parahydroxybenzoates (parabens) as preservatives, to which some patients are sensitive.

## Elastic hosiery

Elastic hosiery performs a similar function to support and compression bandages, but in a more controlled manner. Graduated compression hosiery is designed so that the compression is greatest at the ankle and decreases up the leg. It is classified according to the pressure exerted at the ankle, as shown in Table 19.1.

Compression hosiery is indicated for the treatment of varicose veins, varicose ulcers and venous insufficiency. Class I hosiery is also used prophylactically during pregnancy.

Garments available on the Drug Tariff are below-knee and thigh-length stockings. Anklets and kneecaps are also available in classes II and III. These are used for the support of soft tissue injuries. Each item is subject to a prescription charge, so a pair of stockings would be liable for two charges.

Measurements required for elastic hosiery are:

- circumference of the mid-thigh

| Table 19.1 Classification of graduated compression hosiery | | |
|---|---|---|
| Class | Pressure at ankle (mmHg) | Degree of support |
| I | 14–17 | Light |
| II | 18–24 | Medium |
| III | 25–35 | Strong |

- widest part of the calf
- around the ankle
- length of the foot.

Measurements should be made for each leg early in the day, starting at the top to prevent undue concern.

## Adhesive tapes and dressings

Adhesive tapes consist of a backing material coated on one side with an adhesive mass. The backing material may be fabric or a plastic film. Different combinations of backing material and adhesive give products with different permeabilities:

- permeable – to air, water and bacteria
- vapour-permeable
  - permeable to air and water vapour
  - impermeable to liquid water and bacteria
- occlusive – impermeable.

They are used:

- for securing dressings and appliances
- as skin closures for small incisions
- for covering infected wounds to prevent contamination.

Adhesive dressings have an absorbent pad in addition to the adhesive tape. The pad may be impregnated with a suitable antiseptic, e.g. aminacrine hydrochloride or chlorhexidine gluconate.

## Non-adherent dressings

Non-adherent, or more accurately low-adherent, dressings are either a single layer over which another dressing is placed, or multi-layered with the non-adherent layer in direct contact with the wound.

### Paraffin gauze dressing

Paraffin gauze or tulle gras dressings are made of cotton and/or viscose gauze impregnated with white or yellow soft paraffin. Antimicrobial medicaments, e.g. chlorhexidine, may also be included. Dressings containing antibiotics such as framycetin sulphate and sodium fusidate should be used with caution because of the potential problems of bacterial resistance and skin sensitivity.

Tulle dressings are used mainly to treat partial thickness wounds, where the soft paraffin reduces dehydration of the wound surface. They are also useful in the transfer of skin grafts, when the tackiness of the products is exploited.

### Knitted viscose dressings

Knitted viscose dressings (e.g. N-A Dressing, Tricotex) have an open structure which allows liquid exudate from the wound to pass through to a super-imposed absorbent pad. A medicated version is povidone-iodine fabric dressing (Inadine), where the dressing is impregnated with povidone-iodine ointment as an antiseptic. It may be used on infected superficial burns and other injuries. The orange-brown dressing loses its colour as the iodine is used up, and the decolorized fabric is a visible indication that the dressing needs renewing.

### Perforated film absorbents

Perforated film absorbents consist of three layers with the layer in contact with the wound being a perforated plastic film. The film minimizes adherence to the wound while the perforations allow excess exudate to pass through to the middle absorbent fibrous layer. With type 1 (Melolin), it is important to apply correctly as the outer backing layer of cellulose fibres should not be placed directly onto the wound. In types 2 (Telfa), 3 (Release) and 4 (Skintact), the perforated film on both sides of the dressing alleviates this problem, although type 3 has a join on one side; it is thus recommended that the other side is placed in contact with the wound.

Perforated film absorbents are used for lightly exuding wounds and need to be secured with a bandage or adhesive tape.

## Charcoal dressings

Activated charcoal is used in several dressings (e.g. Actisorb Plus, Carbonet) to adsorb noxious materials and so eliminate offensive odour from infected malodorous wounds.

Actisorb Plus is a microporous activated charcoal cloth, containing silver residues, enclosed in a nylon sleeve. The silver imparts antibacterial properties to the cloth. The dressing may be applied directly to the wound or over a non-adherent dressing. In Carbonet the non-adherent layer is an integral part of the dressing. A charcoal layer is also included in some of the more modern products, such as Lyofoam C and Kaltocarb.

## MODERN WOUND MANAGEMENT PRODUCTS

Many of the wound management products which have been introduced in the last 20 years affect the wound healing process. Most are vapour permeable, so enabling gaseous exchange, but not allowing passage of liquid water or bacteria. This prevents dehydration of the wound surface and so provides a moist environment for the formation of granulation tissue and accelerated epidermal regeneration. The advantages of these products compared to dry permeable absorbent dressings are illustrated in Figure 19.1.

## Vapour-permeable adhesive films

Vapour-permeable films (e.g. Bioclusive, Cutifilm, Opsite Flexigrid, Tegaderm) consist of a thin transparent polyurethane film coated with an adhesive. The main differences between products are their presentation and means of application. For example, Opsite Flexigrid incorporates a grid for monitoring wound size and in Tegaderm the film is enclosed by a paper frame which is removed once the dressing is in place. Applying adhesive films takes some skill as they can easily adhere to themselves. The vapour-permeable properties of these films enable water vapour, but not liquid water, to pass through. This may result in the accumulation of excessive exudate under the film. This can be removed with a sterile syringe and the puncture site covered with a small piece of film, but this does run the risk of possible infection and needle-stick injuries.

Vapour-permeable films are indicated for:

- lightly exuding shallow wounds, such as minor burns
- prevention and treatment of superficial pressure sores
- securing cannulae and catheters
- use as sterile drapes during surgery.

An advantage to medical staff, but not always the patient, is the transparency of the product enabling the wound to be inspected without removal of the dressing.

## Foams

Foam dressings are made of polyurethane (e.g. Lyofoam), or silicone (e.g. Cavi-care). Lyofoam consists of a hydrophobic polyurethane foam sheet, one side of which has been heated under pressure to produce a smooth low-adherent hydrophilic surface. When this smooth surface is placed onto an exuding wound, liquid is absorbed into the 0.5 mm thick hydrophilic layer. As the exudate cannot progress further through the dressing, it maintains a moist

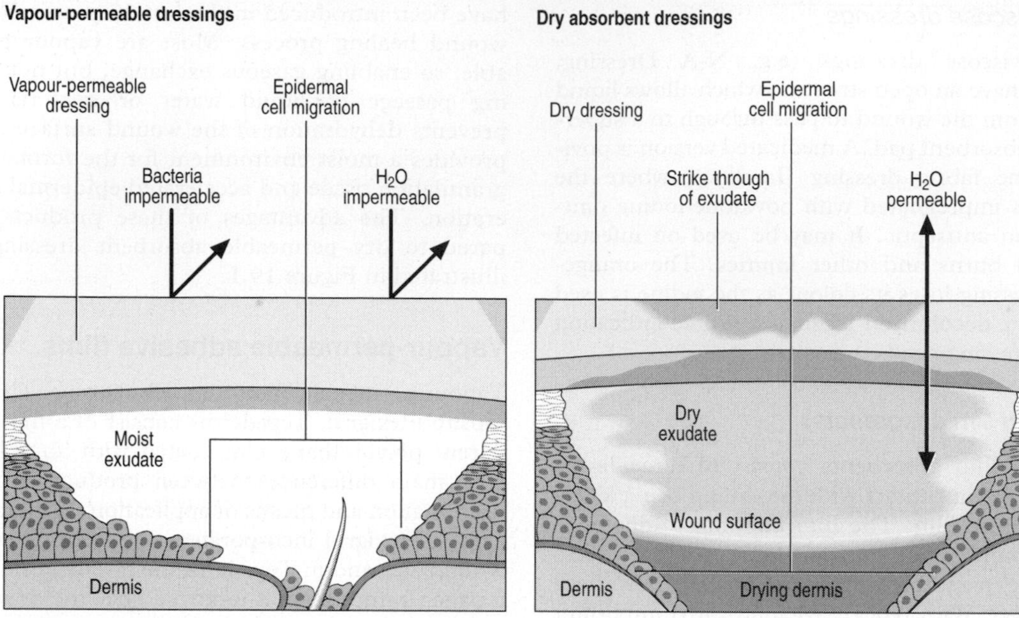

Vapour-permeable dressings

Dry absorbent dressings

**Fig. 19.1** Comparison of the effect of vapour-permeable and absorbent dressings on wounds (after Coloplast Ltd).

wound surface. Eventual lateral strike through indicates the need for a change of dressing. The 8 mm thick hydrophobic layer is vapour permeable and offers good thermal insulation. The dressing is used for lightly to moderately exuding wounds, when it needs to be secured by adhesive tape. This is not necessary with Lyofoam A, which incorporates a self-adhesive surround. Another product, Lyofoam C, contains a layer of activated carbon within the hydrophobic part, and so is useful for malodorous wounds.

Silicone foam cavity wound dressing (Cavi-care) is made in situ by stirring the silicone base with a catalyst for 15 seconds, then pouring into the wound. The foam or 'stent' sets in 3–4 minutes, expanding to about four times its original volume. It forms a hydrophobic membrane over the surface exposed to the atmosphere. However, the foam in contact with the wound remains hydrophilic and is able to absorb exudate from the wound surface. The stent may be removed from the wound twice a day for cleaning, then replaced.

## Foam film dressings

Foam film dressings are multi-layered products consisting of:

- an outer vapour-permeable polyurethane film

- a central absorbent hydrophilic polyurethane foam or membrane
- a low-adherent or adhesive layer.

The Drug Tariff specifies four types as shown in Table 19.2. Allevyn (types 2 and 4) is able to absorb and retain up to 10 times its own weight of fluid within its hydrocellular core and may be used on moderately to heavily exuding wounds. Tielle contains a non-woven wicking layer, which transports excess fluid away from the highly absorbent pad covering the lightly to moderately exuding wound. Allevyn and Tielle may be used under compression bandaging so are useful for exuding leg ulcers as well as pressure sores.

Spyrosorb is a thinner dressing with a central microporous membrane. It is still able to absorb low to moderate exudate, as the vapour permeability of

| Type | Product | Adhesive | Adhesive margin |
|------|---------|----------|-----------------|
| 1 | Spyrosorb | Yes | No |
| 2 | Allevyn | No | No |
| 3 | Tielle | Yes | Yes |
| 4 | Allevyn Adhesive | Yes | Yes |

**Table 19.2  Foam film dressings as classified by the Drug Tariff**

the outer film increases with increasing liquid. A similar product, but without the outer film, is Spyroflex, indicated for lightly exuding wounds.

A foam film dressing designed for deeper wounds is Allevyn Cavity Wound Dressing, made of highly absorbent foam 'chips' enclosed in a non-adherent perforated film. Its circular and tubular shape conforms to the shape of the wound.

## Polysaccharide beads

Polysaccharide dressings (e.g. Debrisan, Iodosorb) are tiny spherical beads of glucose polymers. Debrisan is made of dextranomer, manufactured from a derivative of dextran. Iodosorb is cadexomer iodine, which is a hydrophilic modified starch polymer containing 0.9% iodine. When introduced into an exuding wound the beads exert a capillary action on the exudate. Water is absorbed by the beads, while bacteria and cellular debris become trapped in the spaces between them. The debris is washed away during removal of the dressing.

Beads should not be used on dry or lightly exuding wounds, as they may dry out and be difficult to remove. These products are indicated for infected, sloughy, medium to heavily exuding wounds, especially leg ulcers.

As the slippery beads are difficult to use on some wounds, they are available as alternative formulations:

- a paste
- an ointment
- a paste enclosed in a nylon bag (e.g. Debrisan Absorbent Pad) or gauze (e.g. Iodoflex).

## Alginates

Salts of alginic acid occur naturally in the cell walls of brown seaweeds, whose healing properties have been recognized by sailors for centuries. Only recently has this been exploited in the extraction of alginates and their subsequent use in wound management.

Alginate dressings are made of non-woven fibres of either 100% calcium alginate (e.g. Sorbsan, Tegagel) or 80% calcium alginate and 20% sodium alginate (e.g. Kaltostat, Kaltogel).

When alginates are placed on moist wounds, there is an exchange of sodium ions at the wound surface with the calcium ions of the dressing. The extra calcium ions help to stop any bleeding. The sodium ions convert part of the insoluble calcium alginate dressing into the more water-soluble sodium algi-

nate. In the presence of exudate the sodium alginate forms a hydrophilic gel over the surface of the wound, providing a moist environment for healing. Dressings may be removed by irrigating with sterile saline. Manufacturers claim any fibres trapped in the wound are biodegraded.

Alginate dressings are available as:

- flat non-woven pads – for shallow exuding wounds
- rope – for large, deep, open, exuding wounds
- ribbon – for smaller, deep, moist wounds, especially in awkward places.

A secondary dressing, such as an absorbent pad or vapour-permeable adhesive film, is needed to cover the alginate fibres. The appropriate choice will be governed by the amount of exudate. With some alginate dressings the secondary dressing is incorporated into the one product. Examples are:

- Sorbsan Plus – includes an absorbent viscose pad
- Sorbsan SA – alginate fibres covered by an adhesive polyurethane foam
- Kaltoclude – alginate bonded to an adhesive vapour-permeable film.

Other alginate products are designed for heavily exuding wounds (e.g. Kaltostat Fortex) and malodorous wounds (e.g. Kaltocarb). Calcium alginate is combined with collagen in Fibracol, where the alginate produces a gel at the wound surface, while the gradual breakdown of the collagen component increases deposition of collagen fibres in the wound.

## Hydrogels

Hydrogels are three-dimensional networks of hydrophilic polymers made from materials such as gelatin, polysaccharides and cross-linked synthetic polymers. They interact with aqueous solutions by absorbing and retaining a significant amount of water within their structures, without dissolving. There are two types of hydrogels used in wound management:

- thin flexible sheets (e.g. Geliperm, Vigilon, Spenco Second Skin) – swell as they absorb fluid
- amorphous gels (e.g. Intrasite Gel, Bard Absorption Dressing) – decrease in viscosity as they absorb fluid until the polymer is dispersed.

The high moisture content of hydrogels maintains a moist wound surface. The amorphous gels are particularly useful in rehydrating necrotic tissue and assisting its separation from underlying healthy tissue, and in treating sloughy wounds. Hydrogels are also indicated for lightly to moderately exuding wounds. They cool the wound surface and so reduce pain and inflammation, and unfortunately the rate of healing. They are transparent but do need a secondary dressing.

Intrasite Gel and a partially dehydrated form of Geliperm can act as carriers for water-soluble, low molecular weight medicaments such as metronidazole. These are absorbed in solution into the hydrogel, then released at the wound surface.

## Hydrocolloids

Hydrocolloids (e.g. Granuflex, Comfeel, Tegasorb, Biofilm) are complex formulations containing colloids, elastomers and adhesives. The colloid is the gelling element and absorbent. In most products, it consists of sodium carboxymethylcellulose with some also containing pectin and gelatin. In the sheet form of the dressing, these are present as hydrophilic parti-

cles dispersed in a hydrophobic adhesive. The adhesive is bonded to a vapour-permeable polyurethane film (or polyester sheet in Biofilm), which extends beyond the hydrocolloid part in Bordered Granuflex and Tegasorb. Granuflex also has an outer polyurethane foam.

When a hydrocolloid is placed on an exuding wound, the hydrophilic particles absorb fluid and swell into the wound cavity, forming a moist gel at the surface, as shown in Figure 19.2. When the dressing is removed, part of the gel is left in contact with the wound and may be washed away with saline. The gel often produces an unpleasant odour, about which patients should be warned and reassured.

Hydrocolloids are available as self-adhesive sheets which may be square, oval or triangular. The latter are designed to fit sacral pressure sores. For cavity wounds, hydrocolloid paste, granules or powder are used in conjunction with the sheet form. Comfeel Pressure Relief Dressing combines a hydrocolloid sheet

### 1. Absorption of moisture from wound

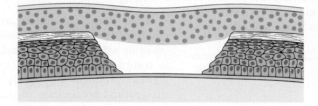

### 2. Swelling and formation of gel

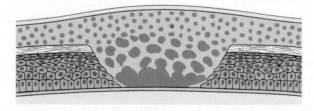

### 3. Removal of dressing

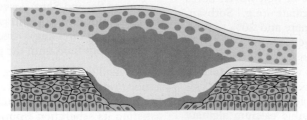

**Fig. 19.2** Effect of a hydrocolloid on an exuding wound (after Coloplast Ltd).

with a flexible foam disc, from which central portions can be removed to alleviate pressure on the wound.

Hydrocolloids are used extensively in the treatment of leg ulcers and pressure sores at most stages in the healing process. They rehydrate hard necrotic tissue, which softens and eventually separates. They also remove dead tissue from sloughy wounds. They encourage granulation, but sometimes produce too much granulation tissue. If this occurs they should be replaced by another type of dressing. Moderately to heavily exuding wounds can be covered by Granuflex or Biofilm, while Comfeel and Tegasorb are indicated for wounds producing a light to moderate exudate.

## SELECTION OF AN APPROPRIATE PRODUCT

From the vast array of products, it is increasingly difficult to select the most appropriate wound management product, especially when other factors such as cost are taken into account. Many hospitals have developed wound management policies in an attempt to rationalize the treatment of wounds and to restrict the number of products available. Table 19.3 summarizes products which may be used to treat various types of wounds.

**Table 19.3  Wound management products for different types of wounds**

| Wound type | Product type | Examples |
|---|---|---|
| Necrotic | Amorphous hydrogel | Intrasite gel, Bard Absorption Dressing (Bard) |
| | Hydrocolloid sheet | Granuflex, Comfeel, Tegasorb, Biofilm |
| Sloughy | Polysaccharide beads | Debrisan, Iodosorb |
| | Amorphous hydrogel | Intrasite gel, Bard |
| | Hydrocolloid – sheet, paste, granules, powder | Granuflex, Comfeel, Tegasorb, Biofilm |
| Granulating cavity | Foam | Cavi-care |
| | Foam film | Allevyn cavity wound dressing |
| | Alginate – rope, ribbon | Sorbsan, Kaltostat |
| | Hydrogel | Granulated Geliperm, Intrasite gel, Bard |
| | Hydrocolloid – paste, granules, powder | Granuflex, Comfeel, Biofilm |
| Granulating and epithelializing | | |
| Heavily to moderately exuding | Foam film | Allevyn |
| | Alginate | Kaltostat Fortex, Sorbsan SA |
| | Hydrogel | Dry Geliperm |
| | Hydrocolloid | Granuflex, Biofilm |
| Moderately to lightly exuding | Foam | Lyofoam |
| | Foam film | Tielle, Spyrosorb |
| | Alginate | Sorbsan, Kaltostat, Tegagel |
| | Hydrogel | Geliperm, Vigilon, Spenco second skin, Intrasite gel |
| | Hydrocolloid | Comfeel, Tegasorb |
| Epithelializing | | |
| Lightly exuding | Paraffin gauze | Jelonet |
| | Perforated film absorbent | Melolin, Telfa, Release, Skintact |
| | Vapour-permeable adhesive film | Bioclusive, Cutifilm, Opsite, Tegaderm |
| | Foam film | Spyroflex |
| Infected | Antibacterial paste bandage | Quinaband |
| | Chlorhexidine paraffin gauze | Bactigras, Clorhexitulle |
| | Povidone-iodine fabric | Inadine |
| | Charcoal dressing with silver | Actisorb plus |
| | Polysaccharide beads with iodine | Iodosorb, Iodoflex |
| | Hydrogels containing metronidazole | Intrasite gel, Dry Geliperm with metronidazole |
| Malodorous | Charcoal dressing | Actisorb plus, Carbonet, Lyofoam C, Kaltocarb |

**Table 19.4  Types of ostomy, effluent and normal type of pouch used for each**

| Ostomy | Type of effluent | Type of pouch |
|---|---|---|
| Colostomy, descending/ sigmoid | Soft to nearly solid | Closed pouch |
| Colostomy, transverse | Semi-liquid to soft | Drainable pouch with open end and clip |
| Colostomy, ascending | Liquid to paste-like | Drainable pouch with open end and clip |
| Ileostomy | Liquid, continuous, includes digestive enzymes | Drainable pouch with open end and clip |
| Urostomy | Urine | Drainable pouch with tap |

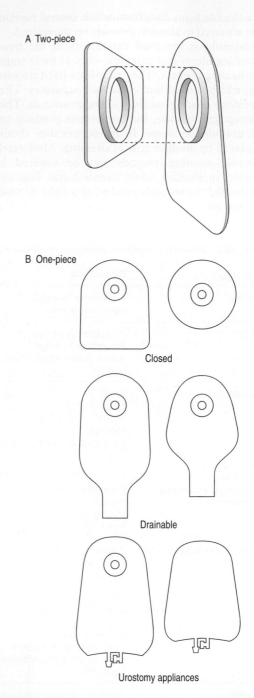

A Two-piece

B One-piece

Closed

Drainable

Urostomy appliances

**Fig. 19.3** The main types of one- and two-piece stoma appliances.

## STOMA

There are three types of stoma, which are created by surgery, namely ileostomy, colostomy and uroscopy. The reasons for their creation vary, as does the type of effluent produced and the type of appliances which will be best suited to their management. These are summarized in Table 19.4.

Two types of appliance are used, one piece or two piece, both being available with closed or drainable pouches. Closed bags are normally used for more solid stools, whilst drainable ones are better with semi-solids or liquids. One-piece products have the skin seal and bag in one item. Holes can be pre-cut or cut to fit the stoma. Two-piece products have a flange attached to the skin onto which the bag is clipped. These require good skin condition and reasonable dexterity. The main types of product are shown in Figure 19.3. Many products are available and take more than 100 pages of the Drug Tariff to detail. Ostomy patients can obtain a prescription charge Exemption Certificate.

### Problems with stoma

Hypoallergenic adhesives are used, but careful skin care is required. Detergents and disinfectants may cause irritation so washing with water is preferred, followed by a dusting powder or barrier cream if required so that the skin is kept as dry as possible. Leaks may occur if the appliance has not been fitted

properly, the skin is uneven or the bag has not been attached properly. Leakage, especially from an ileostomy or urostomy, can damage or irritate skin.

Diet and drugs can affect stoma effluent. A normal, varied diet should avoid too much fibre. Yoghurt and buttermilk may reduce odour and flatus (wind). Filters are also available to reduce odour. Diarrhoea and constipation will need medical supervision to control. Modified-release tablets are not suitable for stoma patients. Absorption may be restricted, so, for example, oral contraceptives are unreliable. Drugs may cause changes in colour and consistency of stools or urine. Pharmacists can offer general advice to stoma patients remembering that stoma patients may be embarrassed or shy. Reassurance of the patient is very important. Where referral is felt necessary, or for further information, there is a network of stoma care nurses.

# INCONTINENCE

Incontinence is the voiding of urine or faeces without control and in a way which undermines dignity. It is very common, but difficult to measure accurately because of social stigma. Estimates suggest about 5% of the population experience incontinence, with two-thirds of these being women. About a third of sufferers are under 65. Any help offered must be discreet.

The different types and causes of urinary incontinence are shown in Table 19.5. Any underlying medical condition requires treatment and some patients may require surgery. Otherwise there are many ways of helping the patient manage the condition.

Pelvic floor exercises are useful and can be taught by continence advisers, nurses, doctors or physiotherapists. Bladder retraining, perhaps combined with drug treatment, can restore an acceptable pattern of micturition. Constipation can cause urinary and faecal incontinence and should be avoided, preferably by diet and fluid control. Laxatives should be avoided if possible. Inadequate fluid intake can increase urinary incontinence.

## Incontinence appliances

A wide range of equipment has been developed to help people where other methods have not prevented their incontinence. Those which are prescribable are detailed in the Drug Tariff; others have to be purchased. Products can be grouped into four types:

- absorbents

- external collectors
- invasive devices
- collection systems.

Selection of a particular aid will be made on the basis of personal preference, nature of incontinence and other personal characteristics such as sex, age, mobility, dexterity and mental awareness.

### Absorbent pads

These can be used by either sex, and may be the only option for many women. Pads are available for different levels of incontinence. Light pads hold 50–100 ml and can be worn inside a user's own pants. Those for moderate urinary incontinence may be specially shaped, whilst heavy incontinence may require elasticated legs, waterproof backs or plastic garments. Bed protection may also be required.

### External collectors

A variety of penile sheaths, dribble pouches and drip collectors are available. Sheaths are made of soft latex and held on the penis by adhesive, the urine being collected in a drainage bag. Different types of bag are available: leg bags, suspensory bags (carried from the waist for larger volumes) and night drainage bags. Users need good eyesight and dexterity.

### Invasive devices

Urethral catheters are more commonly used by women, the urine continually draining into a suitable collecting bag. Indwelling catheters are held in place by a 'balloon' which is inflated after insertion. Intermittent catheterization may be used by patients who wish to retain control over the process. The catheter is inserted several times a day as required. There is an increased risk of bladder infection with catheters and skill is required by the user. With both external collectors and catheters, care is required to ensure connections to the bag are compatible.

### Collection systems

There are some complex body-worn systems, held in place by waist and groin straps, designed to collect urine into a bag. Specialized fitting is required.

**Table 19.5  Different types and causes of urinary incontinence**

| Type | Features | Cause |
|------|----------|-------|
| Stress | Slight leakage on exertion. Normal voiding | Inadequate sphincter. Oestrogen deficiency |
| Overflow | Small, frequent escapes. Slow, difficult, incomplete normal urination | Sphincter pressure too large. Enlarged prostate. Diabetes. Nerve damage |
| Urge | Inability to control passing urine. Nocturnal enuresis | Drugs – diuretics, sedatives. Hypersensitivity. Vaginal atrophy |
| Reflex | No sensation, sudden voiding | Nerve disease (such as multiple sclerosis, cord injury) |
| Continuous | Slow leakage all the time | Fistula. Bladder neck or sphincter open |
| Functional | Inability to reach toilet in time | Disability. Arthritis |

## Other relevant information

Physical changes to the living environment may enable the patient to reach the toilet more quickly. Drugs will affect continence. Those which increase urine flow should be avoided. Drugs which inhibit bladder contractility, such as anticholinergics, tricyclic antidepressants, adrenergic antagonists, have been used in treating incontinence. Skin care is important. Normal, regular hygiene, using simple soaps, should be adequate for most people. Avoid long periods of contact with wet pads or appliances, which will also help reduce odour. Sufferers may find it difficult to talk about their problem. It is best to use the same words to describe the problem as they use. Where a patient first reports faecal incontinence, referral to a GP is advisable in order that the cause can be ascertained. Most regions have continence advisers who can provide further help.

### Key Points

- Wounds may be classified as necrotic, sloughy, granulating, or epithelializing.
- Wounds may become infected and malodorous.

- Wounds can change type as healing progresses.
- Choice of wound management product is influenced by the type of wound.
- Traditional absorbent dressings should not be left in contact with moist wounds.
- Bandages may be medicated or for support, compression or retention.
- Graduated compression hosiery gives the greatest compression at the ankle.
- Measurements for elastic hosiery are the circumference of the mid-thigh, widest part of the calf, ankle and length of the foot.
- Adhesive tapes may be permeable, vapour-permeable or occlusive.
- Non-adherent dressings, which have a low-adherent layer in contact with the wound, include paraffin gauze, knitted viscose dressing and perforated film absorbents.
- Charcoal is used in dressings and stoma appliances to adsorb offensive odour.
- Modern dressings aim to produce conditions which promote wound healing.
- Vapour-permeable adhesive films are transparent and prevent dehydration of the wound.
- Foam dressings have hydrophobic and hydrophilic parts to control moisture at the wound surface.
- Foam film dressings vary considerably in the amount of exudate they can handle.
- Polysaccharide beads may be used on infected exuding wounds.
- Alginate dressings form a gel over moist wounds and provide calcium ions to help stop bleeding.
- Two types of hydrogel are used in wound management: flexible sheets and amorphous gels. The latter are particularly useful in removing necrotic tissue.
- Hydrocolloid dressings contain colloids, elastomers and adhesives, and have a great flexibility of use in treating several types of wounds.
- Stoma appliances may be one or two piece with closed or drainable bags.
- Skin care is important with stoma and incontinence.
- Incontinence is twice as common in women as men.
- There are many self-help techniques which can be used by people with a continence problem.
- Incontinence appliances include absorbents, sheaths, catheters and collection systems.

## FURTHER READING

Anderson R 1994 Pressure sores and leg ulcers. In: Walker R, Edwards C (eds) Clinical pharmacy and therapeutics. Churchill Livingstone, New York, ch 55, pp 769–781

British National Formulary 1996 31st edn. British Medical Association and Royal Pharmaceutical Society of Great Britain, London (use current edition)

British Pharmacopoeia 1993 HMSO, London (use current edition)

Cattell R 1995 Pressure sores in the elderly. Pharmaceutical Journal 255: 583–585

Drug Tariff 1996 HMSO, London (use current edition)

Elcoat C 1986 Stoma care nursing. Baillière Tindall, London

Gartley C B 1988 Managing incontinence. Souvenir Press Educational and Academic, London

Harman R J 1989 Patient care in community pharmacy. The Pharmaceutical Press, London

Mandelstam D 1986 Incontinence and its management, 2nd edn. Croom Helm, Beckenham, Kent

Morgan D 1993 Wound management: which dressing? Pharmaceutical Journal 250: 738–743

Morgan D A 1997 Formulary of wound management products, 7th edn. Euromed Communications, Surrey

Thomas S 1990 Wound management and dressings. The Pharmaceutical Press, London

Thomas S 1993 Bandages and bandaging. Pharmaceutical Journal 250: 744–745

Turner T 1993 The healing process. Pharmaceutical Journal 250: 735–737

Wilson P, Dunn L 1995 The development of Biofilm hydrocolloid dressings – permeability to bacteria. Pharmaceutical Journal 254: 232–235

# 20
# Medical gases

*A. J. Winfield*

After studying this chapter the reader will know about:

**Definition, nature and properties of medical gases**
**Control of medical gases**
**Equipment used with medical gases**
**Identification of medical gases**
**Safety aspects of medical gases**
**The uses of medical gases**
**Counselling of patients receiving domiciliary oxygen.**

## Introduction

A medical gas may be defined as any gas which is inhaled by a patient under the direction of a doctor. The use of gases to treat disease was pioneered in the 18th century, notably by Thomas Beddoes. The hope of these early workers that many diseases could be treated in this way was unfounded, but a number of gases are used in modern medical practice.

Oxygen is provided to patients in their own homes by pharmacies which have a contract with the local health authority or board. Details about this will be discussed later. In hospitals, pharmacists are often involved with the supply of oxygen, nitrous oxide, nitrous oxide/oxygen mixtures, compressed air and vacuum and occasionally more specialized gases. In most hospitals, rather than cylinders being used, a piped system is employed to distribute the gases from a central supply to each bedside. Further details will be given later in the chapter.

## Legal aspects

There are many national and international standards, specifications and codes of practice. In the UK, the manufacture of medical gases is controlled by the Medicines Act 1968, to standards laid down in the *British Pharmacopoeia* and *European Pharmacopoeia*. Ancillary equipment is detailed in British and International Standards (BS and ISO) and various Home Office Specifications. The Drug Tariff details domiciliary equipment and services.

## THE HARDWARE USED WITH MEDICAL GASES

Unless very large quantities are required, medical gases are stored in cylinders. These are made of steel and are designed to withstand pressures of over 200 bar and in the UK must comply with BS 1319 (BSI 1976). Cylinders are filled to a nominal pressure of 137 bar at 14°C. The nominal size of cylinders varies from 36 litre to 5112 litre capacity. The size used for domiciliary oxygen has a capacity of 1360 litres, is 930 mm long and 102 mm in diameter, with an empty weight of about 14.5 kg. The British Standard also gives details of the valves used for closing the cylinders. Three types are used, namely the bull-nosed valve, the handwheel valve and the pin-index or flush-type valve. Other equipment can then be added by means of a standard screw thread. This will always include a device for pressure reduction and flow regulation and may also include flow rate measurement and humidifier before delivery to the patient by mask or nasal catheter.

## IDENTIFICATION OF MEDICAL GASES

A colour coding system for identification was given in BS 1319C, which has been accepted by most countries (ISO 32). In devising the system, the cylinder was divided into two parts, the main body and the shoulder at the valve end. The latter part could be all the same colour, or divided into quarters

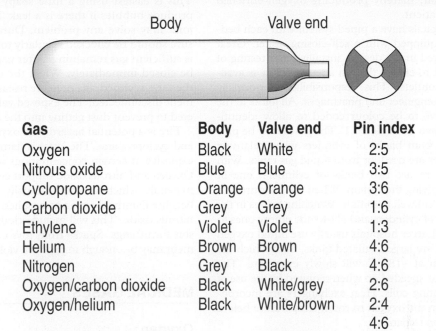

| Gas | Body | Valve end | Pin index |
|-----|------|-----------|-----------|
| Oxygen | Black | White | 2:5 |
| Nitrous oxide | Blue | Blue | 3:5 |
| Cyclopropane | Orange | Orange | 3:6 |
| Carbon dioxide | Grey | Grey | 1:6 |
| Ethylene | Violet | Violet | 1:3 |
| Helium | Brown | Brown | 4:6 |
| Nitrogen | Grey | Black | 4:6 |
| Oxygen/carbon dioxide | Black | White/grey | 2:6 |
| Oxygen/helium | Black | White/brown | 2:4 |
|  |  |  | 4:6 |
| Oxygen/nitrous oxide | Blue | White/blue | 3 |
| Air | Grey | White/black | 1:5 |

Oxygen/helium has two pin indices, where oxygen is less
than 20% 4:6, where oxygen is greater than 20% 2:4

**Fig. 20.1**   Colour code and pin-index methods of identification of medical gas cylinders.

showing alternate colours. When a mixture of gases is in the cylinder, they are indicated by these alternating colours. Details for the common gases are given in Figure 20.1.

The pin-index valve provides an alternative means of identification. Six possible pin positions, relative to the gas outlet, are detailed. A particular gas uses pin positions (usually two) as detailed in BS 1319 (BSI 1970). These are shown in Figure 20.1. In addition, the chemical symbol of the gas is painted onto the cylinder.

Another difficulty with medical gases can be knowing how full a cylinder is. For a permanent gas, the pressure is proportional to the volume, so the use of a pressure gauge is adequate.

Domiciliary equipment is usually calibrated in 'full', 'half', 'quarter'. However, some gases are liquids at cylinder pressures. In these cases, a pressure gauge would only show the vapour pressure of the liquid, which will be constant until the cylinder is virtually empty. This applies to carbon dioxide, nitrous oxide, ethylene and cyclopropane. In these cases, weighing the cylinder is necessary.

## STORAGE AND DISTRIBUTION

Medical gas cylinders need to be stored in cool dry conditions to avoid rusting and damage to the paint. The British Standard of 1976 gave detailed suggestions for rack systems for bulk storage which also allowed for rotation of stock. Pharmacists with contracts to supply domiciliary oxygen must be prepared to deliver cylinders and other equipment to patients' homes and set them up if necessary. Care is required to ensure that there is no confusion between full and empty cylinders. This may be achieved by the use of disposable seals and marking empty cylinders clearly.

Some patients who require large amounts of oxygen may use an oxygen concentrator rather than cylinders. Normally patients considered for an oxygen concentrator would be using oxygen for 15 hours per day or more. Concentrators are not supplied as part of the domiciliary supply system, although they are available on prescription. They operate by using a molecular sieve to remove some nitrogen and other gases from air, thereby producing oxygen-enriched gas for the patient.

Many hospitals have a piped system with each bedside being equipped with a self-closing outlet. Great care is required in the design, installing and testing of the pipework to ensure that an adequate flow is available to all outlets. This responsibility is normally shared by an engineer and pharmacist. All joints in the pipework have to be colour coded to allow identification as shown in Table 20.1. The gases may be provided either from banks of cylinders when relatively small volumes are used, or from liquid gas tanks. With cylinders, there are two banks of cylinders, one of which is supplying the system. When the pressure falls below a pre-set level, automatic switching brings in the reserve bank of cylinders and allows the empty ones to be replaced. Larger hospitals usually use liquid oxygen tanks. These are large insulated tanks, from which the liquid oxygen at −183°C will slowly evaporate. The process can be speeded up when required by the use of electrical heating coils. Heat exchangers are incorporated to warm the oxygen to room temperature before administration to patients.

## SAFE HANDLING OF MEDICAL GAS CYLINDERS

Before use, cylinders should be in a safe position so that they cannot fall over (either in a stand or clamped vertically). When connecting equipment, care should be taken not to grease the joints as this can lead to spontaneous combustion at high gas pressures. Just prior to connecting the equipment, momentary opening of the cylinder valve blows away any dust or particles. This is known as 'snuffing'. On screwing up the joint, do not use excessive force as this might cause damage to the thread. The valve should be turned slowly until fully open, then turned back a quarter turn (to allow another user to recognize that it is open). The key should be left in place if it is a spindle key valve in case an emergency closure is needed. All joints should be checked for leaks.

| Table 20.1 Colour codes used on joints in hospital piped-gas supplies | |
| --- | --- |
| Gas | Colour code |
| Oxygen | White |
| Nitrous oxide | Blue |
| Nitrous oxide/oxygen | Blue/white |
| Carbon dioxide | Grey |
| Air | White/black |
| Vacuum | Primrose yellow |

This is easiest using a little soapy water which will produce bubbles if there is a leak. Reconnecting the joint may solve any problem. During use, the pressure should be checked regularly to ensure that there is sufficient gas remaining. After use the valve should be closed immediately. When the cylinder is empty, the valve is closed, the pressure released and the equipment disconnected. The exposed valve should be covered to prevent dust getting into the mechanism.

Fire is a potential hazard with oxygen, nitrous oxide and cyclopropane. The latter is flammable and can be explosive at certain concentrations with oxygen or air. Oxygen and nitrous oxide support combustion, so that materials which do not normally burn easily may become flammable in an atmosphere rich in oxygen or nitrous oxide. This will include clothing, bedding and soft furnishings. Sparks from toys or electrical equipment may be enough to produce violent ignition.

## MEDICAL GASES

### Oxygen

Oxygen has many therapeutic uses. The main one is treating hypoxia which arises because of under-ventilation of the lungs (such as in bronchitis, pneumonia, acute severe asthma, pulmonary oedema and after general anaesthesia) or where the circulation of the blood is inadequate (as in heart failure). Other situations in which it is used include the treatment of carbon monoxide poisoning, respiratory depression and respiratory failure. High concentrations of oxygen should be reduced as soon as possible owing to its toxic effects. Oxygen can also be used in special chambers at pressures greater than 1 bar (hyperbaric oxygen) for treatment of carbon monoxide and cyanide poisoning and as part of the treatment of anaerobic infections such as gangrene, in radiation therapy and decompression sickness. The use of hyperbaric oxygen in multiple sclerosis is still controversial.

Oxygen can produce respiratory depression and be toxic. Symptoms of toxicity include nausea, mood changes, vertigo, twitching, convulsions and loss of consciousness. Retinopathy of prematurity (retrolental fibroplasia) occurs from an excessive use of oxygen with neonates. This produces blindness and was common in the 1940s and 1950s before the cause was recognized.

Oxygen is produced commercially by fractionation of liquid air. For domiciliary use it is provided in 1360 litre cylinders, although smaller ones are available where portability is important. Such a cylinder provides enough oxygen for 10–12 hours' supply depending on the method of use.

The aim of therapy with oxygen is to increase the amount of oxygen in the lungs without danger to the patient. Most domiciliary apparatus is designed to produce concentrations of up to 28% oxygen in the lungs. There are a number of different ways in which the gas can be given to the patient.

Nasal catheters (or prongs) are moulded plastic devices which introduce oxygen into the nostrils whilst leaving the mouth clear. Oxygen masks come in different designs. Those commonly used in domiciliary oxygen therapy may give either a fixed concentration of oxygen, or may be adjusted to provide different concentrations. The Ventimask MkIV and the Intersurgical 010 Mask both produce 28% oxygen to the patient independently of the patient's pattern of breathing and the flow rate used. It is usual to use a 2 litres per minute flow rate ('medium' on the standard headset). The Intersurgical 005 Mask and the MC Mask give variable performance depending on the flow rate used. At 2 litres per minute it is usually 25–30% oxygen, but at 4 litres per minute ('high' on the standard headset) up to 40% oxygen can be provided, depending on the pattern of breathing. These concentrations tend to be used for patients who require short-term administration, such as acute severe asthma or circulatory failure. Heavy-duty rubber masks are available for more specialized use. Full details of the masks are given in the Drug Tariff.

### Instructions for patients

It is important that pharmacists should give adequate instructions to patients to ensure safe and effective use of their oxygen. The extent of the information presented will vary and be a matter for judgement when a cylinder is delivered. Patients who may have to connect cylinders themselves will require more information than those for whom the pharmacist carries out the operation. Some of the points which may require to be discussed are listed in Table 20.2. Safety has to be a concern because of the risk of explosion and fire. Cards with 'do not' points are available from BOC Gases Medical for attaching to the cylinders.

## Other medical gases

The use of other medical gases is more specialized and so is normally confined to hospital use. A brief summary is given, but further details can be found in Grant (1978) and in pharmacopoeias.

### Nitrous oxide

Nitrous oxide is used for analgesia in midwifery, postoperative pain and procedures such as bronchoscopy and as an anaesthetic in dentistry. It has slight addictive properties. Synthesis is by decomposition of ammonium nitrate at high temperature.

For normal analgesia a 50% nitrous oxide/oxygen mixture is usually adequate. This is readily available commercially as a mixture called Entonox. This mixture remains as a gas down to −7°C, below which the nitrous oxide liquefies and collects at the bottom of the cylinder. When it evaporates, the nitrous oxide remains at the base of the cylinder because of its greater density. Thus storage of Entonox at low temperature must be avoided. Where higher concentrations may be required, oxygen and nitrous oxide are mixed just prior to administration. Some of the equipment allows the patient to control the proportions within externally controlled limits. When inducing anaesthesia, concentrations approaching 100% are sometimes employed. If used for more than a short time this could cause asphyxiation. Nitrous oxide is a non-permanent gas which is present as a liquid in cylinders (critical temperature 36.4°C, critical pressure 72.5 bar). In larger hospitals nitrous oxide may be distributed by a piped system to bedsides. Nitrous oxide is not combustible, but it does support combustion and will, like oxygen, rekindle a glowing split. There is, therefore, a potential fire hazard as with oxygen and similar precautions should be taken.

### Carbon dioxide

This gas is colourless, odourless and tasteless. Commercially it is produced as a by-product from a number of industrial processes. At concentrations

| Table 20.2 | Precautions when using medical gases about which pharmacists may need to inform patients |
|---|---|
| Storage | Avoid extreme heat or cold<br>Dry, clean, well ventilated<br>Away from combustible materials<br>Away from sources of ignition |
| Preparation for use | Never lubricate valve and joints<br>Ensure seal is intact and remove it<br>'Snuff' the joint before connecting<br>Use reasonable force in making connections<br>Open valve fully at first<br>Quarter close during use |
| Leaks | Listen for hissing noise<br>Do not use sealing compounds on leaks<br>Report a leak as soon as possible |
| Use of cylinders | Handle with care, avoid knocks<br>Ensure cylinder cannot fall over<br>Observe no smoking or naked lights<br>Close cylinder valve after use<br>When empty, close valve and replace cap |

up to 5% carbon dioxide is a powerful respiratory stimulant and vasodilator. It finds limited clinical use in treating respiratory depression by drugs such as depressants, hypnotics and anaesthetics and has been used for treating intractable hiccup. At concentrations above 6%, carbon dioxide produces an increasing central depression and acidosis. A ready prepared mixture of 5% carbon dioxide and 95% oxygen is available. Pure carbon dioxide is a nonpermanent gas (critical temperature 31.04°C, critical pressure 73.8 bar) so is present as a liquid in cylinders.

Rapid expansion from the cylinder causes a cooling of the carbon dioxide to below its melting point (−78.5°C) and produces solid carbon dioxide as a 'snow'. This may be collected and shaped for use in cryotherapy of warts, naevi and other skin conditions. Care is required when handling solid carbon dioxide because it 'burns' the skin.

Carbon dioxide dissolves in water to produce carbonated vehicles. These have a sharp taste which has been reported as being useful in masking the unpleasant taste of some liquid medicines.

## Helium

Helium is an inert permanent gas prepared from liquefied air or natural gas. It is used for its physical properties, in particular that it has a very low density (approximately one-tenth of that of nitrogen) which makes it easier to breathe. A 20% oxygen in helium mixture can be used as a substitute for air in patients with acute upper respiratory tract obstruction.

It has a much lower solubility in plasma than nitrogen and so is used in high-pressure diving. Breathing helium increases vocal pitch and distorts the voice.

## Ethylene

This gas, which is produced from petroleum, has properties similar to those of nitrous oxide but its use has declined as a result of its explosive properties. It is liquid in the cylinder.

## Cyclopropane

Cyclopropane is a colourless gas synthesized by reacting zinc with a 1,3-dihalopropane. It is a potent anaesthetic although its use is less widespread than previously. It can form explosive mixtures with air, oxygen or nitrous oxide. It liquefies in the cylinder. Owing to its potency, small quantities only are required and so small cylinder sizes are used.

---

### Key Points

- Medical gases are used in hospital and domiciliary situations.
- The British Standard 1319 gives details of cylinders, valves, colour codes, pin-index identification and storage.
- Colour coding and stencilled chemical symbol are used to identify cylinder contents.
- Mixtures of gases are indicated by alternating colours on the valve end of the cylinder, the body having the colour of the main gas.
- The pin-index valve prevents connection of an incorrect cylinder.
- For permanent gases the pressure is proportional to the amount of gas remaining, but for liquefied gases the pressure remains constant until the cylinder is nearly empty.
- Pharmacists with a domiciliary oxygen supply contract must keep agreed stock levels and assist with delivery and installation.
- Hospital oxygen supplies are designed to avoid any interruption of supply to the patient.
- Medical gases produce fire and explosion hazards which must be minimized.
- Domiciliary patients must be given detailed instructions on the use of oxygen and equipment.
- Oxygen is used to treat hypoxia, carbon monoxide poisoning and respiratory depression and failure.
- Oxygen has the potential to be toxic, so most domiciliary oxygen masks give a maximum 28% concentration.
- Storage of Entonox at low temperature can cause separation of the gases.
- Carbon dioxide is a respiratory stimulant up to 5%, and a central depressant above 6% concentration.
- Helium is used for its low density to aid patients with respiratory tract obstruction.

---

## FURTHER READING

British Pharmacopoeia, current edn. HMSO, London.

British Standard 1319 1976 British Standards Institution, London

Couper I 1994 Medical gases. In: The pharmaceutical codex, 12th edn. The Pharmaceutical Press, London, pp 469–475

European Pharmacopoeia, current edn. Maisonneuve S. A., Saint Ruffine, France

Grant W J 1978 Medical gases: their properties and uses. HM&M Publishers, Aylesbury

# PART 3

# STERILE PRODUCTS

# 21
# Principles of sterilization

*R. M. E. Richards*

---

When you have studied this chapter you should be able to:

**Define: sterility; sterilization; aseptic techniques; sterility testing; disinfection; disinfectant; antiseptic**

**Explain: bioburden; death rates; probability of survival concepts; *D* value; *Z* value; *Q* value**

**Discuss *F* values and the concept of lethality in relation to heat-sensitive products**

**Discuss sterilization in relation to validation and monitoring**

**Describe factors affecting sterilization.**

## Introduction

Pharmaceutical products are generally required to be free from contamination with microorganisms (bacteria, viruses, yeasts, moulds, etc.). Such organisms may cause spoilage by adversely affecting the appearance or composition of a product and may cause serious adverse effects in the patient. Adverse effects are particularly likely if the preparation is introduced into the body via a route which bypasses some of the body's normal defence mechanisms, especially in a seriously ill or immunocompromised patient.

Dosage forms designed for parenteral, ophthalmic or surgical use, as well as irrigation solutions and topical preparations for application to large open wounds, must be free from microbial and particulate contamination. These products are required to be prepared and maintained in a sterile state until used. Some of the terms used in connection with 'sterile pharmaceutical products' are defined below.

### Sterility

Sterility may be defined as the total absence of viable microorganisms and is an absolute state. The production of sterile pharmaceutical products may be achieved by aseptic technique (see Ch. 23) or by means of a terminal sterilization process (see Ch. 22).

### Sterilization

This is the subjection of products to a process whereby all viable life forms are either killed or removed. The sterilization process is usually the final stage in the preparation of the product. The methods of sterilization in regular use include exposure to: saturated steam under pressure, dry heat, ionizing radiation, ethylene oxide or passage through a bacteria-retaining filter. When possible, exposure to saturated steam under pressure is the sterilization method of choice.

### Aseptic technique

This is the preparation of pharmaceutical products from sterile ingredients by procedures that exclude the access of viable microorganisms into the products. It is used for those products that would be adversely affected by being subjected to a sterilization process.

### Sterility testing

Tests for sterility of pharmaceutical products attempt to reveal the presence or absence of viable microorganisms in a sample number of containers taken from a production batch. From the results of such tests an inference is made as to the sterility of the batch.

### Disinfection

Disinfection is a process which aims to reduce the number of harmful (pathogenic) microorganisms in a particular situation. Disinfection will destroy infective vegetative organisms but not necessarily resistant spores, i.e. it is not an absolute process. It often involves the use of chemicals although other means of disinfection may be employed, e.g. the pasteurization of milk is a disinfection process that uses heat.

### Disinfectant

This is a chemical agent used to destroy harmful microorganisms usually on inanimate objects.

### Antiseptic

This is a chemical agent usually applied to living tissues in humans or animals in order to destroy harmful microorganisms.

## STERILIZATION CRITERIA

### The bioburden

In order to select the appropriate parameters for any method intended to kill microorganisms in a given product or associated with a given material, it is necessary to know the initial number of organisms present. That is the 'bioburden' or 'bioload', and the resistance of those organisms to the chosen process. For example, it has been the practice to choose the time and temperature relationship for steam sterilization to ensure that a large number of the known most resistant pathogens would be killed. This treatment would not necessarily be sufficient to kill a large number of the known most resistant non-pathogenic organisms. However, it is extremely unlikely that such an organism would be present. The time and temperature chosen in such a steam sterilization process is also greatly in excess of the treatment necessary to kill the small number of heat-sensitive contaminants likely to be present in pharmaceutical solutions.

### Establishing microbial death

Death in a microbial population is determined by assessing the reduction in the number of viable microorganisms resulting from contact with a given destructive force. Viable organisms are those which when transferred to a culture medium can form a colony. This places the onus on the investigator to provide suitable culture conditions for recovery and growth of any surviving microorganisms.

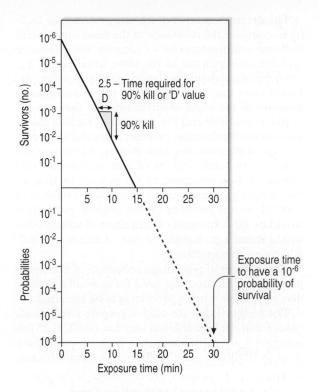

**Fig. 21.1** Microbial survivor curve.

### Death rates

When a population of microorganisms is subjected to a destructive sterilization procedure the order of death is generally logarithmic. That is, a constant proportion of the microbial population is inactivated in any given time interval, approximating to first-order kinetics.

A typical survivor curve is shown in Figure 21.1.

If $N_0$ is the initial number of organisms and $N_t$ is the number of organisms surviving after time $t$, the death rate constant (inactivation constant) $k$ can be calculated.

$$N_t = N_0 e^{-kt}$$
$$\ln N_t = \ln N_0 - kt$$
$$\log_{10} N_t = \log_{10} N_0 - \frac{kt}{2.303}$$

The death rate constant can be calculated as follows from Figure 21.1.

Let $N_0 = 10^6$, $N_t = 10^2$ and $t = 10$

Then:

$$k = 1/10 \ (\log_{10} 10^6 / 10^2)$$
$$= 1/10 \ (6 - 2) = 0.4$$

The determination of death rate provides the facility to compare the resistance of the same organism at different temperatures or to compare the resistance of different organisms to the same lethal agent, e.g. temperature, ionizing radiation, chemical agent, etc. Death rates may also be used to give a quantitative measure of the effect of environmental factors such as pH, osmolarity and the presence of various chemicals on the sterilization process. Since the same percentage of bacteria dies each minute, it is impossible in theory to reach a point of zero survivors. From Figure 21.1 an extension of the process to 30 minutes would give the assurance that the probability of survival of one member of the original population would be $10^{-6}$. In terms of containers of solution this would mean a probability of one container in a million being contaminated.

The concept of percentage reduction of a bacterial population reinforces the need for as small a bioburden as possible when a product is to be sterilized.

The methods that are used to prepare sterile fluids ensure that the bioburden is very low (see Ch. 25). If containers are filled through a bacteria-proof filter prior to sterilization the bioburden is effectively zero.

## D value or decimal reduction time

The death rate can also be expressed as the decimal reduction time or $D$ value. This is the time in minutes at any defined temperature to destroy 90% of viable organisms. In Figure 21.1 this is 2.5 minutes. Numerically it is also the reciprocal of the death rate constant. $D$ values are often given a subscript to indicate the temperature at which they were measured, e.g. $D_{121°C}$. From the $D$ value for a particular combination of organism/time/temperature an 'inactivation factor' (IF) can be calculated, e.g. if the $D$ value of an organism exposed to a temperature of 121°C for 15 minutes was 2 minutes the IF would be $10^{15/2}$, i.e. $10^{7.5}$.

## Z value or thermal destruction value

This relates the heat resistance of a microorganism to changes in temperature. The $Z$ value is the number of degrees of temperature change required to produce a 10-fold change in $D$ value. Bacterial spores have a $Z$ value in the range 10–15°C while most non-sporing organisms have $Z$ values of 4–6°C.

## Q value or temperature coefficient

This also gives a measure of the relative resistance of different microorganisms and describes the change in the death rate over a 10°C change in temperature.

## F values

The $F$ value is a measure of the lethality of the total process of sterilization and equates heat treatment at any particular temperature with the time in minutes at a designated reference temperature that would be required to produce the same lethality in an organism of stated $Z$ value. For a temperature of 121°C and organisms with a $Z$ value of 10°C $F$ becomes $F_0$. Annex 2 of Appendix XVIII of the *British Pharmacopoeia* (BP 1993) contains the following description of $F_0$: 'The $F_0$ value of a saturated steam process is the lethality expressed in terms of the equivalent time in minutes at 121°C delivered by that process to the product in its final containers with reference to microorganisms possessing a $Z$ value of 10°C'.

1 $F$ unit is equivalent to heating the load for 1 minute at 121°C. Mathematically $F$ is defined as:

$$F_0 = 10^{(T_c - 121/Z)} \, dt$$

where $T_c$ = load temperature at time d$t$ and $Z$ = 10°C.

For many years it has been understood that both the heating up and cooling phases of a heat sterilizing cycle contribute to the total lethality of the process. The $F$ principle allows an estimation of the overall lethality by integration of the lethal rates multiplied by the times at discrete temperature intervals (Fig. 21.2).

The total lethality ($F_0$) for the cycle is equal to the sum of the $F_0$ values for each individual time/temperature segment. The accuracy of the estimated $F_0$ is related to the time interval represented by each segment of the profile. Small intervals are conveniently handled by computer. The BP suggests the use of the $F_0$ calculation for the overall lethality delivered to aqueous preparations for a microbiologically validated steam sterilization process. It states that a total $F_0$ value of not less than 8 applied to every container in the load would be considered satisfactory.

Where the product is especially heat sensitive an $F_0$ of less than 8 is deemed justifiable. That is so long as great care is taken to ensure that an adequate assurance of sterility is consistently achieved. In such cases the BP states: 'it is necessary not only to validate the process microbiologically, but also to perform continuous, rigorous, microbiological monitoring during routine production to demonstrate that microbiological parameters are within the established tolerances so as to give a theoretical level of not more

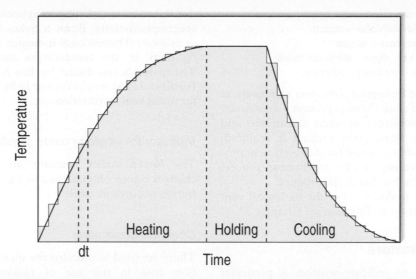

**Fig. 21.2** The time–temperature recording of a typical autoclave cycle showing the method of integration by dividing the time axis into a series of segments (d$t$) (Kirk et al 1982).

than one living organism in $10^6$ containers of the final product'.

Kirk et al (1985) investigated the degradation under autoclaving conditions of 2,4-dihydroxybenzoic acid in aqueous phosphate buffer pH 7. They found those autoclave cycles delivering a standard process lethality ($F_0 = 8$) by means of different holding temperatures caused different degrees of degradation of the chemical. That is high temperature, short time cycles ($121°C/F_0 = 8$) caused approximately 12% degradation but prolonged exposure at a relatively low temperature ($112°C/F_0 = 8$) caused approximately 30% degradation. Thus in the interest of stability these workers suggested that, where other factors permit, the optimum sterilization cycle would consist of the load being subjected to a temperature which continuously increased, no holding phase, until a prefixed $F_0$ had been achieved. The load would then be cooled under controlled conditions and this cooling phase would provide the remaining $F_0$ units required to achieve the predetermined level of sterility assurance.

## STERILIZATION, VALIDATION AND MONITORING

Tests for sterility of the products subjected to a sterilization procedure are discussed in Chapter 30. Whenever possible additional validation and monitoring of the sterilization process is carried out using indicators other than the product. Biological, chemical and physical indicators have all been used.

## Biological indicators

Biological indicators are supplied in one of two main forms, each of which incorporates a viable culture of a stated species of microorganism. One form consists of spores added to a carrier such as a disc or strip of filter paper, glass or plastic, so packaged as to protect the contents before use but to allow the sterilizing agent to reach the spores and exert its effect during use. In the other form the spores are added to representative units of the product to be sterilized or to similar units if it is not practicable to add the spores to selected units of a particular product.

Choice of the biological indicator is critical if the indication given is to be a valid reflection of the efficacy of a sterilization cycle. The viability of the organisms, the storage conditions before use and the incubation and culture conditions after sterilization must be standardized for the result to be meaningful, especially for the less challenging protocols (e.g. $F_0$ values of 8 or less).

The reader is referred to the monographs in the BP (1993) and *United States Pharmacopoeia* (USP 23, 1995) and the Health Technical Memorandum 2010 (1996) for current recommendations.

The organisms used as biological indicators include:

*Bacillus subtilis* var. *niger* – dry heat
*Bacillus stearothermophilus* – steam
*Clostridium sporogenes* – steam
*Bacillus subtilis* var. *niger* – ethylene oxide
*Bacillus pumulis* – ionizing radiation.

In order to use biological indicators effectively in the monitoring of a sterilization process a knowledge of the product bioburden in terms of numbers and resistance to the sterilization method is required. The biological indicator must be so chosen as to provide a greater challenge to the sterilization process than the natural bioburden of the product.

*Sterilization by filtration.* For the biological validation of sterilization by filtration see Chapter 23.

## Chemical indicators

These are used to indicate whether a particular batch of product has been through a sterilization process, they do not generally indicate whether the process was successful. The indicator chosen undergoes some change in physical or chemical nature when exposed to the conditions of the sterilization process.

### Browne's tubes

These are sealed glass tubes (manufactured by A. Browne, Ltd Leicester) containing a red fluid which changes colour through yellow and brown to green on heating at the specified temperature for the appropriate length of time. Various types are available for different sterilization processes, e.g. moist heat and dry heat processes. They should not be used as quantitative indicators.

### Heat-sensitive tape

The Bowie–Dick test is valuable for confirming that steam has displaced all the air from a porous load in a high vacuum autoclave. It consists of using autoclave tape which has heat-sensitive bars, at intervals of about 15 mm, which change colour after contact with steam. The tape is placed suitably wrapped at the centre of a test pack. All the bars on the tape should change colour to demonstrate full penetration of the steam. Duration of exposure or temperature attained is not indicated by this type of indicator.

### Chemical degradation tests

A test has been described which follows the degrada-

tion kinetics of 2,4-dihydroxybenzoic acid by u.v. spectrophotometry. Bunn & Sykes (1981) were able to calibrate Thermalog S indicator strips in terms of $F_0$ units in the temperature range 115–123°C. Thermalog S (produced by Bio Medical Sciences, Fairfield, USA) would appear to be a useful monitor for moist heat sterilization.

### Indicator for ethylene oxide sterilization

The Royce sachet contains an indicator which changes colour on exposure to a given time/concentration of ethylene oxide.

### Chemical dosimeters

These are used to monitor the quantity of the radiation dose in the use of radiation sterilization. Qualitative indicators of exposure to radiation are also available.

## Physical validation and monitoring

In the UK, guidelines on the acceptability of a sterilization cycle are given in the Health Technical Memorandum 2010 (1996) on sterilization. A master process record (MPR) is prepared as part of the validation procedure for a particular autoclave and for each specified product and load configuration. This may then be used as a reference for the process record obtained from a single thermocouple placed in a strategic part of each load (batch process record, BPR).

The MPR should be checked at annual intervals and whenever significant changes occur in the BPR when compared with the MPR.

Microprocessor-controlled sterilization cycles are now a part of modern autoclaves. The microprocessor gives the possibility of a very tight control and description of sterilization cycles.

---

**Key Points**

Factors affecting sterilization:
- Relating to the bioburden:
  - initial number of organisms
  - their heat resistance
  - recovery and growth requirements
- Relating to the sterilization process:
  - method chosen
  - probability of sterilization

- overall lethality
- validation and monitoring
- Relating to the product:
  - solubility
  - pH and nutritive properties
  - heat stability
  - moisture stability
- Relating to the container:
  - suitability to withstand process chosen
  - suitability to protect and not interact with product
  - suitability for transport and storage of product.

## FURTHER READING

British Pharmacopoeia 1993 HMSO, London
Bunn J N, Sykes I K 1981 A chemical indicator for the rapid measurement of $F$ values. Journal of Applied Bacteriology 51: 143–147
European Pharmacopoeia 1996 3rd edn. Maisonneuve S. A., Saint Ruffine, France
Health Technical Memorandum 1996 No. 2010. Sterilization. HMSO London
Kirk B, Hambleton R, Everett M 1982 Computer aided autoclave monitoring. Pharmaceutical Journal 299: 252–254
Kirk B, Hambleton R, Hoskins H T 1985 A model for predicting the stability of autoclaved pharmaceuticals using real time computer integration techniques. Journal of Parenteral Science and Technology 39: 89–98
United States Pharmacopoeia 23 1995 Mack, Easton, PA

# 22

# Methods of sterilization

*R. M. E. Richards*

After studying this chapter you should be able to:

**Explain the moist heat sterilization process for pharmaceuticals, dressings and equipment**

**Explain the dry heat methods of sterilization process for pharmaceuticals and equipment**

**Compare and contrast the advantages and disadvantages of the two heat sterilization processes**

**Explain the functioning of the equipment used in moist and dry heat sterilization**

**Discuss the alternative methods of sterilization available for sterilizing pharmaceuticals, dressings and equipment.**

## THERMAL DESTRUCTION OF MICROORGANISMS

The killing of microorganisms by heat is a function of the time–temperature combination used. If the temperature is increased then the time required for a given kill is decreased. The vital constituents of living matter such as proteins and nucleic acids are denatured with increasing rapidity as the temperature rises above 50°C. Although the mechanism of thermally induced death is not fully understood the traditional theory has been that death results from heat inactivation of vital enzyme systems within the cell.

The consensus of opinion in the literature indicates that bacterial death by moist heat is due to denaturation and coagulation of essential protein molecules, whereas dry heat appears to cause protein denaturation by oxidation processes. The mechanisms of action of dry and wet heat are certainly different. This is emphasized by the finding that

*Bacillus subtilis* var. *niger* spores can resist dry heat at 121°C for nearly 2000 times longer than they resist moist heat at 121°C. However, moist heat only contains approximately seven times more energy than hot air at the same temperature. Thus the factor of 2000 cannot be adequately explained solely in terms of the extra energy content of moist heat.

A prime reference source on sterilization is the latest Health Technical Memorandum 2010 (1996) which provides a comprehensive coverage of the subject in five parts. These are Management policy; Design considerations; Validation and verification; Operational management and Good practice guide.

## MOIST HEAT STERILIZATION

The sterilization method of choice for aqueous preparations and for surgical dressings is heating in saturated steam under pressure. A number of time–temperature combinations have been proposed. The USP 23 (1995) and BP (1993) recommend 121°C maintained throughout the load for 15 minutes as the preferred combination.

### Principles of sterilization by steam under pressure

Pressure itself has no sterilizing power. Steam is used under pressure as a means of achieving an elevated temperature. It is important to ensure that steam of the correct quality is used in order to avoid the problems which follow incorrect removal of air, superheating of the steam, failure of steam penetration into porous loads, etc.

#### Steam production

This may be achieved in two ways. On a small scale, steam may be generated from water within the sterilizer and because water is present the steam is known as wet saturated steam. For large-scale sterilizers, dry saturated steam may be piped from a separate boiler.

## Saturated and supersaturated steam

Steam is described as saturated when it is at a temperature corresponding to the liquid boiling point appropriate to its pressure. Important properties of saturated steam are illustrated by reference to Figure 22.1.

The phase boundary is obtained by joining points representing saturated steam temperatures at different pressures, e.g. 115°C at 172 kPa (1.7 bar), 121°C at 202 kPa (2 bar) and 134°C at 304 kPa (3 bar). If saturated steam at 'A' is isolated from water and heated without change of pressure from 'A' to 'D', or the pressure is lowered without change of temperature from 'A' to 'E', then the steam must become hotter because there is no water from which further evaporation can occur. Therefore it is no longer at the temperature corresponding to the liquid boiling point appropriate to its pressure and it is called superheated steam. Superheat is to be avoided because as steam becomes more superheated it

becomes more like hot air and therefore less effective as a sterilizing medium. Very slight cooling will not make superheated steam condense. Before this can occur the temperature must be reduced to the temperature of the corresponding saturated steam point. That is from 'D' to 'A' or from 'E' to 'F' on the diagram. Superheated steam can arise from several sources but sterilizer jacket heat is the predominant source and is caused when the jacket is hotter than the steam in the chamber. This is a practical consequence of the theory outlined above. In this example the problem arises because the system has, in effect, moved to point 'D' in Figure 22.1. To prevent it, care should be taken to ensure that the jacket and the chamber temperatures are similar.

Now consider again the saturated steam at point 'A'. As soon as the steam is cooled at constant pressure, e.g. from 'A' to 'B', it will deposit water. (The same would happen if the pressure were raised to point 'C' without alteration of temperature.) The condensation of saturated steam on cooling liberates all of its latent heat immediately. This is a very important property in sterilization.

Heat energy in steam is in the form of 'sensible heat' and 'latent heat'. Sensible heat is the heat required to raise the temperature of water, and latent heat (of vaporization) is the amount of heat required to convert water at its boiling point to steam at the same temperature. Table 22.1 illustrates the high percentage of total heat that is latent heat at various temperatures.

The advantages of saturated steam include:

- *Penetration*. It flows quickly to every article in the load (and into porous articles). This is due to its contraction to a very small volume on condensation creating a low-pressure region into which more steam flows.
- *Rapid heating*. It heats the load rapidly owing to the release of its considerable latent heat.
- *Moist heat*. The condensate produced on cool-

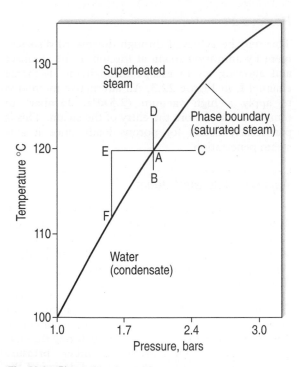

**Fig. 22.1** Phase diagram for water and steam.

| Table 22.1 Heat content of steam at various pressures | | | | | |
|---|---|---|---|---|---|
| Pressure | | Temperature | Heat | | |
| (kPa) | (bar) | (°C) | Sensible | Latent | Latent to total |
| | | | (kJ/kg) | (kJ/kg) | (%) |
| 172 | 1.7 | 115 | 483 | 2216 | 82 |
| 202 | 2.0 | 121 | 505 | 2202 | 81 |
| 242 | 2.4 | 126 | 530 | 2185 | 80 |
| 304 | 3.0 | 134 | 561 | 2164 | 79 |

ing contributes to the lethality by coagulating microbial protein.

- *No residual toxicity.* The product is free from toxic contamination.

### Presence of air

Air occupies the space in the sterilizer before steam is generated or admitted. Air is also present dissolved in water before its conversion to steam. Air allowed to remain in the sterilizer forms a thin layer which clings to every surface on which steam condensation occurs. Since air is a poor conductor it provides a barrier to heat penetration. In small sterilizers turbulence is likely to disperse the air film but in large sterilizers effective air removal is vital.

### Wet steam

Wet steam contains less heat than dry saturated steam and is harmful to dressings.

## THE DESIGN AND OPERATION OF AUTOCLAVES

The word autoclave means self-closing. Originally this referred to the closing of the lid by the excess pressure within the vessel. Modern usage of the word is rather wider and it is often used for modern sterilizing equipment which is not necessarily self-closing.

## Portable autoclaves

These may be used for laboratory work and for small-scale production. They are generally of two types, pressure regulated and temperature regulated.

In a pressure-controlled type the pressure gauge is the sole indicator of the internal conditions and therefore all the air must be removed before the sterilizing exposure time begins.

In the temperature-controlled type shown in Figure 22.2 a thermometer or thermostat is used to indicate or ensure respectively that exposure temperature has been reached and it is less essential to expel the air. The recommended holding time–temperature relationship is 121°C for 15 minutes achieved at a pressure of 202 kPa (2.0 bar). Other recommended time–temperature relationships are listed in Table 22.2.

## Large sterilizers

The essential features of a large sterilizer are shown diagrammatically in Figure 22.3 and will be used in the following general description. While the basic features are common to all types of sterilizer, the manufacturer's literature should be consulted for details of the features of a particular model.

### General procedure

- Load material to be sterilized and close door.
- Remove air.
- Admit dry saturated steam (venting and condensate removal automatic).
- Allow for heating up and expose for required duration.
- Cut off steam supply.
- Allow to cool (or spray cool if appropriate).

These steps are now discussed below in turn.

### Loading

This should be carried out so that heat distribution within the load is optimal and will vary with the type of load, e.g. bottles, plastic containers, dressings, etc.

### Remove air

This may be achieved through downward displacement by admitting steam at the top of the sterilizer and allowing air to escape through the discharge channel L in Figure 22.3. An alternative method is to apply a high vacuum (2.5 kPa, 25 mbar) to remove the air before the entry of the steam. This is particularly useful for porous loads since it aids steam penetration.

### Admit dry saturated steam

In order to reduce the moisture content of steam delivered from the boiler the steam is passed through a separator (B in Fig. 22.3) which collects suspended condensate. The reducing valve, C, lowers the pressure to the required level and in doing so effects further drying.

*Special requirements for plastic containers.* For plastic containers there is an additional requirement for an over-pressure inside the autoclave chamber to prevent the containers from bursting during the sterilization cycle. The excess chamber pressure required will depend on the type and design of the

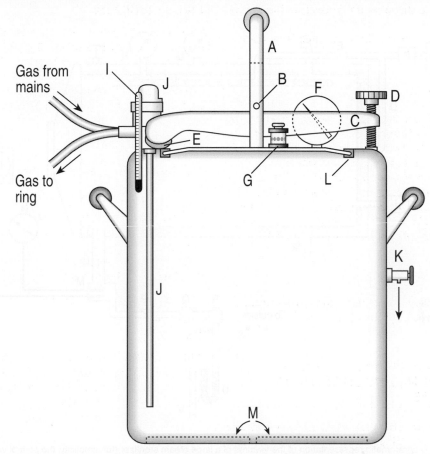

**Fig. 22.2** Temperature-controlled portable autoclave (diagrammatic). A, Handle of lid; B, rivet; C, crossbar; D, thumbscrew; E, pad; F, pressure gauge; G, safety valve; I, thermometer, J, thermostat; K, air vent; L, gasket; M, semicircular plates.

**Table 22.2 Possible time/temperature relationships for saturated steam sterilization**

| Temperature °C | Corresponding nominal pressure | | | Minimum holding time (min) |
|---|---|---|---|---|
| | (kPa) abs | (1bf/in²)g | (bar) abs | |
| 115–116 | 172 | 10 | 1.7 | 30 |
| 121–123 | 202 | 15 | 2.0 | 15 |
| 126–129 | 242 | 20 | 2.4 | 10 |
| 134–138 | 304 | 32 | 3.0 | 3 |

*Note:* Pressures expressed in kgf/cm² and lbf/in² are expressed as 'gauge' (g), i.e. in excess of atmospheric, and in kPa and bar as absolute (abs) pressures.

of condensate are produced, particularly during the heat-up cycle. Condensate runs down to the bottom of the chamber and drains through the same discharge channel as the air (L in Fig. 22.3). A check valve and trap are incorporated to prevent suck-back contamination of the chamber on cooling.

### Exposure for required duration

At least two temperature-sensing devices should be used. One should be placed in the discharge channel and one in a container or in part of the load in a strategic place (i.e. that predicted to be the coolest) in the chamber (see Ch. 21).

container and the amount of air remaining inside the container after filling.

*Automatic removal of condensate.* Large volumes

### Cut off steam supply

This is done by closing the appropriate control valve.

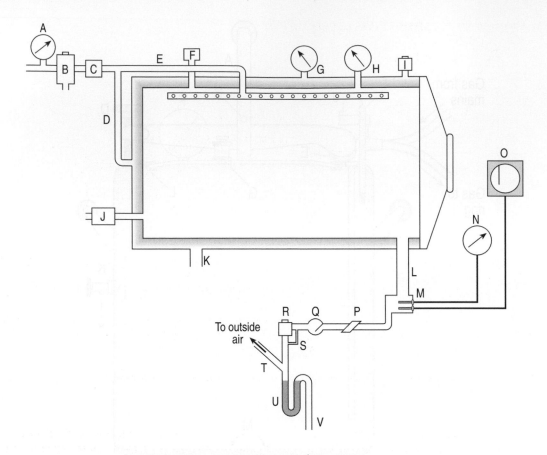

**Fig. 22.3** Diagrammatic representation of the features of a large steam sterilizer (for simplicity, the control valves have been omitted). A, Mains pressure gauge; B, separator; C, reducing valve; D, steam supply to jacket; E, steam supply to chambers; F, air filter; G, jacket pressure gauge; H, chamber pressure gauge; I, jacket air vent; J, vacuum pump; K, jacket discharge channel (detail not shown); L, chamber discharge channel; M, thermometer pocket; N, direct-reading thermometer; O, recording thermometer; P, strainer; Q, check valve; R, balanced-pressure thermostatic trap; S, bypass; T, vapour escape line; U, water seal; V, air-break.

## Allow to cool

The method used for cooling depends on the type of load.

*Fluid containers.* Fluid containers cool very slowly because of their large heat capacity and the containers may burst if the sterilizer is opened at too high a temperature. Cooling time may be reduced by using a very fine mist of cold water (50–100 mμ diameter droplets) sprayed over the containers. Table 22.3 shows the time savings with forced cooling. Compressed air is admitted to the bottom of the chamber to compensate for the pressure drop caused by the condensation of steam. For plastic containers spray cooling must take place with an excess pressure outside the bag in order to avoid bursting. Problems may arise if the spray water is contaminat-

**Table 22.3 Time for contents to fall from 115°C to 95°C**

| Load | Without water cooling | With water cooling |
|---|---|---|
| 24 × 500 ml bottles | 3 h | 10 min |
| 200 × 1 litre bottles | 22 h | 17 min |

ed and/or if the closures of the fluid containers are rendered ineffective by the sterilization process.

Autoclaves have been commissioned in Holland which are heated by very hot water under pressure and cooled by the same recirculating water passing through a suitable heat exchanger. The water is

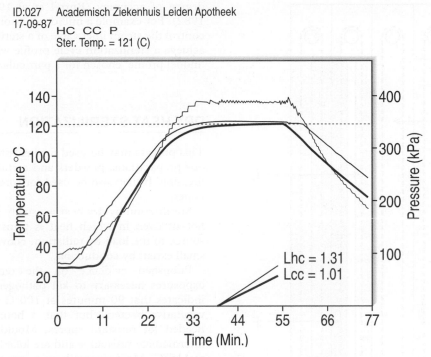

ID:027 Academisch Ziekenhuis Leiden Apotheek
17-09-87
HC CC P
Ster. Temp. = 121 (C)

Lhc = 1.31
Lcc = 1.01

**Fig. 22.4** Record of autoclave pressure and container temperature during a sterilization cycle.

introduced through many small holes at the top of the autoclave and removed from the bottom of the autoclave. The pressure within the autoclave is maintained at a slightly higher pressure than the calculated pressure within the glass bottles or plastic containers. It is important with this type of autoclave to monitor the rate of water flow through the autoclave to check that it is maintained within the desired range.

Figure 22.4 represents the autoclave pressure (highest recorded line on the graph), hottest container temperature (second highest line), coldest container temperature (the lowest recorded line), together with the lethality for each of these temperatures. The record is produced in multicoloured graphical form by a linked microcomputer. This graph then forms the batch record.

*Porous loads.* Porous loads are wet at the end of the exposure period due to absorbed condensate and must be dried. This is best achieved by application of high vacuum. A vacuum pump is used to remove the steam and to reduce the pressure to 2.5 kPa (25 mbar) in about 3 minutes. Under these conditions the moisture content of the dressings is only slightly greater than before sterilization.

The air used for breaking the vacuum after drying must be sterile.

Older methods of drying the load include radiation from the sterilizer jacket, low vacuum with no air and using a steam ejector to suck warm filtered air through the load.

## Hydrostatic continuous sterilizers

The need for the production of large batches of sterilized fluids has led to the development of continuous sterilizers, represented diagrammatically in Figure 22.5.

Containers are fed automatically onto an endless conveyor that carries them up and down a series of towers 17 m high. The containers are subjected in turn to preheating, sterilizing, water cooling and spray cooling before leaving the sterilizer.

## Automatic control of steam sterilizers

Most large sterilizers are operated under automatic control and may offer a series of 'programmes' for different types of load. It is essential that pressure and temperature recordings are checked for each cycle to ensure that no malfunction has occurred and that the selected conditions have been achieved.

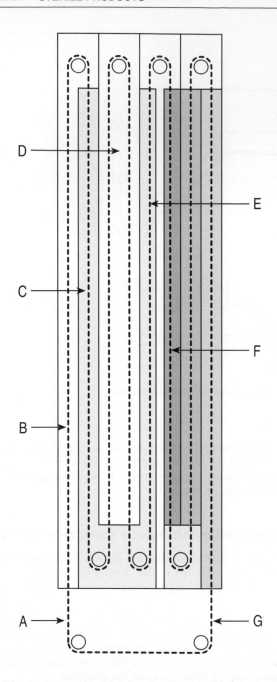

**Fig. 22.5** Hydrostatic continuous sterilizer (diagrammatic). A, Infeed point; B, conveyor; C, hydrostatic preheating leg; D, sterilizing tower; E, hydrostatic cooling leg; F, spray cooling leg, G, discharge point.

*Control by microprocessor*

The microprocessor offers the facility to monitor and to control the steam sterilization process with a high degree of accuracy (Burrel et al 1979, Kirk et al 1982). For example a microprocessor can be used to control the steam inlet valve of a sterilizer in order to achieve a sterilization cycle profile which matches a 'model profile' chosen for a particular type of load.

## DRY HEAT STERILIZATION

This process may be used for heat-stable non-aqueous preparations, powders and certain impregnated dressing. It may also be used for some types of container.

Sterilization by dry heat is usually carried out in a hot-air oven in which heat is transferred from its source to the load by radiation, convection and to a small extent by conduction.

Published evidence on the temperature–time exposures necessary to kill pathogens by dry heat indicates that 90 minutes at 100°C will destroy all vegetative bacteria but that 3 hours at 140°C is needed for resistant spores. Mould spores are of intermediate resistance and are killed by 90 minutes at 115°C. Most viruses have a resistance similar to vegetative bacteria but some viruses are known that are as resistant as bacterial spores, e.g. the virus that causes homologous serum jaundice.

### Recommended time–temperature combinations

Different combinations are required for different products. Cycles recommended in the BP (1993) are:

- a minimum of 180°C for not less than 30 minutes
- a minimum of 170°C for not less than 1 hour
- a minimum of 160°C for not less than 2 hours.

Treatment at 250°C for 45 minutes is a useful method for preparation of glass containers intended for large volume parenteral dosage forms since this is considered to be effective in denaturing pyrogens adsorbed onto the surface of the glassware.

In each cycle it is important to ensure that the whole of the contents of each container is maintained for an effective combination of time and temperature and especially to allow for temperature variations in hot-air ovens, which may be considerable.

### Design and operation of the dry heat sterilizer

Ovens suitable for dry heat sterilization should be

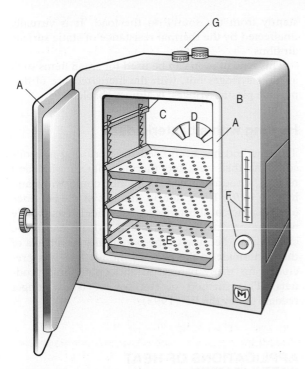

**Fig. 22.6**  Hot-air oven. A, Asbestos gasket; B, outer case containing glass-fibre insulation, and heaters in chamber wall; C, false wall; D, fan; E, perforated shelf; F, regulator; G, vents.

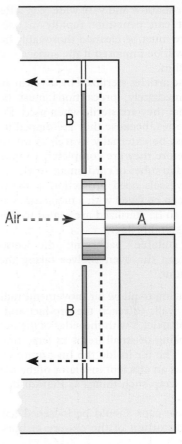

**Fig. 22.7**  Section of rear of an oven showing air circulation produced by a fan. A, Fan; B, false back.

specially designed for the purpose and equipped with forced air circulation (see Fig. 22.6). The Health Services Technical Memorandum 2010 (1996) recommends that the sterilizer be maintained at a positive pressure and all air entering the chamber should be via a bacteria-proof filter. Only a small amount of the heat is transferred from the heat source to the articles in a hot-air oven by conduction, because of the limited pathways and small areas of contact. Convection is responsible for more heat transfer but this is not a very efficient process. Maximum use of the heating capacity of the air is made by circulating it with a fan in order to have the maximum number of air molecules collide with the load and hot chamber surfaces (see Fig. 22.7). In addition, pockets of stagnant cool air are prevented.

Radiation is the chief form of heat transfer and this is why the heaters need to be arranged all round the chamber. It is useful to have the oven fitted with the facility for automatic boost heating to give minimum heat-up times. Accurate temperature control by easily set regulators is essential. The loaded oven temperature variation should not exceed 5°C once the sterilizing temperature is reached. (The temperature variation is usually measured as the difference between the temperature at the centre and any other point; see BS 3421 (1961).)

The method of validating sterilization cycles has been given in Chapter 21.

It is important to reduce the heating-up time to a minimum, partly for economy, but chiefly to prevent excessive overheating of the outer regions of materials and preparations during the time that heat is penetrating to their centres. The best way is to use small containers through which the heat will be transferred quickly, even if the containers are poor conductors. A wise upper weight limit for substances such as powders and oils is 25 g. It is best to load the oven with only one type of material in one size and type of container. The walls of the container should be as thin as practicable and of good heat-conducting material, e.g. metal rather than glass for powders. Tins should be blackened or dull to absorb and not reflect heat and, as a general rule, all containers should be either tall and narrow (e.g. a long cylindrical tin) or shallow and very wide (e.g. a Petri dish) so that heat can penetrate rapidly in one direction. Glassware must be cleaned thoroughly because heat transfer will be impaired if the surface is coated with a greasy film.

Because articles sterilized by dry heat are not often used immediately, precautions must be taken to ensure that they are sterile when used. For example, glass pipettes, because they are dipped in sterile liquids, must be externally as well as internally sterile and therefore they are completely wrapped in paper or packed in tubes of card, metal or glass. Items such as glass vessels need protection at the mouth only and this can be given with a metal cap. Containers of products to be sterilized are sealed with a screw cap having a suitable liner.

After suitable packaging the containers are arranged on the oven shelves taking the following into account.

1. Spacing to allow air movement, radiation from the oven walls to reach the product and to prevent contact of articles with the sides of the oven.

2. Packing of small items in large tins should be avoided. The air inside the tin cannot easily escape and acts as an efficient insulator of the contents. It is better to wrap such things as Petri dishes in twos or threes.

3. Screw caps should be loosened half a turn to prevent distortion of the closure or bursting of the container.

The time is noted when the temperature recorder shows that the oven air has reached the required temperature and the appropriate exposure is subsequently given to include lag time and sterilization time. After switching off, the door is left closed until the temperature has fallen to 40°C in order to prevent breakages. The bottle caps are tightened.

A dry heat oven should have a door lock or accidental openings of the door may occur. Automatic control is easy to achieve consisting of a suitable device to start the timing when the required temperature is reached and to switch off the heating after the appropriate exposure, including lag time, has been given. A record of the temperature and time should be available for each sterilization cycle.

## The infrared conveyor oven

Infrared radiation is thermal radiation, i.e. when absorbed, its energy is converted to heat. It is often known as radiant heat. The infrared conveyor oven makes maximum use of this highly efficient means of heat transfer which is conveyed instantly and con-

stantly from the source to the load. It is virtually unaffected by the thermal resistance of static surface air films.

This type of oven can be used for small items such as glass syringes but, with the increased use of disposable plastic syringes, is almost obsolete.

## Heating with a bactericide

This method has been used for sterilizing aqueous solutions that were too thermolabile to withstand normal autoclaving conditions but could withstand heating to 98–100°C for 30 minutes in the presence of a bactericidal substance. A bactericide compatible with the product, container and closure had to be chosen and, because of the potential toxic effects of the bactericide in the patient, the method was precluded for many parenteral and ophthalmic products. This method of sterilization is no longer recognized by the BP (1993).

## APPLICATIONS OF HEAT STERILIZATION

### Moist heat

Dry saturated steam under pressure is used in the sterilization of the following:

- *Aqueous parenteral solutions and suspensions* – 121°C for 15 minutes is recommended, i.e. a total lethality ($F_0$) of not less than 8 (see Ch. 21).
- *Surgical dressings and fabrics* – 134°C for 3 minutes is recommended.
- *Plastic and rubber closures* – if sterilized separately from the containers.
- *Metal instruments* – immediate drying required to protect against corrosion.
- *Glass apparatus and containers* – if unable to withstand dry heat, e.g. rubber parts.

### Dry heat

Dry heat is used to sterilize:

- *Glassware* – pre-washing in apyrogenic water is required.
- *Porcelain and metal equipment.*
- *Oils and fats* – including oily injections.
- *Powders* – including natural products, e.g. talc, which may contain resistant spores. Severe heat treatment will destroy pyrogens, e.g. in sodium chloride.

| Table 22.4 | Advantages and disadvantages of saturated steam and dry heat sterilization methods | | |
|---|---|---|---|
| **Saturated steam** | | **Dry heat** | |
| Advantages | Disadvantages | Advantages | Disadvantages |
| High heat content plus rapid heat transfer | Unsuitable for anhydrous materials such as powders and oils | It can be used for substances that would be harmed by moisture, e.g. oily materials and powders | Low heat content and low heat transfer |
| Destroys microorganisms more efficiently than dry heat (lethal action of water plus heat) and therefore a shorter exposure at a lower temperature is possible | It cannot be used for thermolabile substances | It causes less damage to glass and metal (except for sharp instruments) than moist heat | Most medicaments, rubbers and plastics are too thermolabile for sterilization by this method |
| It can be used for a large proportion of injections, ophthalmic solutions, irrigants, dialysis, fluids, etc. | It does not destroy pyrogens | It is suitable for sterilizing glass containers and equipment and can be used to destroy pyrogens on materials such as glass | It cannot be used for aqueous solutions |
| It rapidly penetrates porous materials and is therefore very suitable for sterilizing surgical dressings and materials | | It does not contaminate materials with toxic substances | It cannot be used for surgical dressings |
| The process is adaptable for plastic containers and some other special dosage forms | | | Accurate control of the process parameters is more difficult than for dry saturated steam |
| It is more suitable than dry heat for sharp instruments | | | |
| Accurate control and monitoring of the process is possible | | | |
| No toxic contaminants are left in the materials sterilized | | | |

## Advantages and disadvantages of moist heat and dry heat sterilization

As the result of reading this chapter so far you should be able to construct a table summarizing the relative advantages and disadvantages of saturated steam and dry heat for sterilization processes. This is done for you in Table 22.4.

## ALTERNATIVE METHODS FOR THE DESTRUCTION OF MICROORGANISMS

Alternative methods to heat sterilization must be employed for heat-labile materials. Gaseous sterilization and sterilization by ionizing radiations are two possible alternatives. A third option is sterilization by filtration. The latter is really an aseptic process and is discussed in Chapter 23.

## GASEOUS STERILIZATION

### Ethylene oxide

Ethylene oxide is the only gas that is successfully used on a large scale for industrial and medical applications. It is the simplest cyclic ether and has the formula:

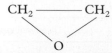

At room temperature it is a colourless gas with a characteristic ethereal odour. It can be liquefied easily and the liquid boils at 10.8°C. The main advantage of ethylene oxide is that many types of materials can be sterilized without damage. Another advantage is its diffusivity. This gives it the ability to sterilize a final product through packaging material and containers and afterwards to diffuse out of the material. However, there are complicating factors to the use of ethylene oxide such as toxicity, combustibility and the need for the correct humidity of the gas–air mixtures. In addition, ethylene oxide is more expensive to use than heat. Toxicity includes inhalation toxicity, which causes nausea and vomiting, and skin toxicity causing irritation or chemical burns. The latter occurs when materials have not been given a sufficient airing and are put into use too soon after sterilization has been completed, e.g. rubber gloves. This type of hazard is overcome by ensuring that those involved with the process are knowledgeable in using ethylene oxide. The inflammability is overcome by preparing special formulations of ethylene oxide mixed with inert gases such as carbon dioxide.

## Antimicrobial activity

Ethylene oxide is active against all microorganisms and there is only a relatively small difference between the concentrations necessary to kill vegetative bacteria and spores in the same exposure time. The ratio is $1:5$ which is much less than the $1:10^3$ ratio for liquid disinfectants. *Bacillus subtilis* var. *niger* is one of the most resistant organisms to the action of ethylene oxide and is used in validating and monitoring ethylene oxide sterilization cycles (see Ch. 21).

## Factors affecting sterilization

Sterilization efficiency is determined by:

- the humidity of the sterilizing atmosphere and in particular the state of hydration of the microorganisms
- the temperature of sterilization
- the concentration of ethylene oxide and time of exposure and the penetrability of the load.

These are discussed below in turn.

### Relative humidity of sterilizing atmosphere

This is the most important parameter affecting the sterilizing efficiency of all gaseous sterilizing agents. Under conditions which allow the materials to equilibrate with respect to the environment a relative humidity (RH) of 33% at 25°C was found to be optimal. In actual practice a higher RH is generally required. This is because sterilization processes are usually carried out at higher than normal room temperatures. If equilibrium with respect to RH has taken place at room temperature and the temperature of the materials to be sterilized is raised, then conditions may be produced which are moisture deficient on the microbial surfaces. Similar moisture-deficient conditions at the active sites may be produced if wrapping materials are used which present diffusion barriers to the moisture. As a result optimum RH is produced only in the environment external to the packaging. Under such conditions the external RH must be in excess of 33% to provide a suitable driving force for the diffusion of moisture across the barrier in order to achieve optimum conditions at the surfaces of the microorganisms. In practice the RH in the chamber atmosphere is usually raised to between 40 and 50%. This allows for absorption of moisture by materials in the load and creates a concentration gradient which increases the rate of diffusion through wrappings.

Moisture is also necessary during the pre-vacuum period of the sterilization cycle. Otherwise when the vacuum is applied dry spores could be dehydrated further and rendered resistant to the action of ethylene oxide.

### Temperature of sterilization

Sterilization can be achieved at room temperature but a long exposure time is necessary. In practice, advantage is usually taken of the decrease in sterilization time with rise in temperature. Within the range 5–40°C this approximates to a halving of the sterilization time for each increase of 17°C. Since gas sterilization is used for thermolabile materials, very high temperatures are impracticable and 60°C can be regarded as the upper limit.

### Concentration of ethylene oxide and time of exposure

Usually concentrations are expressed in mg/litre because the sterilization rate depends on the partial pressure of ethylene oxide which is determined by the amount in the specified volume of the chamber atmosphere. Concentrations used for sterilization range from 250 to 1000 mg/litre. If the concentration is doubled the exposure time necessary is approximately halved.

A manufacturer of ethylene oxide sterilizers recommends, for most purposes, exposure to 850–900 mg/litre for 3 hours, or 450 mg/litre for 5 hours, at 54°C.

### Penetrability of ethylene oxide through the load

Ethylene oxide possesses the ability to penetrate paper, fabrics, a number of plastics and rubber. Therefore materials can be sterilized suitably packaged in appropriate containers. It is, nevertheless, important to ensure that the articles for gaseous sterilization are scrupulously clean. Organic matter reduces the efficiency of the process, but does not prevent it. However, occlusion of organisms within crystals prevents the diffusion of moisture completely. It has been found that spores protected in this way can resist sterilization by exposure to steam, ethylene oxide or dry heat under conditions which would normally effect sterilization. Therefore care needs to be taken to prevent physical protection of microorganisms in gas-impermeable deposits.

In addition to effectively penetrating many materials, ethylene oxide is also strongly absorbed by a wide variety of substances. This means that the sterilized articles should not be used until the absorbed gas has escaped or desorbed. Desorption can be achieved in several ways. Airing the materials in a well-ventilated room for a predetermined time is commonly employed. An alternative is to apply a powerful vacuum immediately after sterilization, e.g. 1.5 kPa (15 mbar) for 2 hours. A third method is to apply a partial vacuum to about 20 kPa (0.2 bar) and then admit sterile air to atmospheric pressure as a flushing agent. This is repeated five or six times.

## Ethylene oxide sterilizers

The following is a general outline of the more important features of sterilizer design and use.

### Design

The features of suitable equipment include:

• An exposure chamber that is gas tight and able to withstand high pressure and vacuum.
• A means of heating the chamber, e.g. a steam or hot water jacket or heating elements clipped to the outside. In some types of sterilizer the load is heated and humidified by injecting steam into the chamber.
• A baffled inlet of the gas mixture, usually at the bottom of the chamber. The baffle protects the contents from liquid ethylene oxide introduced accidentally. The liquid can badly damage certain plastics.
• A method of completely vaporizing the gas mixture and warming it to the sterilizing temperature.
• A means of extracting air before, and the gas mixture after, sterilization. A high-efficiency pump is desirable. It should discharge to the open air.
• A system for adding water to provide the right humidity.
• Provision for the admission of sterile air at the end of the process.
• A safety valve and suitable indicators and recorders of pressure and temperature. Automatic control is advisable because of the significant effects of alterations in temperature and humidity.

As with steam sterilization, the problem of accurate and sensitive measurement of humidity has not been satisfactorily solved.

### Method of use

• The chamber is loaded.
• Sufficient water is introduced to prevent vacuum dehydration of microorganisms. The sterilization time is significantly reduced if the load is humidified prior to gas admission. Hence, if gas and moisture are introduced together sterilization time is lengthened.
• The door is closed and the temperature raised to sterilization level unless exposure is to be carried out at room temperature. When an increased temperature is used the load must be at the correct temperature throughout before the gas is admitted and timing of the sterilization exposure is begun. Steam injection rapidly raises the load to sterilization temperature, but heating up by a steam jacket or by external heaters is very slow.
• The heat-exchanger is raised to a high temperature (about 100°C) because the gas mixture falls to well below room temperature as it leaves the cylinder.
• A high-efficiency vacuum pump is used to reduce the air pressure in the chamber to about 1.5 kPa (15 mbar). On a small scale, the gas may be used to displace the air, but this method is wasteful and insufficiently reliable for large loads.
• If necessary, more water is added to produce a satisfactory exposure humidity.
• The warmed gas mixture is admitted until the correct pressure is reached.

- The exposure time is allowed.
- The gas is desorbed by one of the three methods mentioned previously and in each instance the vacuum is broken by admitting sterile air.

### Control of the process

Methods similar to those for steam sterilization have been used – physical, chemical and biological monitoring of the actual process followed by sterility testing of random samples for each load of sterilized material. The temperature and pressure should be recorded on a chart throughout the sterilization cycle.

However, physical monitoring using conventional instrumentation is not able to provide assurance that each item of the load has been subjected to the predetermined conditions of RH and gas concentration. Chemical monitoring is also inadequate in monitoring the all-important parameter of RH. Therefore the biological monitoring is of major importance. The monitor is in the form of either paper strips impregnated with, or aluminium foil coated with, known concentrations (e.g. $10^6$) of *Bacillus subtilis* var. *niger* spores (USP 23, BP 1993). Usually at least 10 test packages of biological indicator are placed in the least gas-accessible parts of a number of articles and containers situated in different regions of the sterilizer. After exposure they are tested for sterility. A recorded check is made to ensure that all biological indicators have been removed from the load.

## Applications of ethylene oxide sterilization

Ethylene oxide is suitable for sterilizing those powders where it is known that the microorganisms are on the surface of the particles and not embedded inside them.

Equipment, instruments and articles made from plastic, rubber, metal and other materials can be sterilized with ethylene oxide without causing damage. Commercial processes have been developed for catheters and syringes. Other articles which are suitable include intravenous sets, prostheses, blood oxygenators, bottles and vials and polythene-covered stirrers for magnetic mixers.

Some plastics may be damaged. The surface of polystyrene may become crazed if an ethylene oxide/Arcton(s) mixture is used. Damage does not occur with pure ethylene oxide or mixtures with carbon dioxide. Contact with liquid ethylene oxide must always be avoided.

Fragile rubber articles survive more treatments with ethylene oxide than with steam.

Equipment such as cystoscopes, bronchoscopes, ophthalmoscopes and Geiger–Müller counters can also be sterilized with ethylene oxide.

## Advantages of ethylene oxide sterilization

- It is suitable for thermolabile substances because it can be carried out at room temperature or only slightly above.
- It does not damage moisture-sensitive substances and equipment because only a low humidity is required. However, humidification by steam injection, which produces a higher than normal humidity, is inadvisable when such materials and articles are being sterilized.
- Provided the container is made from one of the many materials that are permeable to the gas, it can be used for prepacked articles, because of the great penetrating power of ethylene oxide.
- Although ethylene oxide is a highly reactive compound comparatively few materials are damaged by the process.

## Disadvantages of ethylene oxide sterilization

- It is slow. Long exposures and desorption periods are necessary. Therefore, it is unsuitable in emergencies, or for expensive equipment that must be frequently used.
- Although small batches of materials can be successfully sterilized with simple equipment, large batches require very expensive, elaborately instrumented sterilizers that need skilled and regular maintenance.
- The running costs are high.
- The hazards of inflammability, general toxicity and vesicant action necessitate special precautions.
- Toxic substances, such as ethylene chlorhydrin, are produced in some materials, particularly if, like the flexible PVC used for catheters, tubing and giving sets, they contain free chloride ions. As the amount of free chloride in PVC is increased by exposure to ionizing radiations, it is undesirable to use ethylene oxide for resterilizing previously irradiated PVC articles.

## Conclusions

Ethylene oxide sterilization is less reliable and more expensive than steam sterilization and should not be used when the latter is practicable. To increase its reliability, microbial contamination of articles to be sterilized should be minimized.

## Formaldehyde

Like ethylene oxide this is an alkylating agent but it is generally inferior for use as a sterilizing agent. This is because formaldehyde has poor penetrating power and is readily inactivated by organic matter. Furthermore, high concentrations are difficult to maintain in the atmosphere because it tends to deposit in the form of solid polymers on contact with cool surfaces. Formaldehyde may be used for the fumigation of empty airflow cabinets and rooms to eliminate microbiological contamination from solid surfaces.

Pure formaldehyde cannot be kept at ordinary temperatures and so it is used either as Formaldehyde Solution (Formalin) BP, which is an approximately 37% w/w solution containing stabilizers to prevent deposition of solid polymers, or as tablets of paraformaldehyde. The gas is vaporized from these sources by heating devices or, in the case of formalin for fumigation, by the addition of potassium permanganate which produces heat by oxidation.

*Low-temperature steam with formaldehyde (LTSF).* This is becoming an option for sterilizing thermolabile substances (Health Technical Memorandum 2010, 1996).

## STERILIZATION BY RADIATIONS

Radiations can be divided into two groups – electromagnetic waves and streams of particulate matter. In the former group are infrared radiation, ultraviolet light, X-rays and gamma rays. In the latter group are alpha and beta radiations.

Infrared radiation, ultraviolet light, gamma radiation and high-velocity electrons (a type of beta radiation) are used for sterilization. Infrared radiation has been considered earlier in the chapter.

Ultraviolet light, with a wavelength in the 200–300 nm range, and gamma rays with a wavelength in the range $1-10^{-4}$ nm can both directly damage molecules vital to living cells. High-velocity electrons have a similar effect. As they pass through matter, both types of waves and the high-speed particles are able to excite the planetary electrons surrounding the atomic nuclei. If the electrons acquire sufficient energy they escape from the atoms and ionization results. Both gamma rays and high-velocity electrons have high energy values, over 1.3 million

electronvolts (1.3 MeV) and 4 MeV respectively. Both produce ionization and are therefore called ionizing radiations. Ionizing radiations are very effective sterilizing agents. Although ultraviolet light has relatively low energy (5 eV) and rarely causes ionization, it does cause excitation of the atomic electrons. Excitation is not as potent a lethal effect as ionization but it nevertheless causes the death of microorganisms.

## Ultraviolet light

Only a narrow range of wavelength (220–280 nm) is effective in killing microorganisms, and wavelengths close to 265 nm are the most effective. This is because wavelengths of 265 nm and adjacent wavelengths are strongly absorbed by nucleoproteins.

The main method of generating ultraviolet light for sterilization is by passing a low current at high voltage through mercury vapour in an evacuated tube made of borosilicate glass.

The intensity of ultraviolet radiation is expressed as the energy received by a specified area, usually in microwatts/mm². Intensities of from 10 to 60 $\mu$W/mm², depending on the type of bacterium, will reduce populations of vegetative cells by 90% in a short period of time. However, the most serious disadvantage of ultraviolet light as a sterilizing agent is its poor penetrating power. This is the result of strong absorption by many substances. Applications are therefore limited to the treatment of clean air and water in thin layers and of hard impermeable surfaces in situations where people are not subjected to direct or high-intensity reflected radiation. This latter precaution is necessary because bactericidal ultraviolet light damages the sight and produces erythema of the skin.

Thus, in general, ultraviolet light should not be relied on for sterilization.

## Ionizing radiations

Ionizing radiation suitable for commercial sterilization processes must have good penetrating power, high sterilizing efficiency, little or no damaging effect on irradiated materials and be capable of being produced efficiently. The radiations that best fulfil these four criteria are high-speed electrons from machines and gamma rays from radioactive isotopes.

### High-speed electrons

This type of sterilizing radiation is most widely used in Denmark and the USA. In a machine known as a van de Graaff accelerator electrons are generated from a suitable source and then accelerated along a highly evacuated tube by a tremendous potential difference between the ends. The particles in the emergent beam are travelling at near to the speed of light and, depending on the accelerating voltage, have energies of from 5 MeV to 10 MeV. The beam, which is narrow and intense, is used to irradiate articles on a conveyor belt.

In the UK, the travelling wave linear accelerator, in which a different method of acceleration is used, has been developed.

### Gamma rays

Most gamma-ray sterilization in this country is carried out at specialized irradiation plants. Radiation from the radioactive isotope of cobalt, $^{60}Co$, is used as a source of gamma emission. Most of the disintegrating atoms of this isotope emit two gamma rays in succession (in cascade) which have energies of 1.33 MeV and 1.17 MeV. Therefore irradiated products are treated with gamma radiation having a mean energy of 1.25 MeV.

$^{60}Co$ has a half-life of 5.25 years. It is possible that eventually $^{60}Co$ will be replaced by the radioactive isotope of caesium, $^{137}Cs$, which has a half-life of 30 years. This isotope is a major constituent of spent fuel rods from nuclear reactors. It could be utilized for commercial sterilization rather than being regarded as a waste disposal problem. It emits a gamma ray having an energy of 0.66 MeV. At present $^{137}Cs$ plus other disintegration products are used at Harwell for some commercial sterilization.

Articles for sterilization by radiation are packed in boxes of standard size which are suspended from a monorail and sterilized by slow passages around the gamma ray source (Fig. 22.8).

### Mode of action

Ionizing radiations can cause excitations, ionizations and, where water is present, free radical formation. Free radicals are powerful oxidizing (OH, $HO_2$) and reducing (H) agents which are capable of damaging essential molecules in living cells. Thus all three processes cause disintegration of essential cell constituents such as enzymes and the DNA. This results in cell death.

### Sterilizing dose

The dose is measured in kGy. The gray (Gy) is the SI equivalent to 100 rad. In the UK and the USA the recognized sterilizing dose is 25 kGy. The choice of this value was based on experiments in which test pieces (e.g. paper discs or strips of plastic or foil, heavily contaminated with different types of organisms including vegetative bacteria, spores, pathogens and non-pathogens) were exposed to various doses of radiation. Absence of survivors after treatment with 25 kGy and the high margin of safety of the dose led to its selection. In fact, in North America a sterilizing dose of 18–22 kGy is sometimes used. This is based on a sterility assurance of not more than one item contaminated in one million.

As the inactivation of bacteria by radiation is exponential, the probability of survivors after a particular dose can be calculated. With radiation, the $D_{10}$ value (the decimal reduction dose) is the dose in Gy that reduces the number of viable organisms by a factor of 10. The $D_{10}$ value for *Bacillus pumilis* spores irradiated in air is 1.7 kGy. Therefore, the inactivation factor for the recognized sterilizing dose is $10^{25/1.7} = 10^{15}$ (in the absence of air the factor falls to $10^7$). *Bacillus pumilis* spores have been extensively used for investigating radiation sterilization because they are less susceptible to ionizing radiations than most other commonly occurring microbial cells.

Some non-pathogens show exceptionally high resistance to ionizing radiations. For example *Micrococcus radiodurans* has an inactivation factor of only $10^3$ when exposed in meat to 25 kGy but, because it is harmless and of rare occurrence an increase of the recognized radiation dose is not considered necessary.

It should be noted, however, that in Denmark a sterilization dose of 45 kGy, is recommended. Apparently the evidence for such a high dose was obtained under artificial and not naturally occurring conditions or in practice conditions. For this reason other countries have kept the 25 kGy sterilization dose.

### Sterilization time

The intense beam or pulses of electrons from accelerators can deliver a sterilization dose in a fraction of a second to a few seconds, depending on the size and density of the material or article being irradiated. With isotope sources, because of the diffuse and penetrating nature of their emissions, the dose rate is much less and, therefore, the sterilizing dose has to be accumulated over several days (such as 3 to $3\frac{1}{2}$ days). However, as partial compensation for this, the volume of material that can be exposed at

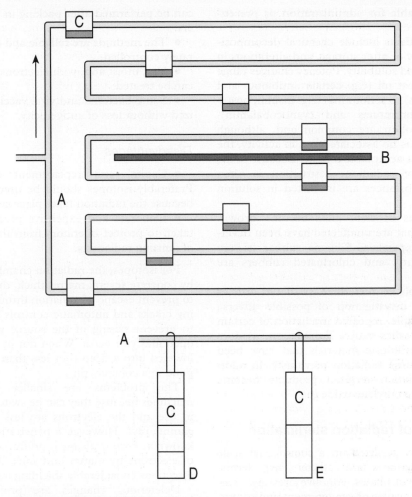

**Fig. 22.8** Monorail system for sterilization by gamma radiation. A, Monorail; B, source plaque; C, packages (shown at only a few positions on the rail) – one side is shaded to illustrate exposure of opposite faces on two sides of the source; D, E, tiers of four and two packages respectively.

the same time is much larger than with accelerators.

*Control of the process*

The actual radiation dose is checked by including dosimeters in packages. The most common type is a Perspex strip or disc containing a radiation-sensitive red dye. Irradiation causes changes in optical density which can be measured in a spectrophotometer and converted to dosage by reference to a calibration curve prepared with a standard source.

It is generally accepted that there is no purpose served in routinely using a biological indicator which

is known to be killed by 25 kGy because this dose is accurately checked by the dosimeter.

*Undesirable effects*

Radiation sterilization appears an attractive method for thermolabile medicaments and equipment because the rise in temperature caused by a sterilizing dose is very small – about 4°C. However, the Association of British Pharmaceutical Industries (ABPI) investigation on the effects of radiation on pharmaceutical products (ABPI Report 1960) led to the conclusion that in many instances 25 kGy produces changes that may make the preparation unacceptable for administration or presentation.

Undesirable effects include chemical decomposition, immediately or after storage, and alterations in colour, texture and solubility. Potency changes range from nil or almost nil (e.g. certain antibiotics and steroid hormones) to serious loss (e.g. insulin, posterior pituitary hormones and cyanocobalamin). Alterations in colour are common and, although sometimes there is no associated loss in activity, the preparation is less acceptable for sale. Because of the indirect effect of radiation, destruction is often greater when substances are irradiated in solution (e.g. heparin).

Ordinary types of clear glass become brown. Special glasses that are unaffected have been developed but are expensive. Silicone rubber is very resistant but butyl and chlorinated rubbers are degraded.

It is inadvisable to resterilize irradiated articles without careful investigation of possible adverse effects. For example, repeated irradiation of certain dressings and plastics causes degradation, as does autoclaving of cellulosic materials that have been subjected to gamma radiation previously. In addition, some radiation-sterilized products become toxic if exposed to ethylene oxide gas.

## Applications of radiation sterilization

Articles regularly sterilized on a commercial scale include plastic syringes and catheters, hypodermic needles and scalpel blades, adhesive dressings, single-application capsules of eye ointment and catgut. Containers made of polythene and packaging materials using aluminium foil and plastic films may also be sterilized by radiation.

A service for hospitals is provided, for example, by the irradiation plant at Wantage. It is for special items that are difficult to sterilize by other methods and not for bulk articles that are readily available from commercial sources.

Radiation sterilization of medicaments is developing slowly because of the adverse effects already described.

### Advantages

● The temperature rise is insignificant.
● The processes can be continuous because exposure is so short (machine generation) or a large amount of material can be treated at once (isotope generation).
● There is no aseptic handling since sterilization can be performed after packing in the final containers.
● The methods are reliable and can be very accurately controlled.
● Dry, moist and, with electrons, frozen materials can be treated.
● Some bacterial and viral vaccines can be sterilized without loss of antigenicity.

### Disadvantages

● Capital and replacement costs are high. Preferably isotopes should be used 24 hours a day because the radiation takes place continuously.
● Elaborate and expensive precautions must be taken to protect operators from the harmful effects of ionizing radiations.

For isotopes, the radiation chamber is surrounded by concrete several metres thick, the door is stepped to prevent escape of radiation through the surrounding cracks and automatic controls are installed, e.g. to prevent raising of the source while the door is open and vice versa. When not in use the source is lowered into a deep (not less than 7 m) water-filled pond in a concrete pit.

The problems are smaller with generating machines because they can be switched off when not in use and the electrons are less penetrating than gamma rays. However, a penetrating form of X-ray known as *bremsstrahlung* is produced by the stopping of electrons by matter and since this escapes in all directions considerable shielding must be provided.

Deleterious changes are produced in many medicaments, fats and foods, Nevertheless, at the dose levels normally used there is no danger of residual radioactivity in irradiated products.

## Key Points

● There are two major means of sterilization:
  – heat sterilization – this consists of moist heat and dry heat sterilization
  – non-heat methods of sterilization – these consist of sterilization by gases and by radiations. Filtration is dealt with in Chapter 23.
● Moist heat sterilization is the method of choice for:
  – heat-stable aqueous preparations
  – surgical dressings.
● Moist heat has the following advantages:
  – penetration – due to contraction on condensing

- – rapid heating – due to the release of latent heat on condensation
- – moisture – the condensate contributes to lethality by coagulation of microbial protein
- – no residual toxicity.
- Autoclaves are used to provide the moist heat sterilization conditions. Each autoclave should be validated before use.
- The USP and BP recommend 121°C maintained throughout the load for 15 minutes as the preferred sterilization time–temperature combination. This is the temperature of saturated steam at 15 lb/in$^2$ (g).
- Dry heat sterilization in the hot air oven is the method of choice for:
  - – heat-stable non-aqueous preparations
  - – powders
  - – certain impregnated dressings
  - – glass containers and certain equipment.
- The BP recommended time–temperature combinations for dry heat sterilization are:
  - – 180°C for not less than 30 minutes
  - – 170°C for not less than 1 hour
  - – 160°C for not less than 2 hours.
- Ethylene oxide is a useful 'non-heat' method of sterilization for suitable materials.
- Factors affecting ethylene oxide sterilization are:
  - – humidity of the sterilizing atmosphere
  - – the temperature of sterilization
  - – the concentration of ethylene oxide (mg/litre)
  - – the time of exposure (several hours)
  - – the penetrability of the load.
- Ionizing radiations are suitable for commercial sterilization of articles which for some reason are not readily sterilized by other methods (plastic containers).

plants. In: Symposium on the sterilization of surgical dressings. Pharmaceutical Press, London, pp 34–35

Burrell R L, Wein R Z, Parisi A N 1979 SCOT (sterilization computer operating terminal) for sterilization control and monitoring. Journal of the Parenteral Drug Association 33: 363–370

Christensen E A, Holm N W, Juul F A 1967 Radiosterilization of medical devices and supplies. In: Radiosterilization of medical products. HMSO, London, pp 265–283

Coles J, Tedree R L 1972 Contamination of autoclaved fluids with cooling water. Pharmaceutical Journal 209: 193–195

Ernst R R, Doyle J E 1968 Sterilisation of ethylene oxide. A review of chemical and physical factors. Biotechnology and Bioengineering 10: 1-31

Higgins D 1972 Contamination of fluids in spray-cooled autoclaves. Pharmaceutical Journal 209: 306

Health Technical Memorandum 1996 No. 2010. Sterilization. HMSO, London

International Atomic Energy Agency (IAEA) 1967 Radiosterilization of medical products. In: Proceedings of a symposium held by the International Atomic Energy Agency. HMSO, London

Kirk B, Hambleton R, Everett M 1982 Computer-aided autoclaving monitoring. Pharmaceutical Journal 229: 252–254

Myers J A, Keall A 1972 MRC bottles for sterile infusion fluids. Pharmaceutical Journal 209: 306–307

Perera R 1972 Autoclaving problems. Pharmaceutical Journal 208: 469

Pharmaceutical Codex 1994 12th edn (incorporating the British Pharmaceutical Codex). Pharmaceutical Press, London

Phillips I, Eykyn S, Laker M 1972 Outbreak of hospital infection caused by contaminated autoclave fluids. Lancet i: 1258–1260

United States Pharmacopoeia 23 1995 Mack, Easton, PA

## FURTHER READING

ABPI Report 1960 Report of a working party established by the Association of British Pharmaceutical Industry and others on the use of gamma radiation sources for the sterilization of pharmaceutical products. Association of British Pharmaceutical Industry, London

British Pharmacopoeia 1993 HMSO, London

British Standard 1752 1963 Laboratory sintered or fritted filters. British Standards Institution, London

British Standard 3421 1961 Performance of electrically heated sterilizing ovens. British Standards Institution, London

Burnard L G 1961 Design and production of irradiation

# 23

# Aseptic technique

*R. M. E. Richards*

---

When this chapter has been completed the reader should be able to:

**Describe the principles of aseptic technique**
**Describe the principles of sterilization by filtration.**

---

## ASEPTIC TECHNIQUES

Aseptic techniques are used to prevent the access of viable microbial and particulate contamination into the following products:

- ophthalmic and parenteral products not intended to be sterilized in the final container
- products sterilized by filtration
- all 'sterile products' undergoing sterility testing.

Applications of aseptic technique include the preparation of intravenous additives (see Ch. 26), the dispensing of cytotoxic agents (see Ch. 26), the compounding of total parenteral nutrition (see Ch. 27) and the production of radiopharmaceuticals (see Ch. 26). The requirements necessary to achieve strict asepsis include:

- sterile starting materials
- sterile equipment
- controlled environment
- sterile containers
- suitable technique by trained personnel.

The methods for sterilizing materials, equipment and containers have been described in Chapters 21 and 22. The design, operation and monitoring of clean rooms and areas suitable for aseptic work are described in Chapter 24. This chapter is concerned with describing good aseptic technique to be followed by the operator in the preparation of sterile products.

## Laminar airflow stations

Filtered laminar airflow (LAF), properly utilized, is a great asset in providing suitable working conditions. Vertical or horizontal laminar airflow (VLAF and HLAF, respectively) can be used to sweep a working area virtually free from microorganisms (see Ch. 24) and to provide a suitable working environment for aseptic procedures.

## Protective clothing

Within the clean room environment, most airborne contamination results from the personnel using the facility. Jansen et al (1974) estimated that in a 24-hour period each person sheds the outermost layer of epithelial cells and MacIntosh et al (1978) indicated that this is about $10^9$ cells per day. Microbes are often associated with whole skin cells or fragments of these cells. The average size of these bacteria-carrying particles is thought to be about 14 μm. They will settle in still air under gravitational forces at a rate of about 0.37 m/min. It has been estimated that male workers can disperse 1000 bacteria-carrying particles per minute. In order to prevent contamination of a work area it is necessary to enclose each person in that area as effectively as possible within appropriately designed sterile, impervious clothing. This includes gloves, footwear and headgear (see Ch. 24).

## Personnel

The numbers of personnel working in a clean area should be as low as possible and the staff involved in aseptic procedures must demonstrate high standards of both integrity and motivation. All personnel should have both formal instruction and suitably validated practical training in the full range of procedures to be undertaken in the workplace. It is important that staff of all levels, including maintenance staff from outside the pharmacy, understand the importance and the significance of the strict controls imposed. Compliance with procedures is likely to be increased if the reason for their imposition is understood.

Clean room personnel should be encouraged to report any minor infections or skin disorders which may render them temporarily unsuitable for aseptic work and regular medical checks should be made.

## Operator technique

Basic rules for effective aseptic processing are:

### Use a 'no touch' technique whenever possible

Handle small articles with sterile forceps and, when sterile apparatus must be touched, handle as distantly as possible from the part of the apparatus which will come into contact with a sterile liquid or solid. For example, the plunger of a syringe must not be touched because it will subsequently come into contact with the inner surface of the syringe barrel and hence with a sterile liquid. This rule applies even when sterile gloves are worn.

### Reduce air disturbances to a minimum

Standard procedure should be designed to minimize movement of personnel within the clean room. Objects should be positioned within reach under the laminar airflow cabinet. Only the hands and arms should be placed into the cabinet area and operators should not position their hands between the source of air and the objects being manipulated. Sharp and sudden movements should be avoided. Poor aseptic technique can easily negate the benefits of the LAF cabinet.

### Consider the arrangement of objects under the LAF

Clean air should not flow over dirty articles to contaminate sterile articles. The cabinet should not be loaded with unnecessary equipment. Materials required should be carefully selected and arranged before beginning the procedure. For example, placement of large objects in the airstream of a LAF cabinet will create downstream turbulence in proportion to the size of the object. If a sufficiently large object is located near the front of a horizontal LAF cabinet, contaminants from the room or from the operator can be drawn into the work area behind the obstruction. Unfortunately a general lack of adherence to

the principles outlined in the above paragraph is quite common. Such lack of discipline is inexcusable.

### Refuse to be distracted

No interruptions should be allowed until a set procedure has been completed.

### Use of the laminar airflow cabinet

The airflow should be switched on and left for 15 minutes before use.

The inner faces of the cabinet should be swabbed with a suitable antimicrobial agent, e.g. 70% IMS. An appropriate swabbing sequence is:

Horizontal LAF – top, sides, work surface
Vertical LAF – back, sides, front, work surface.

All equipment and articles should also be swabbed with 70% IMS before placement in the cabinet. The outer wrapping should be removed from wrapped items.

### Operator tests

Regular tests to ensure the adequacy of the technique of each operator should be carried out. These usually involve serial transfer of a sterile nutrient medium which is subsequently incubated and examined for the presence of turbidity indicating microbial growth. The test should involve both general transfer techniques and specific operations which form part of the daily routine of the operator. Operator tests are discussed in Chapter 24.

## STERILIZATION BY FILTRATION

Sterilization by filtration is a method permitted by the *British Pharmacopoeia* (BP 1993) for solutions or liquids that are not sufficiently stable to withstand the process of heating in an autoclave as described in Chapter 22. Passage through a filter of appropriate pore size can remove bacteria and moulds although smaller microorganisms such as viruses and mycoplasms may not be retained. After filtration the liquid is aseptically distributed into previously sterilized containers which are then sealed. This method has a number of disadvantages and should be used only for those products where sterilization by alternative means is not available.

## Filter media

A sterile filter of nominal pore size 0.22 µm or less is required (DHSS 1983, BP 1993). Filters containing asbestos or any other medium likely to shed fibres or particles may not be used.

## Membrane filters

These are usually the preferred type of filter for sterilization. Membrane filters are made from cellulose derivatives or other polymers and there are no loose fibres or particles. The retention of particles larger than the pore size occurs on the filter surface which also makes this type of filter particularly useful for the detection of bacteria (see Ch. 30).

## Advantages of membrane filters

- Rigid structure – unaffected by bubbles or pressure surges.
- High flow rates – 80% of filter surface consists of pores.
- Non-fibre shedding.
- Minimal absorption – concentration unaffected.
- Minimal wastage – little retention of solution.
- Testable prior to and after filtration.

Although reusable membrane filters are available, the disposable types are generally preferred.

### The use of a pre-filter

Membrane filters are generally blocked by particles which are close in size to the pore size of the filter. Pre-filtration reduces the risk of blockage of the final filter. Since the filtration method of sterilization carries a potentially greater risk of failure than other methods, a second filtration through a sterilized membrane filter provides an additional safeguard.

### Sintered glass filters

Sintered glass filters made from borosilicate glass with an appropriate pore size may be used to sterilize solutions. These have the disadvantages of slowness of filtration, fragility and difficulty of cleaning.

### Other filters

Filter media that have been used in the past as bacteria-proof filters include asbestos pads, ceramic filters and kieselguhr candles.

## Testing of filters

The BP requires that the integrity of an assembled sterilizing filter be verified before use and confirmed after use by means of a suitable test.

### Bacteriological tests

The filter may be challenged by the passage of a diluted 24–48-hour broth culture of *Serratia marcescens*. A sample of the filtrate is collected aseptically and incubated at 25°C for 5 days. This organism is chosen because it has a small cell size (0.3–0.4 µm across). It grows vigorously in aerobic conditions and produces a readily detected red pigment.

### Bubble point test

The bubble point of a test filter is the pressure at which the largest pore of a wetted filter is able to pass air. The pressure varies with the surface tension of the liquid with which the filter is wetted. Details of bubble pressure testing are given in the relevant British Standard (BS 1752; 1983). Sterile membrane filters can be tested before use by a bubble pressure method, usually described in the manufacturer's literature.

### Sterility testing

In-process controls are not generally available for methods of sterilization by filtration. It is therefore advisable to withhold the release for use of products sterilized by this method until sterility data are available (see Ch. 30).

---

### Key Points

- Aseptic technique is necessary for preventing access of viable microorganisms to pharmaceutical products.
- Laminar airflow stations provide an environment in which aseptic technique may be carried out.
- Operator technique involves strict adherence to a few basic rules:
  - using a 'no touch' technique
  - preventing air disturbances
  - keeping the work station uncluttered
  - avoiding distractions
  - regular testing of operator performance.

- Sterilization by filtration is used for liquids which will not withstand heat sterilization methods. It usually involves:
  - 0.22 μm membrane filters
  - validation of the integrity of the filtration system
  - product validation by sterility testing (see Ch. 30).

## FURTHER READING

British Pharmacopoeia 1993 HMSO, London

British Standard 1752 1983 Laboratory sintered or fritted filters including porosity grading. British Standards Institution, London

British Standard 5295 1976 Environmental cleanliness in enclosed spaces. British Standards Institution, London

Department of Health and Social Security (DHSS) 1983 Guide to good pharmaceutical manufacturing practice. HMSO, London

Food and Drug Administration (FDA) 1985 Draft guidelines on sterile drug products produced by aseptic processing. Division of Drug Quality Compliance, FDA, USA

Jansen L H, Hojyo-Tomako M J, Kligman A M 1974 Improved fluorescence staining techniques for estimating turnover of the human corneum. British Journal of Dermatology 90: 9–12

MacIntosh C A, Lidwell O M, Towers A G, Marples R R 1978 The dimensions of skin fragment dispersal into the air during activity. Journal of Hygiene 81: 471–476

Whyte W, Bailey P V 1985 Reduction of microbial dispersion by clothing. Journal of Parenteral Science and Technology 39: 51–60

# 24

# Clean rooms for the production of pharmaceutical products

*D. G. Chapman*

---

After studying this chapter you will know about:

**The requirements for sterile production**
**Grades of clean areas**
**Design and operation of clean areas**
**Isolators**
**Environmental monitoring.**

## Introduction

The production of sterile medicinal products has special requirements. These products must be produced in conditions which ensure that they are pure. They must also be free from viable organisms and have limited or ideally no particulate contamination. It is thus important that only carefully regulated and tested procedures are used to manufacture sterile products.

Owing to their special manufacturing requirements, sterile medicinal products are prepared in special facilities known as clean rooms. These rooms are designed to reduce the risk of microbial and particulate contamination at all stages of the manufacturing process.

The clean area used to produce sterile products is commonly designed as a suite of clean rooms. With this system, the operators enter the clean rooms by way of a changing room. Within this area the operators put on clean room clothing before entering into the clean rooms. The changing room has a lower standard of environmental quality. A clean room with a lower environmental standard is also used to prepare solutions. These solutions are then sterilized by filtration before being transferred into the filling room. The clean room used to fill and seal the product containers is the highest quality of clean room. This will reduce the risk of product contamination.

Sterile products that are marketed in the European Union must be produced in conditions which conform with the details in the revised Annex 1 of Volume IV of 'The Rules Governing Medicinal Products in the European Community'. These manufacturing conditions for sterile products in the revised Annex 1 were implemented in January 1997. It contains the standards to which pharmaceutical clean rooms should be built and used.

## STERILE PRODUCT PRODUCTION

Production of sterile products should be carried out in a clean environment with a limit for the environmental quality of particulate and microbial contamination. This limit for contamination is necessary to reduce the risk of product contamination. In addition, however, the temperature, humidity and the air pressure of the environment should be regulated to suit the clean room processes and the comfort of the operators.

Clean areas for the production of sterile products are classified into grades A, B, C and D. These grades are categorized by the particulate quality of the environmental air when the clean area is operating in both a 'manned' and 'unmanned' state. In addition, these areas are graded by the microbial monitoring of the environmental air, surfaces and operators when the area is functioning. The standards are shown in Tables 24.1 and 24.2.

There are two common procedures used to manufacture sterile products. The first method involves the preparation of products that will be terminally sterilized. The second method involves the aseptic filling of containers which are not exposed to terminal sterilization. Aseptic filling requires a higher environmental quality for the preparation of solutions and the filling of containers. The qualities of the clean rooms used for these production procedures are detailed in Tables 24.3 and 24.4.

**Table 24.1  Airborne particle contamination for manned and unmanned clean rooms**

| Grade | Maximum number of particles per cubic metre equal to or above the size indicated | | | |
|---|---|---|---|---|
| | Clean room at rest | | Clean room operating | |
| | 0.5 µm | 5 µm | 0.5 µm | 5 µm |
| A | 3500 | 0 | 3500 | 0 |
| B | 3500 | 0 | 350 000 | 2000 |
| C | 350 000 | 2000 | 3 500 000 | 20 000 |
| D | 3 500 000 | 20 000 | Varies with procedure | Varies with procedure |

**Table 24.2  Limits for microbial contamination of an operating clean room**

| Grade | Viable organisms per cubic metre of air | 90 mm settle plate per 4 hours | 55 mm contact plate | Glove print (5 fingers) |
|---|---|---|---|---|
| A | < 1 | < 1 | < 1 | < 1 |
| B | 10 | 5 | 5 | 5 |
| C | 100 | 50 | 25 | Not applicable |
| D | 200 | 100 | 50 | Not applicable |

**Table 24.3  Conditions for preparing terminally sterilized products**

| Procedure | Required standard before terminal sterilization |
|---|---|
| Preparation of solutions for filtration and sterilization | Grade C is used for products which support microbial growth. Grade D acceptable if solutions subsequently filtered |
| Filling small and large volume parenterals | Grade C. For products with a high risk of contamination such as wide-necked containers a Grade A laminar airflow workstation with Grade C background |
| Preparation and filling of ointments, creams, suspensions and emulsions | Grade C |

**Table 24.4  Conditions for the production of aseptically prepared products**

| Procedure | Required standard |
|---|---|
| Handling of sterile starting materials | Grade A with Grade B background or Grade C if solution filtered later in production process |
| Preparation of production solutions | Grade A with Grade B background or Grade C if sterile filtered during production |
| Filling of aseptically prepared products such as small and large volume parenterals | Grade A with Grade B background |
| Preparation and filling of ointments, creams, suspensions and emulsions | Grade A with Grade B background |

unit must be separated from the general manufacturing area within the hospital pharmacy or factory. This sterile production unit must not be accessible to unauthorized personnel.

The unit is designed to allow each stage of production to be segregated. It should also ensure a safe and organized workflow. The unit is built and the equipment positioned to protect the product from contamination. The layout must allow efficient cleaning of the area and avoid the build-up of dust. This positioning of the facilities should also reduce the need for personnel to move around the clean rooms. The premises are also arranged to decrease the risk of mix-up or contamination of one product or material by another.

The filling room is typically serviced from an adjacent preparation room. This allows supporting personnel to assemble and prepare materials. These materials are then used by staff within the filling room area. Figure 24.1 shows the layout of rooms for the production of terminally sterilized medicines such as small or large volume injections.

## Design and construction

Access to clean and aseptic filling areas is limited to authorized personnel. Operators enter clean rooms by way of changing rooms. Within the changing room the operators can don and remove their clean room garments.

A low physical barrier, commonly known as a pass-over (or cross-over) bench, extends across the

## PREMISES

High standards are necessary for the manufacture of sterile medicinal products. The sterile production

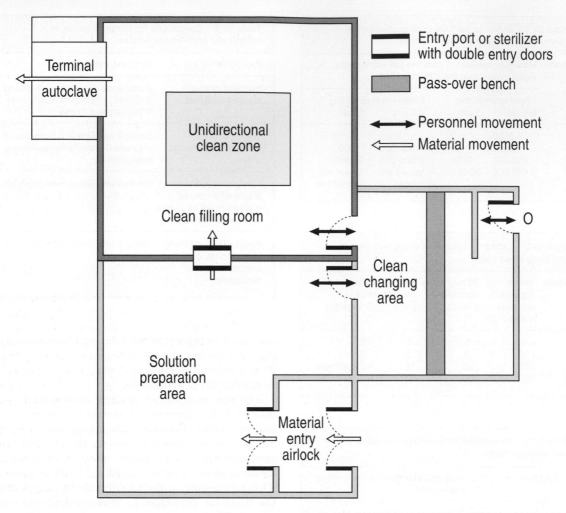

**Fig. 24.1** Rooms for the production of terminally sterilized medicines.

changing room. It forms a physical barrier which separates the different areas for changing by the operators.

Special precautions are needed to avoid contamination of clean and aseptic filling areas when materials are passed through airlocks or hatchways. Thus, sterilizers and entry ports are fitted with double-sided doors. The doors are interlocked to prevent both doors being opened simultaneously.

## Surfacing materials

All clean room surfaces including the floors, walls and ceilings should be smooth, impervious and unbroken. This will decrease the release and build-up of contaminating particles and organisms. The surfaces are made of materials which allow the use of cleaning agents and disinfectants. The ceilings are sealed to prevent the entry of contaminants from the space above them. Uncleanable recesses within the clean room should be avoided. This will reduce the collection of contaminating particles. Thus, the junction between the wall and the floor is commonly coved. The presence of shelves, ledges, cupboards and equipment is minimized. Windows should be non-opening and sealed. This will prevent the ingress of contaminants.

## Services

Piped liquids and gases should be filtered before entering the clean room. This will ensure that the liquid or gas at the work position will be as clean as the clean room air. The pipes and ducts must be positioned for easy cleaning. All other fittings such as fuse boxes and switch panels should be positioned outside the clean rooms.

Sinks and drains must be excluded from areas where aseptic procedures are performed in clean room areas. They should be avoided in the whole unit wherever possible. In areas where sinks and drains are installed they must be designed, positioned and maintained to decrease the risk of microbial contamination. They are thus often fitted with easily cleanable traps. The traps may contain electrically heated devices for disinfection.

There should be a limited number of entry doors for personnel and ports for materials. Entry doors should be self-closing and allow the easy movement of personnel.

Airlock doors, wall ports, through-the-wall autoclaves and dry heat sterilizers should be fitted with interlocked doors. This will prevent both doors being opened simultaneously. An alarm system should be fitted to the doors to prevent the opening of more than one door.

Lights in clean rooms are fitted flush with the ceiling to reduce the collection of dust and avoid disturbing the airflow pattern within the room. Similarly, equipment should be positioned in clean rooms to avoid the distribution and the collection of particles and microbial contaminants.

## ENVIRONMENTAL CONTROL

Potential sources of particles and microbial contaminants occurring within the clean room are:

- the air supply of the room
- inflow of external air
- production of contaminants within the room.

Each of these possible sources can be minimized as described below.

### Air supply

The air supply to a Grade A, B or C clean room must be filtered to ensure the removal of particulate and microbial contamination. This is carried out by filtering the air with high-efficiency particulate air (HEPA) filters. The HEPA filter should be positioned at the inlet to the clean room or close to it. A pre-filter may be fitted upstream of the HEPA filter. This will prolong the life of the final filter. A fan is required to pump the air through the filter.

The HEPA filters use pleated fibreglass paper as the filter medium. The parallel pleats of this filter material increase the surface area of the filter and increase the airflow through the filter. This structure allows the filter to retain a compact volume. Aluminium foil is used to form spacers in the traditional type of HEPA filter. Spacers are not used in the more modern 'mini-pleat' type of filter design. These 'mini-pleat' filters are now widely used. They have a shallower depth in construction than the traditional HEPA filter. Within the structure of the filter, the filter material is sealed to an aluminium frame (Fig. 24.2). At least one side of the filter is protected with a coated mild steel mesh. HEPA filters exhibit:

- a high flow rate
- high particulate holding capacity
- low pressure drop across the filter.

HEPA filters remove larger particles from the air by inertial impaction, the medium-sized particles by direct interception and the small particles by Brownian diffusion. The HEPA filters are least efficient at removing particles of about $0.3\,\mu m$. However, the efficiency of removing particles is affected by the air velocity and the filter packing. Larger and smaller particles will be removed more efficiently.

With a new HEPA filter fitted in a clean room, the air exits from the filter face at a rate of about $0.45\,m/s$ and has a 99.997% efficiency at removing $0.3\,\mu m$ particles. The initial pressure difference across the depth of the filter is about 130 pascals (Pa). At the end of the effective life of the filter the pressure drop across the filter will increase to about 490 Pa. To retain the operating efficiency of the filter, the fan forcing air through the filter must be able to maintain this pressure difference. Sensors are fitted upstream and downstream of the filters to indicate the pressure differential across the filter. An automatic alarm system should be fitted to indicate failure in the air supply or filter blockage.

The HEPA filters for clean room use must conform with the British Standard 5295 (1989) aerosol test. The filters may have faulty seals and can be damaged during delivery or installation. It is thus important that they are tested in situ before use.

The filter material possesses a uniform resistance and is constructed with a large number of parallel pleats. This results in the air downstream of the filter face flowing uniformly with a unidirectional configuration.

The number of air changes in clean rooms is affected by:

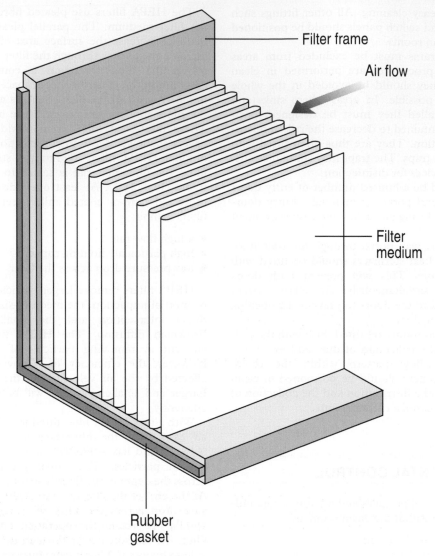

Filter frame

Air flow

Filter medium

Rubber gasket

**Fig. 24.2** Section through a mini-pleat high-efficiency filter, showing its construction.

- the room size
- the equipment in use
- the number of operators in the area.

In practice 25–35 air changes per hour are common. The airflow pattern within the clean room must be carefully regulated to avoid generating particles from the clean room floor and from the operators. The various options for ventilating clean rooms are categorized by the airflow pattern within the room. These are:

- unidirectional airflow systems
- non-unidirectional airflow systems
- combination airflow systems.

### Unidirectional airflow systems

The air enters the room through a complete wall or ceiling of high-efficiency filters. This air will sweep contamination in a single direction to the exhaust system on the opposing wall or floor (Fig. 24.3). In the interests of economy, the exhaust grill may be fitted low down on the wall. The velocity of the air is about 0.3 m/s in downflow air from ceiling filters and 0.45 m/s in cross-flow air. These are highly efficient airflow systems. However, one major disadvantage of these rooms for pharmaceutical use is that they are expensive to construct. They also use much more conditioned air than rooms with non-unidirectional

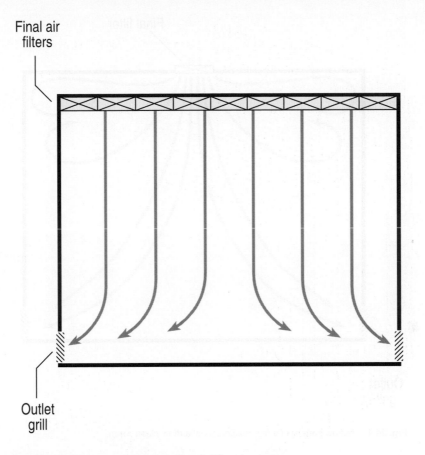

Final air
filters

Outlet
grill

**Fig. 24.3** Airflow pattern in a unidirectional airflow clean room.

airflow. This greatly increases their operating costs. Owing to these factors, unidirectional airflow clean rooms are not often used for pharmaceutical purposes.

### Non-unidirectional airflow systems

The air enters the clean rooms through filters and diffusers which are usually located in the ceiling. The air exits through outlet ducts positioned low down on the wall or in the floor at sites remote from the air inlet (Fig. 24.4). With the use of this system, the filtered inlet air mixes with and dilutes the contaminated air within the room. As the clean room air has been previously heated and cleaned it can be recirculated to save energy, a little fresh air being introduced with each air change cycle.

Various designs of diffuser are used with this ventilation system. These affect the air movement and the cleanliness of the rooms. The perforated plate diffuser produces a jet flow of air directly beneath it. This jet of air will carry contamination at its edges. However,

it does produce high-quality air directly under the diffuser. It is thus important that procedures are located directly below the diffuser. By contrast, the air released from the bladed diffuser will mix with the clean room air. This diffuser thus produces a reasonably constant quality of air throughout the room.

### Combination systems

In many pharmaceutical clean rooms it is common to find that the background area is ventilated by a non-unidirectional airflow system. Meanwhile, the critical areas are supplied with high-quality air from unidirectional airflow units.

The combination airflow system is often selected for pharmaceutical clean room applications as it:

- produces controlled room pressure
- separates the manufacturing process from the general clean room
- is cheaper to use.

Final filter

Outlet
grill

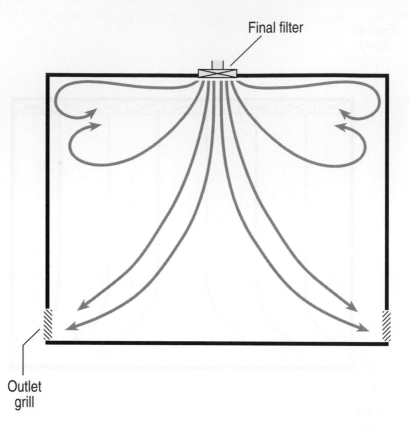

**Fig. 24.4**    Airflow pattern in a non-unidirectional airflow clean room.

Several types of unidirectional flow work stations or benches are used in this combination-type room. Various vertical unidirectional airflow systems are used in combination clean rooms. With one system, the critical area is surrounded by a plastic curtain with vertical unidirectional downflow air 'washing' over the manufacturing process and exiting under the plastic curtains into the general clean room area (Fig. 24.5). An alternative system is often used with the small-scale combination-type clean room in hospital pharmacies. With this system, a horizontal airflow cabinet (Fig. 24.6) is used as the work station. With these cabinets, a fan forces air through a HEPA filter located at the rear wall of the work station. The air which exits from the filter firstly washes over the critical work area before washing over the arms and upper body areas of the operator. Contamination arising from the operator is thus kept downstream of the critical procedures. Grade A environmental conditions are achieved at the critical work area. A similar work station known as a vertical laminar airflow cabinet (Fig. 24.7) could also be used in the combination room. This cabinet passes

air vertically downwards from the ceiling of the cabinet over the critical working area. It produces a Grade A environmental quality. The air exits from the front of the work station.

In recent times, there has been a trend towards protecting the critical procedures within combination clean rooms by using isolator cabinets. The isolator cabinet gives a localized high-quality environment. Isolators give protection from potential contamination in clean rooms as they are positively pressurized with air supplied through HEPA filters. The operator works outside the confines of the isolator using glove ports to perform procedures within the enclosed chamber. The gloved hands of clean room operators can transfer microbial contamination into critical working areas within the clean room. To indicate that the required clean room standards have been achieved (Table 24.2) the fingertips of a gloved hand are depressed onto the surface of a suitable solid growth medium. This medium is incubated to show any contamination.

There is also a need to avoid contaminated external air passing into the clean room environ-

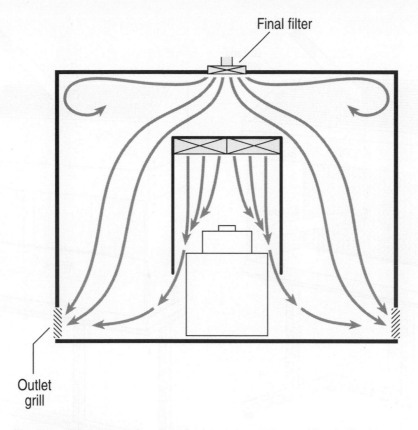

**Fig. 24.5** Airflow patterns in a mixed flow clean room with non-unidirectional airflow background environment and unidirectional airflow protection for a critical area.

ment. Thus, the clean room air pressure must exceed that of the surrounding areas. The pressure differential between different standards of clean room should be 10–15 Pa. This level should be comparatively easy to monitor and will decrease the unregulated outflow of air. The outflow of clean room air and the room pressure are regulated by adjusting grills known as pressure stabilizers located in the walls of rooms. The air moves from an area of high pressure to an area of lower pressure. To maintain the room pressure it is important that the rooms are airtight. However, a small quantity of air will exit from the rooms by way of door spaces.

## Temperature and humidity control

The temperature and the humidity are adjusted to suit the procedures being carried out within the clean room and maintain the comfort of the operators. A target temperature of about 20°C with a relative humidity of about 35–45% are often preferred.

## Personnel

The clean room environment is supplied with high-quality air at positive pressure. The main source of contamination in these areas arises from skin scales which are released by the clean room operators.

To limit clean room contamination by personnel there is a need to:

- restrict the number of operators working in the clean room
- restrict operator conversations
- instruct operators to move slowly
- minimize general movement throughout the room
- avoid operators interrupting the airflow between the inlet filter and the work area.

The clean room operator is constantly shedding dead skin scales from the body surface. Not all of these skin particles are contaminated with bacteria. Males shed more particles which are contaminated with bacteria than females. Individual males and females do show variable rates of bacterial dispersal.

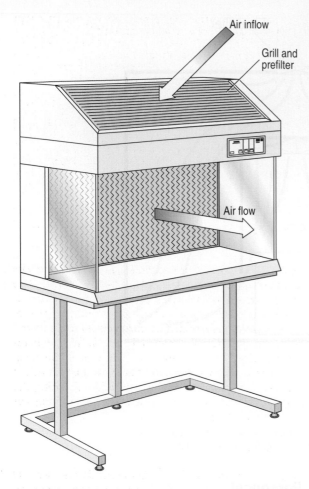

**Fig. 24.6** Horizontal laminar airflow unit (courtesy of John Bass Ltd).

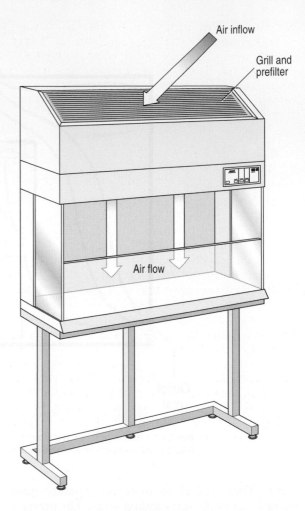

**Fig. 24.7** Vertical laminar airflow unit (courtesy of John Bass Ltd).

This dispersal from the individual is affected by:

● personal characteristics
● general health and skin condition.

Body movements of personnel will increase the number of contaminated particles released from the skin surface. Each individual releases more than $10^6$ skin scales per minute during normal walking movements. There is a need to contain the dispersion of skin particles from the operators in clean rooms and protect both the environment and the product. Containment of particles is achieved by the operators wearing clean room clothing. This clothing is made from synthetic fabrics that filter out particulate and microbial contamination from the operators without themselves releasing contamination. However, this clothing is not absolute and particles can pass through the garments. Although the garments

are close fitting at the neck, wrists and ankles, these sites provide an exit route for particulate matter.

Clean garments should be used for each work session and must provide operator comfort. Disposable single-use garments are available, although most production units employ reusable garments. The clothing is specially laundered in an area with similar standards to those used in the clean room. The garments are laundered by a wet-wash process using particle-free solutions followed by an antibacterial rinse and hot air drying. The garments are then packaged in sealed bags to avoid particulate contamination. This cleaning process fulfils the needs of most pharmaceutical clean room applications which are a balance between cost and acceptability. For a higher level of sterility assurance the garments are gamma irradiated using $^{60}$Co, each garment receiving a Department of Health approved dose of 25 kGy. This treatment is expensive and decreases the life of the garments. The donning of clean room clothing without contaminating the outer surface of the garments is a rather difficult procedure which is performed in the changing room.

*Changing room*

Entry of personnel into clean rooms should be through a changing room fitted with interlocking doors. These doors act as an airlock to prevent the influx of external air. This access route is intended for the entry of personnel only. The changing room is subdivided into three areas. Movement through these areas must comply with a strict protocol. The three areas are often colour coded as black, grey and white, black representing the dirtiest area while white represents the cleanest area.

The black area is where jewellery, cosmetics, factory or hospital protective garments and shoes are removed. Long hair may be contained and a mob cap donned to contain the hair completely. The pass-over bench forms a physical separation between the black and the grey areas in the changing room.

The operator then sits on the pass-over bench, swings the legs over the bench and fits clean room covers over the feet before contacting the floor of the grey area.

The operator then stands up in the grey area. The wrappings on the various garments are opened to avoid contacting the outer surface of the packaging following the hand washing procedure. The operator then washes his/her hands and forearms using an antiseptic solution. Special attention is paid to cleaning the fingernails. The hands are then dried using an automatic air-blow drier as towels shed particles when used for drying hands.

The clothing garments are donned in sequence from head to foot. Throughout this procedure care must be taken to avoid the hands contacting the outer surface of the clean room clothing. Firstly the head and shoulder hood are fitted, ensuring that all the hair is contained within the head cover. A face mask is fitted to prevent the shedding of droplets. The one-piece coverall or alternatively the two-piece trouser suit is put on. Care must be taken to avoid these garments contacting the floor surface. The shoulder cover of the head and shoulder hood is tucked into the coverall. The zip is then closed and the studs fastened. The overboots are then fitted over the clean room shoes. The overboots are kept in position with ties which are suitably fastened for

| Table 24.5 | Clothing for clean room use |
|---|---|
| Clean room grade | Description of clothing |
| A/B | Head cover and face mask<br>Single- or two-piece trouser suit<br>Overboots and sterile powder-free rubber or plastic gloves |
| C | Hair (and beard) cover<br>Single- or two-piece trouser suit<br>Clean room shoes or overshoes |
| D | Hair (and beard) cover<br>Protective suit<br>Appropriate shoes or overshoes |

operator comfort. For entry into aseptic filling rooms an antiseptic cream is applied to the hands. The clean room powder-free gloves are then donned. Care is needed to avoid contacting the outer surface of the gloves. The cuffs of the coverall are secured within the gloves. The gloved hands should be disinfected. The operator now enters into the white clean room area and begins work. The gloved hands of the operators should be regularly disinfected during the work procedures. Key features of the clothing are given in Table 24.5.

## Cleaning

A strict cleaning and disinfection policy is essential to minimize particulate and microbial contamination in the clean room. Microbial and particulate contamination is released within the clean room by operators. These contaminants are mostly deposited onto horizontal surfaces. However, other areas of the clean room can become contaminated due to direct contact with the operators' clothing. It is thus essential that a strict cleaning and disinfection policy is implemented within the clean room to minimize both the particulate and the microbial contamination.

There are two main methods of cleaning. Vacuuming is effective at removing gross particulate contamination of particles greater than 100 μm. However, vacuuming is not very effective at removing smaller particles. The small particles are removed by wet wiping. It is important that the wet wipe is sterile and must not generate particulate contamination. The use of wet wipes involves the use of cleaning agents which will remove particulate contamination and have an antibacterial effect.

The ideal cleaning agent should be:

1. effective in removing undesirable contamination
2. harmless to surfaces
3. fast drying
4. non-flammable
5. non-toxic
6. cost-effective.

The cleaning agents of choice which are commonly used to clean a clean room are usually anionic or cationic surfactants. The disinfectants of choice for clean room use are generally quaternary ammonium compounds, phenols, alcohols and polymeric biguanides. The disinfectant solutions should be freshly prepared before use. Different types of disinfectants should be used in rotation to prevent the development of resistant microbial strains. Most surfactants or detergents will dissipate surface static electricity but the most effective and widely used antistatic agents used in clean rooms are cationic surfactants.

The cleaning of critical clean room areas such as production areas should be stringently performed by trained personnel on a regular basis. A less stringent cleaning protocol is required in the general clean room areas. This applies to the walls and floors where contamination cannot directly contaminate the product. As part of the cleaning protocol regular microbiological monitoring should be carried out to determine the effectiveness of the disinfection procedures.

## ISOLATORS

Isolators are widely used in hospital pharmacy departments as an alternative to clean rooms for the small-scale aseptic processing of sterile products. These devices are selected for aseptic manipulations of sterile products as they are:

- relatively inexpensive
- easily designed for a specific purpose
- capable of providing operator protection from the product.

Isolators are composed of a chamber which controls the environment surrounding the work procedure (Fig. 24.8). The inlet and exhaust air passes through HEPA filters. The airflow pattern within the isolator chamber may be either unidirectional, non-unidirectional or a combination of both. The air within the isolator chamber should be frequently changed to maintain the aseptic chamber environment. If unfiltered air should access the chamber this

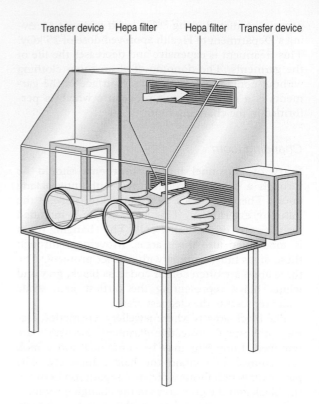

Transfer device    Hepa filter      Hepa filter    Transfer device

**Fig. 24.8** Isolator cabinet.

must be purged from the isolator within a 5-minute period. The particle and microbial contamination of the environment within the isolator chamber must conform with the Grade A standard as detailed in Tables 24.1 and 24.2.

The operator remains outside the isolator chamber environment. To perform manual manipulations within the chamber the operator inserts his/her hands and arms into the chamber. The entry occurs by way of a glove port using either a one-piece full-arm-length glove or a glove and sleeve system. With the glove and sleeve system, the glove is attached to a sleeve which is attached to the wall of the chamber through an airtight seal. Using either of these glove systems the operator is able to perform aseptic manipulations up to a distance of about 0.75 metres within the chamber. The glove system avoids contamination arising from the operator and maintains the integrity of the isolator chamber environment. To perform the work procedure within the chamber, materials must be introduced and prepared products removed without compromising the chamber environment. This transfer procedure is a critical factor in the operation of the isolator and is carried out using a transfer system. The transfer system separates the external environment from the controlled isolator environment. It restricts airflow between these areas while allowing the transfer of materials between them. The transfer system is fitted with an interlocked double door entry system. This will provide an airlock which avoids both doors being opened simultaneously to the external environment. It is preferable if a filtered air inlet and exhaust is fitted to the transfer system.

It is important that the risk of microbial contamination of the product is reduced. The isolator must, therefore, be positioned in a suitable background environment of at least a Grade D classification. This is typically achieved by positioning the isolator in a dedicated room which is only used for the isolator and its related activities.

Isolators are divided into two types: types I and II.

## Type I isolator

This isolator protects the product from contamination arising from an external source and from the aseptic process itself. This isolator operates under positive pressure. It is used for the aseptic preparation of pharmaceutical products.

## Type II isolator

This isolator will protect the product from contamination arising from an external source and from the aseptic manipulation. In addition, however, this isolator should protect the operator from hazardous materials such as cytotoxic preparations or radiopharmaceuticals in the isolator chamber. This type of isolator operates under negative pressure. The exhaust air is ducted to the outside through at least one HEPA filter and through an adsorption material such as activated carbon. Rigid Type II isolators should be used for radiopharmaceutical manipulations. In this situation, the isolator is frequently used with a lead-free vision panel and a lead glass protector around the product. Alternatively, isolators are available with lead acrylic glass windows.

The chambers of isolators are gas sterilized. The ideal sterilant for use in the isolator chamber should have the following properties:

- non-corrosive to metals and plastics
- rapidly lethal to all microorganisms
- good penetration
- harmless.

The sterilants in most general use for pharmaceutical applications in isolators are peracetic acid vapour and hydrogen peroxide vapour. To reduce the risk of chemical contamination of the sterile product, the sterilant contact time should be carefully regulated. The sterilant must be flushed from the isolator before beginning the aseptic manipulations.

Currently marketed isolators are constructed with either a flexible canopy or a rigid containment medium. The rigid type of isolator is often preferred, owing to the reduced risk of puncturing the chamber. This occurs more readily with the flexible canopy design. Rigid isolators are often constructed from a stainless steel frame with a moulded acrylic window. A further isolator known as a half-suit isolator is currently in use. This is a flexible canopy isolator that is made from material such as nylon-lined PVC. Care is needed when using this system to avoid puncturing the chamber walls. It is designed using a half-suit sealed to a wall of the chamber. This system allows the torso of the operator to be introduced into the suit which is located within the chamber of the isolator. To improve visibility, a transparent helmet is sealed to the neck of the suit which is ventilated by a pressurized air supply. This provides operator comfort over prolonged work sessions. The advantage of the half-suit isolator is that the operator can easily access a large area of the chamber and manoeuvre heavier and larger materials. The half-suit isolator is used as dedicated production equipment for the aseptic compounding of products such as total parenteral nutrition (TPN) fluids.

## Isolator tests

Isolators must be tested to ensure that they operate as a sealed chamber. They must also conform with the required level of air quality and surface contamination. They are thus subjected to both physical and microbial tests.

Physical tests include:

- *Integrity tests.* These tests will detect leaks that compromise the integrity of the isolator chamber. The procedure is carried out by sealing the chamber and recording changes in the chamber pressure over time.
- *Glove inspection.* The glove and sleeve are visually inspected for pin holes.
- *HEPA filter test.* The integrity of the HEPA filter should be tested with an aerosol generator and a detector.
- *Airborne particle count.* This is carried out in the isolator chamber and the transfer device using a particle counter.

Microbial tests use microbial growth media suitable for the growth of potential contaminants. The tests include:

- *Active air sampling.* This test determines the number of organisms in the air of the isolator chamber. The procedure uses impact and agar impingement samplers.
- *Settle plates.* 140 mm settle plates containing growth media are exposed in the chamber for 2–4 hours.
- *Surface tests.* Surfaces are sampled using direct contact plates which are then incubated. Following sampling, it is important to remove materials deposited onto surfaces during the test. Alternatively, surfaces are sampled using sterile moistened swabs. The swabs are then streaked onto solid growth media and incubated. Soluble swabs may be dissolved in sterile diluent and the viable count determined.
- *Finger dabs.* The fingertips of the gloved hand are depressed onto the surface of solid growth medium. The medium is then incubated.
- *Broth fill test.* This test challenges both the manipulative procedure of the operator and the facilities. The test simulates routine aseptic procedures by using nutrient media in place of a product to produce broth-filled units. These units are incubated to indicate microbial contamination.

## ENVIRONMENTAL MONITORING

Following construction of a clean room, it must be tested to ensure that it is providing the required quality of environment. These verification tests are rigorously performed and are similar to the tests used to monitor the clean room subsequently. The monitoring tests ensure that the clean room continues to provide satisfactory operation.

To ensure that the pharmaceutical clean room is providing the required environmental standards, the following are determined.

### Air quality

The air supplied to the clean room must not contribute to particulate or microbial contamination within the room. The HEPA filters for the inlet air must be tested to ensure that both the filter fabric and the filter seals are not leaking. This is done by introducing a smoke with a known particle size upstream of the filter. The clean room surface of the filter is then scanned for smoke penetration using a photometer or a particle counter.

### Air movement

Adequate ventilation throughout the clean room can be determined by air movement tests. These are carried out at the time of clean room validation. Air movement within the clean room is determined by measuring the decay profile of smoke particles released into the clean room. Smoke particle release is also used to ensure that a clean area within a unidirectional work station is not being contaminated with air from the clean room environment.

The outflow of air from a clean room with a higher standard of cleanliness to an area with a lower standard is indicated by the pressure differential between the rooms. This is determined using a manometer or magnahelic gauge.

### Air velocity

The velocity of the air at several points in a critical clean room area should be determined. This is done both at validation of the clean room and at timed intervals. The procedure involves the use of an anemometer.

### Airborne particulate and microbial contamination

The particle count and the microbial bioburden of the clean room provide the basis for the air classification system for grading a clean room as detailed in Table 24.1. The points for sampling and the number of samples taken at each position are determined by the size and the class of the clean room. Airborne particles are normally sized and counted by optical particle counters.

### Microbial monitoring

There should be very few viable organisms present in the clean room air. However, operators within the clean room disperse large numbers of skin particles. Many of these particles are contaminated with bacteria. The dispersal of contaminated particles by the clean room operator is greatly decreased by the wearing of occlusive clothing together with appropriate air ventilation. Sampling for microbial contamination is necessary when people are present in the clean room during production. Monitoring of the microbial contamination during production will ensure that the use of clean room clothing by the operators and the air ventilation system are producing the required environmental standards. Air sampling is carried out by volumetric sampling or by the use of settle plates. With volumetric sampling a measured volume of air is drawn from the environment and contaminants are impinged onto a suitable microbial growth medium. The medium is then incubated and the colonies of microbial growth counted. Settle plates rely on bacteria-carrying particles being deposited onto the exposed surface of sterile microbial growth media contained in a 90 or 140 mm diameter Petri dish. When positioning the plates, care is needed to avoid accidental contamination. Owing to the small number of microbial contaminants in the clean room the settle plates are preferably exposed for about 4 hours.

The surfaces of the clean room should also be tested for microbial contamination notably in areas which may be contacted by the clothing of the operators. This is achieved by using contact plates or by using sterile moistened swabs. The contact plates allow a sterile agar surface to be pressed onto the clean room surface. The contact plates are then incubated to reveal microbial growth. Swabbing procedures are carried out as previously detailed in isolator tests.

- Clean room clothing, made from synthetic fabrics, is designed to minimize release of operator contaminants.
- Changing areas are designed and used to minimize the entry of contamination on personnel.
- During cleaning, vacuuming and wet wiping are used to remove large and small particles respectively.
- Isolators give protection to both the product and the operator at relatively low cost.
- Type II isolators protect the operator from hazardous materials in addition to providing the Type I facilities of protection of the product from contamination.
- Isolator interiors are sterilized using a gas sterilant.
- Isolator integrity is tested using physical and microbial tests.
- A range of environmental tests are used in clean rooms to monitor air quality, movement and velocity, airborne particles and microbial contamination.

## Key Points

- Particulate and microbial contamination of sterile products is minimized by preparation in a clean environment.
- Quality of clean areas is graded A, B, C, D in decreasing stringency for particulate and microbial content.
- Premises must allow segregation of stages of production and protect products from contamination by all possible means of design and operation.
- Access to clean areas is restricted and special clothing must be worn.
- Environmental control, particularly of the air supply to the room, is required to ensure a minimal contamination hazard.
- HEPA filters have a 99.997% efficiency at removing 0.3 μm particles, the size at which their efficiency is lowest.
- Airflow may be designed as unidirectional, non-unidirectional or as a combination system.
- In addition to general air quality, localized areas of higher quality can be produced either by airflow design in enclosed areas, or by isolator cabinets.
- The main source of contamination in clean rooms is the skin scales from operators.

## FURTHER READING

Bell N D S 1994 Cleanrooms for pharmaceutical production. In: The pharmaceutical codex, 12th edn. The Pharmaceutical Press, London
British Standard 5295 1989 Environmental cleanliness in enclosed spaces. British Standards Institution, London
Commission of the European Communities 1990 The rules governing medicinal products in the European Community, volume IV: good manufacturing practice for medicinal products. The Commission, Luxembourg
DeVicchi F 1993 Environmental control in parenteral drug manufacturing. In: Avis K E, Lieberman H A, Lachman L (eds) Pharmaceutical dosage forms: parenteral medications, 2nd edn. Marcel Dekker, New York, vol 2
Farquharson G F, Whyte W 1991 The design of cleanrooms for the pharmaceutical industry. In: Whyte W (ed) Cleanroom design. John Wiley, Chichester
Guidance for Pharmaceutical Manufacturers and Distributors 1997 HMSO, London
Lee G M, Midcalf B 1994 Isolators for pharmaceutical applications. HMSO, London
White P J P 1990 The design of controlled environments. In: Denyer S, Baird R (eds) Guide to microbiological control in pharmaceuticals. Ellis Horwood, London

# 25
# Parenteral products

*D. G. Chapman*

---

After studying this chapter you will know about:

**The reasons for parenteral administration**
**The routes available for parenteral administration**
**The various forms and types of parenteral product**
**The design of containers and methods of administration of parenteral products**
**The formulation and uses of parenteral products**
**Pyrogens**
**Tonicity adjustment**
**Large volume sterile products.**

## Introduction

Parenteral products are dosage forms which are delivered to the patient by a route outwith the alimentary canal. The parenteral route of administration is often used for drugs which cannot be given orally. This may be due to patient intolerance, to the instability of the drug, or to poor absorption of the drug if given by the oral route. In practice, parenteral products are often regarded as dosage forms which are implanted, injected or infused directly into vessels, tissues, tissue spaces or body compartments. From the site of administration the drug is then transported to the site of action. With developing technology, parenteral therapy is being used outwith the hospital or clinic environment. It is increasingly being used by patients at home and in the workplace, allowing them to administer their own medication.

Parenteral therapy is used to:

- produce a localized effect
- administer drugs if the oral route cannot be used
- deliver drugs to the unconscious patient

- rapidly correct fluid and electrolyte imbalances
- ensure delivery of the drug to the target tissues.

## ADMINISTRATION

The three major routes of parenteral drug administration are:

- subcutaneous
- intramuscular
- intravenous.

In addition to these, other routes such as intradermal, intra-arterial, intracardiac, intraspinal and intra-articular are also used to deliver drugs by the parenteral route (see Fig. 25.1).

## Subcutaneous injections

These are injected into the loose connective and adipose tissue immediately beneath the skin. Typically, the volume injected does not exceed 1 ml. Injection sites include the abdomen, the upper back, the upper arms and the lateral upper hips. This route is used if drugs cannot be administered orally. The drugs are more rapidly and predictably absorbed than when administered by the oral route. However, absorption of the drug after subcutaneous injection is slower and less predictable than when administered by the intramuscular route.

## Intramuscular injections

Small volume aqueous solutions, solutions in oil and suspensions are administered directly into the body of a relaxed muscle. Several muscle sites are used for these injections including the gluteal muscle in the buttock, the deltoid muscle in the shoulder and the vastus lateralis of the thigh. In adults the gluteal muscle is often used as larger volumes can be tolerat-

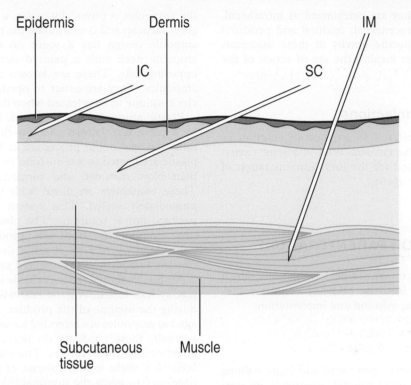

**Fig. 25.1**  Injection routes.

ed. In infants and small children the vastus lateralis of the thigh is usually more developed than other muscle groups and is thus used. For rapid absorption of the medicament the deltoid muscle in the shoulder is often used.

## Intravenous injections and infusions

Small volumes of fluid may be injected intravenously to produce a rapid effect. Large volumes of fluids are infused slowly. The vein which is selected for administering the formulation depends on several factors. These include the size of the delivery needle or catheter, the type and volume of fluid to be administered and the rate of administering the fluid. The fluids are administered into a superficial vein, commonly on the back of the hand or in the internal flexure of the elbow. The intravenous route is widely used to administer parenteral products, but it must not be used to administer water-in-oil emulsions or suspensions.

Other routes of parenteral administration include:

## Intradermal injections

A volume of about 0.1 ml is injected into the skin between the epidermis and the dermis. Absorption from intradermal injections is slow. This route is often used for diagnostic tests for allergy or immunity. It is also used to administer some vaccines.

## Intra-arterial injections

The drug is administered directly into an artery. Owing to the fast flow of blood in the artery it is likely that the drug will be rapidly dispersed throughout the blood system. In addition drugs can be administered by this route to target an organ which is served by the artery.

## Intracardiac injections

These are aqueous solutions which are administered in emergency directly into a ventricle or the cardiac muscle.

## Intraspinal injections

These are aqueous solutions which are injected in volumes less than 20 ml into particular areas of the spinal column. They are categorized as intrathecal, subarachnoid, intracisternal, epidural and peridural injections. The specific gravity of these injections may be adjusted to localize the site of action of the drug.

## Intra-articular injections

These are administered as an aqueous solution or suspension into the synovial fluid in a joint cavity. They are often used for the local administration of anti-inflammatory agents.

## PRODUCTS FOR PARENTERAL USE

Parenteral products are sterile formulations which are administered into the body by various routes including injection, infusion and implantation.

## Injections

These are subdivided into small and large volume parenteral fluids. Small volume parenterals are sterile, pyrogen-free injectable products. They are packaged in volumes up to 100 ml. Small volume parenteral fluids are packed as:

- single dose ampoules
- multiple dose vials
- pre-filled syringes.

### Single dose ampoules

Most small volume parenterals are currently packaged as either ampoules or vials. Glass ampoules are thin-walled containers made of Type I borosilicate glass (Fig. 6.4). Injections packaged in glass ampoules are manufactured by filling the product into the ampoules which are then heat sealed. To achieve the quality required of these products, the packaged solution must be sterile and practically free of particles. These products are typically prepared in clean room conditions (see Ch. 24). However, the great concern with using glass ampoules relates to the hazards of opening them because the product may become contaminated with glass particles. Opening is easier with glass ampoules with a weakened neck. This is achieved by applying a ceramic paint ring to the ampoule neck. The paint, after a process of heat baking, has the effect of weakening the neck. Even though the subsequent opening of

the ampoules is physically easier, a large number of glass particles still contaminate the product. Another ampoule design has a score on the glass at the ampoule neck with a painted dot marker on the opposing side. These are known as one-point cut ampoules. They are easier to open, but glass particles continue to be released when they are opened.

Plastic ampoules are prepared, filled and sealed by a procedure known as blow–fill–seal. This is a four-step continuous procedure in which granules of plastic are heated to a semi-solid state. The plastic is then blow moulded and formed into ampoules. These containers are filled with the product and immediately sealed. This system is only used to package simple solutions. The plastic may take up drug components from the product. When the ampoule is opened by rotating the integral plastic closure, few particles are released into the solution.

Ampoules should have a reliable seal which can be readily leak tested. A good seal will not deteriorate during the lifetime of the product. Medicines packaged in ampoules are intended for single use only. As a result, these products do not contain chemical antimicrobial preservatives. The ampoule must also contain a slight excess volume of product. This is necessary to allow the nominal injection volume to be drawn into a syringe.

### Multiple dose vials

These are composed of a thick-walled glass container which is sealed with a rubber closure. The closure is kept in position by an aluminium seal which is crimped to the neck of the glass vial (Fig. 6.5). These closures are then covered with a plastic cap. The cap is removed before a needle, attached to a syringe, is inserted through the rubber closure to withdraw a dose of product. The contents of the vial may be removed in several portions.

The glass vial packaging system has the advantage of increased dose flexibility and decreased costs per unit dose. There are also certain disadvantages with the use of glass vials. Fragments of the closure may be released into the product when the needle is inserted through the closure. There is also the risk of interaction between the product and the closure. Repeated withdrawal of injection solution from these containers increases the risk of microbial contamination of the product. These products must, therefore, contain an antimicrobial preservative unless the medicine itself has antimicrobial activity. An example of such a multidose product is insulin. Each dose is withdrawn from the vial when required and administered by the patient.

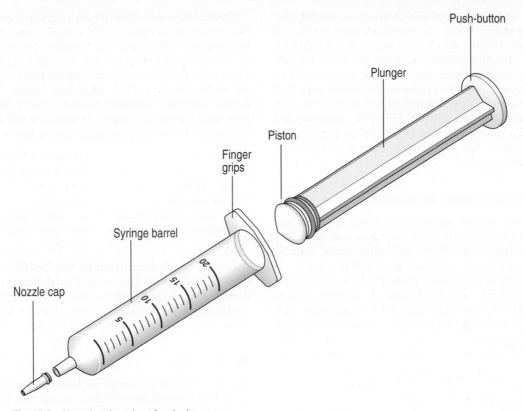

**Fig. 25.2** Hypodermic syringe for single use.

## Prefilled syringes

With these devices, the injection solution is aseptically filled into sterile syringes. The packed solution has a high level of sterility assurance and does not contain an antimicrobial preservative. The final product is available for immediate use. Prefilled syringes are expensive and so only limited products are packaged in this way.

## Administration of small volume parenteral products

Hypodermic syringes and needles are extensively used for administering small volumes of parenteral formulations to the patient. These syringes have been sterilized by ethylene oxide gas or, occasionally, by gamma irradiation following packaging. Various sizes of hypodermic syringes are available. They are composed of a barrel, having a graduated scale, together with a plunger and a headpiece, known as a piston (see Fig. 25.2). These components are often made of polypropylene, although the piston could be made of medical grade rubber.

## FORMULATION OF PARENTERAL PRODUCTS

## Vehicles for injections

The drug is generally present in an injection in low concentration. The vehicle provides the highest proportion of the formulation and should not be toxic nor have any therapeutic activity.

Mains water often contains a wide variety of contaminants such as electrolytes, organisms, particulate matter and dissolved gases, such as carbon dioxide and chlorine. The wide variety of these contaminants causes a problem in the preparation of water for use in injections. This is called water for injections and must be used as the vehicle for parenteral products. It is often used to prepare ophthalmic products but these could be made using purified water.

### Water for injections

Water for injections is the most extensively used vehicle in parenteral formulations. It is well tolerated by the body and ionizable electrolytes readily dissolve in water. Water for injections must be free of pyrogens. It must also have a high level of chemical purity. The *British Pharmacopoeia* (BP 1993) considers that water for injections can only be prepared by distillation in order to produce a consistent supply of the required quality of water. However, the *European Pharmacopoeia*, 3rd edition (EP 1996, implemented in 1997), allows water for parenteral preparations to be prepared by distillation, reverse osmosis or ultrafiltration.

### Preparation of water for injections

The usual method of preparing water for injections is distillation. Whilst other processes can achieve a similar quality of water, these alternative systems cannot produce a consistent quality of product.

The source water used in the preparation of water for injections by distillation is potable water. Nevertheless, this water may be contaminated with suspended mineral and organic substances, mineral salts and chemicals. To improve the quality of the end product the source water may be pretreated by:

- chemical softening
- filtration
- deionization
- pH adjustment.

The conventional still is composed of:

- a boiler containing feed water
- a heater
- a headspace with condensing surfaces known as baffles
- a condenser.

When this still is functioning the water is heated and vaporized in the boiler. The baffles in the headspace return non-volatile impurities to the water. The condenser removes the heat of vaporization and converts the water vapour to a liquid distillate. Only stills designed to produce high-purity water may be used in the production of water for injections. These stills are typically made of stainless steel, although chemically resistant glass could be used.

In operation the first portion of the distillate must be discarded. The remainder is collected in a suitable storage vessel. Conductivity meters are frequently installed at the outlet of the stills to measure the quantity of ionizable materials in the distillate. The conductivity should not be more than $2\,\mu S/cm$. However, the measurement of conductivity alone can be misleading as it does not detect silica in the distillate.

Freshly collected distillate is usually free of microbial contaminants and should contain fewer than 10 bacteria per 100 ml and no *Pseudomonas* species. It must be free of pyrogens with less than 0.25 endotoxin units (EU) per ml as determined by the bacterial endotoxin test. The chemical quality of the freshly collected distillate should comply with the limit tests for purified water. However, it will typically have the following additional quality limits:

| | |
|---|---|
| Chlorides | less than 0.5 parts per million (p.p.m.) |
| Ammonia | 0.1 p.p.m. |
| Heavy metals | 0.1 p.p.m. |
| Oxidizable substances | less than 5 p.p.m. |
| Residues on evaporation | less than 0.001% |
| pH | 5.0–7.0 |

Care is required in handling the freshly collected distillate as it is subject to microbial contamination during storage and distribution. Two systems are commonly used for the storage of water for injections: batch storage and dynamic storage.

### Batch storage

With this system the water for injections is stored as a batch of discrete unit volumes which may be sterilized. Quality control tests are performed on this batch. Only after the batch is identified as being of suitable quality is it released for use. This system provides maximum product accountability before use. It is, however, an expensive storage system.

### Dynamic storage

With this system the storage tank is a surge tank, usually made of quality polished stainless steel. As the level of water for injections in the tank falls then more water for injections is produced and filled into the tank. The fresh water for injections mixes with water remaining in the tank. This system is cheaper and simpler to operate than batch storage. However, it does lack batch accountability and the water may become contaminated through corrosion of the steel tank. Owing to the potential problem with Gram-negative bacterial contamination, it is important that the distillate is stored at 80°C to prevent bacterial growth. Heating the water in the tank is achieved with a steam-heated jacket around the tank.

Surge tanks require sterilization at timed intervals. They are fitted with a filter vent used to equilibrate the tank pressure during filling and emptying the tank. The filter prevents airborne bacterial contamination of the water for injections within the tank.

## Distribution

A loop distribution system may be used to deliver the water for injections to the point of use. The water in the distribution system can become contaminated with organisms. As a result, the water in the stainless steel pipes is constantly circulated from the tank to avoid stagnation and to maintain the temperature. This distribution system has one major disadvantage in that the point of use may not require high temperature water. Thus a cooling system may be fitted close to the point of use. Microbial growth may then occur in the cooled water.

## Sterilized water for injections

This is prepared by packing a volume of water for injections in sealed containers. These containers are then moist heat sterilized which yields a sterile product that remains free of pyrogens.

# Pyrogens

Water is potentially the greatest source of pyrogens in parenteral products. Untreated water is pyrogenic and must be treated to remove pyrogens. This is achieved in the preparation of water for injections by distillation in the UK. Pyrogens are fever-producing substances. The injection of distilled water may produce a rise in body temperature if it contains pyrogens, while water which is free of this effect is described as apyrogenic.

Microbial pyrogens arise from components of Gram-negative and Gram-positive bacteria, fungi and viruses. Non-microbial pyrogens, such as some steroids and plasma components also produce a pyrogenic response if injected. The most important pyrogens in pharmacy products are high molecular weight endotoxins which are found in the outer membrane of Gram-negative bacteria. Therefore, endotoxins potentially exist in all situations harbouring bacteria.

Freshly prepared parenteral products must not be contaminated with organisms which could produce pyrogens. They must be prepared in conditions which reduce microbial contamination because bacteria contaminating aqueous solutions can release endotoxins. Contaminated solutions will become more pyrogenic with the passage of time. Therefore, these products must be sterilized shortly after preparation.

Endotoxins produce significant physiological changes when injected. Their detection and elimination are very important for manufacturers of parenteral products.

## Nature of endotoxins

Endotoxins isolated from the outer membrane of Gram-negative bacteria are composed of three areas. The inner region is composed of lipid A which is linked to a central polysaccharide core. This polysaccharide core is joined to long projections known as the *O*-antigenic side chains. Lipid A is responsible for most of the biological activity of endotoxin. By itself it is not very soluble in water. However, it is joined to a core polysaccharide by an eight-carbon sugar which acts as a solute carrier for the lipid A in aqueous solutions.

The molecular weight of endotoxin is important in determining its biological activity. In a pure aqueous environment, endotoxin has a relative molecular mass of about $10^6$. This is equivalent to the relative molecular mass of a virus particle and is the most common size of endotoxin found in large volume parenteral formulations. In the presence of magnesium and calcium, the endotoxin forms bilayer sheets or vesicles with a diameter of about $0.1\,\mu m$. These small structures can easily pass through a $0.22\,\mu m$ membrane filter. This size of filter is commonly used in the production of pharmacy products.

## Biological activity of pyrogens

The injection of endotoxins and other pyrogens can produce many physiological effects. The most important arising from the use of pharmacy products is the pyrogenic effect, where the lipid A directly affects the thermoregulatory centres in the brain. At high dose levels endotoxin will also:

- activate the coagulation system
- alter carbohydrate and lipid metabolism
- produce platelet aggregation
- produce shock and ultimately death.

As pyrogens can produce these toxic effects they should never be knowingly injected. Their detection and elimination are very important for the production of parenteral products. The contamination of large volume parenteral solutions with pyrogens is especially serious, owing to the large volumes which are administered to seriously ill patients.

Although endotoxins are the predominant pyrogen in parenteral formulations, other pyrogenic substances also exist. These agents include peptidoglycan, from Gram-positive bacteria, and bacterial exotoxins, as evidenced by the erythrogenic response produced by *Streptococcus* group A organisms which causes the skin to turn red. Viruses induce a pyrogenic response which often appears like the fever induced by the common cold virus. Moulds and yeasts also produce a pyrogenic effect following intravenous injection.

## Tests for pyrogens

The rabbit test included in the BP (1993) and in the EP (1996) is very similar to the original rabbit test included in the 1948 edition of the BP. However, in recent times, an alternative test for bacterial endotoxins has been extensively used. While the rabbit test is used to identify the presence of a wide range of pyrogens, the bacterial endotoxin test is a specific test for endotoxins of bacterial origin. Bacterial endotoxin is the main pyrogen found in parenteral products.

### Bacterial endotoxin test

This test, which is commonly referred to as the limulus amoebocyte lysate (LAL) test, uses a lysate of amoebocytes from the horseshoe crab *Limulus polyphemus*. It is an in vitro test for bacterial endotoxins.

Advantages of the LAL test include that it is:

* cheap
* rapid
* simple
* sensitive to low endotoxin concentrations.

The gel clot endpoint test is the method detailed in the BP (1993) for bacterial endotoxins. Other highly sensitive automated kinetic chromogenic and turbidimetric assay methods are used by commercial manufacturers of parenteral products. With the gel clot procedure a solution containing the endotoxin is added to a solution of the lysate. The reaction requires a proclotting enzyme system and a clottable protein coagulogen which are provided by the lysate. The reaction which takes place is shown in Figure 25.3. The rate of this reaction is affected by several factors, including the concentration of endotoxin, the pH and the temperature. Before the test is carried out, it is necessary to determine that:

* the test equipment does not adsorb endotoxins
* the lysate is of suitable sensitivity
* no interfering agents are present.

In the test procedure, the lysate is mixed with an equal volume of the test solution in a depyrogenated container, such as a glass tube. The tube is then incubated undisturbed at 37°C for a period of about

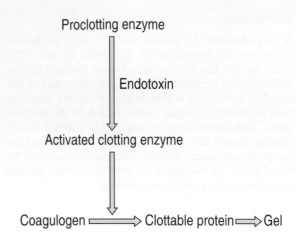

**Fig. 25.3** The lysate clotting mechanism.

60 minutes. The test is a pass or fail test. The end point is identified by gently inverting the glass tube. A positive result is indicated by the formation of a solid clot. This clot does not disintegrate when the tube is inverted. A negative result is indicated if no gel clot has been formed. This LAL test needs appropriate positive and negative controls. For a positive control, a known concentration of endotoxin is added to the lysate alone and then repeated with a product sample. As a negative control, water which is free of endotoxin is added to the lysate. All the controls must produce appropriate results for the test to be valid. The sensitivity of the assay is limited by the sensitivity of the lysate used in the test. The gel clot test will detect between 0.02 and 1.0 endotoxin units per ml.

### Pyrogen testing

The BP pyrogen test involves measuring the rise in body temperature of healthy mature rabbits. This temperature rise is recorded after the rabbits have been intravenously injected with a sterile solution of the test substance. The environment and the equipment used in the test are detailed in the BP (1993). This test can only be carried out where the rabbits can tolerate the test product.

The test itself is preceded by a preliminary test to identify and exclude any animal with an unusual response to the trauma of the injection. With the preliminary test, a warmed pyrogen-free saline solution is injected into the rabbits. The temperature of the rabbits is recorded from 90 minutes before the test to 3 hours after the injection, as specified in the BP (1993). The fever response in the rabbits after the injection with pyrogens follows a biphasic response. After the injection there is a lag time of about 15–18 minutes, which is followed by a rapid temperature rise to a peak within 2 hours. The temperature then falls and is followed by a second rise in temperature. This returns to normal after 6–9 hours. False-positive temperature increases occur with rabbits owing to:

- injury
- badly positioned recording devices
- distress.

The rabbits may develop a resistance to pyrogens. As a result, they are tested at specified time intervals.

## Depyrogenation

The main method of preventing pyrogens contaminating parenteral products is strict control of the ingredients used. That is solvents, raw materials, packaging materials and equipment should not be contaminated with pyrogens.

Depyrogenation is the elimination of all pyrogens, from the production materials, solutions and equipment. It is achieved by either inactivation or removal of the pyrogens.

As pyrogens are non-volatile, the principal method of avoiding contamination of parenteral products is by the distillation of water. This is achieved by positioning a trap, fitted with baffles, in the still. The trap removes the droplets of water by impingement and prevents pyrogens-being carried over into the distillate. However, the freshly collected distillate, which is initially pyrogen-free water, can become contaminated with organisms and pyrogens if stored for more than 4 hours at 22°C. To avoid microbial growth in this water it must be sterilized soon after collection or stored at high temperatures to suppress microbial growth. Pyrogens can be removed from solutions by ultrafiltration. These filters are different from the $0.2\,\mu m$ filters used in pharmacy production. The pyrogens are separated by a process based on their relative molecular mass.

Various methods are used to inactivate pyrogens including heat treatment, acid–base hydrolysis and oxidation. High temperature is widely used to inactivate pyrogens especially for glassware, thermostable equipment and formulation components. Dry heat at 250°C for 30 minutes is normally used. The commonly used dry or moist heat sterilization cycles (see Ch. 22) will not greatly reduce the pyrogen burden of parenteral products.

## Non-aqueous solvents

Water miscible co-solvents, such as glycerine and propylene glycol, are used as vehicles in small volume parenteral fluids. They are used to increase the solubility of drugs and to stabilize drugs degraded by hydrolysis.

Metabolizable oils are used to dissolve drugs which are insoluble in water. For example steroids, hormones and vitamins are dissolved in vegetable oils. These formulations are administered by intramuscular injection.

## Additives

Various additives, such as antimicrobial agents, antioxidants, buffers, chelating agents and tonicity-adjusting agents are included in injection formulations. Their purpose is to produce a safe and elegant product. Both the types and amounts of additives to be included in formulations are given in the appropriate monograph in the BP (1993).

### Antimicrobial agents

These are added to products which are packaged in multiple dose vials. They are not used in large volume injections or if the drug formulation itself has sufficient antimicrobial activity (such as Methohexitone Sodium Injection). Antimicrobial agents are added to inhibit the growth of microbial organisms which may accidentally contaminate the product during use. The antimicrobial agents must be stable and effective in the parenteral formulation. Because they are effective in the free form, their activity can be greatly reduced by interaction with components of the injection. Rubber closures have been shown to take up antimicrobial preservatives from the injection solution. Preservative uptake is more significant with natural and neoprene rubber and much less with butyl rubber closures.

There is concern about the toxic effects of injections containing preservatives. As a result, a low but effective antimicrobial concentration is used in injections. The effectiveness of antimicrobial agents can be tested by challenging the product with selected organisms. The test procedure will evaluate the antimicrobial activity of the preservative in the packaged product. The test procedure is detailed in the BP (1993). Table 25.1 gives details for some commonly used preservatives.

### Antioxidants

Many drugs in aqueous solutions are easily degraded

**Table 25.1  Examples of antimicrobial preservatives used in aqueous multiple dose injections**

| Antimicrobial preservative | Concentration (% w/v) |
|---|---|
| Benzyl alcohol | 1–2 |
| Chlorocresol | 0.1–0.3 |
| Cresol | 0.25–0.5 |
| Methyl hydroxybenzoate | 0.1 |
| Phenol | 0.25–0.6 |
| Thiomersal | 0.01 |

by oxidation. Small volume parenteral products containing these drugs often contain an antioxidant. Bisulphites and metabisulphites are commonly used antioxidants in aqueous injections. Antioxidants must be carefully selected for use in injections to avoid interaction with the active principle. Antioxidants have a lower oxidation potential than the active principle and so are either preferentially oxidized or block oxidative chain reactions. Injection formulations may, in addition to antioxidants, also contain chelating agents. Chelating agents such as EDTA or citric acid, remove trace elements which catalyse oxidative degradation.

## Buffers

The ideal pH of parenteral products is pH 7.4. If the pH is above pH 9, tissue necrosis may result, whilst below pH 3 pain and phlebitis in tissues can occur.

Buffers are included in injections to maintain the pH of the packaged product. pH changes can arise through interaction between the product and the container. However, the buffer used in the injection must allow the body fluids to change the product pH after injection. Acetate, citrate and phosphate buffers are commonly used in parenteral products.

## Tonicity-adjusting agents

Isotonic solutions have the same osmotic pressure as blood plasma and do not damage the membrane of red blood cells. Hypotonic solutions have a lower osmotic pressure than blood plasma and cause blood cells to swell and burst because of fluids passing into the cells by osmosis. Hypertonic solutions have a higher osmotic pressure than plasma; as a result the red blood cells lose fluids and shrink. Following the administration of an injection it is important that tissue damage and irritation are minimized and haemolysis of red blood cells is minimized. Thus,

the BP (1993) states that aqueous solutions for large volume infusion fluids, together with aqueous fluids for subcutaneous, intradermal, and intramuscular administration, should be made isotonic. Intrathecal injections must also be isotonic to avoid serious changes in the osmotic pressure of the cerebrospinal fluid. Aqueous hypotonic solutions are made isotonic by adding either sodium chloride, glucose or, occasionally, mannitol. The latter two agents are incompatible with some active principles. If the solution is hypertonic it is made isotonic by dilution.

Some components of injections, such as buffers and antioxidants, affect the tonicity. Other components, such as preservatives, which are present in low concentration, have little effect on the tonicity.

Injection solutions are often made isotonic with 0.9% sodium chloride solutions. The amount of solute, or the required dilution necessary to make a solution isotonic, can be determined from the freezing point depression. The freezing point depression of blood plasma and tears is −0.52°C. Thus solutions which freeze at −0.52°C have the same osmotic pressure as body fluids. Hypotonic solutions have a smaller freezing point depression and require the addition of a solute to depress the freezing point to −0.52°C.

The amount of adjusting substance added to these solutions may be calculated from the equation:

$$W = \frac{0.52 - a}{b}$$

where:

$W$ = percentage concentration of adjusting substance in the final solution
$a$ = freezing point depression of the unadjusted hypotonic solution
$b$ = freezing point depression of a 1% w/v concentration of the adjusting substance.

An extensive list of freezing point depression values is detailed in Table 6 in the chapter entitled 'Solution Properties' in the 12th edition of the *Pharmaceutical Codex* (1994).

---

**EXAMPLE 25.1**

A 100 ml volume of a 2% w/v solution of glucose for intravenous injection is to be made isotonic by the addition of sodium chloride.

A 1% w/v solution of glucose depresses the freezing point of water by 0.1°C and a 1% solution of sodium chloride depresses the freezing point of water by 0.576°C.

The depression of freezing point of the unadjusted solution of glucose (*a*) will therefore be:

$$2 \times 0.1 = 0.2$$

A 1% w/v solution of sodium chloride depresses the freezing point of water by 0.576°C (*b*).

Substituting these values for *a* and *b* in the above equation:

$$W = \frac{0.52 - 0.2}{0.576} = \frac{0.32}{0.576} = 0.555$$

The intravenous solution thus requires the addition of 0.555 g of sodium chloride per 100 ml volume to make it isotonic with blood plasma.

---

Other methods which are used to estimate the amount of adjusting substances required to make a solution isotonic include:

- sodium chloride equivalents
- molar concentrations
- serum osmolarity.

Details of these methods are given in the chapter entitled 'Solution Properties' in the 12th edition of the *Pharmaceutical Codex* (1994).

## Units of concentration

The concentration of the components in parenteral products may be expressed in various ways:

- *Percentage weight/volume.* Examples include: Magnesium sulphate injection 50%, sodium chloride intravenous infusion 0.9%.
- *Weight per unit volume.* Examples include: Atropine sulphate 600 µg/ml or ephedrine hydrochloride injection 30 mg/ml.
- *Millimoles per unit volume.* Examples include: Potassium chloride solution, strong (sterile) contains 2 mmol each of $K^+$ and $Cl^-$ per ml; Calcium chloride injection BP contains 2.5 mmol of $Ca^{2+}$ and 10 mmol of $Cl^-$ in 5 ml.

During the formulation of injections and infusions the units of interest are the ions of electrolytes and the molecules of non-electrolytes. For molecules, 1 millimole (mmol) is the weight in milligrams corresponding to its relative molecular mass. A mole of an ion is its relative atomic mass weighed in grams. The number of moles of each of the ions of a salt in solution depends on the number of each ion in the molecule of the salt.

---

**EXAMPLE 25.2**

Sodium chloride has one sodium and one chloride ion. Thus, 1 mole of sodium chloride provides 1 mole of both sodium and chloride ions. The weight of sodium chloride which provides a 1 mmol quantity is 58.5 mg. This weight corresponds to its relative molecular mass and provides 1 mmol of both sodium and chloride ions.

Magnesium chloride has one magnesium and two chloride ions. The weight in milligrams which provides 1 mmol of magnesium and 2 mmol of chloride ions is 203 mg. This weight corresponds to the relative molecular mass of this salt. The quantity of salt in milligrams containing 1 mmol of a particular ion can be determined by dividing the relative molecular mass of the salt by the number of the particular ions which it contains. Weights of common salts which provide 1 mmol are given in Table 4 in the chapter entitled 'Solution Properties' in the 12th edition of the *Pharmaceutical Codex* (1994).

---

## Conversion equations

Useful conversion equations include the following:

$$mg \text{ per litre} = W \times M$$

$$grams \text{ per litre} = (W \times M)/1000$$

$$\% \text{ w/v} = (W \times M)/10\,000$$

where:

$W =$ the number of mg of salt containing 1 mmol of the required ion
$M =$ the number of mmol per litre.

---

**EXAMPLE 25.3**

Calculate the quantities of salts required for the following electrolyte solution:

| | |
|---|---|
| Sodium | 12 mmol |
| Potassium | 4 mmol |
| Magnesium | 6 mmol |
| Calcium | 6 mmol |
| Chloride | 40 mmol |
| Water for injections to 1 litre | |

From Table 4 in the *Pharmaceutical Codex* (1994; see above), 4 mmol of potassium ion is provided by $4 \times 74.5$ mg of potassium chloride, which also yields 4 mmol of chloride ions. 6 mmol of

**Table 25.2    The formula for Example 25.3**

| | | Millimoles of: | | | | |
| --- | --- | --- | --- | --- | --- | --- |
| | | Na⁺ | K⁺ | Mg²⁺ | Ca²⁺ | Cl⁻ |
| Sodium chloride | $12 \times 58.5 = 0.702$ g | 12 | | | | 12 |
| Potassium chloride | $4 \times 74.5 = 0.298$ g | | 4 | | | 4 |
| Magnesium chloride | $6 \times 203 = 1.218$ g | | | 6 | | 12 |
| Calcium chloride | $6 \times 147 = 0.882$ g | | | | 6 | 12 |
| Water for injections to 1 litre | | | | | | |
| Total (millimoles/litre) | | 12 | 4 | 6 | 6 | 40 |

magnesium ions is provided by $6 \times 203$ mg of magnesium chloride, which also yields $2 \times 6 = 12$ mmol of chloride ions as there are two chloride ions in the molecule. 6 mmol of calcium ions is provided by $6 \times 147$ mg of calcium chloride, which also yields 12 mmol of chloride ions as there are two chloride ions in the molecule. 12 mmol of sodium ions is provided by $12 \times 58.5$ mg of sodium chloride which also yields 12 mmol of chloride. The formula can, therefore, be shown as in Table 25.2. It should be noted that the charges on the anions and cations are equally balanced.

## EXAMPLE 25.4

Calculate the number of millimoles of dextrose and sodium ions in 1 litre of sodium chloride and dextrose injection containing 5% anhydrous dextrose and 0.9% w/v of sodium chloride.
　　Use the conversion equation for % w/v calculations.

$$\% \text{ w/v} = (W \times M)/10\,000$$

From this equation:

$$M = \frac{\% \text{ w/v} \times 10\,000}{W}$$

**For dextrose**
As dextrose is a non-electrolyte, $W = 180.2$. Thus:

$$M = \frac{5.0 \times 10\,000}{180.2} = 277 \text{ mmol}$$

The 1 litre of solution contains 277 mmol.

**For sodium chloride**

$$M = \frac{0.09 \times 10\,000}{58.5} = 15.4 \text{ mmol}$$

As 1 mmol of sodium chloride provides 1 mmol of both sodium and chloride ions, 1 litre of the solution will contain 15.4 mmol of both sodium and chloride ions.

## EXAMPLE 25.5

Calculate the number of millimoles of magnesium and chloride ions in 1 litre of a 2% solution of magnesium chloride.

$$M = \frac{0.2 \times 10\,000}{203} = 9.85$$

Each mole of magnesium chloride provides 1 mole of magnesium ions and 2 moles of chloride ions. Thus, 1 litre of the solution contains 9.85 mmol of magnesium ions and 19.7 mmol of chloride ions.

# SPECIAL INJECTIONS

These are more complex formulations than solutions for injection.

## Suspensions

Commonly, suspensions for injection contain less than 5% of drug solids with a mean particle diameter within the range 5–10 μm. Owing to the presence of particles in these formulations, these injections are more difficult to process and sterilize than solutions for injection. During the manufacture of suspensions for injection, the components are prepared and sterilized separately. They are then aseptically combined (see Ch. 23). The final product cannot be filter sterilized owing to the presence of particles in the formulation. Powders for use in sterile suspensions can be sterilized by gas, but gas residues must be avoided (see Ch. 22).

## Dried injections

With these products the dry sterile powder is aseptically added to a sterile vial. Alternatively, a sterile filtered solution can be freeze-dried in a vial. The dry drug powder is reconstituted with a sterile vehicle before use.

## Non-aqueous injections

Drugs which are insoluble in an aqueous vehicle can be formulated in solution using an oil as the vehicle. These formulations are less common than aqueous suspensions. Several oils are used in these formulations including arachis oil and sesame oil, which are easily metabolized. These viscous injections give a depot effect with slow release of the drug and are administered by intramuscular injection.

## LARGE VOLUME PARENTERAL PRODUCTS

These are parenteral products which are packed and administered in large volumes. They are formulated as single dose injections which are administered by intravenous infusion. They are sterile aqueous solutions or emulsions with water for injections as the main component. It is important that they are free of particles. During the administration of these fluids additional drugs are often added to the fluids. This may be carried out by the injection of small volume parenteral products to the administration set of the fluid, or by the 'piggyback' method. In this procedure a second, but smaller volume infusion of an additional drug is added to the intravenous delivery system.

Large volume parenteral products include:

- infusion fluids
- total parenteral nutrition solutions
- intravenous antibiotics
- patient-controlled analgesia
- dialysis fluids
- irrigation solutions.

All of these products have direct contact with blood or are introduced into a body cavity. Large volume parenterals are variously formulated and packaged and have been used to:

- restore fluid and electrolyte imbalance in patients suffering from dehydration, shock or injury
- provide nutrition in circumstances where patients are malnourished, e.g. total parenteral nutrition
- act as a vehicle for administration of medicines
- perform dialysis
- allow irrigation of body parts.

Large volume parenterals must be terminally heat sterilized. While water for injections is the main component of these products they also incorporate other ingredients including:

- carbohydrates, for example dextrose, sucrose and dextran
- amino acids
- lipid emulsions which contain vegetable or semi-synthetic oil
- electrolytes such as sodium chloride
- polyols, including glycerol, sorbitol and mannitol.

Most large volume parenteral fluids are clear aqueous solutions, except for the oil-in-water emulsions. The production of emulsions for infusion is highly specialized as they are destabilized by heat. This results in production difficulties, particularly because the size of the oil droplets must be carefully controlled during the heat sterilization.

## Production of large volume parenteral products

The fluids are produced and filled into containers in a high-standard clean room environment. The high standards are required to limit the contamination of these products with organisms, pyrogens and particulate matter. Use of stringent quality assurance procedures is essential to ensure the quality of the products.

In commercial manufacturing facilities large volumes of fluids are used in the production of a batch of product. The fluids are packaged from a bulk container into the product container in highly mechanized operations using high-speed filling machines. Just before the fluid enters the container, particulate matter is removed from the fluid by passing it through an in-line membrane filter. Immediately after filling, the neck of each glass bottle is sealed with a tight-fitting rubber closure which is kept in place with a crimped aluminium cap. The outer cap is also aluminium and an outer tamper-evident closure is used.

When using plastic bags, the preformed plastic bag is aseptically filled and immediately heat sealed.

As an alternative, a blow–fill–seal system can be used. This integrated system involves melting the plastic, forming the bag, filling and sealing in a high-quality clean room environment. Blow–fill–seal production decreases the problems with product handling, cleaning and particulate contamination. Following filling of the product into containers, the fluids are examined for particulate matter and the integrity of container closures established.

Moist heat should be used to sterilize parenteral products, irrigation solutions and dialysis fluids wherever possible. This should be carried out as soon as possible after the containers have been filled. Plastic containers must be sterilized with an over-pressure during the sterilization cycle to avoid the containers bursting.

## Containers and closures

Large volume parenteral fluids are packaged into:

- glass bottles
- PVC collapsible bags
- semi-rigid polythene containers.

The containers and closures which are used for packaging parenteral products must:

- maintain the sterility of the packed fluids
- withstand sterilization
- be compatible with the packed fluid
- allow withdrawal of the contents.

Glass bottles are normally made of Type II glass (Fig. 25.4), but Type I glass is used for products which have a high pH, despite the increased costs. Glass bottles have advantages for packaging these fluids as they are transparent and chemically inert. They may be used for products which are incompatible with plastic containers. Glass bottles also have some disadvantages. They are much heavier than plastic and therefore less transportable. Although they are strong, they are also brittle, and subject to damage during transport and storage. During use they require the use of an air inlet filter device for pressure equilibration within the container. Particles of glass can be released into the injection fluids. Damage to the neck of the bottles may result in contamination of the container contents from the external environment. A further problem with glass containers may occur during moist heat sterilization. This results in contamination of the fluid due to a pressure imbalance between the internal and external environment. Owing to these difficulties with glass containers, plastic containers have become widely used.

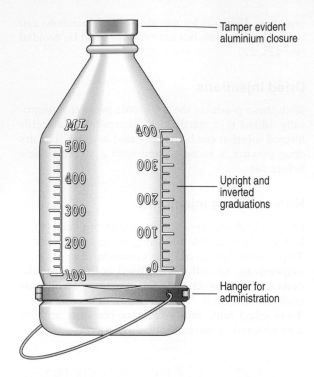

**Fig. 25.4** Glass infusion fluid container.

Labels pointing to the container:
- Tamper evident aluminium closure
- Upright and inverted graduations
- Hanger for administration

PVC collapsible bags are used to package most infusion fluids. They are designed with a port for the attachment of the administration set and an additive port for the addition of small volume parenteral fluids.

PVC collapsible bags are:

- resistant to impact
- flexible and collapse during fluid administration and so do not require an air inlet system.

The disadvantages of plastic bags are that:

- they permit a high moisture penetration
- they adsorb some drugs
- they require an extended sterilization time due to the heat resistance of the PVC
- moist heat sterilization requires air ballasting to avoid pouch explosion.

Semi-rigid plastic containers are used for volumes of 100 ml for electrolyte solutions, 3 litres for total parenteral nutrition solutions and up to 5 litres for dialysis solutions.

Semi-rigid containers:

- are more drug compatible than PVC containers
- are difficult to break
- do not fully collapse

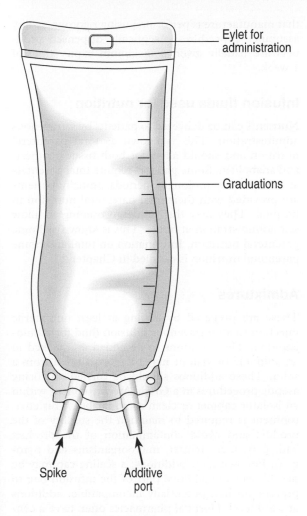

**Fig. 25.5** Semi-rigid infusion bag.

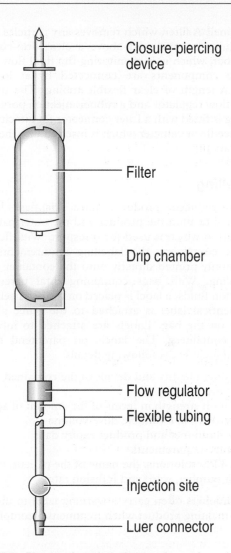

**Fig. 25.6** Diagram of a typical administration set (reproduced by permission from BS 2463: Part 2 1989).

- need extended heat sterilization times
- need air equilibration.

Semi-rigid bags are designed with two ports. One port allows the attachment of the administration set. The other port permits the addition of small volume parenteral products or small volume infusion fluids. These containers are intended for single use. They have a graduated scale which can be read either in an inverted or upright position (Fig. 25.5). To enable containers of large volume parenterals to be suspended from a drip stand for administration, bags are made with an eyelet opening which can be pierced to suspend the bag. Glass bottles are supplied with a plastic band which fits around the container to allow the bottle to be suspended during fluid administration.

## Administration of large volume parenteral fluids

All large volume parenterals are administered to the patient by a parenteral route using a wide variety of administration sets. Most infusion fluids are administered using the standard infusion set specified in British Standard 2463 (Part 2, 1989). These sets are packaged as sterile units intended for single use (Fig. 25.6). Fluid moves through them by gravity, at a rate which is affected by the physical characteristics of the fluid and the fluid pressure, determined by the height of the infusion above the patient. The administration set is made up of a rigid plastic spike which is inserted into the rubber septum of an infusion container. A filter, which removes any particles from the fluid, is positioned above a clear drip-control chamber, which aids monitoring the fluid flow rate. These components are connected by at least a 150 cm length of clear flexible tubing. The tubing has a flow regulator and a rubber injection port. The tubing is fitted with a Luer connector for attachment to a needle or catheter which is inserted into the vein of a patient.

## Labelling

Batch-produced products have identical labels attached to both the product and the outer packaging carton which is used for transport. With flexible plastic containers, the labelling requirements are commonly printed directly onto the container prior to filling. With bags containing total parenteral nutrition fluids, a label is placed on the bag itself and an identical label is attached to the outer plastic cover on the bag. Labels are attached to infusion fluid containers. The labels on parenteral fluids should include the following details:

- product identity and details of the contained volume
- solution strength in terms of the amount of active ingredient in a suitable dose-volume
- batch number and product expiry date
- storage requirements
- for TPN solutions, the name of the patient, the unit number, ward and infusion rate.

Containers often carry a warning label to discard the remaining product when treatment is completed.

## ASEPTIC DISPENSING

Most parenteral fluids are terminally moist heat sterilized. However, some products are aseptically compounded from sterile ingredients in the hospital pharmacy. These products are prepared and dispensed for individual patients. Examples of aseptically prepared products are total parenteral nutrition fluids and the aseptic reconstitution of freeze-dried formulations. These freeze-dried products are often reconstituted using either water for injections or 0.9% sodium chloride injection. Aseptic dispensing is performed in a Grade A clean room environment or Grade A isolator chamber (see Ch. 24). The dispensing of these products relies on good aseptic procedures to ensure the sterility of the product. Owing to the absence of terminal sterilization it is important

that manufacture is performed using rigorous quality assurance procedures. Aseptically dispensed products are usually given a maximum expiry time of 1 week.

## Infusion fluids used for nutrition

Nutrients can be delivered to patients by intravenous administration. This is known as total parenteral nutrition and should allow for both tissue synthesis and anabolism. Some patients require total parenteral nutrition for prolonged periods. Initially patients are provided with their total parenteral nutrition in hospital. They may then undergo training to allow self-administration at home. This is known as home parenteral nutrition. Information on total and home parenteral nutrition is detailed in Chapter 27.

## Admixtures

These are prepared by adding at least one sterile injection to an intravenous infusion fluid for administration. The injections to be added are packed in an ampoule or vial, or may be reconstituted from a solid. These additions should be carried out using aseptic procedures in a Grade A environment within an isolator cabinet or clean room facility. This environment is required to maintain the sterility of the product and avoid contamination of the product with particulate matter, microorganisms and pyrogens. Following the additions, a sealing cap may be placed over the additive port of the infusion bag to prevent further, potentially incompatible, additions at ward level. Hospital pharmacies often have a centralized intravenous additive service (CIVAS) as detailed in Chapter 26. These facilities ensure that additions to infusion fluids are carried out in a suitable environment.

## Novel delivery systems

Special delivery systems are used to facilitate self-medication by patients in a home environment. Some of these delivery systems are described below.

### Infusion devices

There are situations which require strict control of the volume of fluids which are infused into a patient. Accurate flow control with infusion devices is vital for patient safety and for optimum efficacy of the infusion. A range of delivery systems are available which regulate the volume of fluid administered to the patient.

These systems are used both in the hospital and for the self-administration of fluids by patients at home. The selection of an infusion device for the self-administration of medicines by patients requires careful consideration of several factors including:

- delivery volume and control of flow rate
- complexity of the administration procedure
- type of therapy being administered
- frequency of dosing
- reservoir volume available in the infusion device.

Infusion devices available include:

- infusion pumps and controllers
- elastomeric infusers
- electromechanical syringe pumps.

All these devices should be:

- mechanically reliable with accurate flow rates
- able to provide an output pressure which will not damage the injection site
- supported with a back-up power supply if electrically operated
- compact and portable
- simple to operate for hospital staff and home-care patients.

### Infusion pumps

These devices use pressure as the driving force to allow administration of fluids into the patient. Infusion pumps can be divided into those which move fluid by a piston and valve mechanism and those which move the fluid by peristalsis. Infusion pumps are expensive to purchase and operate but allow fluids to be accurately infused into the patient at a slow rate.

### Infusion controller

This is a simple device which can accurately deliver the required fluid volume, although difficulties occur with the administration of viscous solutions. The device relies on gravity moving the infusion fluid down the intravenous administration set. The drop rate in the administration set drop chamber is monitored by a photoelectric mechanism. The device then applies a constriction on the tube of the administration set to give a preselected flow rate.

### Elastomeric infusers

These devices are made of a rigid or flexible outer shell with an inner flexible reservoir (Fig. 25.7). The reservoir inside the device is aseptically filled with the fluid. The elasticity of the filled reservoir exerts a constant pressure. This forces the fluid through an integrated flow restriction device which controls the rate of fluid outflow. The tube from the infuser can be connected to an indwelling cannula in a central vein of the patient. These devices are simple to operate and allow easy home care use.

### Syringe infusers

These devices are used for controlling the delivery of small volumes of intravenous infusions over a predetermined period of time. The syringe driver is widely used as an infusion controller for the administration of intravenous antibiotics and patient-controlled analgesia. They are often powered by mains electricity, or may be battery operated, although clockwork syringe infusers have limited low-risk applications. Syringe infusers move the syringe plunger by a motor-driven screw forcing the fluid into tubing for delivery to the patient. These small lightweight devices allow the administration of precise volumes of fluids. Syringe devices provide good patient home care for patient-controlled analgesia where the drug is often infused over long periods. Patient-controlled analgesia is used by patients to self-regulate the intravenous administration of pain-relieving drugs at controlled intervals. Parenteral administration gives a rapid onset of drug action.

## Irrigation solutions

These solutions are applied topically to bathe open wounds and body cavities. They are sterile solutions for single use only. Examples of irrigation fluids are 0.9% sodium chloride solution or sterile water for irrigation. Most irrigation fluids are now available in rigid plastic bottles. Urologic irrigation solutions are used for surgical procedures; they are usually sterile water or sterile glycine solutions and are used to remove blood and maintain tissue integrity during an operation.

Water for irrigation is sterilized distilled water which is free of pyrogens. The water is packed in containers and is intended for use on one occasion only. The containers are sealed and sterilized by moist heat.

## Peritoneal dialysis fluids

Peritoneal dialysis involves the administration of dialysis solutions directly into the peritoneum by

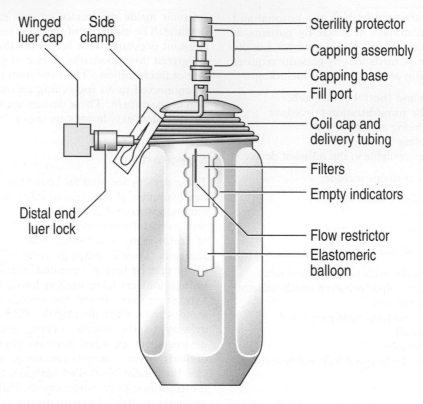

Winged
luer cap

Side
clamp

Sterility protector

Capping assembly

Capping base

Fill port

Coil cap and
delivery tubing

Filters

Empty indicators

Flow restrictor

Elastomeric
balloon

Distal end
luer lock

**Fig. 25.7**  Elastomeric infuser (courtesy of Baxter Healthcare Ltd).

way of an indwelling catheter. The fluid is then drained after a 'dwell-time' to remove toxic waste products from the body. Peritoneal dialysis solutions are sterile solutions manufactured to the same standards as parenteral fluids. The composition of peritoneal dialysis fluid simulates potassium-free extracellular fluid. These fluids are packaged in volumes of 3–5 litres in plastic containers which are similar to the bags used for total parenteral nutrition.

## Haemodialysis

In this dialysis procedure, blood is removed and returned to the patient by way of a catheter, or a double needle arrangement, using a fistula where an artery and vein are joined together. The dialysis procedure involves the use of an artificial disposable membrane within a 'dialyser' machine which acts as an artificial kidney. An electrolyte fluid, simulating body fluid, bathes one side of the membrane with blood from the patient on the other side. There is no direct contact between the blood and the dialyser fluid. Thus fluids for haemodialy-

sis do not require to be sterile or free of pyrogens or particulate matter.

Fluid volumes of 30–50 litres are used daily in haemodialysis procedures. Information on home dialysis is available in Chapter 27.

## Blood products

These products are not usually identified as sterile products although they are commonly packaged as sterile large volume parenteral fluids. These biological products include albumin, human plasma and blood protein fractions. All these products must be treated to inactivate virus contamination prior to packaging. This is usually achieved by specialized heat treatment or filtration. These products are unstable to heat sterilization. Therefore, they are filter sterilized and then aseptically filled into containers in large-scale production facilities. Most of these products are packed as liquids, although a few blood protein fractions such as factor VIII and factor IX are freeze dried. The collection, management and distribution of these products is carried out by the blood transfusion service.

## Key Points

- Convention uses the term 'parenteral' for dosage forms which are placed directly into the body.
- The three main routes are subcutaneous, intramuscular and intravenous, but many others are used in particular situations.
- Parenteral products are sterile forms used for injections, infusion or implantation.
- Glass ampoules are convenient for small volumes, but glass particles can fall into the injection during opening.
- Multiple dose injections must have an antimicrobial preservative.
- Water for injections must be used as the aqueous ingredient in all injections.
- Water for irrigations is used in large volumes to irrigate body cavities and other areas.
- Pyrogens cause fever and must be eliminated from water for injections and water for irrigations.
- Endotoxins, from Gram-negative bacteria, are a major type of pyrogen.
- Bacterial endotoxin is detected using the LAL tests, whilst pyrogens in general are detected by the rabbit pyrogen test.
- Additives to injections include antimicrobial preservatives, antioxidants, buffers, tonicity adjusters and co-solvents.
- Injection solutions for subcutaneous, intradermal, intramuscular, intrathecal and large volume intravenous use should be made isotonic.
- Tonicity calculations are normally based on freezing point depression, but sodium chloride equivalents, molar concentrations and serum osmolarity can be used.
- There is a wide range of large volume parenteral products, including infusion fluids, total parenteral nutrition, dialysis fluids and irrigation solutions.
- All large volume parenteral products must be sterilized after filling into their final containers.
- Large volume parenteral products may be packaged in glass bottles, semi-rigid or collapsible plastic containers.
- When aseptic dispensing is required, rigorous quality assurance is essential and a 1-week expiry date is given to the product.
- A range of infusion devices are available for hospital use and to assist patients' self-administration of infusions at home.
- Sterile solutions have other uses, such as in peritoneal dialysis.

## FURTHER READING

Akers M J 1994 Parenteral quality control: sterility, pyrogens, particulate and package integrity testing. Marcel Dekker, New York

Avis K E, Levchuk J W 1995 Parenteral preparations. In: Gennaro A R (ed) Remington: the science and practice of pharmacy. Mack Publishing Company, Easton, Pennsylvania, USA, Vol II

British Standard 2463 1989 Part 2. British Standards Institution, London

Deeks T 1994 Parenterals. In: The pharmaceutical codex: Principles and practice of pharmaceutics, 12th edn. The Pharmaceutical Press, London

DeLuca P P, Boylan J C 1993 Formulation of small volume parenterals. In: Avis K E, Lieberman H A, Lachman L (eds) Pharmaceutical dosage forms: parenteral medications volume 1, 2nd edn. Marcel Dekker, New York

Demorest L J, Hamilton J G 1993 Formulation of large volume parenterals. In: Avis K E, Lieberman H A, Lachman L (eds) Pharmaceutical dosage forms: parenteral medications volume 1, 2nd edn. Marcel Dekker, New York

Donroe A 1990 Current practices in endotoxin and pyrogen testing in biotechnology. Journal of Parenteral Science and Technology 44 (1): 39–45

European Pharmacopoeia 1996 3rd edn. Bacterial endotoxins. Maisonneuve S.A., Sainte Ruffine, France

Kendall-Smith S C, Marshall I A 1994 Infusion fluids: admixtures and administration. In: The pharmaceutical codex: Principles and practice of pharmaceutics, 12th edn. The Pharmaceutical Press, London

Levchuk J W 1993 Parenteral products in hospital and home care pharmacy practice. In: Avis K E, Lieberman H A, Lachman L (eds) Pharmaceutical dosage forms: parenteral medications, Vol. 1, 2nd edn. Marcel Dekker, New York

Nakata T 1994 Destruction of challenged endotoxin in a dry heat oven. Journal of Pharmaceutical Science and Technology 48 (2): 59–63

Parenteral Society 1996 Tutorial No. 16. Water for injection. The Parenteral Society, Swindon

Pearson F C 1985 Pyrogens: endotoxins, LAL testing and depyrogenation. Marcel Dekker, New York

Turco S 1994 Sterile dosage forms: their preparation and clinical application. Lea & Febiger, Philadelphia, USA

# 26

# Specialized services from a hospital pharmacy

*S. L. Hutchinson and D. Graham*

---

After studying this chapter you will know about:

**The nature and formulation of cytotoxic agents**
**Centralized cytotoxic reconstitution services and the procedures and practices used in them**
**Precautions to be taken when preparing and administering cytotoxic agents**
**Domiciliary chemotherapy programmes**
**Scope, operation and benefits of a centralized intravenous additive service**
**The principles of radiopharmacy**
**Types of radionuclide and their use**
**Production of radiopharmaceuticals**
**The production of $^{99m}$Tc**
**Radiation protection.**

## Introduction

Hospital pharmacies now provide a range of specialized services in the field of parenteral medicines. These will include cytotoxic medicines, i.v. additives and radiopharmaceuticals. Dosage forms requested by medical staff for individual patient requirements are prepared under aseptic conditions in the hospital pharmacy. This chapter outlines the range of services provided in each of these areas and describes the role of the hospital pharmacist in this work.

## PROVISION OF CYTOTOXIC CHEMOTHERAPY

Medicines used in the treatment of malignant disease are cytotoxic in nature. Cytotoxic literally means any substance that is toxic to cells. This cytotoxic effect is not limited to abnormal cells and can

cause harm to healthy cells also. Cytotoxic medicines act by interfering with normal cell division, preventing DNA and RNA replication. The mechanisms of action involved and the relative toxicities of cytotoxic medicines differ from one agent to another. Health care workers involved in handling and administration of cytotoxics must have an understanding of cytotoxic agents and the rationale behind their use in treatment of cancer.

Cytotoxic agents used routinely in treatment of cancer can be divided into five main groups. Classification is based on mechanisms of action. The groups are as follows:

1. *Alkylating agents.* These agents act by forming covalent bonds with molecules such as proteins, amino acids and nucleic acids. They can damage cell membranes, deplete amino acid stores and inactivate enzymes. They stop cell division by forming cross-linkages between DNA chains, thus preventing DNA replication. Examples of alkylating agents are: mustine hydrochloride, cyclophosphamide, ifosfamide, melphalan, chlorambucil, thiopeta, hexamethylmelamine and busulphan.

2. *Antimetabolites.* To allow normal cell division, large reserves of protein and nucleic acids must be built up. For this process to take place, certain essential metabolites must be present. These metabolites form the building blocks for the production of larger molecules. The antimetabolite drugs used in chemotherapy have a similar structure to some of these essential metabolites and can take their place in the nuclear material of the cells inhibiting biological activity. This breakdown in synthesis of essential metabolites and cell components means that cell division will not take place. Drugs in this group include methotrexate, 5-fluorouracil, cytosine arabinoside, 6-mercaptopurine and 6-thioguanine.

3. *Vinca alkaloids.* Their main mode of action is to bind to an intracellular protein, tubulin, which is involved in the process of cell mitosis. These agents

stop cell division at the second phase of mitosis (metaphase) thus preventing cell reproduction. Cytotoxic agents in this group include vincristine, vinblastine and vindesine.

4. *Antimitotic antibiotics.* This is a group of agents used in the treatment of infections, which were in the past found to have an inhibitory effect on dividing tumour cells. Examples of these agents include daunorubicin, doxorubicin and epirubicin.

5. *Miscellaneous agents.* This group of agents does not fit into the other above-mentioned categories very easily. However, they have similar modes of action to some agents, for example cisplatin and carboplatin have similar actions to alkylating agents but vary in cross-linking mechanism of the DNA strands. Other examples in this group include procarbazine, dacarbazine and etoposide.

Cytotoxic agents can be used individually or in combination. Many oncology centres use a combination of medicines, usually denoted by the initial letters of each medicine used in the regimen for example MOPP which stands for mustine, oncovin (approved name vincristine), procarbazine and prednisone. This combined therapy is used for treatment of Hodgkin's disease. Using more than one cytotoxic agent can be more toxic but may produce an enhanced response and an increased chance of survival for the patient.

## DOSAGE FORMS USED FOR CYTOTOXIC MEDICINES

Cytotoxic medicines are available in a range of oral dosage forms including tablets, capsules and paediatric suspensions. Parenteral cytotoxics are available as freeze-dried powders or sterile solutions, both available in sealed vials. The freeze-dried powders are supplied ready for reconstitution with an appropriate diluent. Examples of cytotoxic products include:

● Cyclophosphamide (produced by ASTA Medica Ltd and Farmitalia) is available as a sterile white powder in a vial. It is available in a range of strengths and contains sodium chloride to ensure isotonicity after reconstitution with water for injection.
● Methotrexate (produced by Lederle Laboratories Ltd and David Bull Laboratories Ltd) is available as a clear yellow aqueous isotonic solution for injection or in vials of yellow lyophilized powder of methotrexate sodium ready for reconstitution with water for injection.

● Cisplatin (produced by Farmitalia) is a yellowish white freeze-dried powder which is reconstituted with water for injection and saline solution.

Parenteral cytotoxics can be administered via the following routes:

● by a syringe
● by slow bolus injection into a cannula or the side arm of an infusion
● by addition of a cytotoxic agent directly into an infusion fluid which is then administered over a predetermined infusion period.

Syringe drivers containing cytotoxic medicines are available for use in the community for patients receiving home chemotherapy. This chapter will deal with provision of parenteral cytotoxic medicines for hospital and home patients.

## RISKS INVOLVED FOR HEALTH CARE WORKERS

Over the years there has been concern regarding the handling of cytotoxic agents by health care workers who are involved in the preparation and administration of these medicines. Studies carried out in the past have shown two main areas where health care workers are at greatest risk:

● local effects caused by contact of cytotoxic agents with skin, eyes and mucous membranes
● systemic effects caused by inhalation or ingestion of cytotoxic agents during preparation.

Health care workers handling cytotoxics have in the past experienced symptoms such as dizziness, headaches, light-headedness and nausea. These effects appear to have been caused by inhalation or ingestion of cytotoxic agents during their preparation. However, on these occasions it was noted that procedures were often carried out under unsuitable conditions such as in small poorly ventilated rooms. As yet the long-term effects of cytotoxic inhalation are not fully understood. Systemic effects appear to pose the greatest risk as cytotoxic agents are said to be mutagenic, teratogenic or carcinogenic.

Today, cytotoxic agents are prepared under strict aseptic conditions, in designated areas within a hospital pharmacy, following guidelines published by the Royal Pharmaceutical Society of Great Britain (RPSGB) in 1983. These precautions ensure that the health and safety of all personnel handling cytotoxics are carefully considered. Pharmacy staff preparing cytotoxic agents must be fully trained in the necessary aseptic techniques and must be fully aware of the precautions that are required when handling cytotoxics. Nursing and medical staff must also be taught strict handling and administration techniques to ensure that they do not expose themselves or their patients to any unnecessary risks. All personnel involved in preparing and handling cytotoxic agents should be given an annual health check by the occupational health department in the hospital to ensure their health is not being compromised by working with these agents.

Published guidelines cover the following areas:

- personnel handling cytotoxics and preparation areas used
- techniques and precautions
- dealing with spillage
- disposal of cytotoxics
- labelling, packaging and distribution
- administration of cytotoxics.

Each of these areas will be discussed in more detail.

## PROVISION OF A CYTOTOXIC RECONSTITUTION SERVICE

The guidelines, published in 1983, were intended to give advice to all health care workers handling cytotoxic agents as reconstitution was at that time being carried out by medical staff at a ward level and not in the pharmacy department. The guidelines also advised that the safest option would be to have a centralized cytotoxic reconstitution service.

In the latter half of 1987 into 1988 a group of pharmacists and technicians with a specific interest in this field met together to discuss the idea of setting up a pharmacy-based cytotoxic reconstitution service. This group was known as the Cytotoxic Services Working Group and they made it their aim to produce a manual on how to set up and run a pharmacy-based cytotoxic service. The manual aimed to give information regarding the following areas:

- facilities and equipment required for cytotoxic reconstitution
- training required for staff handling cytotoxics
- documentation required for procedures
- health and safety requirements.

A section giving detailed information on individual cytotoxic agents was also to be included.

By 1990, this original manual became *The Cytotoxics Handbook* and has since been updated and republished (Allwood & Wright 1993) to act as a practical guide for pharmacy staff involved in the reconstitution of cytotoxic agents. *The Cytotoxics Handbook*, together with the RPSGB guidelines, provide the necessary reference material and practical advice to enable hospital pharmacies to set up a cytotoxic reconstitution service.

## Why is the pharmacy department chosen to provide cytotoxic agents?

Pharmacy departments in most of the larger hospitals have existing aseptic dispensing facilities. These facilities may be utilized to provide adequate compounding facilities for reconstitution of cytotoxics provided strict guidelines on preparation are adhered to. Pharmacy staff are already well trained in aseptic dispensing techniques, recording and checking procedures and ensuring that patients receive the appropriate dose regimens. Pharmacists also have the advantage of having a wide clinical knowledge of cytotoxic agents and a unique knowledge of the stability and formulation requirements of such agents.

Prior to setting up a centralized cytotoxic reconstitution service, several factors must be considered. The existing situation must be carefully examined to determine who currently prepares cytotoxic medicines, where they are prepared and how the procedures are carried out. The information gained can be reviewed and compared with the option of providing a centralized service. The rationale behind this service would be to ensure the health and safety of all health care workers involved in handling cytotoxics and to produce a cost-effective service.

## Training required for staff preparing cytotoxics

All personnel involved in preparation and handling of cytotoxics require training in the appropriate techniques. This should include training for pharmacists, pre-registration graduates and all technical staff working in this field. On a practical level, all staff must be aware of the following:

- Procedures required on receipt of a request for a cytotoxic agent.
- How to fill out a worksheet and assemble the required materials for cytotoxic reconstitution.
- Changing procedures required prior to working in a clean room environment.
- General working of laminar airflow cabinets and isolators.

- Cleaning and disposal procedures prior to and following aseptic procedures.
- Storage and transportation of cytotoxics.
- Background information on commonly used cytotoxics.
- Local policies and procedures adopted by the hospital trust or health authority. These should be available for consultation and should be adhered to at all times. They should include: health and safety regulations; safe handling procedures for individual manipulative techniques; procedures for dealing with spillage and disposal; advice on storage and administration.

## Validation of operator techniques

Prior to commencing work on reconstitution of cytotoxics, an operator's competence in this field must be assessed. This is achieved by validating operator techniques. The operator is asked to carry out broth transfer trials where solutions of sterile broth are transferred from one vial or container to another. The aim of the trial is to carry out aseptic transfer techniques which would routinely be used when preparing sterile cytotoxic products. All work is carried out under strictly controlled aseptic conditions. The vials can then be incubated for an appropriate time (5–7 days) and examined for bacterial growth. This procedure can be used in conjunction with observing the operator at work to determine operator competence in aseptic transfer techniques.

Each operator undergoing training is required to undertake a predetermined number of broth transfer trials. Operators must achieve negative results (no growth after incubation) on each occasion before

they are deemed capable of preparing cytotoxic agents. The number of broth trials undertaken can vary from one hospital to another. It can also be dependent on the level of involvement an operator has in this field. Training procedures should be reviewed on a regular basis and retraining and refresher courses made available to all staff.

Certain handling problems can be encountered when dealing with cytotoxic agents. The formation of an aerosol on removing a needle from a vial containing a cytotoxic agent can be a problem. This is known as 'aerosolization'. Operator technique can be assessed by using an inert dye solution such as methylene blue or amaranth in vials instead of the cytotoxic agent. The presence of the dye will clearly indicate any aerosol formation during the procedure. Using this technique, operator handling techniques can be observed and assessed.

## Documentation required for cytotoxics

On receipt of a prescription for a cytotoxic agent a number of procedures must be undertaken. Figure 26.1 shows the areas of work in which a pharmacist may have involvement.

When the prescription is received, it is checked by the pharmacist to ensure that all patient details are in order, dosage calculations are accurate and the dose and presentation are suitable. Drug monographs and data sheets can be consulted to check all details including, for example, shelf life of the reconstituted product and the diluent required. A range of dosage forms are available including syringes, minibags and infusions. The pharmacist in conjunction with medical staff will decide on the most suitable presenta-

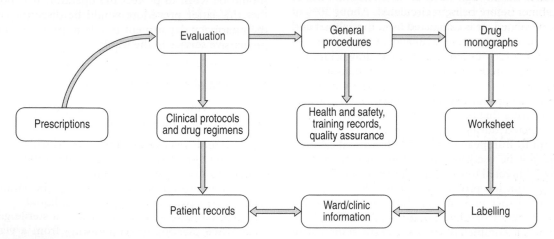

**Fig. 26.1** Documentation required for cytotoxic services. (Reproduced with permission from *Cytotoxics Handbook.*)

tion for the patient. Choice of dosage form will be influenced by the route of administration, the type of cytotoxic agent required and the stability of the final preparation.

Information from the prescription can be transferred to a dispensing worksheet and details of medicine(s) required, diluent, volume for reconstitution and number of vials required are recorded. Details of batch numbers and expiry date for each product used, time and date of preparation and expiry of the final product are also required. Finally a sample label can be attached to the worksheet and the pharmacist will check all details and sign the worksheet. Some cytotoxic agents require protection from light and are sealed in dark-coloured plastic bags to allow protection of the product. In these circumstances labels are required for the outer bag and for the medicine. When the worksheet is complete, the materials required for the reconstitution procedure are collected together and placed in a suitable plastic tray ready for transfer to the designated reconstitution area.

## Personnel handling cytotoxics and preparation areas used

In any hospital setting where large quantities of cytotoxic agents are required on a weekly basis, preparation of cytotoxics takes place in the hospital pharmacy. A designated area is set aside for the preparation of cytotoxics and is used for this purpose only. A vertical laminar downflow safety cabinet sited in a clean room facility can be used for this purpose.

Cabinets can vary in design but the basic principle is that of air being filtered through a HEPA filter and then being passed over the work surface. The air is then directed through vents in the front and back of the cabinet before being recirculated. About 30% of the recirculated air is exhausted from the cabinet and is ducted outside or recirculated in the room. To compensate for this loss, more air is drawn into the cabinet through the front opening. This constant balancing of air creates a negative pressure within the cabinet and produces what is known as an 'air curtain' ensuring that both the operator and the product are protected during working procedures. Cabinets conform to European standards. Horizontal cabinets should not be used for preparation of cytotoxics as airflow is directed towards the operator (see Ch. 24).

Reconstitution procedures can also be carried out using a negative pressure, unidirectional airflow isolator cabinet. Isolators operate on the principle of supplying a completely enclosed work station with filtered air. Materials required for reconstitution procedures are introduced to the isolator via an access port or an airlock. Isolators vary in design and operation but all models are convenient for operator access and still provide a physical barrier to direct contact with cytotoxic agents.

Two main types of isolators exist (see Ch. 24):

• *Rigid isolators*. The cabinet walls are made of a rigid plastic material and operator access is gained via single or double glove ports on the front panel of the cabinet.
• *Flexible film isolators*. These are made of a flexible PVC film on a stainless steel frame. Operator access is achieved by glove ports or personnel wearing a half-suit arrangement and working inside the completely enclosed work station.

The use of isolators for cytotoxic procedures is on the increase as capital and running costs for isolators are less costly than setting up clean room facilities.

## Techniques and precautions

When handling cytotoxics, it is vital that the appropriate protective clothing is worn. Operators using clean room facilities must wear appropriate clean room clothing, with the addition of armlets for extra protection as commercially available suits are known to be permeable to certain cytotoxic agents. When using an isolator cabinet, a full clean room suit is not essential, but appropriate clean room clothing is required. Selection of clothing will be dependent on the background environment in which the isolator is sited. If reconstitution takes place outwith this environment, for example by medical staff at a ward level, goggles, mask, apron, armlets and latex gloves should be worn to protect the operator. It is hoped that this latter procedure would be discouraged as the pharmacy department is able to provide a comprehensive service to the wards.

### Reconstitution procedures

When carrying out reconstitution procedures, certain precautions must be taken:

• Ampoule necks should be covered with a sterile swab before breaking them open and should be broken facing away from the operator.
• Rubber stoppers on vials should be swabbed with a sterile swab prior to removal of liquid.
• Needles should be covered with a sterile gauze swab when piercing or withdrawing from a vial or when air is being expelled.

• Luer lock syringes with wide-bore needles should be used for all procedures to allow more efficient removal of liquid and to prevent the build-up of pressure in the vial.

• Quills can be used to remove liquid from ampoules as they allow faster flow rates than a needle.

• To ensure that no further additions are made to cytotoxic agents outwith the pharmacy preparation area, all completed products in syringe form should be sealed with a blind hub or deadender before removal from the cytotoxic cabinet (see Fig. 26.2). An additive plug must be placed on each minibag once additions are complete.

The vials used to contain cytotoxic agents are effectively a closed system. They are sealed vials which contain either a powder which requires reconstitution with a solvent or a liquid which requires withdrawal from the vial into a syringe. In each case, equalization of pressure within the vial is required to allow withdrawal from it. Reconstitution devices are available to help with the reconstitution process. Some devices consist of a small plastic spike attached to a filter. These devices are useful when repeated volumes of diluent must be measured. However, they are capable of making large holes in the rubber bung of cytotoxic medicine vials thus increasing the risk of leakage of solution from the vial. Another example of a reconstitution devices is a 0.2 micron hydrophobic filter venting needle. The Cytosafe needle (produced by Baxa) is a commonly used example of this type of product. This device consists of a needle which is vented to allow equilibrium of pressure between the vial and the syringe. It is useful for reconstituion of large vials or when more than one vial is required for a dose (see Fig. 26.3). However, care must be taken when withdrawing or adding liquid to a vial as the filter may become blocked.

In the past venting needles (with no filter attached) were used but are no longer recommended due to the risk of leakage of the cytotoxic drug from the vial during reconstitution procedures.

An alternative to using a reconstitution device is to use a 'negative pressure' procedure. This method uses no reconstitution devices and relies solely on the expertise of the operator to ensure proper equalization of pressure within the vial to avoid aerosol formation on withdrawal of the needle. In this procedure the required volume of air for a liquid preparation or solvent for a powder is drawn into the syringe. A small amount of air/solvent is added to the vial and an equal volume of liquid/air is drawn into the syringe. This process is repeated slowly until all the liquid is withdrawn or solvent added. The use of

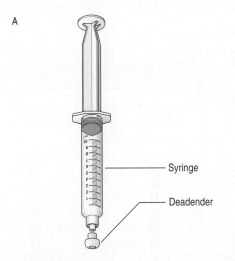

A

Syringe

Deadender

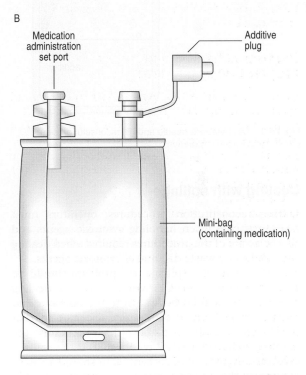

B

Medication administration set port

Additive plug

Mini-bag (containing medication)

**Fig. 26.2** (**A**) Syringe with deadender or blind hub in position. (**B**) Minibag with additive plug.

this method avoids build up of pressure in the vial which may result in leakage through the rubber bung. This process is useful for small vials where there is very little room for large filter needles.

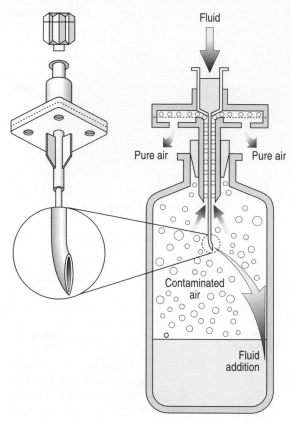

**Fig. 26.3**   (**A**) CytoSafe needle and (**B**) reconstitution set-up (courtesy of Baxa Corporation).

## Dealing with spillage

During reconstitution procedures, operators must take great care when handling cytotoxic agents and also be aware of the procedures required when dealing with spillage or waste disposal of cytotoxic agents.

In the event of a spillage, the problem should be dealt with immediately. A written policy on dealing with spillages should be known to the operator and must be implemented should one occur. A spill kit should be readily available which contains the required materials to deal with a spill. If the spillage involves a liquid, an absorbent cloth should be used to wipe up the spill and the waste materials placed in a cytotoxic hazardous waste bag. Spillage involving a powder should be wiped up using a damp cloth to ensure that inhalation of powder particles does not occur. All surface areas contaminated by the spillage should be washed with copious amounts of water (sterile water is available in the spill kit). In some instances, manufacturers recommend the use of certain chemicals to deal with cytotoxic spillage as a sec-

ondary measure. Manufacturers' literature should be available within the pharmacy and used to obtain appropriate advice in the event of a spillage.

If the spillage has come in contact with the skin, the contaminated area should be washed thoroughly with soap and water. Contact with eyes should be dealt with by irrigation with a sodium chloride eyewash, the incident reported and medical help sought. In the event of a needle-stick injury involving direct contact with a cytotoxic agent, the area should again be thoroughly washed and the operator should receive medical attention. All accidents involving spillage should be reported.

## Disposal of cytotoxics

All cytotoxic waste materials should be placed in a brightly coloured plastic bag, sealed and labelled with a cytotoxic warning label ready for disposal by incineration or degradation by chemical methods.

Sharp objects including needles, syringes, ampoules and vials should be placed in a sharps bin which is made of rigid plastic and does not allow leakage of cytotoxic waste. When the sharps bin is full, it should be sealed with hazardous waste tape and disposed of safely with other cytotoxic waste.

Nursing staff have the problem of handling excreta of patients who have received cytotoxic medicines. The potential risks involved will vary depending on the medicine used, dosage given, route of administration and the type of elimination profile. Reports suggest that excreta should be assumed potentially hazardous for at least 48 hours after cytotoxic administration is complete. Ward staff should be made fully aware of the patients who pose this risk and should always take the necessary handling precautions. For patients on home chemotherapy, family members should be warned about the potential hazards and advised to exercise extreme caution when handling excreta from the patient.

## Labelling, packaging and distribution

Following reconstitution of a cytotoxic agent, the medicine can then be labelled ready for distribution to the ward. Labels must be appropriately designed to show immediately that the container holds a cytotoxic agent.

Labels should include the following details:

- patient's name and ward number
- drug name, quantity and final volume
- vehicle in which the drug is contained (e.g. water for injection)

- batch number, expiry date and storage conditions required
- hospital pharmacy name and address.

Within each hospital, there should be recommended policies for safe transportation of cytotoxics and local procedures implemented for issue and receipt of medicines.

## ADMINISTRATION OF CYTOTOXIC MEDICINES

Medical staff at a ward level are responsible for administering cytotoxic medicines to patients. The pharmacy department can supply the ward with the medicines in a form suitable for convenient administration to the patient. Medical staff will have access to local hospital policies regarding the safe handling and administration of cytotoxics and are required to adhere to these policies at all times. They are held responsible for ensuring the safety of the patient as well as themselves while administering cytotoxic medicines. As a result of this responsibility, staff chosen to carry out these procedures are usually highly trained personnel who have a wide range of experience in this field and have a good working knowledge of cytotoxic agents. They are able to discuss in detail with patients the procedures being carried out, thereby reassuring them about the medical treatment that they are receiving.

On a practical level, medical staff must be capable of setting up infusion sets and syringes to avoid leakage of contents and be proficient in injection techniques to ensure that the patient does not suffer from leakage of cytotoxic medicines outwith the vein. This latter is known as 'extravasation'. In the event of extravasation occurring, medical staff are trained to stop administration immediately, aspirate and carry out locally agreed policies and procedures which involve, for example, the administration of steroids intravenously or subcutaneously and then topically if required. This procedure is used to prevent irreversible tissue damage. Extravasation kits should be available on hand in the ward to deal with this problem.

## PROVISION OF CHEMOTHERAPY AT HOME

Many patients express a desire to have their chemo-

therapy provided at home. This is now possible with the setting up of domiciliary chemotherapy programmes. Patients have more involvement in the administration of their medicines, are able to spend more time with their families and do not require to attend hospital for regular treatment. If their treatment can be managed at home, hospital beds are available to treat other patients, but this can create an increased workload for the pharmacy department.

The implications for a pharmacy department setting up a home chemotherapy service are wide ranging. Many home chemotherapy doses are supplied for a week at a time. There may be a need to employ more staff and to train new and existing staff in the techniques required for filling the ambulatory infusion devices required for home chemotherapy.

In addition, the stability of the formulations must be considered. Stability data on cytotoxic medicines used routinely in chemotherapy are documented in the ABPI data sheet compendium and *The Cytotoxics Handbook* (Allwood, Stanley & Wright 1997). However, fully documented stability data must be obtained for cytotoxic agents administered in home infusion devices before the pharmacy department can take on the responsibility of providing a service to home patients. The pharmacist responsible for the centralized cytotoxics service must have a good working knowledge of appropriate chemotherapy regimens and infusion devices available for home chemotherapy. In certain oncology centres, the pharmacist may also be asked to become involved in training patients in appropriate handling and administration techniques to ensure the health and safety of patients and their carers in the home care environment.

## CENTRALIZED INTRAVENOUS ADDITIVE SERVICE (CIVAS)

Recommendations were made by Breckenridge as early as 1976 that hospital pharmacies should be involved in the provision of i.v. products. However, despite the fact that the preparation of i.v. cytotoxic medicines was taken up, provision of an i.v. additive service did not take place until the late 1980s and then only in a limited number of hospitals.

The setting up of the national CIVAS group in 1991 gave more hospital pharmacists the initiative and support for the provision of a CIVA service. By 1993 a CIVAS manual was produced to provide guidelines for hospital pharmacists setting up a

CIVA service. Today a large proportion of hospital pharmacies in the UK provide a CIVA service.

## Scope of a CIVA service

A CIVA service is set up to provide a range of parenteral dosage forms suitable for administration to patients. The range of dosage forms supplied will be decided by medical, nursing and pharmacy staff involved in patient care in this field. A CIVA service can provide the following:

- i.v. antibiotics
- patient-controlled analgesia
- ambulatory infusion devices for i.v. antibiotic therapy at home.

Often a CIVA service is run in conjunction with services which already exist in the pharmacy (e.g. cytotoxic reconstitution and compounding of parenteral nutrition solutions).

## Setting up a CIVA service

The same principles adopted when setting up a centralized cytotoxic reconstitution service apply when setting up a CIVA service. A working party can be established consisting of representatives from pharmacy, medical and nursing staff and hospital administrators. The current situation can be assessed to determine the amount of i.v. doses currently being used, who prepares them and the conditions under which they are prepared. Information can be provided regarding the benefits of a centralized service and any potential problems identified. Often the pharmacy department will initially carry out a pilot study where a limited number of CIVA doses will be supplied to a particular ward or discipline (e.g. two strengths of an antibiotic supplied when required to surgical wards only). After a predetermined time period, the situation could be evaluated and a decision then made either to implement a CIVA service or to continue with ward staff preparing i.v. doses. If the decision is made to set up a CIVA service, then the pharmacist in charge of this service has a number of factors to consider.

## Role of the pharmacist in the provision of a CIVA service

A study carried out by Needle (1995) suggested that pharmacy managers were the main decision makers in terms of initiating a CIVA service. The pharmacist responsible for setting up the service must assess the current situation, including workload, methods for prescribing, preparation and administration. The pharmacist must look realistically at the potential benefits and problems of providing a CIVA service and the implications this will have for the pharmacy, particularly in relation to cost and staff workload. The ultimate aim of any service provided from a hospital pharmacy should be to improve the quality of health care given to the patient. The potential benefits of providing a CIVA service can include the following:

- improved use of hospital resources
- improved services to the patients
- improved pharmacy control.

Each of these areas will now be discussed.

### Improved use of hospital resources

Pharmacy staff are trained in aseptic procedures and can use their skills to provide a comprehensive range of i.v. products suitable for administration to the patients by medical and nursing staff. This utilizes pharmacy skills to the maximum and at the same time, saves on medical and nursing staff time. Often i.v. doses have to be made up on the ward by nursing staff or junior doctors who have very little experience in this field and have a limited knowledge of calculating appropriate doses, using the required diluent or preparing i.v. medicines. Ward facilities for preparing i.v. medicines are not ideal and increase the risk of the product being contaminated as it is not prepared under aseptic conditions. Using existing aseptic dispensing facilities in the hospital pharmacy ensures that i.v. products are prepared under the highest possible standards. Better control of ward stocks of i.v. medicines can be achieved if the pharmacy provides a CIVA service. Each ward can order i.v. medicines on a daily basis from the pharmacy depending on patient requirements. This reduces the possibility of medicines being kept on the ward and not used before their expiry date.

### Improved services to the patients

When a CIVA service is utilized by the wards, the pharmacy department prepares the doses, sends them to the ward and patients then receive their medication on time. All CIVA doses are clearly labelled with appropriate dosage instructions, ensuring that patients receive the correct medication and that it is administered appropriately. This facility allows medical and nursing staff to spend more time with the patients.

## Improved pharmacy control

If a CIVA service is set up within a hospital, the pharmacy department can be involved from the very beginning. This allows the pharmacist to have a much greater clinical input to the provision of patient care. The pharmacist can be involved in prescription monitoring and checking, recommending appropriate dosage forms and giving advice on stability of preparations.

All procedures used during preparation of CIVA doses will be fully validated and documented. Staff preparing i.v. products will adhere to standard operating procedures (SOPs) and published guidelines. Records will be kept for all i.v. medicines prepared and batch numbers of products used during reconstitution procedures. This ensures that in the event of a product recall or any problems with an i.v. medicine, pharmacy will hold records of all the necessary documentation. Under pharmacy control, a CIVA service can allow standardization of drug concentrations and improved formulary compliance.

## Potential problems of a CIVA service

1. Increased expenditure in the pharmacy including capital expenditure for setting up the service and in provision of staff to prepare the required doses.

2. Pharmacy must ensure that they have adequate storage space for CIVA doses that require refrigeration before being transported to wards. Transportation will require to be organized in such a way as to ensure that CIVA doses are not kept out of the refrigerator for prolonged periods of time.

3. If pharmacy provides a CIVA service, will they be able to provide an out-of-hours service? If they are unable to do so, will i.v. medicines have to be made up in advance for weekends? Can these medicines be given a sufficiently long shelf life? Would pharmacists working at weekends know how to make up i.v. medicines if this is not their normal area for working?

4. Certain wards may be difficult to service, for example Accident and Emergency and Intensive Care, as they may require unusual doses which are not normally provided under the CIVA service. These doses may be required urgently, particularly in an emergency situation. This will put extra pressure on the pharmacy staff and on the facilities, depending on the workload at the time of the request.

5. A further complication is the requirement for individualized doses, for example in paediatrics. A clinical pharmacist who has specialized knowledge of paediatrics may be able to give advice to staff providing the CIVA service to ensure appropriate dosage regimens are prepared.

6. Retrieval and reuse of doses not required by an individual ward can be a problem. Occasionally wards order i.v. drugs and subsequently dosage regimens are changed at a later stage. There has to be a procedure set in place for retrieval of such doses from the ward to prevent drug wastage.

7. Communication requirements must be considered. Good liaison between the clinical pharmacist responsible for the wards supplied and medical staff working in the wards is essential to ensure that orders for CIVA doses are requested on time. Orders for home i.v. doses may require liaison between health care workers in the community and the hospital sector to ensure that home patients receive adequate supplies of medicines.

## Practical considerations when setting up a CIVA service

### Preparation areas

Intravenous products can be prepared under aseptic dispensing conditions either in a designated area using an isolator cabinet or using clean room facilities. Some hospital pharmacies support the use of vertical LAF safety cabinets similar to those used for preparation of cytotoxic medicines. This is to ensure operator safety when handling certain antibiotics and to prevent cross-contamination of i.v. products. Staff working in a clean room environment must wear clean room clothing and carry out all procedures in accordance with SOPS. All materials required for the reconstitution procedures are collected together in the preparation area and transferred to the clean room environment. Procedures used are similar to those adopted for compounding of parenteral nutrition solutions (see Ch. 27).

### CIVA dosage forms

Most hospital pharmacies supply i.v. additives in the form of a preloaded syringe or a minibag. The minibags are small volume infusion bags available in volumes of 50 ml and 100 ml. CIVA doses supplied in minibags are often preferred by medical staff as they are easier to administer than syringes. Reconstitution procedures are often required as i.v. doses can be supplied as sterile freeze-dried powders in sealed vials. These vials are then reconstituted with the appropriate diluent and drawn into a syringe or

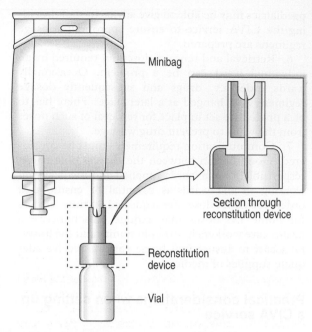

Minibag

Section through
reconstitution device

Reconstitution
device

Vial

**Fig. 26.4** Reconstitution device used for CIVA doses (courtesy of
Baxter Healthcare Ltd).

minibag ready for administration to the patient. If
minibags are used, a reconstitution device can be
used to transfer the diluent into the vial, then, after
vigorous shaking, back into the bag again.
Throughout this procedure the vial and minibag
remain attached via the reconstitution device which
has a double-ended needle. One end of the needle is
placed through the rubber bung of the vial and the
other end is connected into the rubber septum of the
minibag (see Fig. 26.4).

Prior to removal from the LAF cabinet or the isolator cabinet, all prepared syringes are sealed with a
blind hub or deadender and minibags are sealed with
an additive plug. This ensures that no further additions are made to the syringe or minibag outwith the
pharmacy. All products are labelled and sealed into a
bag before being transported to the ward.

### Stability of CIVA doses

Pharmacy departments which have a manufacturer's
licence can prepare i.v. doses for stock and can, in
some cases, give products a 30-day shelf life
(depending on validated stability data). For non-
licensed units the situation is different. Under the
Section 10 exemption in the Medicines Act 1968,
parenteral products can be prepared for stock in
advance of a prescription being obtained, provided

preparation takes place under the supervision of a
pharmacist. Under these circumstances, i.v. doses can
be prepared using aseptic dispensing facilities in the
pharmacy and can be given a shelf life of up to 7 days.
In practice, the shelf life given to individual i.v. medicines will vary. Reference to stability data and manufacturers' guidelines will give detailed information
for each i.v. dose being prepared. Stability data supporting the shelf life must be available for each product being prepared in the pharmacy.

Stability studies have been carried out over the last
few years to determine if the shelf life of i.v. products
can be extended. Published evidence suggests that
chemical stability of i.v. products can be prolonged if
storage temperature is reduced. Studies show that
shelf life of some products can be extended to
6 months or longer if the i.v. product is frozen at
−20°C. However, not all products are stable in this
condition and stability data specific to each product,
including dosage form, diluent and presentation
must all be considered. Intravenous medicines
stored in minibags and then frozen can be very fragile; hence great care must be observed when handling medicines in this form and in packing them in
freezers. Natural thawing time for these i.v. products
will vary and this can be a problem if time is a limiting factor. The use of microwaves to speed up the
thawing time has been suggested, but further work
in this area is required to validate procedures used.

Storage requirements for i.v. doses must be carefully considered. If medicines require refrigeration, a
designated refrigerator should be set aside in the
pharmacy. CIVA doses should be stored there until
they are transported to the wards, where they
should be refrigerated until required. Refrigerators
used in hospital pharmacies are pharmaceutical
grade refrigerators. They should have a temperature recorder and should be fitted with an alarm to
alert pharmacy staff to any changes in storage conditions. Refrigerators used at a ward level should also
be carefully monitored to ensure that adequate storage conditions are achieved. All refrigerated CIVA
doses should be allowed to reach room temperature
prior to administration to the patient.

### Validation of procedures

As with any procedures carried out under aseptic
conditions, routine environmental monitoring must
be undertaken. This will include the use of settle
plates (at least weekly) and contact plates (at least
monthly). Air sampling will also take place routinely
(monthly) and filter checks should be done at least
on an annual basis or in the event of any problems

arising. Validation of operator technique will include the use of broth transfer trials and observation of operator techniques.

## Provision of i.v. doses for home patients

Provision of a CIVA service from a hospital pharmacy will involve a large commitment in terms of staff to ensure that daily requirements are met and that sufficient doses are prepared in advance for an out-of-hours service. However, if provision of i.v. doses for home patients is considered, more staff may be required to provide this service. Many hospital pharmacies initially set up a CIVA service and are then asked to expand the service to provide services for patients in the community. Some have the facilities and resources to provide i.v. doses for home patients, others do not. However, with the advances in home infusion devices and greater emphasis being put on health care at home, hospital pharmacies are under more pressure to provide this extended service.

Provision of i.v. medicines at home using ambulatory devices has meant that pharmacy staff require further training in the filling of these ambulatory devices. A number of different options are available for patients on home i.v. therapy:

- *Single dose infusions*. These are administered in the form of a preloaded syringe or minibag attached to an infusion system which is set at a predetermined flow rate to administer the medicine to the patient. These devices can be used for self-administration by patients three to four times daily.
- *Electronic syringe infusers*. These are electronic or battery-operated infusion devices used in conjunction with a syringe and tubing to deliver the medicine. The infusers are usually small and lightweight allowing the patients to remain mobile during the infusion period.
- *Elastomeric infusers*. These are disposable plastic units which consist of an inner 'balloon' reservoir surrounded by the outer protective shell. They have a medication entry port and permanently attached tubing. The reservoir can be filled using a one-way Luer lock valve. Filling can take place in the pharmacy and, if required, the line can be primed ready for patient use. Flow rates are controlled by an integrated flow-restricting device. Elastomeric devices can be carried by patients in a carrying case or in a pocket.
- *Slow intravenous push*. A needle and syringe are used to deliver the drug by slow intravenous injection over approximately 7 minutes. This is suitable for self-administration by the patient and requires no costly infusion devices.

For all of the above-mentioned methods, the hospital pharmacy can provide the syringes, minibags and elastomeric devices as prefilled products ready for transportation to patients. If large quantities of syringes are required regularly, the hospital pharmacy may use a compounding pump to prepare the quantities required. If hospital pharmacies cannot provide i.v. doses for home patients, commercial pharmaceutical companies can fulfil this role (see Ch. 27).

## RADIOPHARMACY

Radioactivity may be defined as the spontaneous transformation of an unstable nucleus to a more stable nucleus. This transformation involves the release of ionizing radiation which may be in particulate form (e.g. $\alpha$ particles or $\beta$ particles) or may be in the form of electromagnetic radiation (e.g. $\gamma$-rays).

Elements that emit radiation are known as radionuclides and have a number of applications in medicine. Radiopharmacy is concerned with the manufacture of radioactive medicines known as radiopharmaceuticals. These have two main applications in medicine:

- in the treatment of disease (therapeutic radiopharmaceuticals)
- as an aid to the diagnosis of disease (diagnostic radiopharmaceuticals).

Diagnostic radiopharmaceuticals may be classified into two types:

- radiopharmaceuticals used in tracer techniques for measuring physiological parameters (e.g. $^{51}$Cr-EDTA for measuring glomerular filtration rate)
- radiopharmaceuticals for diagnostic imaging (e.g. $^{99m}$Tc-methylene diphosphonate (MDP) used in bone scanning).

In diagnostic imaging, $\gamma$-emitting radionuclides are used since their interaction with tissue is much less than that of particulate emitters and will cause significantly less damage to tissue. Radiopharmaceuticals are administered to the patient, usually by the i.v. route, and distribute into a particular organ. The radiation is then detected externally using a special scintillation detector, known as a $\gamma$-camera. These are used by nuclear medicine departments to image the distribution of the radiopharmaceutical within the patient's body. Using the γ-camera in conjunction with a computer system it is not only possible to produce static images of an organ, but also to examine how the radiopharmaceutical moves through an organ. These dynamic images describe how the organ is functioning. It is also possible to create images in all three planes, a process known as single photon emission computerized tomography (SPECT).

It is important to note that for the safe production of radiopharmaceuticals, the radiopharmacy must be designed to comply with, and procedures must follow, good manufacturing practice and good radiation protection practice. Radiopharmacists working in this field are part of a multidisciplinary team which includes doctors, physicists and nuclear medicine technicians. As part of this team they not only ensure that the radiopharmaceuticals will give high-quality clinical information, but also that they are safe for both patient and user alike.

## RADIONUCLIDES USED IN NUCLEAR MEDICINE

### Alpha emitters

Alpha-decay is the process whereby a nucleus emits a helium nucleus, or α-particle. This commonly occurs with heavy nuclei (e.g. radium-226: $^{226}_{88}Ra \rightarrow$ $^{222}_{86}Rn + \alpha$).

Because they are heavy and positively charged, α-particles travel only short distances in air (~5 mm) and only micrometer distances in tissues. Their ionizing nature would result in a highly localized radiation dose if taken internally and hence they tend not to be used in radiopharmaceuticals.

Some α-emitters (e.g. $^{226}Ra$) when encapsulated are used as sealed sources, emitting X-rays or γ-rays for radiotherapy applications. Here the body is exposed to radiation externally in an attempt to treat malignant tumours.

### Beta emitters

Beta decay occurs in two ways, one that involves the emission of a negatively charged β⁻-particle, or electron, and the other that involves the emission of a positively charged β⁺-particle, or positron.

#### β⁻-emitters

Radionuclides which decay by β⁻-decay tend to have nuclei that are neutron rich. They attempt to reach a more stable state by the transformation of a neutron into a proton with the emission of a β⁻-particle.

Despite β⁻-particles having a range in air of up to several metres, their range in tissues is only a few millimetres. Because of this and their highly ionizing nature, β⁻-emitters tend to be used in therapeutic radiopharmaceuticals (Table 26.1).

The principle of therapeutic treatment with radionuclides is to target the radionuclide to a specific tissue within the body in an attempt to selectively damage or destroy that tissue. Ideally therapeutic β⁻-emitting radionuclides should have energies of 0.5–1.5 MeV and a half-life of several days to provide a prolonged radiobiological effect.

The most widely used example of this is $^{131}I$-sodium iodide which is used in the treatment of hyperactive thyroid disease and in certain thyroid tumours. Here the physiological property of thyroid tissue is exploited to target the radionuclide to the site of action. Since thyroid tissue avidly takes up iodine in the normal synthesis of the hormone thyroxine, radioactive iodine is also taken up and held in the thyroid tissue. Hence the radiation damage is targeted to the thyroid tissue specifically and the normal excretion of any excess iodine results in no significant damage to other organs and tissues.

#### β⁺-emitters

Radionuclides that emit positrons are becoming more widely used in nuclear medicine. In this transformation, a proton-rich nuclide attempts to achieve stability by converting a proton to a neutron with the emission of a positron. The positron is very short-lived, since it interacts with an electron resulting in an annihilation reaction and the conversion of both particles into electromagnetic (EM) radiation. This EM radiation is in the form of two γ-rays, each having an energy of 0.511 MeV, which are emitted at an angle of 180° to each other.

When used in conjunction with a specialized γ-camera with detectors placed 180° apart, it is possible to create images in all three planes with the position of the radiopharmaceutical being very precisely known. This type of imaging technique is known as positron emission tomography (PET).

Radionuclides used in PET (Table 26.1) are radioisotopes of naturally occurring elements and hence the radiopharmaceuticals in which they are synthesized have a biological biodistribution identical to the naturally occurring compound.

The high cost of producing these radiopharmaceuticals, their very short half-life and the expense of

**Table 26.1  Examples of radionuclides used in nuclear medicine**

| Radionuclide | Radiopharmaceutical | Half-life | Clinical use |
|---|---|---|---|
| β⁻-emitters | | | |
| $^{131}$I | Sodium iodide capsules | 8 days | Thyrotoxicosis, thyroid carcinomas |
| $^{32}$P | Sodium phosphate injection | 14 days | Polycythaemia rubra vera |
| $^{90}$Sr | Strontium chloride injection | 50 days | Palliation of pain from bone metastases |
| β⁺-emitters | | | |
| $^{15}$O | $^{15}$O$_2$ gas | 2 min | Brain blood flow imaging |
| $^{18}$F | Fluorodeoxy-glucose injection | 110 min | Brain glucose metabolism |
| Electron capture | | | |
| $^{111}$In | Indium chloride solution | 67 h | Antibody labelling |
| $^{123}$I | Sodium iodide injection | 13 h | Thyroid imaging |
| $^{201}$Tl | Thallous chloride injection | 73 h | Cardiac perfusion imaging |
| Isomeric transition | | | |
| $^{99m}$Tc | Sodium pertechnetate injection | 6 h | See Table 26.2 |
| $^{81m}$Kr | Krypton gas | 13 s | Lung ventilation imaging |

the PET camera, results in this technique being mainly used in medical research.

## Electron capture

Nuclei that are proton rich may, as an alternative to positron emission, capture electrons from the atom's electron orbitals. This process results in the transformation of a proton to a neutron within the nucleus. The subsequent rearrangement of the electrons orbiting the nucleus results in a characteristic emission of X-rays or γ-rays.

Radionuclides which decay by electron capture are useful in diagnostic imaging since they emit γ-rays; examples are given in Table 26.1.

## Isomeric transition

Some radionuclides exist for measurable periods in excited, or isomeric, states prior to reaching ground state. This form of decay involves the emission of a γ-ray and is known as isomeric transition. When radionuclides exist in this transitional state they are known as metastable, which is denoted by the letter 'm' and written thus: $^{99m}$Tc.

A simplified decay scheme for $^{99m}$Tc-technetium is shown in Figure 26.5, where $^{99m}$Tc's parent radionuclide, molybdenum ($^{99}$Mo), decays by β⁻ emission to the ground state $^{99}$Tc either directly or indirectly. The indirect route, which is the most common, involves the isomer $^{99m}$Tc, which in turn decays from this its metastable state to $^{99}$Tc by isomeric transition.

Radionuclides which decay by this process are used in diagnostic imaging since they emit γ-rays (Table 26.1). It should be noted that $^{99m}$Tc is the most widely used radionuclide in hospital radiopharmacy today, making up the radionuclide component of around 90% of the radiopharmaceuticals produced. For these reasons the production processes for $^{99m}$Tc-radiopharmaceuticals will be especially emphasized.

## Facilities required for the production of radiopharmaceuticals

The majority of radiopharmaceuticals are intended for intravenous (i.v.) administration, therefore, it is of paramount importance that these preparations are sterile. They also contain radionuclides with short half-lives that require their preparation and administration on the same day. Because of the constraints of time, it is not possible to use terminal sterilization by autoclaving and hence these injections must be prepared using aseptic techniques. Here highly skilled operators work with sterile ingredients within clean room facilities containing either laminar flow safety cabinets or isolators. Guidance on the facilities required are given in 'Guidance Notes for Hospitals on the Premises and Environment Required for the Preparation of Radiopharmaceuticals' (DHSS 1982) and are more fully described in Chapter 23.

## Principles of radiopharmaceutical production

The physical and chemical properties of $^{99m}$Tc

267

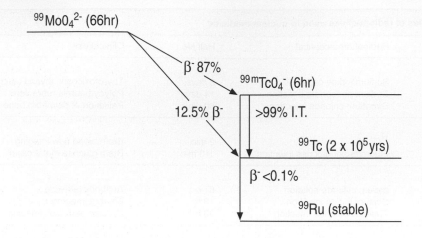

$^{99}MoO_4{}^{2-}$ (66hr)

$\beta^-$ 87%

12.5% $\beta^-$

$^{99m}TcO_4{}^-$ (6hr)

>99% I.T.

$^{99}Tc$ (2 x $10^5$yrs)

$\beta^-$ <0.1%

$^{99}Ru$ (stable)

**Fig. 26.5**  Diagrammatic representation of $^{99}Mo$ decay.

make it nearly ideal for imaging purposes as outlined below.

• It has a 6-hour half-life ($T_{\frac{1}{2}}$); long enough to allow imaging to take place in the working day, whilst also short enough that patients are not radioactive for long periods (in 24 hours, or 4 half-lives, the radioactivity will have decayed by 94%).

• $^{99m}Tc$ emits $\gamma$-rays of 140 keV energy – ideal for use with the modern $\gamma$-camera.

• There are no particulate emissions that, if present, would add to the patient's radiation dose.

• By purchasing a device known as a $^{99}Mo/^{99m}Tc$-generator, $^{99m}Tc$ can be made readily available to the hospital site in a sterile and pyrogen-free form.

• $^{99m}Tc$ has versatile coordination chemistry and will allow a large number of ligands to complex with it. By using different ligands in the radiopharmaceutical's formulation, the radiopharmacist can prepare a wide range of radiopharmaceuticals, providing for the many different investigations carried out in nuclear medicine departments (Table 26.2).

## The production of $^{99m}Tc$ – the molybdenum/technetium generator

Radionuclides with long half-lives (e.g. $^{201}Tl$, $T_{\frac{1}{2}} = 73$ hours) can be easily transported from production site to the user hospital. With shorter half-life radionuclides, for example $^{99m}Tc$, this supply system would be impossible. As a result a device known as the radionuclide generator is used to provide $^{99m}Tc$ to the hospital site.

Radionuclide generators work on the principle that they contain a relatively long-lived 'parent'

radionuclide that decays to produce a 'daughter' radionuclide. The chemical nature of parent and daughter are different, allowing separation of the daughter from the parent.

The molybdenum/technetium generator consists of $^{99}Mo$ absorbed onto an alumina-filled column, the $^{99}Mo$ being present in the form of molybdate ($^{99}MoO_4{}^{2-}$). $^{99}Mo$ decays to its daughter radionuclide $^{99m}Tc$, as pertechnetate, $^{99m}TcO_4{}^-$ (Fig. 26.5). The amount of $^{99m}TcO_4{}^-$ grows as a result of the decay of $^{99}Mo$, until a transient equilibrium is reached. At this point the amount of $^{99m}Tc$ on the column appears to decay with the half-life of $^{99}Mo$ (Fig. 26.6).

By drawing a solution of sodium chloride 0.9% w/v through the column, $^{99m}Tc$ is removed from the column in the form of sodium pertechnetate, $Na^{99m}TcO_4$. This process is known as eluting the generator and the resulting solution as the eluate. The result of this process is a sterile solution of sodium pertechnetate that may now be used to make $^{99m}Tc$-radiopharmaceuticals.

$^{99}Mo$ remains on the column where it decays to produce further $^{99m}Tc$, the equilibrium being re-established about 23 hours after elution. Elution of the generator is repeated daily to provide the radiopharmacy with a supply of $^{99m}Tc$ for 7–14 days, beyond which the yield of $^{99m}Tc$ becomes too small to be useful. Hospital radiopharmacies tend to buy generators on a weekly basis to provide a continuous supply of $^{99m}Tc$.

## Design of a $^{99m}Tc$-generator

The design of a typical generator will be described

**Table 26.2  Examples of $^{99m}$Tc-radiopharmaceuticals**

| Radiopharmaceutical | Organ or tissue of distribution | Main clinical application |
|---|---|---|
| $^{99m}$Tc-sodium pertechnetate | Thyroid | Imaging the thyroid gland and ectopic tissue |
| | Salivary gland | Dynamic images of accumulation and drainage to show gland function |
| | Gastric mucosa | Presence of Meckel's diverticulum containing gastric mucosa |
| $^{99m}$Tc-methylene diphosphonate (MDP) | Skeleton | Bone metastases from carcinoma of lung, breast and prostrate |
| $^{99m}$Tc-macro-aggregates of albumin (MAA) | Lung | Lung perfusion studies most commonly for the diagnosis of pulmonary embolism |
| $^{99m}$Tc-exametazime (HM. PAO) | Brain | Regional cerebral imaging in stroke and tumours Diagnosis of Alzheimer's dementia |
| $^{99m}$Tc-exametazime (HM. PAO) labelled leucocytes | Infection or inflammation | Identification of abscesses associated with pyrexia of unknown origin Extent of inflammatory bowel disease |
| $^{99m}$Tc-tetrofosmin | Heart | Cardiac perfusion imaging |
| $^{99m}$Tc-sestamibi (MIBI) | Heart | Cardiac perfusion imaging |
| $^{99m}$Tc-tin colloid | Liver | Location of hepatic tumours, abscesses and cysts. Detection of cirrhosis |
| $^{99m}$Tc-diethylamine triamine penta-acetic acid (DTPA) | Kidney | Dynamic studies to study kidney function |
| $^{99m}$Tc-dimercapto-succinic acid (DMSA) | Kidney | Static imaging showing the kidney structure |

by reference to the Amersham International generator, Amertec II (Fig. 26.7). The main components of this generator are:

- a 250 ml PVC bag of Sodium Chloride Intravenous Infusion BP 0.9% w/v
- a sterile alumina column to which is bound $^{99}$Mo
- an elution needle
- one 0.22 μm filter and one 0.45 μm filter.

These components are housed within a compact plastic casing. The alumina column is encased in lead to give protection from the radiation.

Operating the generator is fairly straightforward. A sterile evacuated vial, supplied with the generator, is placed in a lead pot designed for the elution process. By placing this on the elution needle, the vacuum draws sterile Sodium Chloride Intravenous Infusion BP 0.9% w/v through the column and into the same vial. When eluate has been collected, air enters the elution vial after first passing through the column. This dries the column as well as removing

excess vacuum in the elution vial. The elution process is now complete and the vial may be removed from the generator.

The sterility of the eluates is maintained throughout the useful life of the generator by the following means:

- The eluting solution is terminally sterilized Sodium Chloride Intravenous Infusion BP 0.9% w/v.
- Air entering the system passes through a 0.22 μm hydrophobic filter.
- A terminal eluate filter is placed between the column and the elution needle.
- Between elutions the needle is protected by a single-use, disposable, sterile needle guard.
- The elution of the generator should be carried out in a Grade A environment (see Ch. 24).

## Preparation of $^{99m}$Tc-radiopharmaceuticals

The daily supply of $^{99m}$Tc is provided by the elution

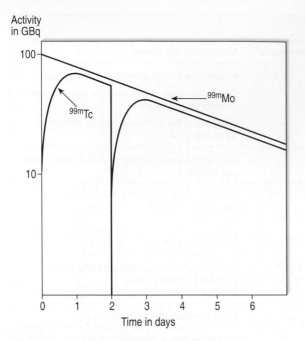

**Fig 26.6**   Radioactivity changes with time in a molybdenum/technetium generator column.

of the generator, resulting in a sterile solution of sodium pertechnetate that is subdivided to provide the activity component of the radiopharmaceutical. Some nuclear medicine investigations use sodium pertechnetate alone as the radiopharmaceutical (Table 26.2). In this case preparation of Sodium Pertechnetate Injection requires only the subdivision from the generator eluate with perhaps some dilution with Sodium Chloride Intravenous Infusion BP 0.9% w/v. Other investigations, and these are in the majority, use radiopharmaceuticals that involve the chemical transformation of the sodium pertechnetate into another radiochemical form.

In order to make the preparation of $^{99m}$Tc-radiopharmaceuticals as simple as possible, commercially available 'kits' are used to manufacture these radiopharmaceuticals. These kits allow the radiopharmacist, in the hospital environment, to transform the pertechnetate, via complex chemical reactions performed within the vial, into the desired radiopharmaceutical. This is achieved by the simple addition of pertechnetate into the vial followed by shaking to dissolve the contents.

A kit consists of a prepacked set of sterile ingredients designed for the preparation of a specific radiopharmaceutical. Most commonly the ingredients are

freeze-dried, enclosed within a rubber-capped nitrogen-filled vial. Normally the kit contains sufficient materials to prepare a number of patient doses. In a typical formulation the following may be found:

- The compound to be complexed to the $^{99m}$Tc. These are known as ligands (e.g. methylene diphosphonate).
- Stannous ions (e.g. stannous chloride or fluoride) which are present as a reducing agent. The reduction of $^{99m}$TcO$_4^-$ to a lower valance state is required to allow the ligands to form a complex with the $^{99m}$Tc.
- Other compounds that act as stabilizers, buffers, or antioxidants.

Given below is an example of how $^{99m}$Tc-radiopharmaceutical production may be performed. The compounding procedures must be carried out within the facilities described in Chapter 24 using aseptic technique and carried out as 'closed' procedures (GMP).

The production method (Figure 26.8) involves two simple steps.

*Step 1.*   The freeze-dried kit is reconstituted by aseptically transferring the necessary activity of sodium pertechnetate using a sterile syringe and needle. This step may also include a further dilution of the eluate with a suitable diluent. The amount of activity withdrawn for the reconstitution of the kit vial depends on two factors:

- The number of patient doses to be manufactured.
- The amount of activity required at injection time for each of the patient doses. The calculation would take into account the decay of $^{99m}$Tc. Manufacturers normally specify a maximum activity that may be added to the vial.

*Step 2.*   The reconstituted kit is aseptically subdivided to provide each patient dose with sufficient activity to allow proper imaging after administration. As in Step 1, a diluent may be added to the final dose to give the desired radioactive concentration.

$^{99m}$Tc-radiopharmaceuticals must be administered on the day of production, for the following reasons:

- *Sterility.* Aseptically prepared pharmaceuticals should ideally be administered within a few hours of production, in accordance with GMP Section 13.
- *Radioactivity.* $^{99m}$Tc has a half-life of only 6 hours.
- *Radiochemical stability.* $^{99m}$Tc-complexes are generally stable for a period between 4 and 8 hours after production.

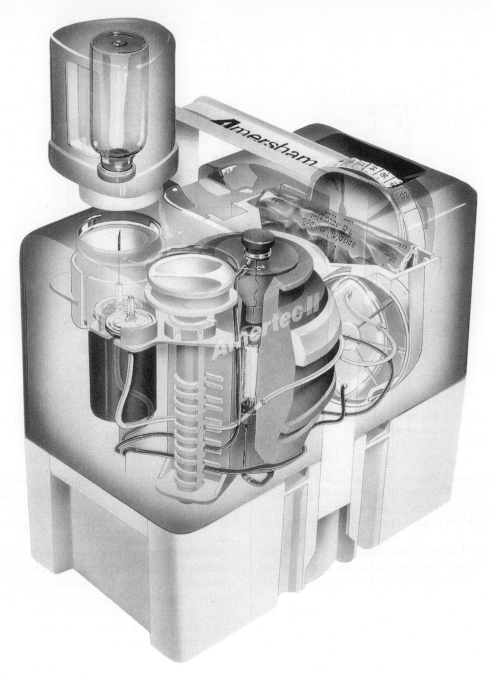

**Fig. 26.7**   The Amertec II $^{99m}$Tc-generator (courtesy of Amersham International plc).

# Radiation protection in the radiopharmacy

There are three basic principles to radiation protection:

- *Shielding*. By placing shielding around the radioactive source the radiation dose rate may be reduced. Materials used as shielding must be appropriate to the type of radiation being emitted by the radionuclide. Plastic, perspex and metals of low molecular weight like aluminium are appropriate materials for shielding $\beta^-$-emitters. For $\gamma$-emitters high

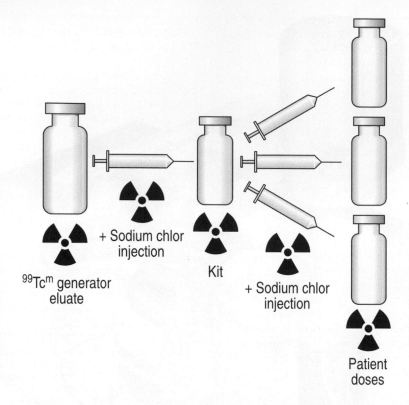

**Fig. 26.8** Schematic representation of the preparation of patient doses of radiopharmaceuticals.

molecular weight metals like lead and tungsten should be used. The thickness of shielding material necessary for $\gamma$-emitters is dependent on the $\gamma$-ray energy – the greater the energy, the thicker the shield required.

- *Distance.* The radiation dose from a radioactive source is inversely proportional to the square of the distance (i.e. by doubling the distance the radiation dose is quartered).

- *Time.* Minimizing the time spent handling a radioactive source will reduce the radiation dose. It is important for new operators to practise the handling operation prior to working with radioactive materials.

In working practice all three of these principles may be used in isolation or together to reduce the radiation dose to the operator. For example in the dispensing operation outlined in Figure 26.8, all vials containing radioactive material would be contained in a 3 mm lead pot. This will attenuate $^{99m}$Tc's $\gamma$-rays by a factor of approximately 1000. The syringes used to carry out the transfers would be

only half full (i.e. 1 ml of radioactive solution would be transferred with a 2 ml syringe) in order to maximize the distance between the operator's fingers and the source, without compromising the accuracy of the dispensing operation.

The syringes, during the operation, should also be contained within a syringe shield. These are made of materials such as lead, tungsten, lead glass or lead acrylic, the latter two being transparent. Lead and tungsten syringe shields have lead glass/acrylic windows incorporated to allow the operator to see the graduations on the syringe. Alternatively the whole syringe shield may be made of lead glass/acrylic which would have the advantage of giving greater visibility.

Handling the vials outwith their lead pots should be carried out using long forceps and not with the fingers. The dispensing process should be carried out over a 'drip tray' that allows easy containment of any accidental spillage. It also should be carried out within a laminar flow safety cabinet or isolator that provides operator protection as well as product protection (see Ch. 23).

The staff working in the radiopharmacy will be constantly monitored to assess their radiation exposure and to ensure compliance with safety legislation. Whole body dose may be monitored with film badges and the radiation dose to the finger pulp with thermoluminescent dosimeters.

## Key Points

- Cytotoxic agents may be alkylating agents, antimetabolites, vinca alkaloids or antimitotics.
- Cytotoxic agents may be given orally (tablets, capsules or suspensions) or parenterally (syringe, slow bolus or i.v. additive).
- There are risks to health care workers who handle cytotoxic agents owing to possible contact with the agent or inhalation of it.
- Use of strict aseptic conditions minimizes the risks during preparation.
- The RPSGB guidelines and *The Cytotoxics Handbook* ensure the health and safety of all personnel, including patients.
- Detailed procedures for preparation and use of cytotoxic agents must be drawn up and followed.
- All personnel involved in provision of a centralized cytotoxic reconstitution service must have full training in procedures, clean rooms, storage and transportation of cytotoxics and all local policies.
- Opening ampoules or the venting or removal of needles from vials carries the risk of escape of cytotoxic material.
- Home chemotherapy services place extra demands on the pharmacy department and could also present drug stability problems.
- A centralized intravenous additive service can provide i.v. antibiotics, patient-controlled analgesia and domiciliary i.v. antibiotics.
- Pharmacy managers are the main decision makers in setting up a CIVAS.
- Potential benefits of CIVAS are improved use of resources, services to patients and pharmacy control.
- A number of problems can arise with CIVAS, such as staffing, storage, distribution, out-of-hours and emergency provision and communications.
- Most doses are provided from CIVAS as preloaded syringes or as a minibag.
- Home i.v. therapy is likely to use single-dose infusers, electronic or elastomeric infusers or a slow i.v. push.

- Radiopharmaceuticals may be used in therapy or diagnosis, the latter either as tracers or in imaging.
- $^{99m}$Tc is the most widely used radionuclide.
- Radiopharmaceuticals are normally administered intravenously and must be produced on the day of use by aseptic techniques.
- A molybdenum/technetium generator will provide a daily supply of $^{99m}$Tc for 7–14 days, as sodium pertechnetate.
- Sodium pertechnetate can be chemically modified by reacting with a suitable ligand.
- Radiation protection should be provided for operators using a combination of shielding, distance and time.

## FURTHER READING

ABPI Compendium of data sheets and summaries of product characteristics 1996 Datapharm Publications, London

Allwood M et al 1997 The cytotoxics handbook, 3rd edn. Radcliffe Medical Press, Oxford

Breckenridge Working Party 1976 Report of the working party on addition of drugs to intravenous infusion fluids. HC(76)9. Department of Health and Social Security. HMSO, London

British Pharmacopoeia, current edn. HMSO, London

Department of Health and Social Security 1982 Guidance notes for hospitals on the premises and environment required for the preparation of radiopharmaceuticals. DHSS, London

Department of Health and Social Security 1983 Guide to good pharmaceutical manufacturing practice, 3rd edn. HMSO, London

Farwell J 1995 Aseptic dispensing for NHS patients. Department of Health, London

MCA 1993 Rules and guidance for pharmaceutical manufacture. HMSO, London

Needle R 1995 A Survey of hospital centralised intravenous additive services. Pharmaceutical Journal 225: 326–327

Pharmaceutical Codex 1994 12th edn. The Pharmaceutical Press, London

Pharmaceutical Society Working Party Report 1983 Guidelines for the handling of cytotoxic drugs. Pharmaceutical Journal 230: 230–231

Sampson C B (ed) 1994 Textbook of radiopharmacy theory and practice, 2nd edn. Gordon and Breach Science Publishers, S.A.

Walker R, Edwards C 1994 Clinical pharmacy and therapeutics. Churchill Livingstone, Edinburgh

# 27

# Hospital at home: the alternative care setting

*S. L. Hutchinson*

---

After studying this chapter you will know about:

**Provision of nutritional support**
**Indications for TPN**
**The nutrition team**
**Components and compounding of a total parenteral nutrition (TPN)/home parenteral nutrition (HPN) formulation**
**Addition of medicines to a TPN or HPN bag**
**HPN training and potential problems**
**Administration of a TPN/HPN formulation**
**The National Total Parenteral Nutrition Group**
**Introduction to home care for patients on dialysis**
**Haemodialysis (HD), peritoneal dialysis (PD), including continuous ambulatory peritoneal dialysis (CAPD), intermittent peritoneal dialysis (IPD) and automated peritoneal dialysis (APD)**
**Dialysis solutions**
**Provision of services from a hospital renal unit, including home dialysis.**

---

## Introduction

Today an increasing number of patients are provided with health care services at home. Such services include provision of home parenteral nutrition and home dialysis. This chapter will explore the provision of parenteral nutrition and dialysis for patients in hospital and will explain how these services can be transferred to the home care setting.

## PROVISION OF NUTRITIONAL SUPPORT

Studies have shown that up to 50% of medical and surgical patients can suffer from nutritional deficiencies. If nutritional support is indicated, enteral feeding is considered as the first option. Patients can receive nutrients orally or via a tube feed, for example by nasogastric feeding. This is only possible if the gastrointestinal tract is functional. If this is not the case, parenteral nutrition may be considered. Short-term (e.g. postoperative) i.v. administration of fluids such as 5% dextrose saline may be sufficient. This could provide the patient with around 500 calories per day but does not provide any protein, vitamins, minerals or trace elements.

For patients requiring longer-term nutrition, total parenteral nutrition (TPN) may be required. TPN is a method of administering adequate nutrients via the parenteral route. The components of a TPN formulation are added to a sterile infusion bag and administered to the patient via a catheter. Administration can be via a peripheral vein or a central vein. However, TPN fluids are normally highly concentrated mixtures which on a long-term basis could cause damage to peripheral veins. For this reason, peripheral veins are only used for TPN administration lasting up to 2 weeks.

If parenteral nutrition is supplied to patients at home, it is known as home parenteral nutrition (HPN). Patients on HPN administer their nutrition via a central vein. A compounding service providing TPN and HPN formulations is now readily available from a large number of hospital pharmacies in the UK. Commercial pharmaceutical companies also provide home care services for HPN patients.

Parenteral nutrition formulations are prepared under strict aseptic conditions following guidelines published by the Medicines Control Agency (MCA) in *Rules and Guidance for Pharmaceutical Manufacturers* (1993) and by the Department of Health in *Aseptic Dispensing for NHS Patients* (Farwell 1995).

HPN is becoming more popular, particularly for patients who require long-term parenteral nutrition. Guidelines have been published by the British Association of Parenteral and Enteral Nutrition (BAPEN) to ensure that adequate provision is made for patients receiving HPN (Wood 1995). Patients who are suitable candidates for HPN will be provided initially with TPN bags in the hospital. Therapy will continue until their medical condition is stabilized. They can then undergo appropriate training to enable them to administer their TPN bags at home. However, HPN patients may still require to return to the hospital for regular check-ups. This means that pharmacists involved in the care of HPN patients will require a working knowledge of the procedures adopted to provide care for patients in hospital and at home. They may also have to liaise with the patient's GP, the community nurse and other health care workers in this field.

This chapter concentrates on the provision of adult TPN in hospital and at home, although neonatal TPN is available.

## INDICATIONS FOR TPN

TPN can be required for finite periods of time or can be required for life. Some of the main indications for TPN are:

- Gastrointestinal disease including: Crohn's disease, ulcerative colitis, pancreatitis and malabsorption syndrome.
- Major trauma including: severe burns, severe septicaemia, intensive care patients and acute renal failure.
- Major abdominal surgery: severely malnourished patients may benefit from early postoperative parenteral nutrition if surgery has resulted in a non-functioning gastrointestinal tract.
- Malignancy of the small bowel.
- Radiation enteritis: TPN is considered if enteritis is severe after treatment of a primary malignancy.
- High-dose chemotherapy, radiotherapy and bone marrow transplantation. Patients are often ill for a limited time (3–6 weeks) and are unable to eat. TPN can be administered during this period to ensure that the patient's nutritional requirements are adequately met.

Several other conditions may require the nutritional support of TPN, for example moderately malnourished patients prior to surgical treatment, patients in a prolonged coma or AIDS patients.

## ASSESSMENT OF THE PATIENT IN HOSPITAL

TPN aims to provide patients with all their nutritional requirements in one formulation which can then be infused directly into the body via a central line catheter into the veins. In order to determine exactly what the patient's nutritional requirements are, clinical and biochemical assessment must take place. A patient history is recorded followed by a physical examination to give a clearer picture of the patient's current medical status. Patients' body weight and height can be recorded and comparison made with their ideal body weight which would be available from standard charts. Some hospitals use nomograms which give an estimation of patients' energy and nitrogen requirements taking into consideration their medical condition and body characteristics.

Biochemical assessment will be undertaken initially by performing a number of routine tests which can then be repeated as necessary during TPN therapy. Factors investigated will include blood counts, 24-hour urine analysis, electrolyte and fluid balance.

Each hospital has its own particular way of designing a TPN regimen. Some hospitals tailor regimes to individual patients and carry out a number of calculations to determine baseline requirements for each component. In this way they can build up a formulation by matching up the patient's requirements to commercially available solutions which contain the required components in the correct proportions. During this process careful consideration is given to the patient's medical condition and the necessary adjustments made.

Other hospitals use a range of standard formulations which are routinely used to treat TPN patients. Standard bags can be altered if the need arises; for example, intensive care patients may require extra nitrogen in the formulation; renal patients may need an electrolyte-free formulation. Further information on specific regimens required for individual patient types can be found in *Clinical Pharmacy and Therapeutics* (Walker & Edwards 1994).

## THE NUTRITION TEAM

In most hospitals where TPN is supplied there will be a nutrition team. This team can include the following people:

- consultant
- senior registrar/registrar
- pharmacist
- nutrition nurse(s)
- dietitian(s)
- biochemist(s).

The role of these individuals in provision of patient care can vary from one hospital to another. In general, the consultant is responsible for prescribing the TPN formulation and liaising with the patient's GP to provide care for HPN patients.

The pharmacist can provide information on aseptic techniques for handling and setting up TPN bags, formulation requirements, potential complications or stability problems and storage conditions required. In some hospitals, the pharmacist's role can be extended to include the following:

- training nursing staff in the techniques required for i.v. administration of TPN fluids
- helping with patient training for HPN
- monitoring of patients in HPN clinics.

The nutrition nurse and dietitian will together give advice on a day-to-day basis regarding the nutritional status of the patients and advise on necessary dietary requirements. The nutrition nurse can also be responsible for training patients for HPN.

The biochemist can supply results of daily or weekly analysis of patients' urine and electrolyte levels and alterations can then be made to the TPN formulation if required. The nutrition team can meet on a weekly basis to discuss the requirements of patients currently receiving TPN both in hospital and at home.

If HPN is supplied by the hospital pharmacy, patients can be provided with the support of a small group of people, some of whom may be part of the nutrition team. This group usually includes the nutrition nurse, the hospital pharmacist and the patient's GP.

Commercial companies supplying home care services have a nutrition nurse who provides medical care, support and advice (on a 24-hour basis if required); a patient coordinator who deals with the ordering of HPN bags and ancillaries; and a designated delivery person who will supply the necessary equipment and HPN bags to the patient's home.

## COMPONENTS OF A TPN FORMULATION

TPN formulations can contain the following components:

- water
- protein source
- energy source – carbohydrate and possibly fat
- electrolytes
- trace elements
- vitamins and minerals.

## Baseline water requirements

Water accounts for over 50% of the body weight. To prevent patients becoming dehydrated, daily water losses and gains must be carefully considered. Water can be lost through urine and faeces and through 'insensible losses' through skin and lungs.

Several methods are available for estimating daily fluid requirements, but most take into consideration body weight and measured urine output, and an allowance is made for insensible losses. The average adult requires between 1500 and 3000 ml of fluid per day. A TPN regimen will require to provide this volume of fluid on a daily basis.

## Protein source

Protein requirements vary from one patient to another and are highly dependent on the metabolic status of the patient. Undernourished patients requiring parenteral nutrition are generally said to have a negative nitrogen balance. This means that the amount of nitrogen excreted in urine and faeces is greater than the nitrogen administered.

Lack of nitrogen in the body can result in poor wound healing and interference with body defence mechanisms. To overcome this problem, a utilizable source of nitrogen must be administered to the patient. This is achieved by administering amino acid solutions in a TPN formulation. These solutions act as a source of nitrogen and are said to be the building blocks for the formation of proteins in the body. Nitrogen requirements can be estimated from a 24-hour urine collection. This done by analysing the total amount of urea excreted and by considering the individual patient's body weight and clinical 'type'.

---

### EXAMPLE 27.1

A postoperative surgical patient requires 0.2 g/kg/24 h of nitrogen. The patient weighs 47 kg.

Nitrogen requirement per day = 0.2 × body weight
= 0.2 × 47 kg
= 9.4 g nitrogen

This requirement can then be matched up to commercially available solutions. Each gram of amino acid nitrogen is equivalent to 6.25 g of protein. Vamin 9 (produced by Pharmacia) contains 9.4 g of nitrogen. This is equivalent to 60 g of protein and will provide the patient with the required daily nitrogen intake. However, care must also be taken when selecting an amino acid

---

solution for inclusion in a TPN formulation as most commercially available solutions are hypertonic in nature and have a pH between 5 and 7.4. The pH of the amino acid solution may have an effect on the overall stability of the formulation and must be considered carefully.

## Energy sources

Carbohydrates and fats are chosen to provide optimal energy sources for TPN patients. The relative proportions of each will be dependent on the clinical requirements of the patient and formulation considerations. The carbohydrate of choice is normally dextrose and is available in solution with concentrations ranging from 5–70% w/v. Like amino acid solutions, dextrose solutions are hypertonic and have a low pH (3–5). If dextrose is required in large quantities (greater than 300–400 g per day), insulin can be administered in the TPN formulation to increase the uptake of dextrose into the body tissues from the bloodstream and to reduce the risk of hypoglycaemia at the end of the infusion period.

The fat component in a TPN formulation is administered in the form of an oil-in-water emulsion. Fat emulsions are isotonic with plasma, have neutral pH and provide a high calorie source in a low volume. As a result, they are often used in combination with dextrose to provide the necessary calorie content thereby avoiding the potential problems encountered with excessive dextrose administration.

Fat emulsions provide the patient with essential fatty acids and also act as a vehicle for fat-soluble vitamins which may be required in the TPN formulation. Fat is not required in every TPN formulation, but fat deficiency can occur in patients who do not receive fat components for periods greater than 1 month. Depending on individual requirements, patients on long-term TPN may require fat added to their TPN bag daily, on alternate days or two or three times weekly.

Commercially available preparations are based on soya bean oils and are composed of varying combinations of long and medium chain triglycerides. Energy content of commercially available solutions for both carbohydrates and fats is expressed in kcal/litre, for example Intralipid 10% Novum (produced by Pharmacia) provides 550 kcal/500 ml; Dextrose 5% provides 210 kcal/500 ml.

## Electrolytes

The main electrolytes of clinical significance in a TPN formulation include sodium, potassium, magnesium, calcium, phosphate and chloride. The requirement for electrolytes can be met in the form of injectable solutions of varying percentage content. Electrolyte content of each is expressed in terms of mmol/litre. The individual role of each electrolyte in a TPN formulation is given in Table 27.1.

## Trace elements

Trace elements act as metabolic cofactors and are said to be essential for the proper functioning of several enzyme systems in the body. Despite being termed essential, they are only required in very small quantities, expressed in micromoles. The main trace elements required in a TPN formulation are zinc, copper, manganese and chromium. More details on trace element requirements are given in *Clinical Pharmacy and Therapeutics* (Walker & Edwards 1994).

## Vitamins and minerals

Vitamin requirements fall into two categories, fat soluble and water soluble. Four fat-soluble vitamins (vitamins A, D, E and K) and nine water-soluble vitamins (vitamins $B_1$, $B_2$, $B_3$, $B_5$, $B_6$, $B_{12}$, C, folic acid and biotin) are said to be essential.

Vitamins and minerals are normally included in foods taken in orally and must therefore be included in TPN formulations for patients on long-term parenteral nutrition. They are required for several body processes and act as essential coenzymes in carbohydrate metabolism and amino acid and DNA synthesis. Commercially available solutions include Multibionta, Parentovite, Solivito N and Vitlipid N Adult.

## COMPOUNDING OF TPN AND HPN FORMULATIONS

Compounding can take place within a hospital pharmacy using aseptic dispensing facilities within a clean room or within a designated compounding unit in a commercial pharmaceutical company.

## Preparation and training

For patients in hospital, the consultant will prescribe a suitable TPN regimen. On receipt of the prescription, the pharmacist checks the suitability and compatibility of the formulation, the required volume of

Table 27.1 Role of electrolytes used in TPN formulations (reproduced by permission from Walker & Edwards 1994)

| Electrolyte | Principal function | Daily intravenous requirement | Symptoms of deficiency | Symptoms of excess | Common sources |
|---|---|---|---|---|---|
| Sodium | Main extracellular cation<br>Regulation of water balance<br>Neuromuscular contractility | 1–2 mmol/kg | Weakness, lethargy, confusion, convulsions, appetite, nausea and vomiting | Lethargy, coma, convulsions, muscle rigidity, thirst | Sodium chloride<br>Sodium acetate<br>Sodium phosphate |
| Potassium | Main intracellular cation<br>Regulation of acid–base balance<br>Neuromuscular contractility | 1–2 mmol/kg | Muscle weakness, ileus, arrhythmias, alkalosis | Muscle weakness, paraesthesia, bradycardia, nausea and vomiting | Potassium chloride<br>Potassium phosphate |
| Magnesium | Cofactor for enzyme systems<br>Neuromuscular contractility | 0.1–0.2 mmol/kg | Lethargy, cramps, tetany, paraesthesia, arrhythmias, neuromuscular excitability, hypokalaemia, hypocalcaemia | Decreased muscular activity, lethargy, respiratory depression | Magnesium sulphate<br>Magnesium chloride |
| Calcium | Mineralization: bones + teeth<br>Neuromuscular contractility | 0.1–0.15 mmol/kg | Paraesthesia, tetany, fitting, confusion, arrhythmias | Nausea, anorexia, lethargy, muscle weakness, confusion | Calcium gluconate<br>Calcium chloride |
| Phosphate | Main intracellular anion<br>Acid–base balance<br>Energy | 0.5–0.7 mmol/kg | Weakness, tingling | Non-specific effects on calcium balance | Phosphate salts of sodium and potassium, hydrogen |
| Chloride | Main extracellular anion<br>Acid–base balance | 1–2 mmol/kg | Alkalosis | Acidosis | Chloride salts of above cations |

each component is calculated and details are transferred to a worksheet. Patient details can be entered into a computer and labels generated for the worksheet and the final product. In the preparation area items required for the compounding process can be collected together in an appropriate tray ready for transfer to the clean room facility. Batch numbers for each product used are recorded on the worksheet. All details, including calculations, are checked by the pharmacist before the compounding procedure begins.

Compounding of a TPN formulation is carried out under strict aseptic conditions (in a Grade A environment) using a laminar airflow (LAF) cabinet within a clean room facility. Chapter 24 gives details regarding clean room facilities, gowning-up procedures for entry to clean rooms and working procedures for using LAF cabinets. Standard operating procedures (SOPs) should be available for all staff carrying out aseptic dispensing procedures. Operators will undergo appropriate training includ-

ing validation of operator techniques by broth fill tests (see Ch. 24) prior to commencing work in this field.

## TPN/HPN bags

The components of a TPN formulation are sterile and are prepared under sterile conditions as the formulation is eventually infused directly into the bloodstream of the patient. It is therefore essential that the bags used to hold the TPN formulation are also sterile. In the past, only polyvinyl chloride (PVC) bags were used for TPN formulations. However, because of to problems of leaching of plasticizers from PVC bags containing a fat component, ethylvinyl acetate (EVA) bags (which contain no plasticizers) are now more commonly used. However, EVA bags have been shown to be permeable to oxygen; hence multilayer EVA bags are now available for formulations requiring prolonged storage. These bags are made of layers of plastic with an inert inner layer made of EVA. This arrangement reduces oxygen permeation to a minimum.

Bags are usually supplied with a pre-mounted sterile filling set attached. The filling set consists of a number of hollow plastic tubes (up to six) with a plastic spike attached to the end of each. The spikes are used to pierce the rubber septum of the bottles and bags of amino acids, glucose and fat emulsion to enable filling of the components into the TPN bag. Clamps fitted with air vents are attached to each filling tube to clamp off the source bottles and bags when they are empty. Filling sets are used for compounding purposes only and are disconnected and replaced with a sterile hub before being sent out to the patient. Every HPN bag is supplied with a sterile giving set which allows the bag to be infused into the patient.

TPN bags vary in size, ranging from small 250 ml bags used for neonatal TPN up to 3-litre bags for adult TPN. Bags used for HPN patients are identical to those used for TPN in hospitals. Figure 27.1 shows a TPN bag with filling set attached.

## Addition of components to a TPN bag

Components are added into the TPN bag in a strictly defined procedure. Small volume additives can be added directly into large volume fluids (but not directly into the fat component) or directly into the additive port on the bag (depending on manufacturers' recommendations). Amino acid solutions and glucose are added into the bag first, followed by any fat emulsion if required. To prevent precipitation of vitamins, they are generally only added immediately before administration.

Filling of the TPN bags can be achieved under gravity. The bag is placed on the floor of the LAF cabinet and the solution components suspended from a retort stand, enabling the solutions to flow freely into the bag. If several bags require to be compounded in a limited time period, the bag can be placed in a vacuum chamber to speed up the filling process. Electronic devices, known as compounders, are also available. They are usually under microprocessor control and can be preprogrammed to fill TPN bags with set volumes of individual components. They can be used to achieve rapid filling of a number of TPN bags and are useful devices for compounding neonatal TPN bags where strict control of fluid volumes is required.

When all the components are added, the bag can be clamped off and the filling set removed. A sterile hub replaces the filling set to prevent any further additions being made to the bag outwith the sterile

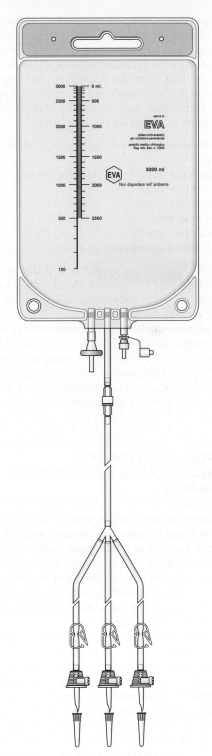

**Fig 27.1** A TPN bag with filling set attached.

production area. The bag is shaken vigorously to ensure adequate mixing of all components. The TPN bag and compounding materials are transferred back to the preparation area. A visual inspection of the bag is made, including checking of the additive port, for integrity. All necessary documentation is completed and the TPN bag is labelled. Details to be included on the label are:

- patient name (ward and unit number if hospital patient)
- components of the bag (expressed in mmol)
- total volume (ml)
- energy content (kcal)
- nitrogen content (g)
- infusion rate (ml/h)
- expiry date and storage conditions.

The TPN bag is then sealed into a dark-coloured outer plastic bag (to protect the formulation from light) and an outer label attached identical to the label on the bag itself.

To maintain stability of the formulated product, it is refrigerated until required. All TPN and HPN formulations must be stored in a designated pharmaceutical grade refrigerator. Coolboxes packed with ice packs can be used for transportation of TPN formulations to the ward or the patient's home.

## COMPOUNDING OF HPN FORMULATIONS BY COMMERCIAL COMPANIES

A designated compounding unit is used for preparing HPN formulations. Conditions used will be the same as those used in the hospital sector (aseptic dispensing facilities in a clean room). If the commercial company does not have its own compounding facilities it may utilize the services of a hospital pharmacy or another industrial pharmaceutical company to compound the HPN bags.

Regardless of the compounding arrangements, the commercial company providing the home care service must be in receipt of a prescription for the HPN formulation prior to compounding. The prescription will be the same formulation which the patient initially had during his/her stay in hospital.

However, when the health care is transferred to the home care setting, in Scotland, the patient's GP will take on the responsibility for supplying the HPN prescription. In England and Wales the health authority is responsible for providing the HPN prescription. Subsequent prescriptions will then be forwarded to the commercial company in advance of the patient's requirements. Orders for sundries and ancillaries such as pumps, dressings, needles, etc. will be dealt with by the patient coordinator.

Realistic annual costs for a patient receiving HPN are in the region of £35 000 for an adult and £42 000 for a paediatric patient. These figures can be broken down into individual costs; for example, up to £100 a day for the HPN formulation, £5 to £20 per day for ancillaries, and pump hire at £85 to £150 per month. Patients are not required to pay these costs as funding is achieved from the GP or the health authority.

## POTENTIAL COMPLICATIONS ARISING DURING COMPOUNDING AND ADMINISTRATION OF TPN FORMULATIONS

The components of a TPN formulation will individually and collectively contribute to the overall stability of the resulting formulation. However, with several hospitals now using standard TPN formulations, many of these problems can be overcome. For hospital pharmacies which have a manufacturing licence, standard bags can be made up in advance of requirements and stored in a refrigerator for periods of 30 days or more. Shelf life given to individual formulations must be based on validated stability studies previously carried out on the formulation.

Individual components of the formulation such as vitamins, electrolytes and fat can cause formulation complications. Vitamin stability is very poor particularly in the presence of light and with extended storage time. Stability is also affected by solution pH, hence the need for careful consideration of the overall formulation.

The requirement for administration of calcium and phosphate in a formulation can lead to precipitation of calcium phosphate. This reaction is said to be affected by factors such as the relative amounts of each component present, solution pH, concentration of amino acid solutions present and the mixing process used. To overcome this type of problem, manufacturers of parenteral nutrition fluids can supply tables which give details of the amount of each component which can be safely combined to ensure stability of the formulation is maintained. These tables are specific to an individual formulation and details cannot be interchanged between formulations.

The presence of fat in a TPN formulation can

cause stability problems. As storage time increases, the fat component of the formulation becomes less stable, resulting in a process of 'cracking' where the oil and water phases of the emulsion separate out. If the formulation is administered to the patient in this unstable condition, this can lead to potentially dangerous fat deposits arising in the lungs and other body tissues.

The factors a pharmacist must consider when formulating a TPN bag with a fat component are:

- the order in which components are added to the bag
- the types of electrolytes present and their relative proportions – divalent and trivalent cations reduce stability
- pH of the resultant mixture – higher pH improves stability
- conditions arising during storage and administration
- the type of plastic bag used – EVA bags preferred.

## ADDITION OF MEDICINES TO A TPN OR HPN BAG

Stability studies have been carried out on a number of medicines to determine their compatibility and stability in a TPN bag. So far, studies have confirmed the suitability of only a limited range of medicines which includes: heparin, insulin, aminophylline, cimetidine, famotidine, ranitidine and certain antibiotics. Reference to manufacturers' literature and compatibility studies will provide current recommendations.

## ADMINISTRATION OF TPN/HPN FORMULATIONS

For TPN administration lasting longer than 2 weeks, central venous access is required. During their stay in hospital, patients have a catheter inserted into the subclavian vein under anaesthesia. It has an exit site on the lower chest wall, allowing patients easy access for care of the catheter site.

Catheters can be made of materials such as polyvinyl chloride or silicone. For long-term feeding a permanent catheter (a Hickman catheter or a portacath) is used. It is held in place by a Dacron cuff (an internal woven plastic used to connect arteries and veins under the skin). Good aseptic techniques

are essential to ensure that the catheter site does not become contaminated. Infection around the catheter site can be difficult to treat successfully and may eventually result in removal of the catheter and replacement at another site.

Catheter sites should only be used for administration of TPN fluids and not for blood sampling or administration of other medicines. However, in exceptional circumstances (where venous access is limited) the TPN line may have to be used for these purposes. In some instances, a triple lumen catheter can be used with one line being kept for administration of the TPN bag only. To infuse the TPN formulation into the patient, the catheter is connected via an extension set to a volumetric infusion pump. These devices use positive pressure as the driving force to allow accurate infusion at pre-set rates (see Ch. 25).

Adult TPN formulations can have a volume ranging from about 1500 ml to 3000 ml. The infusion period varies from 24 hours in hospital to around 8–12 hours for home patients (as HPN can often be administered overnight). Infusion rate can be calculated by dividing the total volume of the infusion (ml) by the infusion period (hours) giving a rate of ml/hour. Most pumps now have the ability to be programmed to give an infusion rate which 'steps up' at the beginning and 'steps down' at the end of the infusion period, avoiding potential problems with high concentrations of dextrose in the formulation. They are also fitted with an alarm which will alert the patient if a technical fault arises.

## POTENTIAL PROBLEMS FOR HPN PATIENTS

### Mechanical problems

Problems of pneumothorax, or air embolism, are more likely to occur in the hospital environment in the early stages of catheter placement and are dealt with before the patient commences on HPN. However, daily connection and disconnection of the catheter hub may result in cracking and possible leakage of the HPN fluid. Repair kits are available and if used promptly when the problem first arises, catheter replacement may not be necessary.

Internal blockage of the catheter can arise. Patients are taught to flush out the catheter port with heparinized saline to prevent thrombus formation. Blockage of the line arising during administration of the HPN fluid can cause changes in flow rate which are recognized by the pump and the alarm is activated.

## Metabolic problems

Metabolic complications include problems with electrolyte levels leading to conditions such as hypernatraemia or hyponatraemia, with glucose levels leading to hyperglycaemia or hypoglycaemia, and in balancing of fluid intake (to ensure adequate hydration is achieved). The majority of the metabolic complications which can affect HPN patients can be overcome by careful monitoring of the patient initially in hospital and with regular check-ups and home visits by the nutrition nurse.

## Catheter-related complications

Catheter-related infections can arise as a result of poor management of the catheter exit site. Infection is distinguished by pain, redness and tenderness around the site. To minimize such infections, staff in the hospital are trained to use strict aseptic procedures when changing TPN bags and use of the catheter port is restricted to administration of the TPN bag only. HPN patients are taught the same aseptic techniques and are required to carry out these procedures at all times when changing bags at home. Home care patients are also taught to be aware of their own physical condition and alert to any deterioration in their medical condition at the earliest possible time. Patients are asked to contact their nutrition nurse if they experience any signs or symptoms of infection around the catheter site.

## Psychological and social problems

Patients receiving TPN in hospital or at home must learn to adapt to the changes occurring in their lifestyle. Some patients have, over a prolonged period of time, suffered from a general deterioration in their health and as a result adapt well to the initiation of parenteral nutrition as it improves their quality of life. Other patients require TPN as a result of major trauma and these patients find the dramatic changes in their lifestyle very difficult to cope with.

While in the hospital receiving treatment, patients have the constant support of medical and nursing staff who can help them to cope with any practical difficulties encountered. When patients return to the home care setting they need continued support to enable them to cope with their HPN therapy on their own. The ability of patients to adapt to HPN is highly dependent on a number of factors:

- Patient's underlying medical condition.
- Physical ability and capability of the patient.
- Training and counselling prior to leaving hospital.
- Home circumstances, particularly support from family members and the patient's GP.
- Ability to deal with physical and emotional changes in lifestyle, for example dependence on others, potential for mood swings and clinical depression. Disruption to normal sleeping pattern during administration of the HPN bag overnight and loss of 'social' eating can be difficult for many patients, particularly in the initial stages of HPN.

To enable a smooth transition from hospital to home to be achieved, patients require the services of the nutrition nurse and other health care workers to teach them the necessary skills required for handling, setting up their HPN bags and disconnecting them once the procedure is complete.

## TRAINING FOR HPN PATIENTS

Health care which can be provided at home has a number of advantages. Patients have a better quality of life and can become more independent as their confidence in providing self-care increases. However, motivation and confidence to carry out the required manipulations at home are essential. Thus training in the hospital environment is required to build up the necessary skills and techniques.

When a patient has been selected for home care a nutrition nurse will begin a training programme with the patient to teach the practical skills required for safe and effective administration of the TPN bag at home. A discharge plan is required for each patient working towards home care. The British Association of Parenteral and Enteral Nutrition (BAPEN), a registered charity formed in 1992, has laid down guidelines for the provision of nutritional care at home. Individual hospitals will develop their own guidelines based on the advice given by BAPEN. The scope of BAPEN includes guidelines on the following matters:

- details which should be included in a patient discharge plan
- knowledge and practical skills which must be achieved by patients prior to discharge
- guidelines for GPs on the provision of HPN
- advice on how to liaise with the patient's GP to ensure that everyone is aware of their responsibilities
- information regarding the supplier of the HPN

bags and equipment and how this service will be provided

- details of appropriate people who patients can contact for advice and help with any problems they have.

The length of time required for training can vary depending on the patient's underlying medical condition and personal approach to training. Patients must be taught aseptic techniques and the importance of ensuring that they are carried out correctly. They must demonstrate their skills and competence on several occasions prior to leaving the hospital. Training will take place during the day initially then, as the patient becomes more confident with the techniques, overnight feeding will be started. This allows the patient to lead as normal a life as possible and allows some patients to return to a working environment. Areas covered during the training period include:

- aseptic techniques for setting up and disconnecting the HPN bag
- care of the catheter site
- how to deal with problems of the catheter blocking
- setting the pump for infusion of the HPN bag
- dealing with simple mechanical problems with the pump.

Information booklets on HPN and educational videos can be used with patients to reinforce the training received in hospital.

## SERVICES PROVIDED BY HOME CARE COMPANIES

Patients receiving home care will require certain practical arrangements to be put in place before HPN can be initiated. Home care companies who provide services to HPN patients normally provide the following items for patient use: a refrigerator for storing HPN bags; a trolley for patients to set up their HPN bags aseptically; a drip stand and an infusion pump. Patients are required to have adequate storage space to keep any extra components which may be required for HPN administration and easy access to hand washing facilities for use prior to setting up their HPN bag.

## SUPPORT SERVICES PROVIDED FOR HPN PATIENTS

Patients will be metabolically stable prior to transfer

to the home care setting, hence frequency of monitoring will be reduced to a minimum. Patients can have monthly check-ups at the hospital initially, reducing to 3-monthly as they adapt to life on HPN. During visits, patients may be seen by the consultant and the nutrition nurse, possibly at a lipid clinic. Routine monitoring can be carried out during these visits including the following:

- checking the patient's underlying medical condition
- reviewing the patient's nutritional status, particularly in relation to his/her weight
- routine haematological and biochemical tests
- checking for any cardiovascular complications
- reviewing the patient's psychological status.

The nutrition nurse will make home visits if required to check on aseptic techniques and any practical difficulties being encountered by patients and/or their partner or carer.

Patients on HPN can benefit from the support of others undergoing nutrition therapy at home. This is made possible by an organization called 'PINNT' (Patients on Intravenous and Nasogastric Nutrition Therapy). This is a charitable organization which aims to support and bring together people who have similar medical conditions and could benefit from the moral support of others who understand the problems they face. PINNT provides practical help in areas such as provision of portable equipment for people on HPN who wish to go on holiday; help with holiday arrangements including appropriate travel insurance; and general advice on benefits available to HPN patients. A newsletter is produced on a regular basis and close links are kept between PINNT and BAPEN to ensure that patient needs are adequately met.

## THE NATIONAL TOTAL PARENTERAL NUTRITION GROUP

Pharmacists in the UK can keep up to date with the working of organizations like PINNT and BAPEN by joining the National Total Parenteral Nutrition Group (NTPNG). Currently NTPNG has approximately 160 members most of whom are hospital pharmacists working in the NHS. However, membership also includes dietitians, nutrition nurses, research workers and members of commercial companies who work in the field of TPN and HPN. The NTPNG exists to further the practice of TPN through a number of activities including research, contributing to the work of BAPEN and arranging symposia on practical and scientific developments in the field. This group is also one of five constituent groups which make up BAPEN. Hence good communication is achieved between the different sectors of health care who provide care for home and hospital patients receiving nutrition support.

## INTRODUCTION TO HOME CARE FOR PATIENTS ON DIALYSIS

Like HPN, dialysis at home is now a regular occurrence. Patients requiring dialysis at home are those who require treatment for end-stage renal disease (ESRD) or renal failure. For such patients their options are dialysis in a hospital renal unit, home dialysis or a transplant. However, because there are insufficient kidney donors, patients can require dialysis for prolonged periods.

## WHAT IS DIALYSIS?

In a healthy individual the kidney acts as a crude filter removing toxic waste products such as creatinine and urea from the body, whilst retaining the essential components required to maintain the body's natural homeostatic balance. This process is often referred to as an 'ultrafiltration' process. If renal function is impaired water and electrolyte balance is disturbed, toxic waste products build up in the blood and the patient suffers from fluid overload. An artificial method of allowing this ultrafiltration to take place must be adopted. This is where dialysis can be used.

Dialysis can never completely replace renal function but can be used as a way of removing toxic metabolites, correcting acid–base balance and avoiding fluid overload. The process of dialysis is dependent on the use of a semipermeable membrane which can allow the separation of a mixture of blood and dialysis fluid as it passes over the membrane. Such a membrane is only permeable to water and small ions but is not permeable to blood cells, plasma proteins or lipids (fats). As the dialysis fluid moves over the membrane it removes water and waste products from the blood restoring the homeostatic balance. Two main types of dialysis exist:

- haemodialysis (HD)
- peritoneal dialysis (PD).

Both HD and PD can be carried out in a hospital renal unit or in the patient's home. Patients are constantly monitored and readings of blood pressure and body weight recorded before, during and after dialysis periods.

### Haemodialysis (HD)

In HD blood is removed from the patient's body and filtered by passing it over an artificial semipermeable membrane known as a 'dialyser' before being returned to the patient's body again. To allow HD to take place an access point into the patient's body is required. This is achieved using a surgical procedure whereby a fistula is created. This involves joining an artery and a vein together to allow blood at arterial pressure to enter the veins near the skin surface. This allows access to the body circulation. Over a period of weeks the walls of the fused artery and vein dilate creating an access point to enable dialysis to take place. The fistula is usually created in the forearm of the non-dominant arm. Usually two needles with a length of tubing attached are inserted into the fistula; one for transportation of blood to the dialyser and the other to carry purified blood back to the patient. Heparin is normally added to the dialysis fluid to prevent the blood clotting.

To achieve HD the patient's blood must pass over a membrane with a large surface area. This allows solutes to be exchanged between the blood and dialysis fluid. Dialysis membranes are sterile disposable membranes made of cellulose or polycarbonate materials. (In some renal units, dialysis membranes are being recycled by sterilizing them with ethylene oxide.) Pressure is applied to the blood to induce the ultrafiltration process and allow removal of excess water. Dialysis machines have preprogrammed cycles to allow dialysis to be achieved as quickly and efficiently as possible.

HD will initially take the form of short dialysis periods which will be repeated on a regular basis to resolve the fluid overload problem. Once the situation is under control, HD sessions can take place at least three times weekly and will last approximately 4 hours.

HD is a much more efficient way of treating renal failure than peritoneal dialysis (PD) and can correct the fluid overload and electrolyte imbalance more rapidly. However, a number of factors make it a more complicated procedure for home patients:

- Training for patients can be time consuming and complicated. Specially trained staff are required to teach aseptic techniques for handling the fistula site and administering i.v. medicines.

● Patients must have a restricted diet and fluid intake as urine output between dialysis sessions is minimal.

● Blood loss can arise during dialysis resulting in a 'washed out' feeling and possibly anaemia.

● A fine balance is required to achieve the correct dialysis concentration to allow sufficient removal of excess fluids. Hypotension can be a problem if short intensive dialysis periods occur too often.

## Peritoneal dialysis (PD)

In PD the dialysis fluid is passed directly into the patient's body and no blood removal occurs. Dialysis is achieved by passing the dialysis fluid directly into the peritoneum-lined abdominal cavity, leaving it in situ for a predetermined period and draining it back out again. This is known as the 'dwell time'. During this time, the peritoneal membrane acts as a semipermeable membrane allowing exchange between the blood and the dialysis solution. This enables removal of excess water and waste products from the blood, restoring the body's homeostatic balance. This cycle of filling and draining can be repeated up to five times daily.

Fluids are introduced into the body via an indwelling sterile silicone catheter, known as a Tenckhoff catheter. The catheter is inserted under anaesthesia using surgical procedures. The catheter is held firmly in position by two Dacron cuffs. The distal end of the catheter has tiny holes in it to allow the dialysis fluid to flow freely into the peritoneal cavity. Patients and medical staff are taught strict aseptic techniques to ensure that the catheter site remains sterile and free from infection.

With PD, the ultrafiltration process is achieved by an osmotic effect created by the presence of high concentrations of glucose in the dialysis fluid. Glucose concentrations can be adjusted to achieve the required removal of the excess fluid from the patient.

Three main types of PD exist:

● continuous ambulatory peritoneal dialysis (CAPD)
● intermittent peritoneal dialysis (IPD)
● automated peritoneal dialysis (APD).

CAPD is the procedure which is most widely used by home dialysis patients. When CAPD is initiated, no dialysis machines are required. Dialysis fluids are warmed to body temperature using a bag warmer and allowed to flow into the peritoneal cavity under the influence of gravity. The fluid bag is attached to a drip stand and is suspended approximately 1 metre above the patient's body. Once the fluid is completely drained from the bag into the peritoneum, it remains there for approximately 4–8 hours. The bag can be disconnected and a sterile Luer lock cap placed over the outer catheter site to avoid the risk of contamination. (Special 'Y' connectors can be used, one for filling and the other for draining.) During this time, patients can carry on with their normal daily routine. When the dwell time is over, an empty sterile dialysis bag is reconnected to the catheter site, the bag placed on the floor and the dialysis fluid drained off. Once the process is complete, a new bag is set up. Each cycle of filling and draining is known as an 'exchange'. Patients on CAPD are recommended to carry out between three and five exchanges per day. The longest dwell time can be 8–10 hours overnight.

IPD involves the use of a 'cycling' machine which automatically repeats the fill and drain sequence, avoiding the need for patients to manually change the dialysis bags. The machine can be loaded with a number of dialysis bags, providing a reservoir of dialysis fluid which can be warmed and delivered into the patient in pre-set volumes. Dwell times can vary (20 minutes or more) but in general, the patient is connected to the machine for approximately 12 hours. Patients can carry out IPD overnight at home or within a hospital dialysis unit. The process is generally repeated two to four times weekly. For home IPD patients a special room must be set aside to accommodate machinery and dialysis fluids. IPD can be costly to set up at home and is not used as a home dialysis method in preference to CAPD. Patient mobility is also restricted owing to the machinery involved; hence IPD is not as popular with patients.

APD or continuous cycle PD (CCPD) involves the use of a machine to perform the dialysis overnight. The machine utilizes a pump delivery system which warms the dialysis fluid prior to administration and delivers a carefully selected volume of dialysis fluid which exchanges throughout the infusion period overnight. The home patient is required to set up the machine every night by connecting it to the catheter site. The main advantage of this type of dialysis is that the patient is free to continue with a normal daily routine and carry out the dialysis overnight. APD is becoming more popular with patients as procedures used do not require constant bag exchanges. However, it still remains a more costly procedure than CAPD for home patients.

Using CAPD as a technique for home dialysis has a number of advantages:

• CAPD is used continuously (dialysis fluid kept in contact with blood for longer periods) hence there is less disruption to the body's electrolyte balance and fluid and dietary restrictions are limited.

• Blood loss is avoided, hence this is a safer technique for anaemic patients.

• CAPD is a relatively simple process to teach patients as no complicated equipment is required.

• It is a useful technique for children as they have a large peritoneal cavity relative to their body mass.

• Blood sugar levels in diabetic patients can be well controlled by the addition of insulin added to dialysis fluids if required.

However, CAPD also has a number of disadvantages:

• CAPD is not as efficient a process as clinicians would desire. Patients can suffer from nutritional problems due to the peritoneum allowing the loss of large protein and amino acid molecules through the membrane. As a result, CAPD patients can require high dietary input to make up for daily protein losses.

• Obesity can be a problem with some patients due to large quantities of glucose being absorbed from the dialysis fluids. This gives the added complication of potential cardiovascular problems.

• CAPD is contraindicated in patients who have recently undergone abdominal surgery or those with severe pulmonary disease as dialysis can compromise lung function.

• Peritonitis can develop in CAPD patients.

Home dialysis patients are taught to recognize the signs and symptoms of peritonitis developing, for example cloudiness in the dialysis fluid being drained out, abdominal pain, redness or swelling around the catheter site. They are requested to contact the CAPD nurse or the renal unit immediately. If the infection is caught in the early stages, antibiotic treatment can be initiated and may prevent the complications of catheter replacement. If peritonitis becomes a recurring problem, the patient may have to revert to HD.

## DIALYSIS SOLUTIONS

Dialysis solutions used for both HD and PD have similar constituents. They are required to contain electrolytes in concentrations similar to those found in normal extracellular body fluid.

Composition of solutions can vary, but in general they contain sodium, calcium, magnesium, chloride ions and a source of bicarbonate ions (usually from lactate or acetate). Glucose is included as a component of dialysis fluids to achieve the necessary osmotic effect during dialysis. Potassium is normally only incorporated into HD solutions, but can be added to PD solutions if required. Owing to the large volumes of fluids required for HD, solutions are normally prepared in the form of a concentrate which can then be diluted with water prior to use.

HD solutions are not required to be sterile as the membrane within the dialysis machine does not permit the passage of bacteria. All PD solutions require to be sterile and are prepared using aseptic techniques and terminally sterilized by autoclaving. Dialysis fluids are compounded by commercial pharmaceutical companies who supply them directly to hospital renal units or to home dialysis patients. Solutions are supplied in sterile plastic bags (similar to EVA bags used for TPN formulations). Bags are available in a range of sizes from 2 to 7 litres. Drainage bags used in CAPD must be of larger capacity to accommodate excess fluid removed during dialysis.

## PROVISION OF SERVICES FROM THE HOSPITAL RENAL UNIT

Within the unit there will be a multidisciplinary team of people who are responsible for making decisions regarding the treatment required by patients, for providing medical care and support and training patients for home dialysis. This group can meet at least once or twice weekly to discuss the needs of patients in hospital and at home. The following people can be included in this team: consultant, registrar, pharmacist, renal nurses, dietitian, social worker and renal technician. The renal team members will all have individual responsibilities similar to those in the nutrition team:

• The consultant/registrar is responsible for prescribing during dialysis and monitoring the patient's clinical condition.

• The pharmacist can have involvement in a number of areas including: advice on aseptic handling techniques and catheter care; clinical assessment of patients; provision of drug information (particularly bioavailability of renally excreted drugs) and ordering and supplying dialysis fluids and ancillaries to home dialysis patients.

• Renal nurses can be responsible for providing

nursing care; monitoring the patient's condition and training patients for home dialysis.

- The dietitian can provide patients with detailed information on necessary dietary requirements, food and fluid restrictions.
- A social worker is included in the renal team to provide the necessary advice and practical help for patients at home, for example housing requirements, care of other family members particularly children, benefits available for patients unable to work while on dialysis.
- The renal technician is responsible for day-to-day functioning of dialysis machines and advising on dialysis fluid concentrations.

## TRAINING FOR HOME DIALYSIS PATIENTS

Training is carried out by a member of the renal team, usually a CAPD nurse as the majority of patients on home dialysis are CAPD patients. The CAPD nurse will provide the training in hospital and can also act as a point of contact for patients once they are home. Patients will have regular home visits from the CAPD nurse to ensure that they are coping with their dialysis at home. A training room will be used to set up CAPD or HD to allow patients to practise their techniques and build up the necessary confidence to carry out their dialysis at home. Educational videos and literature can be used with patients to reinforce practical skills learned within the hospital. The length of time required for training will vary depending on the capabilities of individual patients and the techniques being taught.

HD training can take longer than for CAPD as patients have to be taught a wide range of procedures including:

- aseptic techniques for handling the fistula, checking to ensure that it is in working order and keeping it free from contamination
- how to connect up the fistula lines to the dialysis machine and set it up for dialysis (including adding dialysis fluid and setting up the dialysis cycle)
- injection techniques for administration of medicines and anaesthetics required during dialysis procedures
- use of heparin to maintain patency of the line and to prevent blood clotting during dialysis.

Many patients find these procedures too complicated to learn and to carry out on a long-term basis.

They also require the constant support of another family member to help with the day-to-day practical issues of carrying out the dialysis.

## SUPPORT AND SERVICES FOR HOME DIALYSIS PATIENTS

Like HPN patients, home dialysis patients can be provided with their dialysis fluids, equipment and ancillaries by the hospital pharmacy or a commercial home care company. If the pharmacy provides the service, the pharmacist may be responsible for ensuring that all dialysis fluids and ancillaries are ordered and delivered to the patient on time. If the service is provide by a home care company, each patient will be allocated a patient coordinator whom the patient will telephone to order dialysis supplies. A designated delivery person will deliver dialysis fluids to the patient's home and rotate stock to ensure that it is used in appropriate date order. Companies can also provide a nutrition nurse to give 'on call' advice to patients, but patients are still free to contact their dialysis unit at any time.

Dialysis is expensive. A cost of £30 000 per annum, including the cost of home visits, has been given for home HD and £16 000 for CAPD in 1997.

Each individual hospital will be affiliated to the Kidney Patients' Association and will encourage patients and their carers to attend regular meetings to provide practical support for home dialysis patients.

---

### Key Points

- Up to half of medical and surgical patients can have nutritional deficiencies.
- TPN/HPN formulations are prepared under strict aseptic conditions.
- Before starting TPN a full assessment of the patient's nutritional needs must be made.
- The nutrition team contribute their expertise to provide good patient care by meeting regularly to monitor patient needs.
- A TPN formulation may contain water, protein, carbohydrate, fat, electrolytes, trace elements, vitamins and minerals.
- Most TPN patients have a negative nitrogen balance and so require amino acids.
- Care must be taken when administering dextrose in a TPN/HPN formulation to prevent problems of hyper- or hypoglycaemia.

- Strictly defined procedures are followed when adding ingredients to TPN bags during preparation.
- Stability of TPN formulations is one of the major issues which must be carefully considered.
- Incompatibilities, such as that between calcium and phosphate, can be minimized by controlling quantities.
- TPN bags containing a fat component become less stable on prolonged storage and could result in fat deposits arising in lungs and capillaries if administered in this unstable condition.
- For TPN lasting longer than 2 weeks a central vein should be used.
- A number of problems can arise during TPN/HPN administration. For HPN patients, adequate training to deal with problems arising at home is essential.
- HPN patients require to make psychological and social adjustments, but can also have an improvement in quality of life.
- BAPEN has laid down standards for home nutritional care which are used as the basis for patient training prior to discharge.
- Dialysis is used to remove toxic metabolites, correct acid–base balance and avoid fluid overload.
- In haemodialysis, the patient's blood is passed over a semipermeable membrane to allow exchange of small solutes with dialysis fluid.
- Peritoneal dialysis uses the peritoneal membrane as the semipermeable membrane, the dialysis fluid staying in the peritoneal cavity during the exchange.
- CAPD has a number of advantages and disadvantages for patients.
- HD solutions do not require to be sterile, but PD solutions must be sterile and aseptic technique used in handling.
- Home dialysis patients will require training and support. Patients are encouraged to join the Kidney Patients' Association.

Medicines Control Agency (MCA) 1993 Rules and guidance for pharmaceutical manufacture. HMSO, London

Pharmaceutical Codex 1994 12th edn. The Pharmaceutical Press, London

Walker R, Edwards C 1994 Clinical pharmacy and therapeutics. Churchill Livingstone, Edinburgh

Wood S (ed) 1995 Home parenteral nutrition: quality criteria for clinical services and the supply of nutrient fluids and equipment. British Association for Parenteral and Enteral Nutrition, Maidenhead

## FURTHER READING

Farwell J 1995 Aseptic dispensing for NHS patients. Department of Health, London

Harman R 1989 Patient care in community practice. The Pharmaceutical Press, London

# 28
# Ophthalmic products

*R. M. E. Richards*

After studying this chapter the reader should be able to:

**Discuss the formulation, preparation and uses of single and multiple dose ophthalmic solutions**
**Discuss the formulation, preparation and uses of ophthalmic ointments**
**Explain the packaging and labelling requirements for ophthalmic preparations**
**Describe the anatomy and physiology of the eye in relation to the administration of medication and the wearing of contact lenses**
**Explain the properties of contact lenses in relation to their physicochemical composition**
**Discuss the wearing of and caring for contact lenses and the various products available to facilitate comfort, effectiveness, convenience and safety**
**Highlight the role of antimicrobial preservatives in ophthalmic products with particular reference to the high-risk microbial contaminants.**

## Introduction

The human eye is an amazing organ and the ability to see is one of our most treasured possessions. Thus the highest standards are necessary in the compounding of ophthalmic preparations and the greatest care is required in their use. It is necessary that all ophthalmic preparations are sterile and essentially free from foreign particles.

These preparations may be categorized as follows:

- eye drops including solutions and suspensions of active medicaments for instillation into the conjunctival sac

- eye lotions for irrigating and cleansing the eye surface
- eye ointments, creams and gels containing active ingredient(s) for application to the lid margins and/or conjunctival sac
- contact lens solutions to facilitate the wearing and care of contact lenses
- parenteral products for intracorneal, intravitreous or retrobulbar injection
- solid dosage forms placed in the conjunctival sac and designed to release active ingredient over a prolonged period.

Medicaments contained in ophthalmic products include:

- anaesthetics used topically in surgical procedures
- anti-infectives such as antibacterials, antifungals and antivirals
- anti-inflammatories such as corticosteroids and antihistamines
- antiglaucoma agents to reduce intraocular pressure, such as beta-blockers
- astringents such as zinc sulphate
- diagnostic agents such as fluorescein which highlight damage to the epithelial tissue
- miotics such as pilocarpine which constrict the pupil and contract the ciliary muscle increasing drainage from the anterior chamber
- mydriatics and cycloplegics such as atropine which dilate the pupil and paralyse the ciliary muscle and thus facilitate the examination of the interior of the eye.

## Anatomy and physiology of the eye

Figure 28.1 gives an indication of the relevance of the external structures of the eye and the structure of the eyelids to the application of medication and the wearing of contact lenses.

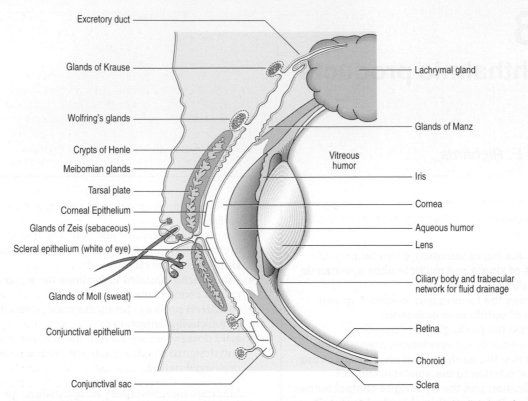

**Fig. 28.1** Section of the eye showing the glands which produce the fluids that form the tears, the epithelial sites of drug absorption and the internal sites of pharmacological action.

## FORMULATION OF EYE DROPS

The components of an eye drop formulation are given below:

- active ingredient(s) to produce desired therapeutic effect
- vehicle, usually aqueous but occasionally may be oil e.g. tetracycline hydrochloride
- antimicrobial preservative to eliminate any microbial contamination during use and thus maintain sterility
- adjuvants to adjust tonicity, viscosity or pH in order to increase the 'comfort' in use and to increase the stability of the active ingredient(s)
- suitable container for administration of eye drops which maintains the preparation in a stable form and protects from contamination during preparation, storage and use.

The single most important requirement of eye drops is that they are sterile. During the 1940s and 1950s there were several instances reported where microbially contaminated eye drops were used and consequently introduced infection into the eyes being treated. The results were particularly damaging when the contaminating organism was *Pseudomonas aeruginosa* which is difficult to treat successfully and can cause loss of the eye.

## Antimicrobial preservatives

It is essential that multiple dose eye drops contain an effective antimicrobial preservative system which is capable of withstanding the test for efficacy of preservatives of the *British Pharmacopoeia* (BP 1993). This is to ensure that the eye drops are maintained sterile during use and will not introduce contamination into the eyes being treated. Normal healthy eyes are quite efficient at preventing penetration by microorganisms. Eyes that have damaged epithelia have their defences compromised and may be colonized by microorganisms. This has to be guarded against. The lack of vascularity of the cornea and certain internal structures of the eye make it very susceptible and difficult to treat once infection has been established.

| Table 28.1 Preservatives suitable for specific eye drops | | |
|---|---|---|
| Preservative | | |
| Benzalkonium chloride (BZK) 0.01% w/v | Chlorhexidine acetate (CHX) 0.01% w/v | Phenylmercuric nitrate* (PMN) 0.002% w/v |
| Atropine sulphate | Cocaine | Amethocaine |
| Carbachol | Cocaine and | Chloramphenicol |
| Cyclopentolate | homatropine | Fluorescein[†] |
| Homatropine | | Hydrocortisone |
| Hyoscine | | and neomycin |
| Hypromellose | | Lachesine |
| Phenylephrine | | Neomycin |
| Physostigmine | | Sulphacetamide |
| Pilocarpine | | Zinc sulphate |
| Prednisolone | | Zinc sulphate and adrenaline |

*The acetate may also be used.
[†]This is preferably used as single dose preparations.

No single substance is entirely satisfactory for use as a preservative for ophthalmic solutions. The systems that have been used, based on work of the author and others in the 1960s, have seemingly been effective.

It should be noted that eye drops supplied for use during intraocular surgery should not contain a preservative because of the risk of damage to the internal surfaces of the eye.

Preservatives which are suitable for a selection of eye drops are given in Table 28.1.

## Benzalkonium chloride

This quaternary ammonium compound is the preservative of choice if not otherwise contraindicated for reasons of compatibility or patient sensitivity. It is present in over 70% of commercially produced eye drops and over a third of these also contain disodium edetate, usually at 0.1% w/v.

Rather surprisingly benzalkonium chloride is not a pure material, but is a mixture of alkylbenzyl-dimethyl ammonium compounds. This permits a mixture of alkyl chain lengths containing even numbers of carbon atoms between 8 and 18 and results in products of different activities. The higher the chain length the greater the antibacterial activity but the less the solubility. Therefore the manufacturer should seek to maximize the activity within the con-straints of solubility. This means maximizing the proportions of $C_{12}$, $C_{14}$ and $C_{16}$. It should be noted that Benzalkonium Chloride BP contains 50% w/v benzalkonium chloride.

Benzalkonium chloride is well tolerated on the eye up to concentrations of 0.02% w/v but is usually used at 0.01% w/v. It is stable to sterilization by autoclaving. The compound has a rapid bacteri-cidal action in clean conditions against a wide range of Gram-positive and Gram-negative organisms. It destroys the external structures of the cell (cell envelope). It is active in the controlled aqueous environment and pH values of ophthalmic solutions. Activity is reduced in the presence of multivalent cations ($Mg^{2+}$, $Ca^{2+}$). These compete with the antibacterial for negatively charged sites on the bacterial cell surface. It also has its activity reduced if heated with methylcellulose or formulated with anionic and certain concentrations of nonionic surfactants. Benzalkonium chloride is incompatible with fluorescein (large anion) and nitrates and is sorbed from solutions through contact with rubber.

The antibacterial activity of benzalkonium is enhanced by aromatic alcohols (benzyl alcohol, 2-phenylethanol and 3-phenylpropanol) and its activity against Gram-negative organisms is greatly enhanced by chelating agents such as disodium edetate. These agents chelate the divalent cations, principally $Mg^{2+}$ of Gram-negative cells. These ions form bridges and bind the polysaccharide chains which protrude from the outer membrane of these cells. Thus the integrity of the membrane is compromised and the benzalkonium chloride activity enhanced. This is particularly valuable in preserving against contamination with the most feared bacterial contaminant *P. aeruginosa*.

The surface activity of benzalkonium chloride may be used to enhance the transcorneal passage of non-lipid-soluble drugs such as carbachol. Care must be taken since the preservative can solubilize the outer oily protective layer of the precorneal film. This film has an internal mucin layer in contact with the corneal and scleral epithelia, a middle aqueous layer and an outer oily layer. The oil prevents excessive aqueous evaporation and protects the inner surface of the lids from constant contact with water. The blink reflex helps maintain the integrity of the precorneal film. It is important not to use benzalkonium chloride with local anaesthetics. The combination of the anaesthetic abolishing the blink reflex and the preservative solubilizing the oily layer results in drying of the eye and irritation of the cornea.

### Chlorhexidine acetate or gluconate

Chlorhexidine is a cationic biguanide bactericide with antibacterial properties in aqueous solution similar to benzalkonium chloride. Its activity is often reduced in the presence of other formulation ingredients. It is used at 0.01% w/v. Its antibacterial activity against Gram-negative bacteria is enhanced by aromatic alcohols and by disodium edetate. Activity is antagonized by multivalent cations. Stability is greatest at pH 5–6 but it is less stable to autoclaving than benzalkonium chloride. Chlorhexidine salts are generally well tolerated by the eye although allergic reactions may occur.

### Chlorbutol

This chlorinated alcohol is used at 0.5% w/v and is effective against bacteria and fungi. Chlorbutol is compatible with most ophthalmic products. The main disadvantages are its volatility, absorption by plastic containers and lack of stability at high temperatures. For example at autoclaving temperatures it breaks down to produce hydrochloric acid which produces solutions of pH 3–4. Although chlorbutol is more stable at low pH such solutions are not desirable for eye drops.

### Phenylmercuric salts

Phenylmercuric acetate and nitrate are organic mercurials and are used in the concentration range 0.001–0.04% w/v. They are slowly active over a wide pH range against bacteria and fungi. Activity is increased by phenylethanol and decreased by disodium edetate. Incompatibilities include halides. Absorption by rubber is marked.

Opinion is against using heavy metals as preservatives if there are suitable alternatives. The organic mercurials should not be used in eye drops which require prolonged usage because such use can lead to intraocular deposition of mercury (mercurialentis).

### Thiomersal

This is another organic mercurial and is used at a concentration of 0.005–0.01% w/v. Its action is bacteriostatic and fungistatic. Allergy to this preservative is possible.

## Tonicity

Where possible eye drops are made isotonic with lachrymal fluid (approximately equivalent to 0.9% w/v sodium chloride solution). In practice the eye will tolerate small volumes of eye drops having tonicities in the range equivalent to 0.7–1.5% w/v sodium chloride. Nevertheless it is good practice to adjust the tonicity of hypotonic eye drops by the addition of sodium chloride to bring the solution to the tonicity of the lachrymal fluid. Methods for calculating the amount of sodium chloride required are given in the *Pharmaceutical Codex* (1994). Likewise non-essential increases in the tonicity of hypertonic solutions should be avoided. Some preparations are themselves hypertonic and this cannot be avoided.

If the physiology of the eye is adversely affected, such as when tear film is deficient, or even where hard contact lenses are worn, then the eye surface is more sensitive to variations in tonicity and eye drops should be as near as possible isotonic.

## Viscosity enhancers

There is a general assumption that increasing the viscosity of an eye drop increases the residence time of the drop in the eye and results in increased penetration and therapeutic action of the drug. Most commercial preparations have their viscosities adjusted to be within the range 15–25 millipascal seconds (mPas). It should be noted that gently pressing downwards on the inside corner of the closed eye restricts the drainage channel into the nasal cavity and prolongs contact time. Under normal conditions a large proportion of a typical 50 μl drop will have drained from the conjunctival sac (capacity 25 μl) within 30 seconds. There will be no trace of the drop after 20 minutes.

Viscolizing agents include methylcellulose derivatives and polyvinyl alcohol.

### Hypromellose

The hydroxypropyl derivative of methylcellulose is the most popular cellulose derivative employed. It has good solubility characteristics (soluble in cold but insoluble in hot water) and good optical clarity. Typical concentrations in eye drop formulations are 0.5–2.0% w/v. Higher concentrations tend to form crusts on the eyelids.

### Polyvinyl alcohol

This is used at 1.4% w/v. It has a good contact time on the eye surface and good optical qualities. As well as withstanding autoclaving, it can be filtered through a 0.22 μm filter.

| Table 28.2 Buffers suitable for some specific eye drops | | |
|---|---|---|
| Borate buffer (boric acid/borax) pH range 6.8–9.1 | Phosphate buffer (sodium acid phosphate/sodium phosphate) pH range 4.5–8.5 | Citrate buffer (citric acid/sodium citrate) pH range 2.5–6.5 |
| Chloramphenicol eye drops BP 1993 – pH 7.5 | Neomycin eye drops BPC 1973 – pH 6.5 | Benzylpenicillin eye drops – pH 6.0 |
| Hypromellose eye drops BPC 1973 – pH 8.4 | Prednisolone sodium phosphate eye drops BPC 1973 – pH 6.6 | Idoxuridine eye drops – pH 6.0 |

Polyvinylpyrrolidone, polyethylene glycol and dextrin have also been used as viscolizing agents.

## pH adjustment

The best compromise is required after considering the following factors:

- the pH offering best stability during preparation and storage
- the pH offering the best therapeutic activity
- the comfort of the patient.

Most active ingredients are salts of weak bases and are most stable at an acid pH but most active at a slightly alkaline pH.

The lachrymal fluid has a pH of 7.2–7.4 and also possesses considerable buffering capacity. Thus a 50 μl eye drop which is weakly buffered will be rapidly neutralized by lachrymal fluid. Where possible very acidic solutions, such as adrenaline acid tartrate or pilocarpine hydrochloride, are buffered to reduce stinging on instillation. Suitable buffers are shown in Table 28.2.

## Antioxidants

Reducing agents are preferentially oxidized and are added to eye drops in order to protect the active ingredient from oxidation. Active ingredients requiring protection include adrenaline, proxymetacaine, sulphacetamide, amethocaine, phenylephrine and physostigmine. With physostigmine, the antioxidant is purely cosmetic as the initial breakdown product is formed by hydrolysis. The antioxidant only prevents the subsequent discoloration of this product produced by oxidation.

### Sodium metabisulphite and sodium sulphite

Both may be used as antioxidants at 0.1% w/v. The former is preferred at acid pH and the latter at alkaline pH. Both are stable in solution when protected from light. Sodium metabisulphite possesses marked antimicrobial properties at acid pH and enhances the activity of phenylmercuric nitrate at acid pH. It is incompatible with prednisolone phosphate, adrenaline, chloramphenicol and phenylephrine.

## Chelating agents

Traces of heavy metals can catalyse breakdown of the active ingredient by oxidation and other mechanisms. Therefore chelating agents such as disodium edetate may be included to chelate the metal ions and thus enhance stability. It is seen that disodium edetate is a very useful adjuvant to ophthalmic preparations at concentrations of up to 0.1% w/v to enhance antibacterial activity and chemical stability. It has also been used at higher concentrations as an eye drop for the treatment of lime burns in cattle.

## Bioavailability

The effect of pH on the therapeutic activity of weak bases such as atropine sulphate has already been indicated under the section on pH adjustment. At acid pH these bases exist in the ionized hydrophilic form. In order to penetrate the cornea, the bases need to be at alkaline pH so that they are in the unionized lipophilic form. Thus at tear pH (7.4) they are able to penetrate the outer lipid layer of the lipid–water–lipid sandwich which constitutes the physicochemical structure of the cornea. Once inside the epithelium the undissociated free base will partially dissociate. The water-soluble dissociated moiety will then traverse the middle aqueous stromal layer of the cornea. When the dissociated drug reaches the junction of the stroma and the endothelium it will again partially associate forming the lipid-soluble moiety and thus cross the endothelium. Finally the drug will dissociate into its water-soluble form and enter the aqueous humor. From here it can diffuse to the iris and the ciliary body which are the sites of its pharmacological action (Fig. 28.1). Thus it is seen that the most effective penetration of the lipophilic–hydrophilic–lipophilic corneal membrane is by active ingredients having both hydrophilic and lipophilic forms. For example, highly water-soluble steroid phosphate esters have poor corneal penetration but the less water-soluble, more lipophilic steroid acetate has much better corneal penetration.

This also explains why the more lipophilic dipivaly-ladrenaline 0.1% w/v is as active as 2% w/v of the more hydrophilic adrenaline.

## Storage conditions

To minimize degradation of eye drop ingredients storage temperature and conditions must be considered at the time of formulation. The stability of several drugs used in eye drops is improved by refrigerated storage (2–8°C) and the following eye drops are recommended for such storage in *Medicines, Ethics and Practice* (1996): Chloramphenicol, Eppy, Minims, Mydrilate, Neosporin, Otosporin, Sno-Phenicol and Sno-Pilo.

## Containers for eye drops

Containers should be regarded as part of the total formulation. They should protect the eye drops from microbial contamination, moisture and air. Container materials should not be shed or leached into solution neither should any of the eye drop formulation be sorbed by the container. If the product is to be sterilized in the final container all parts of the container must withstand the sterilization process used.

Containers may be made of glass or plastic and may be single or multiple dose. The latter should not contain more than 10 ml.

### Single dose containers

The 'Minims' range manufactured by Smith & Nephew Pharmaceuticals Ltd is the most widely used type of single dose eye drop container in the UK. It consists of an injection-moulded polypropylene container which is sealed at its base and has a nozzle sealed with a screw cap. This container is sterilized by autoclaving in an outer heat-sealed pouch with peel-off paper backing.

### Plastic bottles

Most commercially prepared eye drops are supplied in plastic dropper bottles similar to the illustration (Fig. 28.2). The bottles are made of polyethylene or polypropylene and are sterilized by ionizing radiation prior to filling under aseptic conditions with the previously sterilized preparation.

### Glass bottles

Most extemporaneously prepared eye drops are sup-

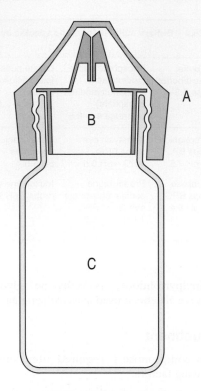

**Fig. 28.2**   Plastic eye drop bottle. A, Rigid plastic cap; B, polythene friction plug containing baffle that produces uniform drops; C, polythene bottle.

plied in 10 ml amber partially ribbed glass bottles as defined by British Standard 1679: Part 5 (1973, amended 1974).

The components of the eye dropper bottle are illustrated in Figure 28.3.

The important information to know about the bottle is the glass composition. The bottle is made of either neutral glass or soda glass which has had the internal surfaces treated during manufacture to reduce the release of alkali when in contact with aqueous solutions. The former bottles can be autoclaved more than once but the latter can only be autoclaved once.

Likewise it is necessary to know whether the teat is made of good quality natural or synthetic rubber. The former will withstand autoclaving at 115°C for 30 minutes but will not withstand the high temperatures of dry heat sterilization. The latter teats, made from silicone rubber, will withstand dry heat sterilization and are suitable for use with oily eye drops. Surprisingly silicone rubber is permeable to water vapour which was not realized initially. As a result aqueous suspensions sometimes became solid cakes! For this reason aqueous eye drops having silicone

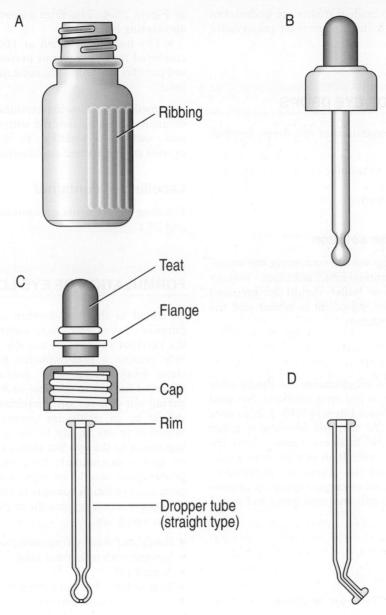

**Fig. 28.3** Eye dropper bottle to BS 1679; Part 5 (1974): (**A**) bottle; (**B**) assembled closure; (**C**) components of closure; (**D**) dropper tube (angled type). (Reproduced by permission of the British Standards Institution (complete copies can be obtained from BSI at Linford Wood, Milton Keynes, MK14 6LE).)

rubber teats are given a limited shelf life of 3 months. This can be lengthened by supplying the sterile eye drops in an eye drop bottle sealed with an ordinary screw cap together with a separately wrapped and sterilized silicone rubber dropper unit. The dropper is carefully substituted for the cap when the eye drops are about to be used.

Teats and caps are used once only. All components are thoroughly washed with filtered distilled or deionized water, dried and stored in a clean area until required.

Rubber teats sorb preservatives and antioxidants during autoclaving and storage. Generalized quantitative relationships for this process do not exist and it is necessary that individual studies are undertaken during formulation to help counteract preservative and antioxidant loss.

## PREPARATION OF EYE DROPS

Extemporaneous preparation of eye drops involves the following:

- preparation of the solution
- clarification
- filling and sterilization.

### Preparation of the solution

The aqueous eye drop vehicle containing any necessary preservative, antioxidant, stabilizer, tonicity modifier, viscolizer or buffer should be prepared first. Then the active ingredient is added and the vehicle made up to volume.

### Clarification

The BP has stringent requirements for the absence of particulate matter in eye drop solutions. Sintered glass filters or membrane filters of 0.45–1.2 µm pore sizes are suitable. The clarified solution is either filled directly into the final containers which are sealed prior to heat sterilization or filled into a suitable container prior to filtration sterilization. Clarified vehicle is used to prepare eye drop suspensions which are filled into final containers and sealed prior to sterilization.

### Sterilization

This can take the form of:

- Autoclaving at 115°C for 30 minutes or 121°C for 15 minutes.
- Heating at 98–100°C for 30 minutes together with either benzalkonium chloride 0.01% w/v or chlorhexidine acetate 0.01% w/v or phenylmercuric acetate or nitrate 0.002% w/v or thiomersal 0.01% w/v. This method is described in the BP (1980) but is no longer a pharmacopoeial recommended method.
- Filtration through a membrane filter having a 0.22 µm pore size into sterile containers using strict aseptic technique. Filling should take place under Grade A laminar airflow conditions. A suitable filter holder for extemporaneous preparation is illustrated

in Figure 28.4. The filter assembly is sterilized by autoclaving before use.

- Dry heat sterilization at 160°C for 2 hours is employed for non-aqueous preparations such as liquid paraffin eye drops. Silicone rubber teats must be used.

Immediately following sterilization the eye drop containers must be covered with a readily breakable seal, such as a viskring, to distinguish between opened and unopened containers.

### Labelling of container

Labelling requirements are summarized in Tables 28.3 and 28.4.

## FORMULATION OF EYE LOTIONS

As stated in the introduction to this chapter the purpose of eye lotions is to assist in the cleaning of the external surfaces of the eye. This might be to help remove a non-impacted foreign body or to clean away conjunctival discharge. Eye lotions intended for use in surgical or first-aid procedures should not contain antimicrobial preservatives and should be in single-use containers. There is no intention to use an eye lotion to deliver any active ingredient to the eye but rather to remove unwanted gross contaminants from the eye. Thus these preparations should be very simple and the most common eye lotion consists of sterile normal saline. This preparation typifies the requirements of an eye lotion which are:

- sterile and usually containing no preservative
- isotonic with lachrymal fluid
- neutral pH
- large volume but not greater than 200 ml
- non-irritant to ocular tissue.

### Labels

These should include:

- title identifying the product and concentration of contents
- 'Sterile until opened'
- 'Not to be taken'
- 'Use once and discard the remaining solution'
- expiry date.

Preserved eye lotion would need the additional labelling:

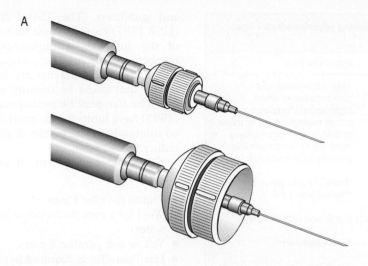

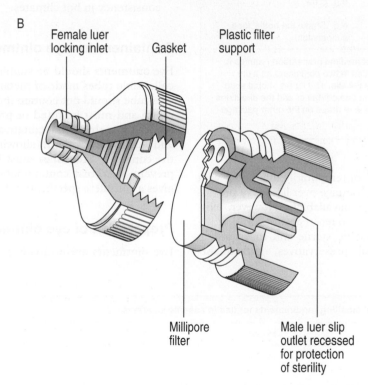

Female luer
locking inlet    Gasket

Plastic filter
support

Millipore
filter

Male luer slip
outlet recessed
for protection
of sterility

**Fig. 28.4** Swinnex holders for bacterial filters: (**A**) 13 mm and 25 mm types fitted to syringes; (**B**) cutaway view of 25 mm type (courtesy of Millipore (UK) Ltd).

- 'Avoid contamination of contents during use'
- 'Discard remaining solutions not more than 4 weeks after first opening'.

The lotions should be supplied in coloured fluted bottles and sealed to exclude microorganisms.

## FORMULATION OF EYE OINTMENTS

Eye ointments are popular and duplicate many of the therapeutic options offered by eye drops. Ointments

**Table 28.3    General labelling requirements for eye drop containers**

| Requirement | Include on label |
|---|---|
| Fully identify the product | Title: either name and concentration of active ingredients or reference to official monograph giving these details. If monograph allows more than one concentration then state the one used |
| Specify storage conditions | 'Store in a cool place' or 'Protect from light' |
| State product expiry date | Month and year of expiry |
| Warning label | 'Not to be taken' |
| Specify volume | e.g. '5 ml' |
| Ensure correct use | e.g. 'Shake the bottle' for a suspension |

*NB:* When the stability of the final preparation requires it, eye drops may be provided in two containers as a dry powder and an aqueous vehicle. The labels should state 'Powder for eye drops' on one container and the directions for the preparation of the eye drops on the other package or container.

and stabilizers. The *United States Pharmacopoeia* (USP 1995) requires these ointments to contain one of the following antimicrobials: chlorbutol, the parabens or the organic mercurials. It is necessary also that such ointments are free from particulate matter that could be harmful to the tissues of the eye. The *European Pharmacopoeia* (EP 1996) and BP (1993) have limits for the particle size of incorporated solids which will be met if all particles have been reduced to <25 µm.

The basic components of an eye ointment are given below:

- Liquid paraffin 1 part
- Wool fat 1 part (to facilitate incorporation of water)
- Yellow soft paraffin 8 parts
- Hard paraffin as required to produce required consistency in hot climates.

## Containers for eye ointments

Eye ointments should be supplied in small sterilized collapsible tubes made of metal or a suitable plastic. The tube should not contain more than 5 g of preparation and must be fitted or provided with a nozzle of a suitable shape to facilitate application to the eye and surrounds without allowing contamination of the contents. The tubes must be suitably sealed to prevent microbial contamination. BS 4230 (1967) gives a complete specification for metal tubes.

## Preparation of eye ointments

Eye ointments are normally prepared using aseptic

have the disadvantage of temporarily interfering with vision, but have the advantage over liquids of providing greater total drug bioavailability. However, ointments take a longer time to reach peak absorption.

Eye ointments must be sterile and may contain suitable antimicrobial preservatives, antioxidants

**Table 28.4    Additional labelling requirements for use in specific locations**

| | Hospital | | | Domiciliary |
|---|---|---|---|---|
| All locations | Wards | Operating theatres | Clinics | |
| Include concentration of active ingredient and name and concentration of any antimicrobial present | Patient's name. The eye to be treated.* Date of opening bottle and/or date to discard (7 days later) | Single dose for once-only use. Marked with indication and concentration of active ingredient according to approved code BP 1993 A204. No preservative. Outer package fully labelled | Single dose or multidose used once only | 'Avoid contamination of contents during use' 'Discard 4 weeks after opening' 'Keep out of the reach of children' Plus instructions on how to use, e.g. 'Add one drop to each eye morning and evening |

*If both eyes are to be treated a separate bottle is supplied for each eye and labelled accordingly.

techniques to incorporate the finely powdered active ingredient or a sterilized concentrated solution of the medicament into the sterile eye ointment basis. Immediately after preparation the eye ointment is filled into the sterile containers which are then sealed so as to exclude microorganisms. The screw cap should be covered with a readily breakable seal.

All apparatus used in the preparation of eye ointments must be scrupulously clean and sterile.

Certain commercial eye ointments may be sterilized in their final containers using ionizing radiation.

### Preparation of eye ointment basis

The paraffins and the wool fat are heated together and filtered, while molten, through a coarse filter paper in a heated funnel into a container which can withstand dry heat sterilization temperatures. The container is closed to exclude microorganisms and together with contents is maintained at 160°C for 2 hours (BP 1993, Appendix XVIII).

## Labelling

This includes the following:

- the names and percentages of the active ingredients
- the date after which the eye ointment is not intended to be used
- the conditions under which the eye ointment should be stored – normally at a temperature not exceeding 25°C
- the name and concentration of any antimicrobial preservative or other substance added to the preparation
- a statement to the effect that the contents are sterile providing the container has not been opened.

## CONTACT LENSES AND THEIR SOLUTIONS

The ready accessibility of the eye and its external structures not only facilitates the use of topical medications in the conjunctival sac and on the anterior surface of the eye but also facilitates the fitting and wearing of lenses on the precorneal film and on the surface of the eye.

## Popularity, problems, risks

The popularity of contact lenses results from their cosmetic appeal, optical advantages and their usefulness in sporting activities. Many prefer extended-wear soft lenses to daily-wear soft and hard lenses because of their relative convenience.

The problems that occur with the wearing of contact lenses result from inadequate education of the wearer about lens care. Extended-wear lenses in particular have been marketed in a manner which maximizes the volume of sales at the expense of adequate consumer education. That is, the marketing of lenses has overemphasized the convenient and carefree aspects of overnight lenses to the extent of trivializing the wearing of contact lenses. This has often resulted in poor patient compliance with suggested regimes of lens wear and care. It is estimated that more than 50% of those who wear contact lenses care for them unhygienically.

The risks associated with the wearing of contact lenses include recurrent corneal abrasions, corneal scarring and corneal vascularization. However, the most dreaded complication is microbial ulcerative keratitis or corneal ulcer, caused by bacterial invasion of the cornea. Left untreated this can lead to loss of vision. Fortunately the natural defences of the cornea are very effective and the normal cornea resists bacterial infection as long as the surface epithelium is intact.

It has been shown that the risk of corneal ulcers is 9–15 times greater for extended-wear lenses worn overnight than for daily-wear soft lenses worn only during the day. The risk increases with the number of consecutive days that lenses are worn without removal.

A serious, but fairly rare, complication that can arise from using non-sterile water in the care of lenses is infection with *Acanthamoeba* which is hard to diagnose and to treat and can lead to serious loss of vision.

The aim of formulators and providers of contact lens systems must be to supply the safest possible system with known and acceptable risks; that is, convenience and safety must be the aim.

## Relevant properties of the eye

### Anatomy and physiology

Figure 28.1 indicates the structures of the eye which are particularly relevant to the use of topical medications, contact lenses and contact lens products. Firstly, it is important to note that the cornea, the lens and the humor compartments are avascular and that this property facilitates the transmission of light and vision. Secondly, exchange of nutrients and waste products in these situations takes place almost entirely by diffusion processes through the aqueous humor, through the lens and cornea and through the lachrymal fluid. Contact lenses reduce the diffusion of oxygen to the cornea and thus can affect corneal metabolism.

### Secretions

The secretions of the eye have an important role and influence on the wearing of contact lenses. Tears perform the important functions of lubricating, hydrating, cleaning and disinfecting the anterior surface of the eye. The latter function is performed by the enzyme lysozyme (1,4-*N*-acetylglycosaminidase) which catalyses the hydrolysis of 1,4-glycosidic linkages between *N*-acetyl muramic acid and *N*-acetyl-glucosamine in the peptidoglycan layer of the bacterial cell wall. The peptidoglycan layer of Gram-positive cells is accessible to the action of lysozyme.

### Lachrymal fluid

The fluid forming the precorneal film is produced by differing groups of glands. It contains mucus (Henle and Manz), water (Krause and Wolfring) and oil (Meibomian, Moll and Zeis). These fluids are stratified in three distinct layers. The surface-active mucoid layer spreads on the corneal surface and associates with the intermediate aqueous layer externally. The aqueous layer is surfaced with an oily layer which lubricates and protects the mucous membranes of the internal lid surfaces.

### Tear electrolyte content

This is broadly similar to that of serum except that the potassium ion is approximately four to six times greater (24 milliequivalents/litre compared with 4–6 mEq/l in serum). The protein content of tears is mainly albumin and globulin and is approximately a tenth of that in serum (0.7% compared with 7%).

### Tear production

Tears are produced in response to four distinct types of stimuli: emotional via psychological factors, sensory via external irritants, continuous via automatic nervous control and systemic via chemicals in the bloodstream affecting the nerves innovating the lachrymal glands.

### Tear pH

This is slightly alkaline at 7.2. Tears have sufficient buffering capacity to adjust rapidly the pH of small volumes of weakly buffered solutions to pH 7.2.

### Eyelids

These perform a protecting and a cleaning function. The outer margins of the eyelids close slightly before the inner margins and sweep the fluids across the eye towards the lachrymal duct at the inner angle of the eye and into the nasal chamber. Systemic absorption of excess eye medicament may take place via the nasal mucosa through this mechanism. Conversely, by gentle pressure with the tip of a finger, the lachrymal duct may be closed temporarily and eye medicament maintained in contact with the eye surface for a longer period.

### Bacterial flora

There is a common misconception that lachrymal fluid is sterile. It has been known since 1908 that staphylococci and diphtheroids can be found regularly in normal conjunctiva. Gram-negative enteric bacilli have also been isolated from the conjunctivas and lids of about 5% of people. This shows that care is necessary when wearing contact lenses to avoid abrading the corneal epithelium.

## CONTACT LENSES

Sir John Herschel used a refractive glass shell in 1823 to protect the cornea from a diseased lid. The term 'contact lens' was first used by Dr Eugen Fick, a Swiss physician, in 1887. Fick's blown glass lenses were intended to correct defective vision. In 1948 Tuohy introduced the hydrophobic hard plastic corneal lens and in 1962 soft pliable lenses were introduced as the result of work in Prague University. These lenses have been very popular. Gas-permeable hard lenses have also been introduced which allow oxygen perfusion to the cornea. These lenses are more comfortable than the original hard lenses.

The aim in making contact lenses is to produce lenses which will:

- correct the patient's vision
- maintain their position on the eye
- allow respiration of the cornea
- permit free flow of tears round or through the lens

- not release toxic substances
- not introduce microbial contamination
- be wearable throughout the day
- be easy to handle and economical to use.

## Hard lenses

Methacrylic acid is esterified to produce the basic monomer methyl methacrylate which is polymerized using benzoyl peroxide as catalyst to produce poly-methyl methacrylate. This is popularly called 'Perspex' and has optical properties similar to specta-cle crown glass. Polymethyl methacrylate has hydrophobic properties conferred by the large proportion of methyl groups compared to hydrophilic carboxy ester groups. This means that lachrymal fluid does not readily wet lenses made of this material. Therefore the lenses need to be wetted before mounting on the precorneal film to reduce or eliminate patient discomfort. Hence the need for a wetting solution to facilitate wear and the need for a storage, hydrating, decontaminating solution to facilitate care of the lenses when not being worn. The original hard lens composition had some major disadvantages for the wearer. Free passage of oxygen and carbon dioxide to and from the corneal epithelium could not take place. Corneal oedema and distortion were a common result. Thus modern lenses have been designed to be gas permeable. These lenses are physiologically more user-friendly and have greater wearer acceptance.

The original gas-permeable lenses consisted of cellulose acetate butyrate (CAB) which was readily wettable and proved quite acceptable. More recently lenses based on silicone and fluorine have been produced which have greater gas permeability. Silicone methacrylate copolymers are very popular. The silicone composition controls the permeability properties and the polymethyl methacrylate composition controls the degree of rigidity. Similarly fluorosilicone methacrylate copolymers which have very high oxygen permeability properties and good wetting properties are proving to be popular. These gas-permeable lenses are cared for using hard lens solutions. These lenses are less subject than soft lenses to deposits of lipids, protein and other substances from the lachrymal fluid. They also have better optical qualities and are generally easier to care for.

## Soft lenses

The hydroxyethyl ester of polymethacrylic acid (poly-HEMA) is prepared. The large number of polar hydroxyl groups confer hydrophilic properties to the polymer. Poly-HEMA is flexible and can absorb about 47% of its own weight of water. Thus lenses of this material are comfortable and easy to wear but more difficult to care for than hard lenses. A particular problem is uptake of antibacterial preservatives and subsequent release and irritancy during wear. Although a wetting solution is not needed, cleaning, storing, hydrating and decontaminating functions are required of solutions.

Copolymers of poly-HEMA with vinylpyrrolidine (VP) are also produced which can absorb up to 80% by weight of water depending on the HEMA/VP ratio. The higher water content lenses have the advantage of greater gas permeability and comfort than the poly-HEMA lenses which may occasionally cause corneal oedema. However, they are more fragile and difficult to care for than poly-HEMA, have a greater tendency to attract deposits, more solution problems and less precise optical properties.

## Disposable lenses

It is argued that lens design, life span and manufacturing problems can be overcome by the introduction of disposable lenses. Disposable lenses may be discarded after 1 month, 1 week or even 1 day. The latter would obviate the need for the use of solutions and theoretically increase the safety and acceptability of lens wear. However, the original intention of these lenses was for extended wear without removal. It has already been pointed out that the additional risks associated with extended wear makes this an unattractive and even dangerous practice. These lenses would seem to offer the greatest advantage to those people who wear lenses on an irregular basis for social and sporting activities and for those children who may need soft lenses.

## HARD LENS SOLUTIONS

A 'wetting solution' and a 'soaking/storing/decontaminating solution' are required for the wear and routine care of hard lenses. The first is suitable for placing in the eye but the second must not have contact with the eye.

### Wetting solution

*Purpose*

- Achieves rapid wetting by the lachrymal fluid and thus promotes comfort.
- Facilitates insertion of lens.

- Provides cushioning and lubricating.
- Enables cleaning after removal.
- Must be non-irritant during daily use.

*Formulation*

- Wetting and viscolizing agents – polyvinyl alcohol and hypromellose.
- Viscosity 15–20 mPas for comfort.
- pH 6.8.
- Tonicity ≡ 0.9–1.1% sodium chloride.
- Antimicrobials – benzalkonium chloride 0.004% plus disodium edetate 0.1%.

## Storing solutions

*Purpose*

- Achieves cleaning and microbial inactivation.
- Hydrating.

*Formulation*

- Surface-active agent not inactivating antimicrobials.
- pH 7.4.
- Antimicrobials – benzalkonium chloride 0.01% plus disodium edetate 0.1%.

# SOFT LENS SOLUTIONS

## Cleaning solutions

*Purpose*

- To remove deposits such as lipoprotein adhering to the lens after wear.

*Formulation*

- Viscolizing surface-active agent such as hypromellose to enable suitable gentle friction with fingertips.
- Antibacterial – fast-acting benzalkonium chloride 0.004% may be used if contact time is only 20–30 seconds.

## Storing solutions

*Purpose*

- Hydrating.

- Cleaning.
- Inactivation of microbial contamination.

*Formulation*

- Isotonic ≡ 0.9% sodium chloride.
- Antibacterial – 3% hydrogen peroxide for 30 minutes followed by suitable inactivation with sodium pyruvate, or platinum catalyst, or other suitable method to facilitate subsequent safe wearing of lens. Hydrogen peroxide has the additional advantage of good activity against *Acanthamoeba* contamination.

## Enzyme protein digest

*Purpose*

- Occasional cleaning procedure followed by suitable washing and cleansing before wear. Frequency will vary with the individual and his/her state of health. Influenza or hay fever for example will increase the need.

*Formulation*

- Proteolytic enzyme, such as papain, as a solution tablet to produce a suitable solution when dissolved in a stated volume of aqueous vehicle.

Lipid digest or combined protein and lipid digest systems are also available.

## All-purpose solutions

These have been available for hard lens wearers who have found compliance with a two-solution regimen difficult to adhere to. The all-purpose solutions have represented a compromise and have not been as effective as two-solution regimens, but have been far superior to using no solution. Single-solution lens care systems are now available for soft lenses. The majority of such all-purpose soft lens solutions incorporate polyhexamide (polyhexamethylene biguanide) 0.00006–0.0004% as the antimicrobial agent. It is reported to be active against a wide range of bacteria and against *Acanthamoeba*. Such solutions would appear to be gaining in popularity.

## Containers

Contact lens solutions are usually packed in plastic containers. It is imperative that the low concentrations of antimicrobials present in these products are not reduced to ineffective levels due to sorption effects with the plastic.

Contact lens storage cases are also of importance to the contact lens wearer. It is important that these containers are kept in a hygienic condition by keeping them scrupulously clean and using the disinfecting/storage solutions strictly in accordance with the manufacturers' instructions.

## Advice to patients

Contact lens wearers presenting at the pharmacy with a persistent red eye indicating an infection should not be recommended Brolene eye drops. They should be referred to an ophthalmologist. This is to guard against the possibility that the person might have an infection with *Acanthamoeba*. Such an infection would be more difficult to diagnose after treatment with preparations containing propamidine isethionate.

### Information sheets on contact lens products

The Medicines (Contact lens fluids and other substances) (Advertising and Miscellaneous amendments) regulations 1979 (SI 1979 No. 1760) define the type of information to be provided on information sheets for these products.

### Effect of medication and physical condition

It should be noted that certain medication can affect the eye surface and lachrymal fluid production and thereby influence the comfort of contact lens wear. Medication having anticholinergic properties such as sedative antihistamines (chlorpheniramine), antispasmodics (hyoscine), tricyclic antidepressants and neuroleptics can all reduce lachrymal fluid production. The consequent lack of lubrication may cause lens discomfort from lack of lubrication and increased lens deposits.

Oral contraceptives may cause corneal oedema, decreased aqueous and increased mucus and protein production and thus lead to lens intolerance.

Pregnancy may also be associated with increased lens awareness and discomfort possibly associated with reduced tear flow and changes in corneal thickness and the curvature of the eye.

Disease states leading to a dry eye syndrome such as Sjögren's syndrome which is mostly confined to menopausal women having osteoarthritis will also adversely affect the ability of a person to wear contact lenses.

Oral administration of certain medication such as labetalol, nitrofurantoin, phenolphthalein, rifampicin, sulphasalazine and tetracyclines may cause lens discolouration via the lachrymal fluid.

The pharmacist should be aware of these various possibilities when discussing customers/patients' questions.

---

### Key Points

- Ophthalmic preparations must be sterile.
- Eye drops contain:
  - active ingredient
  - liquid vehicle free from particulate matter
  - antimicrobial preservative
  - adjuvants: tonicity, viscosity, pH, antioxidants, chelating agents.
- Eye drops are contained in a glass or plastic bottle.
- Eye lotions are:
  - isotonic
  - neutral pH
  - large volume but not greater than 200 ml
  - non-irritant
  - contained in a fluted, coloured bottle.
- Eye ointments contain:
  - semi-solid base
  - active ingredient
  - antimicrobial preservative
  - adjuvants: antioxidants, stabilizers.
- Eye ointments are:
  - free from harmful particulate matter
  - contained in a metal or plastic tube.
- Properties of the eye affecting formulation of products include:
  - anatomy and physiology
  - secretions
  - lids
  - bacterial flora.
- Contact lenses may be:
  - hard lenses including gas permeable
  - soft lenses including disposable.
- Contact lens solutions may be:
  a. Hard lenses:
     - wetting and cleaning
     - storing and disinfecting
     - all purpose
  b. Soft lenses:
     - cleaning
     - storing and disinfecting
     - all purpose .
- Enzyme cleaning agents are required for all lenses

---

# FURTHER READING

British Pharmacopoeia 1993 HMSO, London

British Standard 1679 1973 Specification for containers for pharmaceutical dispensing Part 5. Eye dropper bottles (amended 1974). British Standards Institution, London

European Pharmacopoeia 1996 3rd edn. Maisonneuve S.A., Saint Ruffine, France

Medicines, Ethics and Practice – a guide for pharmacists 1996 The Royal Pharmaceutical Society of Great Britain, London (Updated twice yearly – use current edn)

Pharmaceutical Codex 1994 12th edn. The Pharmaceutical Press, London

The Medicines (Contact lens fluids and other substances) (Advertising and Miscellaneous amendments) regulations 1979 (SI 1979 No. 1760)

United States Pharmacopoeia 23 1995 Mack, Easton, PA

# 29

# The principles of quality assurance

*D. G. Chapman*

---

After studying this chapter you will know about:

**Terminology and definitions associated with quality**
**The nature of quality assurance systems**
**Application of quality assurance to**:
  Good manufacturing practice
  Quality control
  Standards
  Personnel and 'qualified person'
  Premises and equipment
  Documentation
  Production
  Complaints and product recall
**Quality audits**
**Sterile product manufacture**.

## Introduction

Very complex and potent medicines have been developed in recent times. These medicines have very high research, development and production costs. The special nature of these products requires a high level of product consistency. The medicines are produced by highly regulated processes. The consumers of these medicines, namely the patients, also have a high expectation of product quality. They also have a right to expect quality. All of these factors have resulted in the need for advanced quality assurance systems in the batch production of medicines.

### Useful definitions

*Quality assurance.* All systems which ensure that manufactured products are of the required quality for use.

*Good manufacturing practice.* Ensures that products are consistently produced. The standard of quality must be suitable for use.

*Quality control.* Ensures that a satisfactory quality of materials and products is used. This will involve sampling, testing, documentation and release procedures. Only when materials and products are of a satisfactory quality are they released for use.

*Product design.* All factors involved with the design of the product must be selected to achieve a quality product.

*Process development.* The production process must be designed to produce a quality product. It must allow for any deviations which arise in the production process.

*Validation.* The procedure which is used to prove that the various production procedures, equipment and materials will produce accurate results.

## A QUALITY ASSURANCE (QA) SYSTEM

In the large-scale production of medicines quality is not achieved by accident. It is the result of a carefully constructed quality assurance system. This system must ensure that each medicinal product conforms with its intended use. This applies in terms of safety, therapeutic effectiveness and acceptability. It is important that quality is built into the product. This applies at all stages of the manufacturing process. It is not adequate that the product is only tested retrospectively at the end of the manufacturing process.

A quality assurance system is constructed by merging a series of actions. These actions collectively ensure product quality. As a result, the quality assurance system must:

1. establish specific activities before production begins
2. control factors during production
3. evaluate results following production.

The quality assurance system in a pharmaceutical production unit can be likened to the railings on a

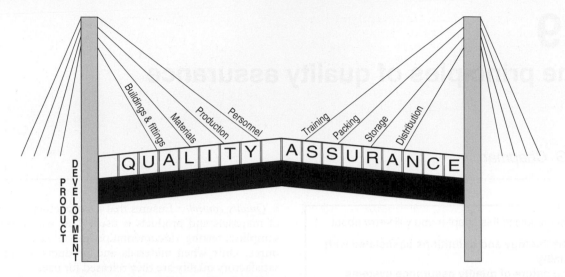

**Fig. 29.1** The production bridge (adapted from Goldberger 1991).

suspension bridge (Fig. 29.1). The bridge spans the production process from the initial stages of product development to the final marketing of the product. The span of the bridge is supported by suspension wires. These wires represent a range of production functions carried out in the manufacturing plant. Collectively the functions form the complete production process.

The senior management of a manufacturing facility is responsible for obtaining a quality product. However, to obtain total control of quality requires an organized effort. This is required by the entire production workforce. It is also required by the suppliers of materials and by the final product distributors. It may be beneficial if the manager of quality assurance is involved with the production team as a coach, counsellor, or teacher. This is carried out in the interests of acceptability by the workforce. By adopting these various roles, the manager is promoting quality assurance in the workplace. This ultimately results in an improved quality of product.

Differences exist in the organization of a quality assurance system in each manufacturing facility. However, there are certain fundamental features of any quality system. These features include:

- a quality policy which defines the purpose and objectives of the pharmaceutical manufacturing facility; it also outlines the ways in which these objectives will be achieved
- resources which include materials, equipment and personnel

- documentation which includes procedures and standards
- an audit process to provide assurance that procedures have been complied with; this process can also be used to improve the quality system.

In a pharmaceutical production process, quality assurance is involved in the following activities:

| | |
|---|---|
| purchasing | dispatching |
| warehousing | operational protocols |
| manufacturing | training |
| quality control | validation. |
| packaging | |

Rigorously designed procedures must be used to achieve a quality system for each of these activities. Each system must be detailed and monitored both during and after the activity. The systems for each of the listed activities must provide:

- assurance that materials, product, labelling and storage have conformed to an established programme of operation
- monitoring to ensure that the system is complied with or updated.

With a system of quality assurance integrated into a manufacturing process, simply making a product well is insufficient. The production processes must be carried out according to good manufacturing practice. All processes must be monitored. This applies both during and after the activity. Details of the manufacturing procedures must be entered onto documents known as records. Records must account for all the procedures which have been carried out during manufacture. The records form a history of the production process. These records are available for further study. Any changes to the manufacturing processes and procedures must comply with specified procedures. As a result of these actions in the production process, the quality assurance system will:

- ensure quality
- provide evidence
- generate confidence.

Implementing a quality assurance system in a manufacturing facility is expensive. However, these costs are greatly outweighed by the benefits of a quality assurance system. The benefits of a quality assurance system include:

- higher standards of production
- compliance with regulatory requirements
- reduced waste
- less risk of product defects.

Quality assurance is an all-embracing function. The concept includes not only manufacturing but all the other factors which affect the quality of the manufactured product. This extends from the initial stages of product development to the final stages of product distribution. With the manufacture of medicines, the quality assurance system is also involved with product recall from the market place.

Quality assurance must be distinguished from quality control which is concerned with specifications, sampling and testing. On its own, quality control cannot provide the necessary assurance of product quality. Quality control is only one component of the multi-component quality assurance system.

Quality assurance in pharmaceutical manufacturing is concerned with good manufacturing practice and quality control systems. It is also involved with product design and process development. Ultimately, all these areas contribute to assuring product quality. The concepts of good manufacturing practice, quality control, product design and process development are interrelated and encapsulated by the term 'quality assurance'. This concept is illustrated in Figure 29.2.

Quality assurance is involved with product design. This begins in the initial stages of product development. Factors such as the route of administration, formulation and packaging are incorporated into product design. All these factors must be carefully considered to produce a quality product. In addition, the product must be designed to allow for process development. Manufacture of a batch must

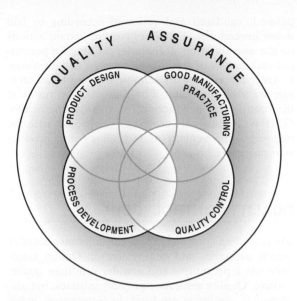

**Fig. 29.2** Relationships within quality assurance in pharmaceutical manufacturing.

ensure that each product, e.g. each tablet, exhibits a consistent quality. To achieve this objective, the manufacturing systems must have some flexibility. This will allow for variables which may arise during the production process, yet produce a consistent quality of product.

Within the European Union a system of marketing approvals is designed to ensure that all medicinal products are assessed by a competent authority. These medicines must be produced by authorized manufacturers. Within the UK this competent authority is the Medicines Control Agency. This agency ensures the safety, quality and efficacy of the product. A licence to manufacture is required by manufacturers of medicines in the European Union. This applies to products sold either within or outside Europe.

## GOOD MANUFACTURING PRACTICE FOR MEDICINAL PRODUCTS (GMP)

The principles of GMP are applied to the manufacture of medicines for both human and veterinary use. The principles of GMP also apply in the hospital production of medicines for use in clinical trials and for wholesaling.

GMP ensures that manufacturing processes are

defined, validated and reviewed according to laid down procedures. This does require certain actions by the manufacturer. It includes training for personnel and the use of suitable equipment and premises. Correct materials with suitable transport and storage are also necessary. These procedures result in the consistent production of quality medicines. GMP is continuously evolving. This occurs with the ongoing improvement of technology and production processes.

## QUALITY CONTROL (QC)

There is often confusion about the difference between quality assurance and quality control. Quality assurance has a preventive and a wider role than quality control. Quality assurance not only initiates, but also promotes, quality in products. In comparison, quality control carries out an analytical function. It is involved with controlling the quality of components and products. To perform this function, quality control uses physical, chemical and other test methods. In effect, quality control has a verifying role. It acts after an event, but does not prevent errors or poor manufacturing practices occurring in the workplace. For example, quality control must identify a faulty batch of product and avoid its distribution for use. To achieve this, tests must be carried out. As a result of these tests, quality control must provide a verdict on the batch of product by passing or failing it. Quality assurance is involved with quality control in exactly the same way as it is involved with other functions. It approves test methods and standards and ensures that high standards, which must conform with good laboratory practice, are being maintained within the quality control facility.

In small organizations a single manager may be responsible for both quality control and quality assurance. However, workers in the production facility may have trouble accepting the situation where the person who controls quality also assures quality. In the larger organization there may be a separate manager for each of these roles.

## STANDARDS

In 1991 the European Union issued directives which laid down principles and guidelines of GMP for medicinal products for human and veterinary medicines. The directive on human medicines came into force on 1 January 1993. The veterinary directive was implemented on 23 July 1993.

The directive for the production of human medicines is detailed in Volume IV of the Rules Governing Medicinal Products in the European Community (Commission of the European Communities 1992). It is entitled 'Good Manufacturing Practice for Medicinal Products'. It is a statutory requirement that manufacturers in the European Union must ensure that medicines are made, packaged and distributed according to the these rules. The European document has been incorporated into the 1997 publication from the Medicines Control Agency. This document is entitled *Rules and Guidance for Pharmaceutical Manufacturers*. As with previous editions, this text is bound in an orange cover. It has thus become known as the 'Orange Guide'. The 'Orange Guide' contains the main regulations, directives and guidance that a manufacturer is expected to follow when making a medicine.

## PERSONNEL

Everyone involved with the manufacture of a medicinal product must have quality at the forefront of their thinking. They must build quality into every aspect of their work – 'Quality Rules – OK!'. Each individual must ensure that every step and every component involved with the manufacturing process is rigorously performed. This will help to ensure that the required quality is contained within the product. Most defects in manufactured medicinal products arise through human error or carelessness. This is a clear indication of the need for quality procedures by the workforce. The personnel involved with the production of medicines should be aware of the principles of GMP that affect them. They should be given initial and continuing training to suit their working procedures. Details of the training which the workforce receive should be documented.

All new personnel should receive a medical examination. Persons with potentially infectious diseases or open wounds should not be involved with the manufacture of medicinal products. Appropriate garments should be worn by personnel working in the manufacturing areas. Care should be taken to avoid contact between the hands of personnel and the exposed product or the equipment which may contact the product. Unhygienic practices by personnel within the production areas must be avoided. Food, drink or smoking materials are excluded from the production areas.

There are three important personnel employed in a manufacturing unit. These are the production manager, the quality control manager and the qualified person. The production manager and the quality control manager must be different individuals. They must act independently of each other.

## The qualified person

The qualified person, commonly known as the 'QP', is the individual who is ultimately responsible for ensuring that each manufactured batch of product has been suitably produced and tested. The QP is responsible for releasing each batch of product for use. It is important that the actions carried out by the QP are detailed on records. Within a manufacturing unit there must be sufficient QPs to carry out all the tasks which are the responsibility of the manufacturer.

## PREMISES AND EQUIPMENT

The premises and equipment must be designed and constructed to suit the manufacturing operations. The premises must also be suitably maintained for the production processes. Both the premises and the production equipment should be designed and positioned to minimize the risks of errors during the manufacturing process. The cleaning and maintenance of the production equipment and premises should be easy. This will reduce the risk of cross-contamination and the build-up of dust. As a result of these actions there should be less risk of adverse effects which could affect the quality of the manufactured products.

## DOCUMENTATION

Good documentation of the procedures involved with the production of pharmaceutical products is an essential part of a quality assurance system. All documents involved with the manufacture of medicines must be clearly written. They must also be set out logically and be free of errors. The documents must be approved, signed and dated by authorized personnel such as the head of production. The documents used in the manufacture of medicines provide details of:

• Specifications. These documents detail the

materials to be used during the procedures. They will also specify the packaging materials.
• Manufacturing formulae and instructions for processing and packaging.
• Procedures for carrying out processes such as the operation of equipment and the sampling and testing of materials. These documents are commonly known by the self-descriptive term: standard operating procedures (SOPs).
• Production records such as batch manufacturing records and batch packaging records. These documents form a record of the appropriate activity.

The use of these documents avoids potential errors which could arise from verbal communication. The documents used in the manufacturing process should be reviewed and updated at timed intervals such as every 1 or 2 years. The timing for the review is frequently specified on the document. When a document has been revised, it is important that the superseded document is not used. A system should exist to continuously overcome this potential problem.

During the manufacturing processes, it is imperative that the required details are entered onto the appropriate documents at the time of the event and not entered subsequently. With this system of entering data onto a document, the information is then available for subsequent inspection. The entries on documents act as a history of the production process. If a change is required to an entry on a document, the original entry must remain visible. The change must be signed and dated. The reason for the alteration must also be noted on the document.

The documents used in the manufacturing process must be kept for at least 1 year beyond the expiry date of the product. However, manufacturers frequently keep their documents for a longer period.

As an alternative to paper documentation, manufacturing facilities are increasingly using electronic data processing systems. However, it is important that only authorized personnel should be able to access or modify the data contained in the electronic storage system. Access to the electronic data system, which usually employs computer facilities, is frequently regulated using a password entry system. The use of a password also restricts both the type and the amount of data accessible to the operator using the electronic storage system. As with paper documents, any changes to the electronically stored information must be recorded.

## PRODUCTION

Production operations must follow clearly defined procedures. The operations must comply with the principles of GMP. This is necessary to produce the required quality of product and comply with the manufacturing and marketing authorizations. The measures taken to prevent cross-contamination of starting materials and products should be regularly assessed. Validation studies are used to reinforce GMP and are carried out according to specified procedures.

Guidelines are detailed for the purchase, delivery, labelling, and storage of starting materials. The purchase, handling and control of starting materials, including primary packaging and printed packaging materials (see Ch. 6), should be carefully examined. The processing and packaging operations are carried out according to defined procedures. Following production, the finished products are held in a pre-release store, also known as 'quarantine' by some manufacturers. The products will remain in the pre-release store until they are released for use or sale. These products must fulfil all the conditions which have been set up by the manufacturer. They are then released for use by the manufacturer.

Rejected materials and products should be clearly identified as 'rejected'. They must be separated from the materials which are suitable for use. This is necessary to avoid mix-up between the rejected materials and the materials or the products which are suitable for use.

Rejected materials should either be returned to the suppliers or, where appropriate, reprocessed or destroyed.

## QUALITY CONTROL IN PRACTICE

Each manufacturing facility which has a manufacturing authorization should have a quality control department. This department should be independent of other departments. The quality control department operates under the authority of an experienced manager. However, quality control personnel will need to access production areas for sampling and investigation. Certain test procedures may be carried out during production processes by personnel involved with the manufacturing operation, such as 'positioning' settle plates in clean rooms to establish the microbial contamination of the environment. However, the procedures which these operators carry out must conform with methods that have been approved by quality control.

As detailed above, quality control is concerned with sampling, specifications and testing. It is also involved with the organization, documentation and release procedures. These procedures are established to ensure that the necessary tests are performed.

The tests carried out by quality control ensure that the materials are suitable for use and the products are suitable for sale or supply. All of these quality control tests are carried out according to written procedures using analytical methods that have been validated. The results of these tests require to be detailed on records. Sampling of products or materials for quality control tests should be carried out according to approved written procedures. It is important that the samples of the packaged product should be representative of the entire batch of product. Samples of the product may be tested before release for use. In addition, product samples are stored in their final container in suitable conditions. These samples are kept for at least 1 year after the product expiry date. Samples of the materials used in the production process should be placed into containers which are suitably labelled. Stable sample materials are kept for at least 2 years after release of the product.

## COMPLAINTS AND PRODUCT RECALL

All complaints and other information regarding potentially defective products must be reviewed according to written procedures. These complaints should be handled by a designated person. Records of complaints should be kept and regularly reviewed. Deficiencies arising during the manufacturing process should be reviewed. These deficiencies have narrowly avoided errors in the production process. They are often known as 'near hits'. Both the QP and the quality control manager should be informed of all complaints and deficiencies.

A procedure should be designed to recall products from the market. These products may be either defective or potentially defective. The method of recalling these products is carried out and coordinated by a designated person. Within the manufacturing facility, this person should operate independently of both sales and marketing. Following recall, the products should be identified and stored in a secure area. These products are kept in storage until a decision is made about their fate. The progress of the recall process is recorded and a final report issued. Both the QP and the quality control manager should be aware of all recall operations.

## INSPECTIONS

Inspections are carried out as internal quality audits of the manufacturing system. The manufacturer may also carry out external inspections. External inspections are typically carried out with suppliers of materials. Inspection is also carried out with contract manufacturers, packagers and contract warehouse and distribution systems.

Internal inspections are carried out at regular time intervals as part of the quality assurance system. They are carried out in an independent and detailed manner by competent personnel from the manufacturer. Independent audits by external experts may also be performed. The inspection will check that the principles of good manufacturing practice are being carried out throughout the production facility. Information about each self-inspection should be recorded as a report. This report must detail the observations made during the inspections. The report also gives proposals for corrective measures. The actions which were implemented as a result of the report should be documented. Internal inspections will:

* determine the level of compliance
* generate confidence in good manufacturing practice and the quality assurance system
* promote interdepartmental understanding
* identify necessary procedures to improve production standards
* recommend and monitor improvements.

In addition to the functions of the internal inspection, the external inspection will:

* establish and monitor the capability of suppliers and contractors to deliver suitable goods and services
* promote understanding between the manufacturer and suppliers of materials or services.

## MANUFACTURE OF STERILE MEDICINAL PRODUCTS

Quality assurance is very important in the manufacture of sterile products owing to the need to avoid particulate and microbial contamination. The manufacture of these products must be carried out using carefully established and validated procedures. The skill, training, and attitudes of the personnel involved with the manufacture of sterile products are important. The manufacture is carried out according to established and validated procedures in clean areas as detailed in Chapter 24. Methods of sterilizing these products are detailed in Chapter 22. It is important for the manufacture of sterile products that the method of sterilization is validated.

Samples of the product which are used in a sterility test should be representative of the entire batch. However, it is important that any areas of the batch considered to be at most risk of contamination should be included in the sampling programme. Sterility testing of the finished product is only the last in a series of control measures which give assurance of product sterility. Parametric release, arising through the implementation of quality assurance procedures, has superseded sterility testing in some situations (see Ch. 30).

> **Key Points**
> * QA systems ensure that medicinal products conform with intended use.
> * A quality assurance system will normally include a quality policy, resources, documentation and audit.
> * Making a product well is insufficient to ensure quality – GMP must be followed.
> * GMP ensures quality, provides evidence and generates confidence.
> * QC alone cannot assure quality.
> * Quality begins with product design.
> * Manufacturing procedures must be capable of allowing for variables and still produce consistent quality.
> * In the UK, the Medicines Control Agency grants licences to manufacture.
> * GMP is evolving as technology advances.
> * QC has the role of verifying quality.
> * The 'Orange Guide' contains regulations, directions and guidance which a manufacturer is expected to follow.
> * Errors by people are the cause of the majority of defects which occur.
> * All personnel need to be trained for their part in the production process.
> * The production manager and quality control manager should be different individuals.

- A wide range of documentation is required as part of QA, covering specifications, formulae, procedures and production records.
- Documents may be paper based or electronic.
- Quality control is concerned with sampling, specifications and testing and with release procedures.
- Procedures must exist for systematically dealing with complaints and effecting product recall if this is required.
- All procedures need to be audited on a regular basis.
- QA is particularly important in producing sterile products.

## FURTHER READING

Commission of the European Communities 1992 The rules governing medicinal products in the European Community, volume IV: good manufacturing practice for medicinal products. The EU Commission, Luxembourg

Goldberger F 1991 Pharmaceutical manufacturing quality management in the industry. Ebur, Evreux, France

Huxsoll J F 1994 Organization of quality assurance In: Huxsoll J F (ed) Quality assurance for biopharmaceuticals. John Wiley, New York

Medicines Control Agency 1997 Rules and guidance for pharmaceutical manufacturers. HMSO, London

Willig S H, Stoker J R 1997 Good manufacturing practices for pharmaceuticals: a plan for total quality control, 4th edn. Marcel Dekker, New York

# 30
# Sterility testing

*R. M. E. Richards*

---

After studying this chapter the reader should be able to:

**Discuss the role and the limitations of the sterility test**
**Explain the factors affecting the growth of bacteria**
**Describe the phases of growth of bacteria**
**Explain the factors affecting the growth of moulds**
**Explain the reasons for the various media used in sterility testing**
**Discuss the properties required of a medium used in sterility testing**
**Describe the two test methods – membrane filtration and direct inoculation**
**Discuss the interpretation of the results of the test for sterility**
**Discuss the issues involved in the selection of samples for sterility testing**
**Describe the main differences in the USP sterility test from the sterility test of the BP and EP.**

## LIMITATIONS OF THE TEST

Sterility testing of pharmaceutical preparations purporting to be sterile is a procedure that has limitations both inherent (technical and biological) and imposed (numerical and economical), which means that it can only provide partial answers to the state of sterility of the product batch under test.

The *European Pharmacopoeia* (EP 1996) introduces the section on sterility testing with the following comments.

*The test is applied to substances, preparations or articles which, according to the Pharmacopoeia, are required to be sterile. However, a satisfactory result only indicates that no contaminating microorganism has been found in the sample examined in the conditions of the test. The level of assurance provided by the absence of contaminated units in the sample as applied to the quality of the batch is a function of the efficiency of the adopted sampling plan. The extension of the test result to the whole of a batch of a product requires the assurance that the product was produced under homogeneous conditions. Clearly this depends on the precautions taken during manufacture. In the case of products sterilized in their final sealed containers, physical proofs, biologically based and automatically documented, showing correct treatment throughout the batch during sterilization are of greater assurance than the sterility test. The sterility test is the only analytical method available for products prepared under aseptic conditions and furthermore it is, in all cases, the only analytical method available to the authorities who have to examine any product for sterility.*

Thus it is acknowledged that sterility testing is inadequate as an assurance of sterility for a terminally sterilized product. This is because the level of probability of an accidental microbial contaminant in an aseptic process is one in a thousand ($10^{-3}$) but the probability of a microbial survivor in a terminal sterilization process is only one in a million ($10^{-6}$). Nevertheless, the test is still a regulatory test in most countries. However, there appears to be a trend towards exempting from the test products prepared by manufacturers who provide evidence of good manufacturing practice combined with properly validated and controlled sterilization cycles. This has been referred to as 'parametric release' of parenteral solutions sterilized by moist heat sterilization. The parameters for release are the initial validation data and physical and biological data routinely collected in process (see Ch. 21). On the other hand, sterility testing has valuable application in aseptic processes such as filtration.

Stated very simply, sterility testing attempts to reveal the presence or absence of viable microorganisms in a sample number of containers taken from a batch of product. Based on the results obtained from testing the sample a decision is made as to the sterility of the batch. Great care is taken to try to eliminate false positives which might arise from technician error. Recently this has led to some major pharmaceutical companies introducing robotics. Initial experience has shown that robotic sterility testing can reduce false positive rates quite markedly. This may lead to the increased use of robotics in sterility test procedures in the pharmaceutical industry (Zlotnick & Franklin 1987).

Major factors of importance in sterility testing include: the environment in which the test is conducted; the quality of the culture conditions provided; the test method; the sample size and sampling procedure.

## STERILITY TEST CONDITIONS

### Environmental conditions required for the test

The basic requirement of the facility used for carrying out sterility testing is that it should be designed to provide conditions which avoid accidental contamination of the product during the test. A suitable environment is a Grade A laminar airflow cabinet located in a Grade B clean room (see Ch. 24). Regular microbiological monitoring with contact swabs, settle plates, etc. should be carried out.

Chemical antimicrobial agents should be used with care. There must be no possibility of such an agent adversely affecting either microorganisms which may be present in the sample under test or the culture medium subsequently inoculated with the test sample.

### Culture conditions

Sterility testing involves testing for viable microorganisms which are likely to have been damaged by the sterilization process. Consequently it follows that appropriate conditions for growth of any surviving organisms should be provided by the culture media selected.

The following account of factors affecting the growth of microorganisms indicates the importance of selecting the most appropriate culture conditions for sterility testing.

## FACTORS AFFECTING GROWTH OF BACTERIA

Nutrition, moisture, air, temperature, pH, light, osmotic pressure and the presence of growth inhibitors are all important factors which affect the growth of bacteria.

### Nutrition

All bacteria need mineral salts and sources of carbon and nitrogen. Some, like the denitrifying bacteria, can use very simple materials, e.g. carbon dioxide as the source of carbon and ammonium salts or nitrates as the source of nitrogen. Most, including the pathogens, must be provided with much more elaborate compounds, e.g. carbohydrates or organic acids as carbon sources and proteins or, more often, their degradation products, as sources of nitrogen.

The synthesis of bacterial protoplasm is the result of chains of chemical reactions. Certain compounds, known as essential metabolites, form vital links in these chains and therefore growth stops if they are not available. As some bacteria cannot synthesize these substances they must be included in the growth medium and are then known as growth factors. Important examples are para-aminobenzoic acid, thiamine hydrochloride (vitamin $B_1$), cyanocobalamin (vitamin $B_{12}$) and folic acid.

Thus it can be seen that to produce vigorous growth of bacteria, suitable and adequate sources of carbon, nitrogen, mineral salts and growth factors must be present in the culture medium.

### Moisture

Bacteria require moisture in order to utilize the aforementioned food substances. Usually a medium for the growth of bacteria must contain at least 20% of water. In the absence of moisture, bacteria cease to multiply but spore-bearing forms may continue to exist in spore form for many years.

### Air

Many bacteria will grow in the presence of air and are called 'aerobes', e.g. *Pseudomonas aeruginosa*; others can multiply only in the absence of oxygen and are known as 'anaerobes', e.g. *Clostridium tetani*. A third group, 'facultative anaerobes', are able to grow with or without air, e.g. *Escherichia coli*.

Anaerobic bacteria may be cultivated successfully

either by providing an oxygen-free atmosphere or by adding reducing substances to the growth media.

The state of oxidation or reduction of a medium can be measured and is known as the oxidation–reduction potential.

## Temperature

Most pathogenic bacteria multiply best at normal human body temperature, i.e. approximately 37°C. However, some common and serious contaminants of wounds, eye drops and injections (e.g. *Pseudomonas* spp.) have an optimum growth temperature of about 30°C and may not be detected at 37°C. The *United States Pharmacopoeia* (USP 1995), EP 1996 and *British Pharmacopoeia* (BP 1993) all recommend an incubation temperature of 30–35°C.

Some saprophytes have an optimum range of 55–80°C and are known as 'thermophiles'. The spores of some species, e.g. *Bacillus stearothermophilus*, are extremely heat resistant and are used to test the efficiency of heat sterilization processes.

At temperatures approaching 0°C and below most organisms stop multiplying, but they remain alive, and this behaviour is utilized in the preservation of cultures of microorganisms by freeze-drying.

Temperatures above 50°C are harmful, particularly if moisture is present. All vegetative cells are killed by exposure to dry heat at 100°C for 1.5 hours or moist heat at 80°C for 1 hour. Spores are more resistant.

## pH

The optimum pH for growth is about 7.4, although this varies with different organisms. Growth is less rapid as the liquid is made more acid or more alkaline. Solutions that are strongly acid or alkaline are bactericidal.

## Light

Exposure to sunlight in the presence of air has a harmful action on bacteria and may inhibit growth or destroy the organism. It is for this reason that the incubators used for growing bacteria have no windows. The damage is caused chiefly by light waves from the ultraviolet region. This explains the occasional use of ultraviolet lamps for reducing the contamination of atmospheres and surfaces.

In addition to its action on bacteria, light may also produce changes in the medium in which the bacteria are growing and render it unsuitable for supporting growth. Hence it is important to store culture media in the dark and to use them as soon after preparation as possible.

## Osmotic pressure

Bacteria respond rather slowly to changes in osmotic pressure, but they are plasmolysed by strongly hypertonic solutions and they swell and may burst when placed in hypotonic medium. Suspensions of bacteria used for test purposes should be suspended in diluents of optimum osmotic pressure. When used in sterility testing the inhibitory effect of strongly hypertonic solutions must be allowed for.

### Growth inhibitors

Many substances can inhibit the growth of bacteria. Substances that prevent the growth of bacteria without destroying them are called 'bacteriostats' while substances that kill bacteria are called 'bactericides'. However, substances can be bacteriostatic at low concentrations and bactericidal at high concentrations and bacteria may die if subjected to prolonged contact with bacteriostatic concentrations.

Bactericides are extensively used in injections as preservatives.

## Application to sterility testing

Consideration of the foregoing factors is necessary to establish the most suitable conditions for the growth of bacteria. Thus to produce the rapid and luxuriant growth required in the preparation of bacterial cultures, or testing for sterility, it is necessary to provide ample nutrients, sufficient water and a suitable hydrogen ion concentration. The temperature will also need to be maintained in the optimum region by using an incubator which will exclude light. For anaerobes precautions must be taken to ensure a low oxidation–reduction potential. In all cases the presence of excessive quantities of substances having bacteriostatic or bactericidal action must be avoided.

Multiplication of organisms may be prevented by maintaining them in complete dryness, by cold storage, by adjustment of the pH to an unsuitable value for growth and/or by adding a suitable bactericide. With solutions to be injected it is not usually possible to control all these factors and the course normally adopted to prevent multiplication of organisms inadvertently introduced during use is the addition of a bactericide. However, it should be borne in mind that the medicament itself may in some cases produce a solution having a pH or tonicity unfavourable to the growth of bacteria.

## PHASES OF BACTERIAL GROWTH

Four distinct phases of growth are exhibited when bacteria are freshly inoculated into a satisfactory liquid medium and incubated under optimal conditions (Fig. 30.1).

### Lag phase

Immediately after inoculation there is an interval of rest during which the bacteria seem to rejuvenate themselves. This is followed by a period of considerable growth activity in which, although there is no cell division, the cells increase in size and metabolism is very high. Towards the end of the lag phase multiplication begins and soon increases in rate.

This phase usually lasts 2–3 hours but its length is affected by a number of factors, of which the following are of particular importance in sterility testing.

#### Inoculum size

The smaller the inoculum the longer the lag. It appears that before an organism can make use of certain nutrients in the culture medium it must convert them into more suitable forms and it does this by liberating enzymes. If the number of cells in the inoculum is very small these enzymes, together with

the products of their activity, may be rapidly dispersed and diluted by diffusion. In these circumstances the bacteria fail to multiply and the lag phase is lengthened and may be indefinitely prolonged. On the other hand, if a large inoculum is transferred the necessary concentration of suitable metabolites is quickly built up. Another factor is that in a large inoculum it is likely that part of the inoculum will consist of medium containing the metabolites. Furthermore part of the inoculum will probably consist of dead cells which will break down and release metabolites. Thus the viable cells in the large inoculum start reproducing fairly quickly and the lag phase is short.

Pharmaceutical products are tested for sterility by incubating samples in culture media. Only rarely will these samples be heavily contaminated. Therefore there is a danger that the small numbers of bacteria present may not multiply sufficiently to produce the detectable turbidity used as an indicator of contamination. Consequently the sample of product taken for the test should be as large as other factors allow to ensure that as many organisms as possible are transferred to the culture media.

#### Sensitivity of medium

Some culture media contain nutrients that are very easily metabolized by bacteria which renders them more sensitive or conducive to promoting the growth

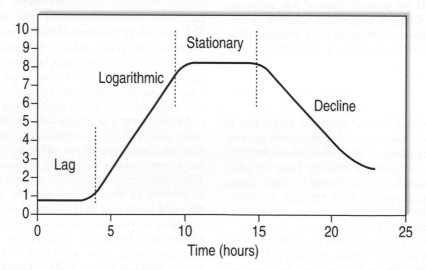

**Fig. 30.1** Phases of bacterial growth.

of small inocula than others. Such media are essential for sterility testing.

### Previous history of organism

Bacteria that are rapidly multiplying under ideal conditions when transferred will have a short lag time, but organisms suffering from the toxic effects of a previous environment will take longer to recover and a prolonged lag will result.

Bacteria in pharmaceutical preparations will most probably have been subjected to adverse conditions such as heat treatment, long contact with a bactericide or a solution of unfavourable pH. Therefore they may show a long lag time even in an optimal medium. For this reason incubation times of at least 7 days are prescribed for sterility tests.

## Logarithmic phase

This follows the lag phase and usually lasts for about 6 hours. During this period growth is at its maximum and the number or bacteria increases logarithmically; that is, the graph obtained by plotting the logarithm of the number of bacteria per millilitre against the incubation time is a straight line. The number of organisms required to render the medium turbid varies slightly with the size of the organisms but turbidity can usually be detected when about 10 million organisms/ml are present. The time at which detectable turbidity is produced depends upon the size of the original inoculum, the nutritive properties of the medium, the incubation temperature and the rate of multiplication of the cells. Under ideal conditions the rate of multiplication of a given strain of bacteria is reproducible, but different species of bacteria have varying rates of multiplication.

## Stationary phase

In this phase division is slower and a point is reached where the number of new bacteria formed is approximately balanced by the number dying. The reasons for the decreased reproduction rate include depletion of essential nutrients and, in some cases, the accumulation of toxic by-products.

## Decline phase

The stationary phase proceeds into one in which the number of organisms dying increasingly outnumbers the newly formed bacteria. Division ultimately ceases due to lack of nutrients and the accumulation of toxic waste products.

## FACTORS AFFECTING GROWTH OF MOULDS AND YEASTS

Although there is an overlap in the growth requirements of moulds and yeasts with those required by bacteria, there are also some differences. The similarities and differences are pointed out in the following comments on the factors affecting the growth of moulds and yeasts.

### Nutrition

Moulds and yeasts require the same classes of nutrients as bacteria but the carbohydrate and nitrogen sources are particularly important.

A supplementary source of carbohydrate must be added to most media because a high concentration is essential; examples are 2% dextrose, 3% sucrose and 4% maltose.

Extracts are used as nitrogen sources and are often obtained from vegetable materials, such as malt and potato extracts. However, the pathogenic fungi grow better in media containing extracts from animal sources. Thus the soyabean casein digest medium used in the fungal sterility test of the USP, EP and BP contains tryptone (a pancreatic digest of casein) as well as the vegetable extract (soya peptone). Peptones are often used to supplement or replace extracts. Special mycological grades have been developed and give rapid and luxuriant growth of moulds and yeasts.

Some moulds, like certain bacteria, grow profusely in stored distilled water.

### Air

The common saprophytic moulds are strongly aerobic but yeasts can grow both aerobically and anaerobically. For example, anaerobic growth can occur deep in large containers of unpreserved syrups, or syrupy preparations, producing alcohol and carbon dioxide, which may eventually expel the stopper or burst the container. However, special anaerobic media are unnecessary.

### Temperature

The optimum temperatures for the growth of most moulds and yeasts lie between 20°C and 25°C. As many moulds grow rather slowly, tests should be incubated for at least 7 days.

Cultures may be freeze-dried but in general mould spores are more sensitive to heat than bacterial spores. Exposure to dry heat at 115°C for 1.5 hours is reported to kill all mould spores and they are rapidly killed by moist heat at 100°C.

## pH

Moulds and yeasts prefer a pH well on the acid side of neutrality. Test media are usually adjusted to between pH 5 and 6. A pH of less than 5 is avoided when the medium contains agar because this is hydrolysed, with consequent loss of gel strength, if autoclaved at low pH. If a higher acidity is essential it is obtained by adding sterile acid after sterilization.

## Light

Most moulds and yeasts grow equally well in the light and dark. Since incubators are not made with windows it is more convenient to incubate in the dark.

## Osmotic pressure

Moulds and yeasts are more tolerant of high osmotic pressure than bacteria and are often found as contaminants of unpreserved syrups, semi-solid creams and ointments. Additional sodium chloride is unnecessary in mould media.

## Growth inhibitors

Substances used to prevent the growth of moulds and yeasts are known as 'fungistats' while substances used to kill them are called 'fungicides'. These must be neutralized or 'diluted out' in sterility testing.

## CULTURE MEDIA FOR STERILITY TESTING

Culture media suitable for sterility testing must be capable of initiating and maintaining the vigorous growth of a small number of organisms. These organisms may consist of aerobic and anaerobic bacteria and the lower fungi. The former include common saprophytes, pyogenic cocci (*Staphylococcus aureus* and *Streptococcus pyogenes*, Group A) and spore-bearing bacteria pathogenic to man. The lower fungi include yeasts and moulds responsible for spoilage.

The BP (1993) suggests the use of two dual-purpose or joint media. These are fluid mercaptoacetate medium (fluid thioglycollate medium) and soyabean casein digest medium.

## Fluid mercaptoacetate medium

The fluid mercaptoacetate medium is intended primarily for the culture of anaerobic bacteria but will also sustain the growth of aerobic bacteria. The formulation contains a number of ingredients and some have a specific role. For example, reducing conditions are promoted by mercaptoacetic acid and glucose. Resazurin is included as an oxidation–reduction indicator and agar is present to increase the viscosity and thus reduce the inward diffusion of oxygen into the medium.

The nutrients include sodium chloride, glucose and pancreatic digest of casein. Yeast extract is present as a growth factor and the amino acid L-cystine is included to encourage the growth of certain clostridia.

The formulation is suitable for the detection of anaerobes if not more than the upper 30% of the medium in the container, such as a 100 ml bottle, has been oxygenated. This is indicated by a green coloration of the medium. If necessary, reducing conditions can be restored immediately before using by heating the medium in a water-bath, until the green colour disappears, and then cooling rapidly. However, repeated reheating can give rise to toxic degradation products.

A medium with the top 10% oxygenated is very suitable for use because aerobic growth will be more quickly initiated under such conditions and anaerobic growth will also take place.

## Soyabean casein digest medium

The soyabean casein digest medium is intended primarily for the growth of aerobic bacteria but also supports the growth of fungi. Owing to the inclusion of tryptone (from casein) and soya peptone, this medium is particularly supportive to injured or fastidious aerobic bacteria that grow slowly in fluid mercaptoacetate medium (especially if trapped in the anaerobic region), because of the low oxidation–reduction potential. In addition, it has given good results in the membrane filtration method of sterility testing.

Other media may be used provided that they have been demonstrated to support the growth of a wide variety of organisms. The media used must also be shown to comply with certain tests. These tests must be either carried out previous to, or in parallel with, the sterility test on the product being examined. They should be designed to demonstrate the sterility of the medium, its nutritive properties and its effectiveness in the presence and absence of the preparation being examined.

The explanations that follow relate to the tests described in the BP (1993) and the EP (1996). It is important to note the periods of incubation. Where there is a need to establish the absence of microorganisms a minimum period of 7 days is suggested. Where there is a need to demonstrate the provision of adequate growth conditions then a maximum incubation period to 7 days is recommended. An emphasis on the early detection of growth is also made.

## Sterility of the media

Assurance that the media to be used in the sterility test are sterile is necessary in order to eliminate the possibility of false positives arising from contaminated media. This assurance is obtained by incubating portions of the media at appropriate temperatures for not less than 7 days. Media intended for detection of bacteria are incubated at 30–35°C and media intended for detection of fungi are incubated at 20–25°C. Sterility is confirmed by the absence of microbial growth.

## Nutritive properties of the media – fertility control

Tubes of the chosen media are individually inoculated with 100 viable microorganisms of one of a selection of culture types. These organisms are representative of the various types of contaminant that the test is seeking to detect. The BP (1993) suggests the use of *Staphylococcus aureus*, NCTC 7447 (an aerobe), *Bacillus subtilis*, NCIMB 8054 (a spore-forming aerobe), *Clostridium sporogenes*, NCTC 532 (an anaerobe) and *Candida albicans*, NCYC 854 (a fungus).

Incubation at the appropriate temperature for bacteria and fungi is for not more than 7 days. Early and copious growth of the microorganism confirms the suitability of that medium.

## Effectiveness of media under test conditions – growth control

This test is to demonstrate whether or not culture conditions are satisfactory in the presence of the product being examined or a membrane filter, where applicable. This should be repeated for culture media for aerobic bacteria, anaerobic bacteria and fungi. A control set of cultures is included to provide a means of comparing the rate of onset and the density of growth in the presence and absence of the material being examined. The initial inoculations should be carried out in a separate laboratory.

## Aerobic bacterial test

An appropriate sample, as used in the test for sterility, of the preparation being examined is added to at least two containers of selected medium. Each container is then inoculated with 0.1 ml of a suspension of a suitable aerobic organism, such as *Staphylococcus aureus*, diluted to contain approximately 1000 viable organisms/ml. It should be noted that if the preparation being examined is an antibiotic then the organism used must be sensitive to that antibiotic.

A control set of containers is prepared without the addition of the product being examined. All containers are incubated at 30–35°C for not more than 7 days.

## Anaerobic bacterial test

This is performed in a similar manner to the aerobic bacterial test except that a suitable strain of anaerobic organism (such as *Clostridium sporogenes*) and a suitable medium for anaerobic organisms are used.

## Fungal test

The test is carried out similarly to the aerobic bacterial test except that a suitable strain of a fungus (such as *Candida albicans*) and a suitable medium for fungi are used. Incubation is at 20–25°C for not more than 7 days.

If cultures containing the preparation being examined show equivalent growth to the cultures in the absence of the preparation, it indicates that the preparation has no antimicrobial action under the conditions of the test. Therefore the test for sterility of the preparation may be carried out without modification. If weaker growth, delayed growth or no growth occurs in the presence of the preparation compared with the control cultures, then the material being examined has antimicrobial action. This must be eliminated before or during the test for sterility of the preparation. Suitable methods may be neutralization, dilution or filtration. Whichever way is chosen it must be demonstrated as being effective by repeating the foregoing test procedure.

## TEST METHODS FOR TESTING THE STERILITY OF THE PRODUCT

Two methods are described in the BP (1993) and the EP (1996). The methods are referred to as the membrane filtration method (Method I of the BP) and the direct inoculation method (Method II of the BP). The EP (1995) introduced the two tests as follows.

*The test may be carried out using the technique of membrane filtration or by direct inoculation of the culture media with the product to be examined. The technique of membrane filtration is to be preferred whenever the nature of the product permits, that is, for filterable aqueous preparations, for alcoholic or oily preparations and for preparations miscible with or soluble in aqueous or oily solvents which do not have an antimicrobial effect in the conditions of the test.*

### Membrane filtration

Membrane filters having a nominal pore size of 0.45 μm and whose effectiveness in retaining microorganisms has been established are recommended for this method. Filters of the appropriate composition for filtering the various solvents are available; for example, cellulose nitrate filters for aqueous, oily or weakly alcoholic solutions and cellulose acetate for strongly alcoholic solutions.

Filter discs commonly used are about 50 mm in diameter and the technique described in the BP (1993) and EP (1996) is based on this size of filter. For filters of different diameter, the volumes of dilutions used may have to be adjusted.

The filtration system and membrane are first sterilized by appropriate means. They should be so designed that solutions to be examined are introduced and filtered under aseptic conditions. One of two procedures may then be followed. Either the membrane is removed intact (or divided into two) and aseptically transferred to one (or two) containers of appropriate culture medium. Alternatively, culture medium is passed through the closed system to the membrane which is then incubated in situ in the filtration apparatus. The latter technique may be conveniently performed with one of the commercially available systems, for example the Sartorius system which consists of a multiple suction filtration device. The system is capable of being sterilized by autoclaving at 121°C for 30 minutes (a deliberate excess) prior to use.

Millipore produce a transparent blister-packed system which has been sterilized by ethylene oxide.

The system known as Steritest uses a peristaltic pump to provide pressure filtration. After completion of the test the plastic test system is disposed of suitably.

Various fully automatic systems have also been developed.

### Aqueous solutions

Each membrane is prepared by moistening with a small quantity of suitable sterile diluent such as 0.1% w/v neutral solution of meat or casein peptone. This renders the membrane less liable to damage and reduces the retention of inhibitors.

The quantity of the preparation to be examined depends on the end-use of the product. Tables 30.1 and 30.2 summarize the BP and EP requirements.

The appropriate quantity is transferred from the container or containers to be tested to the membrane or membranes. If necessary, dilution is made to about 100 ml with a suitable sterile diluent and

**Table 30.1  Minimum samples to be used in each culture medium in the test for sterility of parenterals (based on the BP 1993 and the EP 1996)**

| Liquids | Volume in container (ml) | <1 | 1–<4 | 4–<20 | 20–100 |
|---|---|---|---|---|---|
| | Sample volume | All | Half | 2 ml | 10% |
| Solids | Weight in container (mg) | <50 | 50–<200 | 200 or more | |
| | Sample weight | All | Half | 100 mg | |

**Table 30.2  Quantities to be combined and quantities to be used in the test for sterility of ophthalmic and other non-injectable preparations (based on the BP 1993 and the EP 1996)**

| Type of preparation | Quantity to be combined | Quantity to be used for each culture medium |
|---|---|---|
| Solutions | 10–100 ml | 5–10 ml |
| Preparations soluble in water or appropriate solvents | 1–10 g | 0.5–1 g |
| Insoluble preparations, creams and ointments (suspend or emulsify) | 1–10 g | 0.5–1 g |

| Table 30.3 Inactivating agents for selected antimicrobials | |
|---|---|
| Antimicrobial | Inactivating agent |
| Alcohols | None (dilution 1 to 50) |
| Arsenic compounds | Thioglycollate (<0.5%) |
| Cephalosporins Cephaloridine Cephalotin | Cephalosporinase |
| Hydroxybenzoates | Polysorbate 80 (1%) or (dilution 1 to 50) |
| Mercury compounds | Cystine (0.1%) or thioglycollate (0.05%) + polysorbate 80 (3%) |
| Penicillins Ampicillin Carbenicillin Penicillin G Penicillin V Phenethicillin Propicillin | Penicillinase |
| Phenols, cresols | Polysorbate 80 (1%) or (dilution 1 to 50) |
| Quaternary ammonium compounds | Polysorbate 80 (3%) + lecithin (0.3%) |
| Sulphonamides | p-aminobenzoic acid (25 mg will neutralize up to 5 g sulphanilamide) |

filtration is carried out immediately. For those solutions being tested that have antimicrobial properties, the membrane is immediately washed with three successive 100 ml quantities of the chosen diluent. Where necessary, a suitable antimicrobial inactivating substance is added to the diluent or to the medium (Table 30.3).

A membrane is transferred to each of the culture media or each medium transferred onto a membrane in the sealed apparatus. The media are incubated for not less than 7 days at 30–35°C for the detection of bacteria and 20–25°C for the detection of fungi.

Alternatively, the combined quantity of the material being examined for all media is transferred to the membrane – diluting, filtering and washing as previously described. The membrane is then aseptically cut into the appropriate number of equal parts. One of the parts is transferred to each medium. Incubation is then carried out for not less than 7 days at the appropriate temperatures as just described.

### Soluble solids

For each medium the appropriate quantity (indicated in Tables 30.1 and 30.2) is dissolved in a suitable solvent such as 0.1% w/v neutral solution of meat or casein peptone. The test is then followed as

described for aqueous solutions. If non-aqueous solvent is used it may be necessary to use membranes made of a material other than cellulose nitrate.

### Oils and oily solutions

At least the quantities indicated in Tables 30.1 and 30.2 are used for each medium. Using a dry membrane, oils and oily solutions may be filtered without dilution. Isopropyl myristate, or some other suitable diluent having no antimicrobial activity under the conditions of the test, is used to dilute viscous oils. In fact heat-sterilized isopropyl myristate should be used.

After the oil has been in contact with the membrane and has penetrated the membrane by gravity then filtration should be commenced by applying either pressure or suction gradually. The membrane is then washed at least three times with 100 ml quantities of sterile solution containing a suitable surface-active agent. Neutral meat or casein peptone 0.1% w/v containing either 1% w/v polysorbate 80 or 1% w/v (4-tert-octylphenoxy)-polyethoxyethanol are suitable washing fluids. The divided membrane, or whole membranes, is then transferred to the appropriate culture media. Alternatively the culture media are transferred to the membranes as described for the aqueous solutions. Incubation is also as described in the procedure for aqueous solutions.

### Ointments and creams

The minimum quantities for each medium are shown in Table 30.2. Again isopropyl myristate forms a suitable diluent and it can be used to dilute ointments in a fatty base or water-in-oil emulsions to 1%. If necessary gentle heat may be used up to a maximum of 40°C, followed immediately by filtration, as described under oils and oily solutions. Both the BP (1993) and the EP (1996) permit heating to not more than 45°C in exceptional cases but the test is reaching the limits of credibility under such conditions.

Any antimicrobial activity in the product to be tested must be neutralized by inactivation or by dilution in a suitable quantity of culture medium before incubation.

After filtration, washing and incubation procedures are carried out similar to those described for the oils and oily solutions.

## Advantages of the filtration method

1. Wide application. It can be used for:

a. solutions with or without inhibitory properties
b. soluble solids with or without inhibitory properties
c. insoluble solids without inhibitory properties
d. oils
e. ointments, provided a non-inhibitory solvent or dispersing medium can be found
f. articles, such as syringes, that can be rinsed with a sterile fluid
2. A large volume can be tested with one filter. Therefore the method is applicable to the testing of poorly soluble solids.
3. A much smaller volume of broth is required than for testing by direct inoculation into culture media.
4. It is applicable to substances for which no satisfactory inactivators are known, e.g. certain antibiotics.
5. Some strongly adsorbed antibacterial agents, such as the mercurials and quaternary ammonium compounds, can be inactivated on the filter by treatment with the appropriate neutralizing solution.
6. Subculturing is often eliminated, e.g. for oils and oily preparations and substances that, like the barbiturates, give precipitates in broth.

## Disadvantage of the filtration method

An expensive facility, highly trained staff and a consistently high level of operation are required. However, there is no easy alternative.

## Direct inoculation method

The quantity of the preparation to be examined (as shown in either Table 30.1 or 30.2) is transferred directly into the appropriate culture medium. Antimicrobial properties are neutralized as previously described in the membrane filtration method (see p. 320).

To ensure that the sample does not excessively dilute the ingredients and so impair the growth-promoting properties of the medium, the volume of culture medium must be at least 10 times the liquid sample volume. For solids it is recommended that the proportion of medium to sample is 100 to 1 in order to negate any effect of the dissolved solid on the nutritive properties of the medium. However, when the volume of sample is large, it is difficult for bacteria and yeasts to produce a detectable turbidity in the correspondingly large volume of medium within the incubation period of the test. Therefore in such circumstances it is better to use a concentrated medium

which when diluted with sample gives the correct strength of medium. Where appropriate the concentrated medium may be added directly to the preparation in its container.

### Oily liquids

When oily liquids are being examined it is necessary to add to the media used an appropriate emulsifying agent which has no antimicrobial activity under the conditions of the test. The two agents described under the membrane filtration test are suitable, i.e. 1% w/v polysorbate 80 or 0.1% w/v (4-tert-octylphenoxy)-polyethoxyethanol.

### Ointments and creams

The sample is diluted 10-fold in a suitable sterile diluent (0.1% w/v neutral solution of meat or casein peptone) containing the chosen emulsifying agent. The emulsified diluted product is transferred to medium not containing an emulsifying agent.

Incubation for the direct inoculation method is for not less than 14 days at 30–35°C (mainly for the detection of bacteria) and 20–25°C (mainly for the detection of fungi). The longer incubation time, compared with membrane filtration, is a disadvantage. The cultures are observed periodically throughout the incubation period, preferably every day. This is because some bacteria produce a detectable turbidity at first which later settles as an insignificant deposit at the bottom of the tube or bottle and leaves clear, apparently uncontaminated medium above. Therefore it is advisable to swirl containers gently before examination to stir up any sediment. It is also necessary to gently shake media containing oily products daily. However, great care must be taken with the mercaptoacetate medium not to destroy the anaerobic conditions at the base of the medium.

Daily examination of the medium also means that repeat tests (where these are permitted) can be commenced immediately contamination is detected.

## Interpretation of the results

The batch passes the test for sterility if there is no sign of growth in any of the test media. When microbial growth is present then the sample fails the test for sterility. In such a situation the media showing growth are kept to one side. If it can be demonstrated that there was a breakdown in the aseptic technique, then the test is declared invalid and the initial test may be repeated. Where there is no evidence that the test was invalid, it is possible to proceed to a retest to demonstrate whether or not the growth obtained originated from the product under test. Should the retest have no growth in any of the containers then the batch passes the test for sterility on the evidence of the retest. However, if the retest also results in growth of microorganisms, then tests are undertaken to determine whether or not the microorganisms which grew in both tests are similar or quite distinct. If in fact the microorganisms growing as the result of the two tests are readily distinguishable, then a second retest is allowed by both the BP and the EP using twice the number of samples. No evidence of microbial growth occurring as a result of the second retest allows the product being examined to pass the test. However, should there be evidence of growth of any microorganism in the second retest then the preparation being examined fails the test for sterility. The interpretation of the results is set out in Figure 30.2.

It is recognized that there will be a low incidence of accidental contamination or false positives obtained during sterility testing of a sample that is actually sterile. This is especially the case when a number of manipulations are required for testing as in the membrane filtration technique. It will also depend on the testing personnel and the environmental conditions during the test. Avallone (1985) stated that the incidence of false positives should not exceed 1% and pointed out the value of reviewing the type of organism which caused the growth. The type of organism, together with an assessment of its ability to survive the manufacturing process to which the product being examined has been subjected, could provide valuable information as to whether it was in fact likely to be a false positive or not. The example was given that *Escherichia coli* would not be expected to be present in a sterility testing environment. Thus if growth in the media was due to *Escherichia coli* then it would not be interpreted as a false positive. On the other hand, if the growth was due to *Staphylococcus epidermidis*, which is also found to be readily killed by the preservative used in the product being examined, then it could not be interpreted as originating in the product under test. Rather it would appear to have originated as a skin contaminant from an operator involved in conducting the test for sterility. Therefore there would be justification for classifying the *Staphylococcus epidermidis* as a false positive.

Nevertheless the current situation allows different manufacturers to interpret their results obtained from testing for sterility in widely different ways. This is undoubtedly an unsatisfactory aspect of the

interpretation of the test. For example, Avallone (1985) reported the case of a manufacturer who, if on the first test found either 'mold or Gram-negative bacilli', failed the batch on this evidence alone. The opposite extreme was also reported where a manufacturer accepted a batch 'which had an initial contamination of a mold, a Gram-negative bacillus and a Gram-positive cocci'.

Some manufacturers include a product known to be sterile in their testing procedure. This is referred to as a 'negative control'. The negative control may be an ampoule or ampoules of sterile medium or media. On the other hand, the negative control may be samples of the product being tested, e.g. antibiotic powder, which has been terminally sterilized. The negative control is of assistance in interpreting false positives and provides a check on operator technique.

## Applications of the test

Guidelines are necessary for those faced with the task of testing for sterility for a wide range of sterile products and materials. The BP (1993) and the EP (1996) contain advice on how to apply the test to injectables, ophthalmic products and other non-injectables and also to surgical dressings, catgut and other surgical sutures.

### Injections

With the membrane filtration method it is best to use the whole contents of the container whenever possible; otherwise the quantities indicated in Table 30.1 are used. Where it is necessary to dilute the sample, it is diluted to about 100 ml with a suitable sterile solution (e.g. 0.1% w/v neutral meat or casein peptone).

With the direct inoculation method the quantities shown in Table 30.1 are used.

The tests to detect bacterial and fungal contamination are carried out on the same sample of the product being examined. In the situation where the amount contained in a single container is insufficient to carry out the test, then the contents of two or more containers are combined and used to inoculate the different media. In those cases where the contents of the container exceed 100 ml the membrane filtration method is the procedure of choice. The total volume to be filtered through one membrane filter should not exceed 1000 ml.

### Ophthalmic and other non-injectable preparations

For these products the contents of an appropriate

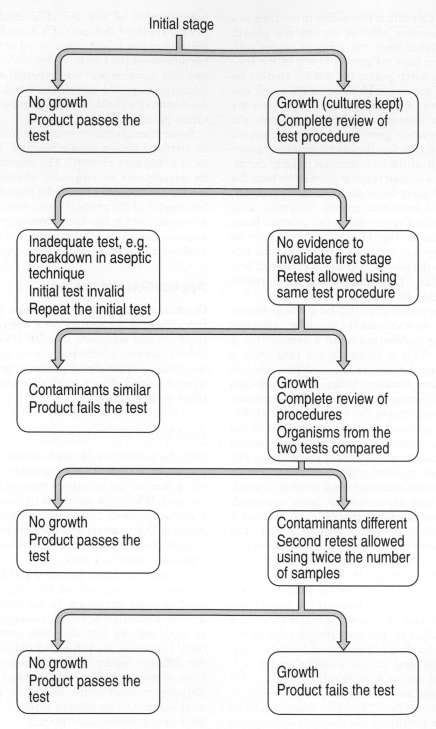

**Fig. 30.2** Interpretation of results obtained with the EP (1996) and BP (1993) test for sterility.

number of containers are combined to provide not less than the minimum and not more than the maximum quantities shown under 'Quantity to be combined' in Table 30.2. Then, from the well-mixed sample, the amount shown under 'Quantity to be used for each culture medium' in Table 30.2 is used.

### Surgical dressings

The procedure for surgical dressings follows a similar pattern to previous tests. That is, the test is carried out in a microbiologically controlled environment. The sealed package is opened using aseptic precautions and appropriate portions are removed from three different parts of the package. For absorbent cotton wool 1 g portions are used and for woven materials 10 cm² portions are considered appropriate. For gauze compresses, whether individually wrapped or not, three complete compresses are taken from different parts of the pack. Portions from each location of the pack, three in all, are used for each culture medium. The quantity of medium used should be sufficient to cover the selected portions of dressing (20–150 ml).

In the membrane filtration method, the test portion is shaken for 10 minutes together with at least 50 ml of sterile nutrient broth containing 0.07% w/v lecithin and 0.5% w/v polysorbate 80 as a combined antimicrobial inactivating and washing solution. Then, as quickly as possible, the washings are filtered through a membrane filter previously moistened with a small amount of culture medium. Subsequent to filtration the membrane is rinsed with at least three successive 50 ml quantities of the chosen diluent. The membrane is then transferred to the appropriate culture medium or the medium is transferred to the membrane as previously described under 'Aqueous solutions' above.

In the direct inoculation method three test portions are transferred to separate containers of each type of medium.

### Catgut and other surgical sutures

The direct inoculation method is used into medium in wide-mouthed containers. The test sample consists of whole strands from freshly opened packages, usually containing one strand per package. Five strands are transferred to a separate container of 20–150 ml of each type of culture medium. If the sutures are present in multistrand packages then the five strands must be taken from five different packages.

The growth control test must be carried out to show

that small numbers (about 100) of selected organisms are able to grow satisfactorily in the presence of the sample of product under examination. If the sample inhibits growth then the antimicrobial activity has to be inhibited and the growth control test repeated.

Incubation, at the specified temperatures for bacterial and fungal media, should be for not less than 14 days. This longer incubation time is necessary for the following reasons. Catgut is made from the intestines of sheep which in the slaughterhouses often become heavily contaminated with the spores of dangerous pathogens such as *Clostridium tetani* and the *Clostridium* spp. responsible for gas gangrene. During manufacture these may be trapped deep inside the threads, and as it is essential to detect any that escape sterilization, the incubation period of the sterility test is lengthened. This gives time for the culture medium to permeate the threads and the organisms to recover and multiply into detectable turbidity.

If it is necessary to carry out a retest, or a second retest, for any of these surgical dressings, catgut or other surgical sutures, then the same number of test portions is used as in the original test and each must be taken from a separate freshly opened package.

## Sampling

The selection of samples and the number of samples to be taken from any given batch of sterile product or materials is obviously an important aspect of testing for sterility.

### Selection of the samples

Samples must be representative of the whole of the bulk material and each batch of final containers.

For the bulk, the material must be thoroughly mixed before the sample is taken.

For the final containers, the sample must be selected at random, but:

1. When a load from a heat sterilization process is being tested, samples should be taken from every shelf and from any parts of the sterilizer in which less satisfactory conditions are believed to exist.

2. For aseptically processed preparations, samples must be taken throughout the filling operation. The USP 23 defines the latter as a period not exceeding 24 consecutive hours during which no interruptions or changes affecting the integrity of the filling assembly have occurred and in which an identical group of containers has been filled with the same product from the same bulk lot.

3. For articles sterilized by a continuous process,

such as radiation sterilization, samples are selected from the total number of similar items subjected to uniform sterilization during an appropriate period which the USP 23 suggests should not exceed 24 consecutive hours.

### Sample size

There has been much debate on sample size. This has involved statistically based arguments related to the lack of assurance that the test for sterility will detect low levels of contamination. The present situation, however, has changed to where the test is seen as part of a total process aimed at providing assurance of sterility. This has reduced the reasons for criticism of the test. The test is not expected to 'stand alone' as an assurance of the sterility of a product. In fact it may be omitted in some cases. For example, the USP 23 states:

> If data derived from the manufacturing process sterility assurance validation studies and from in-process controls are judged to provide greater assurance that the lot meets the required low probability of containing a contaminated unit (compared to sterility testing results from finished units drawn from that lot), any sterility test procedures adopted may be minimal, or dispensed with on a routine basis.

The EP (1996) and the BP (1993) suggest minimal sample sizes for various products. These are sum-marized in Table 30.4. This is by way of guidance to manufacturers who have to include in their decisions on the size of samples such factors as: the environmental conditions of the manufacture, the volume of preparation per container and any other special considerations applying to the preparation concerned. The suggestions summarized in Table 30.4 assume that the preparation has been manufactured under conditions designed to exclude contamination.

## Sterility test record

An example of the type of records that need to be kept on each test for sterility that is carried out is given in Figure 30.3.

## USP sterility test

The USP 23 has a very similar sterility test procedure to that which has been described and which is based on the EP (1996) and the BP (1993). Differences that do occur relate to the following.

The anaerobic bacterium suggested for the test is *Bacteroides vulgaris* but *Clostridium sporogenes* is suggested as an alternative if a spore-forming organism is desired. *Staphylococcus aureus* is not used but *Bacillus subtilis* is the aerobic test organism suggested, with *Micrococcus luteus* as an alternative if a spore-forming organism is not wanted. *Candida albicans* is the recommended fungal test organism.

The inoculum for the 'fertility control' and the

| Table 30.4 Minimum sample size related to batch size (based on the BP 1993) | | |
|---|---|---|
| Product | Batch* size (containers/packages) | Minimum sample size (containers/packages) |
| Injectables | ≤100<br>>100 but <500<br>>500 | 10% or 4 whichever is the greater<br>10<br>2% or 20 whichever is the lesser |
| Ophthalmics and other non-injectables | ≤200<br>>200 | 5% or 2 whichever is the greater<br>10 |
| Surgical dressing | ≤100<br>>100 but ≤500<br>>500 | 10% or 4 whichever is the greater<br>10<br>2% or 20 whichever is the lesser |
| Catgut and non-absorbable surgical sutures | ≤100<br>Each additional 1000 | 2% or 5 whichever is the greater<br>Add 2 up to ≤40 strands |
| Bulk solids | <4<br>4 to ≤50<br>>50 | Every one<br>20% or 4 whichever is the greater<br>2% or 10 whichever is the greater |

*Batch = homogeneous collection of sealed containers so prepared that the possibility of microbial contamination is uniform.

**Sterility test record** Direct inoculation method

Date test commenced ___ First test ___ Retest ___ Second retest ___

Product ___ Batch no. ___ Method of sterilization ___

Vol/wt. in each container ___ Vol/wt. of sample ___ No. tested ___

Antimicrobial and conc. ___ Inactivator/diluent ___

Results of incubation. Day number 1,2,3,4,5,6,7, 14

| | Mercaptoacetate medium 31°C | | Soya bean casein digest medium 25°C | |
|---|---|---|---|---|
| | Anaerobic | Aerobic | Aerobic | Fungal |
| Test | | | | |
| Control organisms | Cl. sporog. | S. aureus | S. aureus | C. albicans |
| Density of growth Scale 1–3 — 'Fertility' | | | | |
| 'Growth' | | | | |
| Controls — 'Negative' | | | | |

Conclusion: Sample passed ___ Batch passed ___

Sample failed ___ Retest allowed ___

Sample failed ___ Batch failed ___

Signed ___ Date completed ___

**Fig. 30.3** Sterility test record: direct inoculation method. 'Fertility control' = media + organism; 'Growth control' = media + organism + product and for the membrane filtration method + membrane; 'Negative control' = sterile media, or terminally sterilized product + media. This latter control is to check the operator technique and should be negative. *Note:* The same sterility test record format can be used for the 'Filter membrane method' noting the difference in the 'Growth control'.

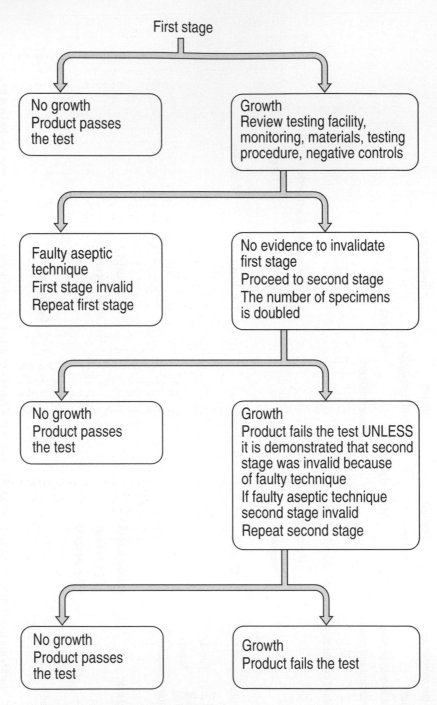

**Fig. 30.4** Interpretation of results obtained with the USP 23 sterility test.

'growth control' is recommended to be within the range 10–100 viable organisms which should result in a slightly lower inoculum than with the EP and the BP tests.

Two types of thioglycollate media are suggested in the USP. The medium that is different from the EP and BP is called the 'alternative thioglycollate' medium and does not contain agar or resazurin sodium.

This medium must be freshly prepared or heated in a steam-bath and allowed to cool just prior to use. It is useful for testing devices which have a narrow lumen into which the more viscous thioglycollate medium will not enter.

The number of representative containers selected to be tested is standardized as 20 for each medium used. This is independent of the batch size and for small batches will represent a larger test sample than that required for the EP and BP test.

When isopropyl myristate is used as a solvent for ointments and oils it is specified that the isopropyl myristate used must have a pH of water extract not less than 6.5. It must be sterilized by filtration through a 0.22 μm membrane filter.

The maximum temperature allowed for melting an ointment or warming a solvent is 44°C.

Interpretation of results is a little different. The USP refers to the initial test for sterility as the 'first stage'. The product tested passes the test for sterility if no growth is observed in the test samples at this stage. If microbial growth is found in the sample of product under examination and it can be shown by review of testing facility, monitoring, materials used, testing procedures and negative controls that the test was inadequately performed, then the first stage can be repeated (as a first stage test). This is equivalent to the repeat of the initial test in the EP and BP procedure.

The second stage is carried out if a review of procedures gives no ground for invalidating the first stage. For the second stage the minimum number of specimens of product is doubled. Thus this is different from the retest of the EP and BP which uses the same number of specimens as in the initial test.

If no microbial growth is found at the second stage then the product passes the test for sterility. The presence of growth confirms the failure of the article to pass the test for sterility. However, if it can be demonstrated that the second stage was invalid because the aseptic technique was inadequate, then the second stage may be repeated. This is set out in Figure 30.4.

Thus the main difference between the USP test on the one hand and the EP and BP test on the other, is in the number of samples selected for testing. That is, the number of samples taken from the batch of product in the first instance and the number of samples required for the second-stage test of the USP, differ from the equivalent retest stage of the BP and the EP.

The inclusion of samples known to be sterile, as negative controls to evaluate operator technique, provides very useful information to assist with deciding whether a particular test is valid or not.

## Key Points

- The sterility test has limitations related to:
  - sample size – cannot guarantee to detect a small level of contamination
  - the possibility of false positives – due to the fallibility of the test conditions and/or operator technique.
- Sterility test conditions need to be controlled and these include:
  - environmental conditions of the test laboratory
  - general culture conditions for the microorganisms
  - species and strains of the test microorganisms.
- The phases of bacterial growth have particular relevance to the successful culture of contaminants. The four phases are:
  - lag phase
  - logarithmic phase
  - stationary phase
  - decline phase.
- Bacteria and moulds have different specific culture requirements and need their own specific culture media, incubation temperature, and length of incubation. Examples of sterility test media are:
  - fluid mercaptoacetate medium – primarily for anaerobic bacteria but also sustains growth of aerobic bacteria
  - soyabean casein digest medium – primarily for aerobic bacteria but will also support the growth of fungi.
- There are two methods recommended in the BP and EP for testing the sterility of the product. The methods have to be followed in exact detail if they are to have the possibility of success. The two methods are:
  - membrane filtration – the method of choice where applicable
  - direct inoculation.
- The tests specify:
  - inactivating agents which are effective for a range of antibacterial agents contained in the product
  - sample sizes to be tested in relation to the original manufacturing batch size of the product
  - how the results obtained are to be interpreted with regard to passing or failing the test or whether a retest is allowed.

## FURTHER READING

Avallone H L 1985 Control aspects of aseptically produced products. Journal of Parenteral Science and Technology 39: 75–79

British Pharmacopoeia 1993 HMSO, London

British Standard 5295 1976 Environmental cleanliness in enclosed spaces. British Standards Institution, London

Brown M R W, Gilbert P 1977 Increasing the probability of sterility of medicinal products. Journal of Pharmacy and Pharmacology 27: 434–491

Department of Health and Social Security 1983 Guide to good pharmaceutical manufacturing practice. HMSO, London

European Pharmacopoeia 1996 3rd edn. Maisonneuve S.A., Saint Ruffine, France

United States Pharmacopoeia 23 1995 Mack, Easton, PA

Zlotnick B J, Franklin M L 1987 A robotic system for the sterility testing of injectables. Pharmaceutical Technology 11: 59–64

# PART 4

# FROM THEORY TO PHARMACEUTICAL CARE

# 31

# Clinical pharmacy practice

*J. A. Cromarty, J. G. Hamley and J. Krska*

---

After studying this chapter you will know about:

**The development of clinical pharmacy**
**The care of patient groups**
**Prioritizing care**
**Assessing patients**
**Planning care**
**Monitoring patients**
**Transferring care**
**Assessing clinical pharmacy practice**.

## Introduction

The practice of clinical pharmacy aims to help maximize drug efficacy, minimize drug toxicity and promote cost-effectiveness. In order to achieve this, pharmacists require to work as fully integrated members of the health care team. Both as team members and members of their own professional body, pharmacists are accountable to patients for the services which they provide.

Patients' rights, expectations and needs should be considered when planning and assessing services. Pharmacists are required to respect the confidentiality of information relating to a patient and the patient's family. Patients should be consulted about the types of services which they require. They should also be involved in assessing their quality.

Pharmaceutical care has been defined by Hepler and Strand (1990) as 'the responsible provision of drug therapy for the purpose of achieving definite outcomes that improve a patient's quality of life'. The term is used also to refer simply to the contribution to patient care resulting from the practice of clinical pharmacy (Clinical Resource and Audit Group 1996). Both indirect and direct patient care activities are involved. Influencing prescribing is an example of the former. Direct patient care activities include responding to symptoms, medication review and patient counselling.

In the hospital service, participation in drug and therapeutics committees, ward rounds and other clinical meetings is common practice. Clinical pharmacists may be ward based or spend most of their time at ward level. Access to other members of the health care team and participation in team activities are taken for granted. The pharmacist's contribution to patient care is generally welcomed by other health care staff. Most established hospital clinical pharmacy services are now well developed. They have been shown to improve prescribing, patient outcomes and cost-effectiveness.

In primary care, a growing number of pharmacists work within, or in association with, general practice surgeries. Some work on a sessional basis whilst others are employed full time. They work closely with medical and nursing staff. Indirect patient care activities include promoting generic prescribing and devising or reviewing local formularies and treatment protocols. Pharmacists may also have responsibility for reviewing the therapy of patients with certain chronic diseases. Examples of target patient groups are asthmatics and patients with upper gastrointestinal disease. The experience of hospital pharmacists helped to establish pharmacist-led anticoagulant clinics in a number of practices. Early studies have suggested that significant savings and benefits accrue from these activities. This is currently being tested in randomized controlled trials.

Ready access to other health care team members may prove to be more difficult for pharmacists based within community pharmacies. It is within community pharmacies, however, that the general public, including patients, has its greatest accessibility to any health care professional. With this comes the profession's greatest opportunity to practise clinical pharmacy. Responding to symptoms, the effective use of patient medication records and the provision of counselling and advice on medicines are key functions of community pharmacists. Uniquely, they can ensure compatibility between prescribed medicines and those purchased over the counter (OTC). This role is likely to increase as more potent medicines are deregulated. The increased emphasis on a primary care-led NHS strengthens the need for better integration of the community pharmacist into the primary care team. Effective referral systems between members of the team are required. As we move into the 21st century, the challenge for clinical pharmacy practice will be to deliver quality pharmaceutical care to patients, irrespective of their location. Continuity of care must be maintained as patients transfer from one health care environment to another.

This chapter sets the scene for Part 4 of the book. It describes briefly how modern clinical pharmacy practice developed. Indirect patient care activities, described under 'Care of patient groups' (p. 336), set in place safe systems of work. Their objectives are to facilitate rational and cost-effective prescribing and to ensure the appropriate use of medicines. A systematic approach to clinical pharmacy practice then ensures that drug therapy for individual patients is optimal. This is the main focus of the chapter. Finally, the need for continuous quality improvement is emphasized in the section 'Assessing clinical pharmacy practice' (p. 351).

## THE DEVELOPMENT OF CLINICAL PHARMACY

Modern clinical pharmacy practice in the hospital service has its roots in the mid-1960s. However, pharmacists have been practising what is now called clinical pharmacy for centuries. They did this first as apothecaries and later as chemists and druggists. Responding to symptoms appropriately and advising patients on the correct use of their medicines are very important clinical functions. Taken in its broadest sense of pertaining to a patient, 'clinical' has always described the work of pharmacists practising in the community. However, until recently, there was reluctance on the part of the medical profession to accept that pharmacists had a clinical role. There was also reluctance by some pharmacists to further develop that role. There can be little doubt now that the evolution of hospital-based clinical pharmacy practice did a great deal to consolidate the role. It also served to facilitate the acceptance of the pharmacist as a valued member of the health care team.

Purchasing, manufacturing and supplying medicines occupied the majority of hospital pharmacists until the mid-1960s. They had much less contact with patients than their counterparts in the community. A combination of factors stimulated change. The need for a better system of prescribing and administering medicines was highlighted by studies on medication errors at ward level (Vere 1965). This led to the development of prescription and drug administration records (Crooks et al 1965). The need to avoid either the transfer of these records from the wards to the pharmacy, or their transcription by nursing staff was recognized. Consequently, pharmacists started to visit the wards. At the same time, the range of potent new medicines was increasing. The associated demand for independently evaluated drug information provided pharmacists with another reason for visiting the wards. The concept of ward pharmacy in the UK was born. First reports came from opposite ends of the country: Calder & Barnett (1967) in Aberdeen, and Baker (1967) in London.

Early ward pharmacy activities focused on reviewing prescription charts mainly for the purposes of stock control and medicine supply. New treatments were also checked for accuracy and completeness. Pharmacists looked for drug incompatibilities and checked doses. In carrying out these activities pharmacists were available at ward level to answer drug-related enquiries. The demand for such information grew and led to the establishment of drug information centres at area or regional level (Rogers & Barrett 1972). These centres provided vital drug information support to ward pharmacists and other health care professionals. In 1976 they were linked by a National Drug Information Network (see Ch. 36).

Another key factor in the development of clinical pharmacy was the provision of postgraduate courses. Early Masters' Degree courses were in Hospital Pharmacy (e.g. Heriot-Watt University in Edinburgh 1969, and University of Manchester 1971) or Biopharmacy (e.g. Chelsea College, London 1966). These paved the way for the development of Masters' Degrees in Clinical Pharmacy (e.g. University of Strathclyde 1976, and University of London 1980). There followed many postgraduate diploma and degree courses in Clinical Pharmacy. These courses, leading to a formal postgraduate qualification, were complemented by in-service education and training courses at hospital level (e.g. Hope Hospital, Salford 1978) and at regional level (e.g. North West Thames Regional Clinical Pharmacy Training Scheme 1983). Indeed, a number of postgraduate diploma and degree courses emanated from these in-service courses.

This battery of education and training provision

did much to effect the transition from ward pharmacy to clinical pharmacy. However, the process took time. Some of the earlier postgraduate courses lacked input from teachers with experience of clinical pharmacy practice. In addition, not all graduates of these courses were given carte blanche to practise clinical pharmacy. Inevitably, there was some resistance to change both from within and outwith the profession. Early surveys demonstrated widespread variation in levels of clinical pharmacy development (e.g. Hospital Pharmacists' Group Policy Statement 1981, and DHSS 1984 ORS 60/84).

By the mid-1980s a reasonable number of key teacher–practitioner posts had been established between universities and health authorities/boards. More courses were generating larger numbers of clinically trained pharmacists. These 'clinical pharmacists' had the important task of consolidating and extending the pioneering work of the 1960s and 1970s.

The art of prescription monitoring in hospitals had by this time given way to a more thorough assessment of the patient. Direct access to patients was required initially for drug history taking and patient counselling. Pharmacists were also able to assess the pharmaceutical needs of patients through access to medical notes and by participating in selected medical rounds. Interaction with other members of the health care team increased. All of this enabled pharmacists to make a more comprehensive assessment of medication and individual patient risk factors. Pharmacists became better equipped and more adept at providing advice both to the health care team and to patients. Hospital pharmacists were now in a better position to optimize the therapeutic management of individual patients.

At the same time as developing these skills in direct patient care, hospital pharmacists were increasing their influence on prescribing for patient groups. Many played key roles in drug and therapeutics committees and formulary committees. Formularies are summarized under 'Care of patient groups' (p. 339) and described more fully in Chapter 34. Medicines resource management aims to optimize the use of medicines to obtain maximum therapeutic benefit within available resources. By identifying and improving patterns of prescribing and medicines use, pharmacists contribute to this important multidisciplinary activity. This subject is dealt with in more detail in Chapter 35.

In parallel with the development of generic skills in clinical pharmacy practice were developments in

specialist areas. Good examples of combining traditional skills with new clinical skills were the development of total parenteral nutrition and therapeutic drug monitoring services. These services utilized respectively the pharmaceutical and analytical expertise of pharmacists. In some cases, the analytical expertise and the drug assay service were provided by biochemistry departments. As well as the development of these specialist services, pharmacists were gaining experience in the provision of clinical pharmacy services within many clinical specialities. For example, clinical pharmacy services became established in mental health, care of the elderly, oncology/haematology, intensive care, paediatrics and renal units. The growth of clinical pharmacy practice was gaining momentum.

The profession was to gain further support from two important sources. First, an independent Committee of Inquiry was appointed by the Nuffield Foundation in October 1983. Its terms of reference were 'To consider the present and future structure of the practice of pharmacy in its several branches and its potential contribution to health care and to review the education and training of pharmacists accordingly'. The 'Nuffield Report', as it became known, was published in January 1986. This comprehensive document made 96 main conclusions and recommendations. 'Clinical pharmacy should be practised in all hospitals', concluded the Report which also recommended that there 'should be a general statement of the clinical pharmacy service that should be provided in all hospitals'. Other aspects of the Nuffield Report are dealt with in Chapter 1.

The Government responded to Nuffield's recommendation with the publication of a health service circular entitled 'The Way Forward for Hospital Pharmaceutical Services'. In England this was issued as DHSS Circular HC(88)54. In Scotland and Wales, similar NHS Circulars, 1988(GEN)32 and WHC(88)66, respectively, were issued. These circulars called for action by health authorities and health boards. They were to review their pharmaceutical services and plan for the implementation of clinical pharmacy and formulary management systems. This was to be included in their planning programme for 1989/90.

Forward plans were established in response to these circulars by the Regional Pharmaceutical Officers (RPhOs) in England (1989) and by the Scottish Chief Administrative Pharmaceutical Officers (CAPOs) in Scotland (1990). The RPhOs issued a Statement on Clinical Pharmacy (1989) and the CAPOs produced a plan: 'Implementation of Clinical

Pharmacy in the Scottish Hospital and Community Health Service'. The latter was also referred to as the 'CAPOs' Implementation Plan 1(90)'.

The RPhOs' Statement made the following recommendations:

1. Drug and therapeutics committees and formulary management systems were to be actively supported.
2. Resource levels required to provide standards for pharmaceutical services were to be quantified.
3. Staff were to be redeployed.
4. Staff training requirements were to be recognized.
5. Activity data were to be collected with a view to the development of performance indicators.

The CAPOs' Implementation Plan 1 (90) set time scales for each of the following recommendations:

1. Pharmaceutical aspects of patient care were to be reviewed (by Autumn 1990).
2. Clinical pharmacy services were to be planned (by Spring 1991).
3. Clinical pharmacy services were to be implemented (by Autumn 1991).

In addition, it was recommended that the CAPOs' Group should initiate a system to monitor and coordinate progress with implementation.

The main areas identified in the plan were as follows:

1. identification of pharmaceutical needs
2. resources and the provision of education and training
3. implementation, monitoring and review of formulary management systems
4. approach to practice.

The extent to which hospital clinical pharmacy services developed in Scotland was evaluated by postal questionnaire in 1993 and reported in 1994. This was a joint initiative between the Scottish Management Efficiency Group (SCOTMEG) and the Clinical Resource and Audit Group (CRAG). The project reviewed progress with the CAPOs' Implementation Plan 1 (90) in Scotland's 46 NHS Trusts/Directly Managed Units with a pharmaceutical service. The SCOTMEG/CRAG Project Report on Clinical Pharmacy Services indicated that 'definite progress' had been made (Cromarty et al 1996). It also identified considerable variation in the extent of clinical pharmacy development. This variation occurred not only between but within hospitals. The Report indicated a need to strengthen the man-

agement framework supporting clinical pharmacy services. Clear 'service specifications' and objectives should be agreed. Standards of performance should be monitored through programmes of professional and service evaluation. Information systems were required to document and collect data to support clinical pharmacy and drug use evaluation. At UK level, a survey investigated the range of clinical pharmacy services provided in hospitals throughout the country (Cotter et al 1994). A comparison of the Scottish and UK surveys indicates that clinical pharmacy services are often provided by pharmacists with a postgraduate qualification. Of the 'local best practices' in Scotland, 73% were provided by such pharmacists. 66% of clinical pharmacy services in Scotland were provided by pharmacists with MSc degrees. This compared with a UK figure of 53%. A more marked difference existed in relation to the taking of medication histories. This was carried out in 36% of hospitals in Scotland compared with a UK average of 16%. The Scottish figure for patient counselling (in 74% of hospitals in Scotland) compared with a UK average of 60%. Both the above surveys captured subjective data on a self-reporting basis. However, they were useful in that they highlighted aspects of hospital clinical pharmacy services in need of further development.

A joint working party on the future role of community pharmaceutical services was set up by the Department of Health and the pharmaceutical profession in 1990. Its report, entitled 'Pharmaceutical Care: the Future for Community Pharmacy', was published in 1992 by the Royal Pharmaceutical Society of Great Britain. The Report made 30 recommendations on how NHS community pharmaceutical services might be developed to increase their contribution to health care. It complemented the Nuffield Inquiry Report (1986) and the government White Papers 'Promoting Better Health' (1988) and 'Working for Patients' (1989). Together, these reports and white papers recognized ways in which pharmacists' skills could be used more effectively in community practice. Reasonable progress has been made in implementing many of their recommendations.

A number of key innovators in community pharmacy have led the way. Although not widely adopted as yet, one of the most important developments to have taken place was a brave departure from tradition. In Clare Mackie's pharmacies in Glasgow, the patient medication record (PMR) system was relocated. Instead of being in the dispensary, the system, along with the pharmacist, is located in the front shop. This move was designed to facilitate a number of the pharmacist's key functions. It enables the pharmacist to be involved in every patient consultation. An open counselling area beside the PMR system can be used by the pharmacist to obtain relevant aspects of the patient's medical history. The pharmacist can assess the appropriateness of the new prescription. The prescription can then be entered into the PMR system in the usual way. This generates the labels on the printer in the dispensary. In such a situation, technicians can then perform the supply function. The pharmacist hands out every prescription and counsels every patient. The location of the system and pharmacist also means that the sale of OTC medicines can be directly supervised. This has two important consequences. First, the pharmacist can directly assess the appropriateness of OTC medicines in relation to the patient's history and his prescribed medicines. Second, OTC sales can then be recorded in the PMR system. This development has considerably enhanced the pharmacist's professional role. It has also made patients very much more aware of it.

Developments have not been restricted to improving practice in the more traditional aspects of the pharmacist's role. Some studies have investigated the provision of parenteral nutrition and therapeutic drug monitoring services by community pharmacies. Domiciliary pharmaceutical services and services to nursing and residential homes have been developed and assessed. An increasing number of studies are investigating collaborative working with general practice surgeries. These have ranged from assistance with the interpretation of prescribing data through repeat prescribing/dispensing systems to individual patient medication review.

Programmes of continuing pharmaceutical education throughout the UK have greatly facilitated these developments. Formal postgraduate diploma and degree courses are responding to the need for change in community pharmacy practice. A Specialist Interest Group in Primary Care Pharmacy has been formed within the United Kingdom Clinical Pharmacy Association. Its growing membership indicates the level of interest and involvement in clinical pharmacy practice within primary care.

A good foundation for the development of clinical pharmacy has been established over the last 30 years. As we move into the next century, pharmacy and pharmacists face exciting challenges. The need to demonstrate cost-effectiveness in medicines resource management will grow as expenditure on health care continues to rise. The requirement for quality of pharmaceutical care and value for money will become ever more apparent. The expectations both of society and of government require to be met.

## CARE OF PATIENT GROUPS

The rational use of medicines aims to ensure cost-effectiveness. There is a need to manage the limited resources available within existing health care systems to maximize benefits for the majority of the population. Inappropriate or unnecessary use of medicines should be avoided as it may lead to increasing costs of illness. This applies not only to the cost of the medicines themselves, but also to the much greater costs of potential adverse effects, hospital admission, corrective treatment and loss of employment. Failure to treat some patients in the most cost-effective way may compromise the financial ability of the health care system to treat other patients. Everyone who has influence over medicines use therefore has a responsibility to ensure that they are used optimally.

Pharmacists play a major role in determining the use of medicines, both those which are prescribed and those which are used for self-medication. Much of the work of a clinical pharmacist is directed towards individual patients. Unfortunately, however, not all patients are able to benefit from clinical pharmaceutical expertise. There are two main and related reasons for this. First, there is a shortage of clinically trained pharmacists. Second, patients in need of clinical pharmaceutical expertise may not have access to it. Housebound patients send representatives to collect their prescriptions. A proportion of patients obtain their medicines from dispensing doctors and never see a pharmacist. However, pharmacists can help to ensure the rational use of medicines in many more patients than they see individually. This can be achieved by influencing the prescribing and use of medicines in particular patient groups. Clinical pharmacists are involved in the development, implementation and monitoring of methods designed to promote the rational use of medicines. Community and hospital pharmacists both play an important part in these activities. Pharmaceutical prescribing advisors are also active contributors.

### Needs assessment

There are many diverse groups of patients for whom health care must be planned. This requires that the needs of these groups must be assessed. Needs assessment is a multidisciplinary activity, involving social services as well as health care services personnel. The involvement of pharmacists is essential, since needs assessment must include patients' pharmaceutical needs. This refers not only to patients' needs for prescribed medicines, but also to their need for other pharmacy services. Access to pharmacies for their self-medication facilities and general advice on health care is important. Counselling and advice on prescribed and purchased medicines should be available, as should compliance aids, where necessary. Particular community pharmacies may be a source of specially manufactured products, e.g. TPN bags, or special services, e.g. harm minimization services for drug misusers. Patients in residential and nursing homes may have unrecognized needs which could only be met through a visit by a pharmacist.

Determining the needs of different patient groups enables pharmaceutical services to be planned for. This is different from providing pharmaceutical services in response to a demand which may not equate to need. Patients in need of particular services may not be fully aware of these needs. Conversely, those who request services are not always those in greatest need. A simple example is housebound patients with chronic diseases for which they are prescribed regular medication. Neighbours may be willing to collect dispensed medicines for these patients, but the patients may need pharmaceutical advice about whether the medicines are appropriate and how to use them optimally. If these patients never visit a pharmacy and a pharmacist never visits the patients, their pharmaceutical needs may not be determined. Thus patients should have a right of access to pharmaceutical assessment, irrespective of their location.

## Groups of patients with pharmaceutical needs

The population can be divided into groups by many different methods. Here the division is for the purposes of determining pharmaceutical needs and of planning the delivery of the services required. It is therefore built around medicines use. The groups are:

- patients suffering from a particular condition or group of conditions
- patients in particular age groups
- patients treated with a particular drug or group of drugs
- patients taking medicines for chronic diseases
- patients cared for within a particular health care setting
- patients transferring from one health care setting to another
- patients who self-medicate.

Each of these groups will have different needs. Consequently, the role which the pharmacist plays in their care will differ. Some of these differing roles are now described.

### Patients suffering from a particular condition or group of conditions

Examples of this type of group are those suffering an acute myocardial infarction, those with chronic pain, those with mental health problems or those with learning difficulties. Each of these will require different types of pharmaceutical services.

Patients who have had a myocardial infarction need to be admitted to hospital rapidly. They should receive the optimal treatment to minimize adverse consequences of their condition and to prevent a recurrence. Thus a policy is required which ensures this. Pharmacists should be involved in developing, implementing and monitoring such a policy. These patients will probably also require advice about their condition, the drug therapy which they receive and their lifestyle. There are many other examples of particular clinical conditions for which policies about medicine use and advice are needed. Very often such policies are achieved through local treatment protocols (see p. 340). These may be based on nationally agreed clinical guidelines (see p. 339).

Patients who have chronic pain are often in the community and may have mobility problems. It can often be difficult to relieve pain. Patients may have to adapt their lifestyle to cope with their condition. Pharmaceutical advice on optimizing therapy is likely to be needed on an individual basis. Policies may also be needed for the treatment of subgroups of patients with chronic pain. An example of such a subgroup would be patients with rheumatoid arthritis. These patients need a multidisciplinary service. This may involve occupational therapists, physiotherapists, nurses and medical practitioners, as well as pharmacists. Rheumatoid arthritis patients will often wish to consult other practitioners and may derive benefit from complementary methods of treatment. For example, some of these patients use acupuncture, aromatherapy or chiropractic. Thus the pharmacist must be able to work as part of a team. In this way, the patients in this group are able to receive optimal care including rational drug therapy.

Patients with mental health problems constitute a diverse group. Problems may range from the acutely ill psychotic in a hospital ward to the patient with depression who is living at home. This group of patients needs specialized pharmaceutical input. A considerable degree of collaboration with other health care and social services workers is required. As an integrated member of the team, the pharmacist is better able to understand the complex needs of this group of patients. Other members of the team also require to be fully appraised of the risks and benefits of drug therapy for this group of patients.

Patients with learning difficulties have special requirements with regard to their medicines. Various social, clinical and pharmaceutical factors may render this group of patients vulnerable to medicine-related problems. Patients discharged from long-stay care may be at particular risk. Their pharmaceutical needs require to be assessed in the context of their social support. Carers and patients may require advice and counselling on their medication. As with the mental health group, effective liaison between health care sectors and social services is essential.

### Patients in particular age groups

The very young and the elderly have special pharmaceutical needs. This is due mainly to alterations in pharmacodynamics and/or pharmacokinetics, compared to the normal adult population. In addition, the elderly are more likely than younger patients to have multiple medical conditions and multiple drug therapy. Thus they are at greater risk of adverse drug reactions. Patients aged 75 years and over living at home must have an annual assessment, which may be carried out by a nurse or health visitor. Many such patients have multiple pharmaceutical needs. It may be necessary therefore to train nurses and health visitors to identify pharmaceutical needs. Alternatively, and preferably, pharmacists should become involved routinely in such assessments. Elderly patients are likely to have considerable needs for counselling and advice about their medicines. It may be sensible therefore to adopt a structured guidelines-based approach to patient counselling (see Ch. 37). The same principle applies at the other end of the age spectrum. Where possible, therefore, a structured guidelines-based approach should be taken in caring for neonatal and paediatric patients. This minimizes the risk of medication-related problems in these vulnerable patient groups.

### Patients treated with a particular drug or group of drugs

Certain types of pharmaceutical services may be needed by patients who are prescribed particular medicines. For example, patients taking certain drugs with narrow therapeutic indices, e.g. gentam-

icin, may require a therapeutic drug level monitoring (TDM) service. Antibiotic use within hospitals is nearly always controlled by a policy. Similarly, the operation of a TDM service may be subject to a hospital policy. The use of highly expensive drugs, expensive drugs in common use, or those with a narrow therapeutic index is usually controlled by policy. Thus patients treated with ulcer-healing drugs or non-steroidal anti-inflammatory drugs (NSAIDs) should be treated according to appropriate policies. As well as dealing with drug choice within a group of drugs, policies should specify the need to review therapy. This may include specific guidelines on monitoring for efficacy and toxicity. Pharmacists should be involved in the development, implementation and monitoring of these policies.

### Patients taking medicines for chronic diseases

Patients in this group are most likely to be living at home and, generally, will receive most, if not all, of their medicines from their general medical practitioner (GP). General practice surgeries have repeat prescribing systems which facilitate this. Policies are required to ensure regular review of these long-term medicines and to prevent abuse of the system. Increasingly, pharmacists are becoming involved in improving these repeat prescribing systems. In due course, pharmacists are likely to assume responsibility for more of the repeat prescribing itself. This will also involve pharmacists in the regular review of patients. GPs face increasing demands for medicines from their patients. Government pressure is being placed upon GPs to prescribe rationally and cost-effectively. At the same time, they are being asked to provide an increasing range of services. Better systems are required therefore for the management of medicines for patients with chronic diseases. Where there exist valid and reliable indicators of disease progress, drug efficacy and drug toxicity, it seems likely that pharmacists could best fulfil this role. They could take responsibility for monitoring these indicators and taking action according to an agreed protocol (Clinical Resource and Audit Group 1996). Of course, there would have to be effective liaison and referral systems between pharmacists and GPs. In continuing a patient's medication, the pharmacist would have to be assured on a number of points. Essentially, these relate to indication, concordance, efficacy and toxicity.

### Patients cared for within a particular health care setting

Although the majority of patients are living at home,

many will at some time experience a hospital stay. Others will be in residential or nursing homes, in sheltered housing or in other community-based settings. These patients will experience varying degrees of care. Within a hospital, there are different groups of patients, each with different needs. Patients may be grouped according to their major disease state or according to their age. For example, patients may be located in renal or in neonatal units, respectively. The pharmaceutical needs of these different groups determine how pharmaceutical services are divided between different units within a hospital.

Pharmaceutical services to patients in residential homes will also differ from those provided to patients in nursing homes. In the latter, medicines administration is undertaken by nursing staff. Local policies concerning medicines use in both types of home require pharmaceutical input (see Ch. 40).

### Patients transferring from one health care setting to another

Admission to hospital or discharge from hospital can substantially change patients' pharmaceutical needs. The same may be generally true of transfer from one health care setting to another. Patients may require additional medicines, fewer medicines or changes in their drug regimen. Some may also require support on discharge in order to manage their medicines. However, at least some long-term medication will usually need to be continued. Information about these medicines, the patient's progress with therapy and any other special requirements about the medicines should be transferred with the patient. Those responsible for the patient's care in the community should also be informed about any changes to therapy made during the admission. Similarly, they need to be made aware of any new medical conditions which have developed and any new pharmaceutical needs which have been identified. In other words, all relevant information must be transferred with patients when they cross health care boundaries (see 'Transferring care', p. 349). Clearly, pharmacists have a major role to play in this transfer process. Effective communication between pharmacists across health care boundaries is essential. So too is communication between pharmacists and other members of the health care team.

### Patients who self-medicate

An increasing number of people self-medicate for a variety of conditions. Many of these are patients receiving prescription medicines as well.

Pharmacists have a responsibility to ensure that they provide for the pharmaceutical needs of the population no matter which medicines people may be taking. This may include medicines which are available from outlets other than pharmacies. Uniquely, the community pharmacist has the opportunity to ensure compatibility between prescribed medicines and those purchased over the counter. This role is likely to increase as more potent medicines are released from the POM to the P category. Every pharmacy must have a protocol to be followed when a medicine is supplied or when advice is sought about treatment of a medical condition. In addition, pharmacists should be involved in the development of local guidelines. These may relate to which medicines should be sold for particular conditions or about when to refer patients to their GP.

## Methods of ensuring rational use of medicines

In providing for the pharmaceutical needs of patient groups, a few key tools are essential:

- formularies
- clinical guidelines
- local policies and protocols
- evaluated prescribing information
- evaluated drug information.

Some of these are discussed in greater detail elsewhere in this book. However, an overview of how they are integrated to provide pharmaceutical care for patient groups is discussed below.

### Formularies

Formularies are lists of recommended drugs which may be prescribed. They are devised by local multidisciplinary groups, taking into account the principles of rational prescribing. Formularies may apply to prescribed medicines or to medicines for self-medication. They may list drugs to be used in a hospital or in the community. Ideally, they should list drugs for use in both settings within a locality. A formulary may list sufficient drugs to serve the needs of much smaller groups of patients, for example those in one unit of a hospital. Within particular drug groups, formularies recommend drugs of choice. Thus the care of patients being treated with certain groups of drugs may also be facilitated.

### Clinical guidelines

Clinical guidelines are statements which help clinicians to decide how to treat specific clinical conditions. Their purpose is to improve the effectiveness and efficiency of clinical care. Many guidelines are produced at a national level by the most eminent clinical practitioners in the relevant field. For example, the British Thoracic Society produced national clinical guidelines on the treatment of asthma. National clinical guidelines on the treatment of myocardial infarction are produced by the British Heart Foundation Working Group.

In Scotland, a multiprofessional group produces evidence-based clinical guidelines. This group, SIGN – Scottish Intercollegiate Guideline Network – includes pharmacists as well as clinicians, nurses and dentists. The guidelines produced by SIGN are based on systematic literature reviews, as all guidelines should be, although a number of guidelines are still developed by expert groups without formal literature reviews. For SIGN guidelines, various levels of evidence are obtained from the literature for particular therapies in different clinical conditions. SIGN ranks these different types of evidence. Meta-analysis of randomized controlled trials is the highest level of evidence. This is followed by evidence from at least one randomized controlled trial and so on. Evidence obtained from expert committee reports or opinions and/or clinical experience of respected authorities is the lowest level. Similar grading of literature evidence prior to guideline development is undertaken in other countries. This process is essential. It serves to qualify the evidence-base and to prevent guidelines from recommending ineffective or inefficient practices.

As with formulary development, a sense of ownership is needed to promote the use of guidelines in practice. Consultation is therefore essential at an early stage in their development. Local factors must also be taken into account during implementation. Local development, for example, within a hospital unit or a general practice surgery, may result in modifications which help the guidelines to fit the population being served. In Scotland, SIGN has a role in facilitating the implementation of local arrangements.

Audit of guideline use is also essential to ensure that guidelines are being followed and to monitor outcomes. This should identify the need for clinical guidelines to be updated and for methods of implementation to be modified if necessary.

## Local policies and protocols

Local protocols for the treatment of specific clinical conditions may be developed from national guidelines. Many local policies are devised without such help, for example antibiotic policies. It is essential in devising such a policy that local microbial sensitivity patterns are used. A local prescribing policy may also be developed from a local formulary. This can be achieved by adding information about when and how the formulary drugs should be used.

There are many other examples of local protocols for the care of particular patient groups. Shared care protocols devised jointly by practitioners working in primary and secondary care are increasing in number. These help to define the roles and responsibilities of the various health care professionals involved. For example, they may define when patients should be referred to hospital by GPs. They may also state who is responsible for the monitoring of which therapeutic outcomes. Pharmacists should be involved in the development of these, since they often apply to patients on long-term medication.

Many pharmaceutical services to patient groups would benefit from local policies. Examples include the supply of repeat medicines and the provision of services to drug misusers.

## Evaluated prescribing information

Information about individual or practice prescribing is available to most prescribers in the UK. It does not identify individual patients and so is relevant to the care of patient groups. This information needs to be evaluated before it can be of use in ensuring rational prescribing. Pharmacists are frequently called upon to carry out evaluation of prescribing data. This can help to identify ways in which prescribing quality can be improved and/or cost savings can be made. One method of evaluation is the COMPASS system in Northern Ireland (see Ch. 34). This system identifies areas of sub-optimal drug prescribing. Having identified such an area, it is then necessary to carry out a more detailed investigation. Methods such as drug use review and peer review can be used to identify causes and solutions. Ultimately, this should result in the development and implementation of local policies to improve the prescribing.

Prescribing advisors have access to prescribing data for large populations and can identify trends in prescribing. For example, prescribing in a local area or even within a particular general practice surgery could be compared with national trends. Prescribing databases can also be used to monitor the uptake of novel formulations and new products. For example, it would be easy to detect any increase in the prescribing of a novel product following intensive marketing by its manufacturer.

Various prescribing parameters have been proposed as indicators of 'good' prescribing, which relate to particular patient groups. An example is inhaled steroids and cromoglycates as a percentage of the use of inhaled steroids, cromoglycates and beta$_2$-adrenoceptor agonists. Such indicators raise questions about specific aspects of prescribing. Caution should be exercised in attaching clinical significance to some of these indicators. Variations in comparative 'performance' must be considered against the background of differences between practices. Such differences relate mainly to the demographics of patient populations, e.g. age/sex profile, morbidity, mortality and deprivation. Prescribing indicators also take no account of the indication for therapy, where more than one indication pertains.

### Evaluated drug information

Practitioners are inundated with information about medicines. This comes directly from manufacturers or pharmaceutical industry representatives, from journal articles, editorials and advertisements, and via the media. If prescribing is to be rational, the information on which it is based must be as good as possible. This means that clinical practice must be based on the results of well-designed clinical studies. Such data should be published in respected, peer-reviewed professional journals. Independently evaluated information, based on published data which have been critically reviewed, is therefore of great importance. Sources of this information are journals such as the *Drug and Therapeutics Bulletin, Evidence-based Medicine* and bulletins from drug information centres or from the Medicines Resource Centre. The use of data from these sources can help in the development of formularies and local protocols.

## DIRECT PATIENT CARE

## Prioritizing care

Whether in hospital or community pharmacy practice, pharmacists interact with a large number of patients and/or customers. Time does not permit, nor would it be appropriate, to allocate the same degree of attention to each person. It is important, therefore, that pharmacists consider how they can use their time most effectively.

The previous section of this chapter summarizes the pharmacist's involvement in formularies, guidelines, policies and protocols. Such activities ensure an appropriate pharmaceutical input to the care of patient groups. Potentially, this type of input makes efficient use of pharmacists' time. In the case of individual patients, it is not always possible or necessary for the pharmacist to deal with each patient or customer. What is important is that systems are in place to identify those patients in need of the pharmacist's attention.

In hospitals, prioritization should be based on assessment of the needs of different patient groups. This is normally achieved by discussion amongst managers, clinical directors and pharmacists. The level of priority or service to be given to each group is then specified within service level agreements. Pharmacists working within general practice surgeries also tend to target particular groups of patients. This may be according to selected disease states or drug therapy. Other target groups in this situation may be elderly patients on polypharmacy or patients receiving repeat medication. For example, some general practice surgeries have established pharmacist-led anticoagulant clinics.

Within community pharmacies the situation is more complex. Whilst there is some scope for targeting particular groups of clients, pharmacies may have little or no control over their client base. There is also no control over the number requiring attention at any one time. Thus there is a need for some form of screening to identify those patients who need to see the pharmacist. This may also apply within the targeted patient groups in hospitals and general practice surgeries. The processes of *targeting* and *screening* are described below (p. 342).

Irrespective of their location, pharmacists provide care to patients as members of teams. This may be the community pharmacy staff team, the primary care team or the health care team in the hospital. All members of these teams should be clear about their role, which should reflect their particular knowledge and skills. It is important that an appropriate skill mix is utilized. This applies both amongst pharmacy staff and within the health care team.

In hospitals and increasingly in community pharmacies, the responsibility for technical tasks such as dispensing is being devolved to dispensers and technicians. This process of change is not always easy. There is some resistance to it from within the profession. Some community pharmacists hang on to their traditional dispensing role. Others have difficulty in obtaining competent, trained dispensers and technicians. The move is essential if pharmacists are to further develop their clinical role. Both in hospital and community the devolvement of routine administrative and technical functions frees pharmacists' valuable time. The system used in Clare Mackie's pharmacies (see p. 335) is very successful in this respect. It frees the pharmacist to review every prescription, counsel every patient and record relevant information on the PMR.

In addition to dealing with prescribed medicines, it is important to have safe systems in place for OTC medicines. The pharmacist cannot be available to deal with every OTC transaction. The Council of the Royal Pharmaceutical Society has issued supplementary statements to its Code of Ethics. Since 1 January 1995, there should be a written protocol in each pharmacy covering procedures for the supply of a medicine. The protocol should also define the procedure for when advice on treatment for a medical condition is sought. Since 1 July 1996, staff regularly selling medicines in a pharmacy must have completed or be undertaking a prescribed course (Royal Pharmaceutical Society, 1996). These measures help to ensure that pharmacy staff are trained and have procedures to follow. They can then deal appropriately with certain customers' needs and know when to refer the patient to the pharmacist. In this way the pharmacist can prioritize his or her time. Patients in real need of the pharmacist's attention get it.

In the hospital pharmaceutical service skill mix varies both between and within hospitals. This has an obvious influence on prioritizing care. For example, hospital pharmacists' roles in the management of pain may vary widely, depending upon the relative knowledge and skills of the respective team members. In a particular ward the pharmacist may be given responsibility for development of an analgesic protocol and for training junior medical and nursing staff in its use. In a hospice, where medical and nursing staff are highly proficient in the principles of pain management, the pharmacist's involvement might be low. In another situation, the pharmacist may be the most experienced member of the team in the management of pain. In such a case, that aspect of patient care may be devolved to the pharmacist.

## Targeting and screening

Prioritization of care can be achieved by adopting a systematic approach to practice. The targeting of patient groups and screening of patients within these groups are the first steps in a systematic approach.

The principle of targeting should be apparent from the beginning of this section. It is the process of selecting patient groups to receive particular clinical pharmacy services. An assessment of the needs of different groups should form the basis of pharmaceutical resource allocation. In hospitals, this should be agreed with management, clinicians and patient representatives. The type of patient, the nature of care provided and the duration of stay are all factors which feature in the allocation of priorities. As a group, long-stay elderly patients without active care plans often receive lower priority than, for example, patients admitted to a general medical ward with acute renal failure. The high risk of adverse effects associated with cancer chemotherapy is usually reflected by the extent of pharmaceutical input to oncology units.

Many community pharmacists are geographically isolated from the rest of the health care team. Thus, many determine their own priorities for particular patient groups. These priorities should be based upon a combination of professional judgement and current evidence on best practice. Wherever possible, these priorities should reflect the views of other health care professionals and of patients. For example, time might be allocated to counsel all patients newly commenced on metered-dose inhalers. Similarly all patients with comprehension difficulties might be targeted to receive compliance aids.

This process of targeting groups of patients for particular attention is a tool to guide the most appropriate use of resources. However, it should always be remembered that pharmacists have a duty of care to each and every one of their patients and customers.

The screening process involves a quick assessment of the individual patients within a targeted group. Not all patients within a targeted group will require the attention of a pharmacist. This process identifies those patients or customers who do require the pharmacist's immediate attention. For individual patient records, it is important to document the outcomes of the screening process. Such a record may also prove useful for management information purposes. Patients screened out at this stage should be subject to periodic review. Their need for a pharmacist may change. The processes of targeting and screening are summarized in Figure 31.1.

The experienced hospital clinical pharmacist has an in-depth knowledge of a particular area of practice. This enables the pharmacist to recognize the common presenting signs and symptoms of major diseases and to understand their treatments. Priorities of the health care team are understood and the pharmacist has a knowledge of the particular areas of expertise of the various team members. This allows the pharmacist to screen groups of patients and to select those individuals who, potentially, are most in need of pharmaceutical care.

The skills required to screen groups of patients

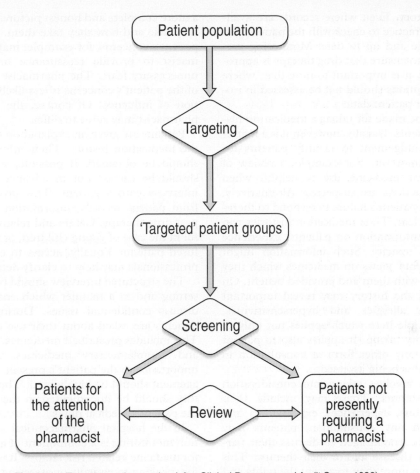

**Fig. 31.1** Targeting and screening (after Clinical Resource and Audit Group 1996).

develop with experience. Criteria used to screen patients or customers are based upon an assessment of potential risk and benefit to the individual. Some criteria relate to the medicine, others to the patient or customer. Examples include the number of medicines prescribed and purchased, the potential for adverse drug reactions, the use of unlicensed or newly marketed medicines, medicines with a narrow therapeutic index, unusual formulations and specialized administration devices. Other criteria are linked with the patient's physical, mental and social condition.

## Assessing patients

Targeting particular patient groups and screening patients within these groups identifies patients with *potential* medicine-related problems. Subject to the availability of relevant clinical information on patients, the pharmacist can make a more detailed assessment. Information from a variety of sources is assimilated and analysed. Sources of information include the patient, the prescription, computerized records, medical case notes, patient medication records and other health care professionals. The purpose of this assessment is to identify patient and medication risk factors. The patient's pharmaceutical needs are confirmed and *actual* medicine-related problems are identified.

In most cases pharmacists will have access to a minimum of two of the above sources of information. The patient and prescription are usually available. In addition, many community pharmacists have a PMR on the majority of their patients. Hospital pharmacists have access to patients' case notes. Maximum use should be made of what is available. Unless dealing with a carer or representative, the pharmacist may choose to obtain a medication history directly from the patient. Of course, some carers and representatives may be able to provide a good history. Even where records are available, it is good practice to check with the patient that they are accurate and up to date. Monitoring prescriptions helps to ensure that drug therapy is appropriate. However, it is important to note that, where possible, prescriptions should not be assessed in isolation from other patient data.

A case could be made for taking a medication history from all patients. Usually, however, it is a matter of professional judgement to identify patients for whom this is important. For example, a review of past and current medicine use is helpful when adverse drug reactions are suspected. Alternatively, the reasons for a patient's failure to respond to therapy may not be clear. Thus medication histories can produce useful information on patients' experience of efficacy and toxicity. Such information might include the patients' views on medicines which they feel have agreed with them and provided benefit. On the other hand, the history may reveal important information on allergies and hypersensitivities. There is a principle here which applies not only to medication history taking. It applies also to patient counselling and any other form of consultation in which the patient is being assessed.

The principle involves taking into consideration the views of patients. These may include their beliefs, perceptions, experiences, expectations and wishes. Thus in any consultation, patients may reveal, or may be encouraged to discuss their perceptions of their disease and/or their therapy. This approach does no more than to accept the rights and the autonomy of individual patients. However, it is of fundamental importance, as it enables pharmacists and physicians to form a therapeutic alliance between themselves and their patients. This concept has been described as concordance in a recent working party report (Royal Pharmaceutical Society of Great Britain & Merck, Sharp & Dohme 1997). It has been proposed as an alternative model of the consultation between prescriber and patient. It applies equally to the relationship between pharmacist and patient. Rather than assuming the patient's role in the consultation to be passive, there should be respect for the patient's agenda. The intention is to create openness in the relationship. In the concordance model, the consultation is a negotiation between equals.

Applying the concept to medication history taking is likely to increase the usefulness of the information obtained. For example, patients may be more inclined to participate and contribute information if they perceive that their views will be listened to, respected, and taken into account. This may lead to a more complete and honest picture of the medicines they take and how they take them. A picture of the patient's concerns, for example, may allow the pharmacist to provide reassurance or to dispel any unnecessary fears. The pharmacist who is unaware of the patient's concerns is less likely to be in a position of influence. Of course, the patient and the pharmacist may agree to differ.

Patients are given an explanation of the purpose of the medication history. Their informed agreement should be obtained. If possible, some preparation should be carried out in advance of a structured interview with a patient. This involves compiling, from patient records, information on current and past drug therapy. Carers and relatives may be helpful in the case of young children, or forgetful or confused patients. Equally, access to other health care professionals may help to clarify details.

The structured interview should be conducted in a setting and in a manner which enables patients to discuss confidential issues. During the interview patients are asked about their use of all medicines. This includes prescribed medicines, OTC medicines and complementary medicines. Any factors of importance to the patient's present and future management should be highlighted. The medication history should be documented in the PMR and/or in the patient's medical notes.

In the hospital pharmaceutical service, prescription monitoring is a component of assessing patients for medicine-related risk factors. It is not a substitute for speaking to patients or assessing other sources of patient information. When monitoring antibiotic therapy, the hospital pharmacist will usually have easy access to relevant clinical information. Used in context, prescription monitoring assists in a complete and continuous assessment of patients' needs for pharmaceutical care. For example, it may enable the pharmacist to judge the appropriateness of dose, route and frequency of administration. In the case of gentamicin, however, this would only be possible if the pharmacist also had access to the patient's age, weight and renal function.

In a community pharmacy, the appropriateness of a prescription for ciprofloxacin may be more difficult to discern. The pharmacist would wish to consider whether this was the drug of choice for the indication involved. However, information on the exact indication and any results from culture and sensitivity testing may not be available to the pharmacist. On the other hand, the pharmacist may be aware of the clinical circumstances in which the GP prescribes ciprofloxacin. Indeed the pharmacist may have been involved in helping the general practice surgery to produce its formulary. The community pharmacist would also wish to consider the patient's concomitant drug therapy. This could be established from the pharmacist's PMR or from the patient. If necessary, the pharmacist may have to contact the prescriber to avoid the possibility of a serious drug interaction, e.g. with theophylline.

Having accessed and evaluated all the requisite information which is available, the patient's pharmaceutical needs are identified. The pharmacist then confirms those needs with the patient and the health care team. Actual medicine-related problems are identified. A decision is made as to which of these require to be addressed by the pharmacist. Other members of the team may also be involved. In hospi-

tal practice, typically, this might be achieved during a ward round. In community practice, it may necessitate a telephone call or referral to the patient's GP. The hospital pharmacist also requires to consider at this early stage of assessment, the patient's discharge plan. Early consideration is designed to accommodate the patient's anticipated pharmaceutical needs and problems on discharge. This is part of a systematic approach to individual patient care (Fig. 31.2). It requires pharmacists to continuously address the changing pharmaceutical needs and medicine-related problems of patients.

Information on patient and medication risk factors and medicine-related problems should be recorded. This initiates a patient medication profile. These

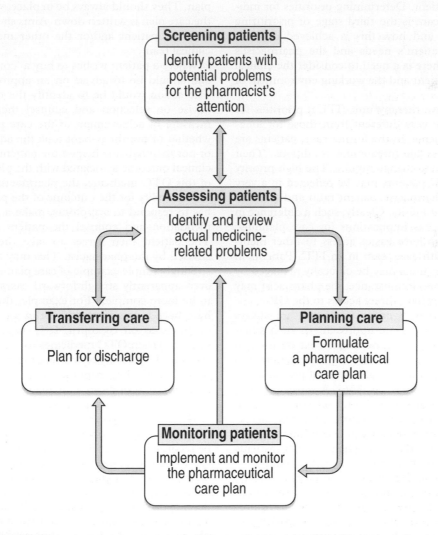

**Fig. 31.2** A systematic approach to individual patient care (after Clinical Resource and Audit Group 1996).

profiles may be recorded within paper-based or electronic record systems. This can be done as a separate pharmacy record or as part of the overall patient record system. Such records are updated as necessary to provide a continuous means of identifying potential medicine-related problems.

## Planning care

Targeting patient groups and screening patients within them are the first two stages of prioritizing care. These processes identify those patients potentially in need of the pharmacist's attention. The pharmacist then needs to assess them (see above) and plan their care. This requires to be achieved within the context of the overall clinical management of the patient. Determining priorities for individual patient care is the third stage of prioritizing care. Whether and how this is achieved depends both on the patient's needs and the pharmacist's opportunity. There is a need to consider the clinical status of the patient and the working environment of the pharmacist.

In an intensive therapy unit (ITU), priorities for patient care are very different from those for long-stay elderly patients. In the former case, patients are being treated for life-threatening conditions. Their clinical status may change rapidly. The high priority attached to ITU patients may be reflected in a very much higher pharmacist:patient ratio and a higher frequency of ward visits. Clearly, such a difference in patients' needs has implications for care planning. Pharmacists also have easier access to other members of the health care team in an ITU. Patients in long-stay elderly units may be clinically managed by their GPs. In this circumstance, the pharmacist may only occasionally have direct access to the GP.

Some issues which occur frequently are always managed using the same approach. In such situations the pharmacist's time might best be used to facilitate the development and implementation, and to monitor the use of a local treatment protocol (see 'Care of patient groups', p. 336). A sepsis protocol can guide appropriate antibiotic selection prior to receiving the bacteriology report. Similarly, agreement may be reached between a community pharmacist and local GPs over when to refer patients with symptoms of dyspepsia for a medical opinion.

As described under 'Prioritizing care' (p. 341), other staff may be trained to manage some commonly occurring medication-related issues. Appropriately trained counter assistants guide patients in selection of medicines for many common conditions. Nurses may be trained to assess patients' use of their inhalers and to identify those requiring to be counselled. In such situations the pharmacist must ensure that staff are appropriately trained and that procedures are followed correctly. This represents appropriate and judicious use of policies, protocols and other trained staff. It creates time for the pharmacist to focus on planning care for those patients most in need of their attention.

### Formulating a pharmaceutical care plan

In all interactions with patients, pharmacists must be able to describe an aim (what they wish to achieve), an action (how they intend to achieve the aim) and a measure that tells them that their aim has been achieved. These are the basic elements of a care plan. They should always be in place, whether or not the care plan is written down. Aims should be agreed with the patient and/or the other members of the clinical team.

Where a patient wishes to buy a 'cough bottle' the aim should be to advise on an appropriate choice. The action would be to identify the type of cough, advise on selection and counsel the patient. The measure of achievement of the care plan would be whether or not the patient took the advice. Whether or not the medicine helped the patient would be the clinical outcome associated with the plan. In the case of this OTC medicine, the pharmacist has a shared responsibility for the outcome of the plan. He or she has to respond to symptoms, make a sound recommendation and counsel the patient appropriately. The patient then agrees to take the medicine as advised by the pharmacist. This may appear to be a strikingly simple example of care planning. However, even apparently straightforward cases can turn out to be more complex. For example, the cough could have been a persistent dry one in a patient recently commenced on captopril. It is important prior to sales of certain OTC medicines to establish from the PMR or the patient, concurrent disease states and/or drug therapy. For example, some cough medicines may be contraindicated in diabetic patients or in those taking monoamine oxidase inhibitors.

When providing care in a team situation (e.g. in a hospital ward) the pharmaceutical care plan should be recorded. This enables the actions of the pharmacist to be coordinated with those of other members of the team. Preferably, aims should be stated as measurable end-points to be achieved within a definite time scale. For example, the aim might be to advise on the selection of a non-stock medicine. The pharmacist may wish to see it prescribed and administered by the next drug administration round.

Alternatively, an aim may be to ensure that a patient understands his new inhaler. Prior to discharge, the pharmacist would aim to have the patient demonstrate his inhaler technique.

The above aims relate to the advising of prescribers and the supplying, administering and taking of medicines. Aims may also be expressed in terms of achieving specified levels of improvement in laboratory or clinical markers of diseases. An aim to prevent drug toxicity may be to ensure that a particular laboratory value remains within a specified range. For example, the plan might be to measure, at specified intervals, urea and electrolyte levels in a patient prescribed a high dose of frusemide.

In considering the most appropriate actions to achieve their aims pharmacists should take account of the following:

• Local formularies or protocols which could assist in the selection of the most cost-effective therapy. For example, formularies may provide advice on the choice of non-steroidal anti-inflammatory agents for use in the elderly.

• Any underlying disease states, or concomitant drug therapy which could affect the choice or dosage of medicine. For example, the dosage of digoxin in a patient with renal impairment.

• Any previous adverse drug reactions, including drug allergies or hypersensitivities. For example, the proposed use of a cephalosporin in a patient with a history of penicillin sensitivity.

• Any requirement of the patient for health promotion (see Ch. 38). For example, a patient who wishes to purchase an antacid for heartburn may require advice on posture and eating habits.

• The patients' knowledge and understanding of their medicines and their ability to use them correctly. For example, the geriatric patient on seven medicines being discharged to sheltered housing.

• The patients' level of domestic and/or social independence or support. For example, the blind patient who obtains assistance with her medicines from her partially sighted husband. This will necessitate the use of some form of compliance aid. In such circumstances, effective transfer of information to carers, community-based health care professionals and/or social workers is essential (see 'Transferring care', p. 349).

The pharmacist's record of an individual patient's medicine-related problems and aims, together with the proposed actions, form a documented pharmaceutical care plan. This allows pharmacists to report on their actions. This is very important for three reasons. Firstly, it provides a medico-legal record.

Secondly, it supports continuity of care. This applies whether patients remain in one care environment or transfer from one care environment to another. Finally, it provides a basis for peer review (see 'Assessing clinical pharmacy practice', p. 351).

Increasingly, there will be attempts to standardize care plans for patients with certain diseases. This is in response to the production of national clinical guidelines. Their purpose is to improve the effectiveness and efficiency of clinical care. This is achieved through the identification and promotion of evidence-based clinical practice. Such guidelines, or protocols derived from them, define the aims of therapy and the actions required to achieve good clinical outcomes. They tend to focus on those areas where effective care is not at present being delivered uniformly. Thus they facilitate the prioritization of pharmaceutical care.

As standard care pathways emerge, pharmacists will be encouraged to address the needs of individual patients within agreed protocols. However, adherence to guidelines and protocols may not be in the best interests of all patients. For some patients, deviations are justified on grounds of contraindications arising from concurrent disease states or concomitant drug therapy. The particular needs of the individual patient should always take priority.

## Monitoring patients

Various health care professionals monitor patients to assess their progress with drug therapy. Most commonly this involves doctors, pharmacists or nurses. Ideally, the process should be a structured one involving care plans with specified targets and review dates. This requires a systematic approach supported by effective communication and collaboration between the health care professions involved.

In both primary and secondary care some pharmacists are well integrated into the health care team's activities. In these situations pharmaceutical care planning may be a routine activity. Implementation of the care plan involves the pharmacist in agreeing with the health care team time scales for monitoring or reviewing the patient. The pharmacist then coordinates his or her actions with those of the patient and the other members of the team.

Various indicators may be used to monitor a patient's progress against the aims stipulated in the care plan. These include clinical signs and symptoms, biochemical and haematological parameters and, for certain medicines, serum drug levels. Where appropriate, clinical assessment should be used in conjunction with objective measures. In the absence of objective indicators, the pharmacist relies on the clinical assessment of the patient by other members of the health care team. Where there are valid objective measures of the therapeutic or adverse effects of drugs, the pharmacist may assume responsibility for monitoring them and taking appropriate action. This is usually achieved within a jointly agreed treatment protocol or care plan.

Monitoring patients may be carried out for one or more of the following reasons:

- to monitor health promotion measures
- to monitor the progress of disease
- to monitor for drug efficacy and/or drug toxicity
- to monitor the patient's satisfaction with drug therapy.

### Monitoring health promotion measures

Health promotion activities may be directed at preventing disease in healthy subjects or minimizing harm in patients with disease. This is dealt with in more detail in Chapters 38 and 42. Monitoring patients addicted to nicotine, alcohol or opiates can help them get the best use from any medicines used in their management. Of equal importance is lifestyle counselling and monitoring in patients with certain chronic conditions. For example, patients with ischaemic heart disease should be encouraged to adopt a healthy lifestyle in relation to their diet and exercise. If relevant, they should be monitored and supported through a smoking cessation programme. Some of these patients may also require assistance in reducing their intake of alcohol.

### Monitoring the progress of disease

Both drug choice and the drug regimen may be affected by the severity and nature of particular disease states. For example, some drugs are contraindicated in renal impairment (e.g. metformin) and others require dosage reduction (e.g. atenolol). Patients with deteriorating renal function therefore require close monitoring of their disease.

### Monitoring for drug efficacy and/or drug toxicity

In some cases the efficacy or toxicity of a drug will require to be determined by the assessment skills of a particular clinician. For example, the efficacy of an antidepressant agent may be assessed by a psychiatrist. Confirmation of possible visual disturbance due to ethambutol may require the expertise of an ophthalmologist. However, the efficacy or toxicity of many drugs is readily detected through routine laboratory investigations. Careful and timeous monitoring of appropriate biochemical/haematological parameters may confirm efficacy and/or prevent drug toxicity. Thus blood glucose is monitored in diabetic patients to inform the dosage adjustment of insulin or of oral hypoglycaemic agents. Blood counts are monitored in AIDS patients receiving ganciclovir for the treatment of cytomegalovirus. Leucopenia and thrombocytopenia are ganciclovir's most frequently observed side effects.

Patients can play an important role in monitoring for toxicity themselves. This requires that they are provided with a knowledge and understanding of the possible side effects of their medicines. Thus the patient on warfarin therapy should be asked to report any signs of unusual or excessive bruising. Patients should be encouraged to be vigilant, even where objective measures of potential toxicity are available to the health care professional. In the case of warfarin, the risks and benefits may be monitored by examining prothrombin times. The therapeutic aim may be to achieve an International Normalized Ratio (INR) of between 2.0 and 3.0. This could be confirmed when the patient is monitored at an anticoagulant clinic. However, the time between visits to an anticoagulant clinic, coupled with many factors which can affect anticoagulant control, could render the patient at risk of a serious bleed prior to the next appointment. In such a situation the patient's informed vigilance could be potentially life saving.

For a small number of drugs it may be inappropriate or potentially dangerous to monitor patients through clinical signs or symptoms alone. There may be no appropriate biochemical or haematological indicators of efficacy or toxicity. The use of serum drug levels is appropriate for such drugs with a narrow therapeutic index and a well-defined target serum concentration range. Interpretation of drug levels should always be made with a knowledge of medication and dosage history, sampling times and relevant clinical details of the patient. Targeting particular drug levels by the application of pharmacokinetic principles can often result in a quicker and safer route to efficacy than that achieved by clinical assessment alone. This activity is known as therapeutic drug monitoring (TDM). For example, in the case of certain anticonvulsants, efficacy could be monitored by fit frequency alone. To do so, however, puts the patient at risk. A TDM service facilitates the achievement of effective serum levels of these anticonvulsants whilst minimizing the risk of toxicity.

A more detailed consideration of the prevention,

detection, monitoring and reporting of adverse drug reactions is provided in the next chapter.

### Monitoring the patient's satisfaction with drug therapy

Asking patients how they are getting on with their medicines encourages patients to express their views. This approach is useful whether within or outwith a formal structured approach to care planning. The patient's response to this open question may express satisfaction and/or concern. A patient's level of satisfaction need not parallel responses to drug therapy indicated by more objective measures. However, it is of equal importance. Patients may be dissatisfied with their drug therapy for what they perceive to be good reason. They may feel sufficiently dissatisfied to cause them to stop taking their medicine. This may be through a lack of obvious response or through suspected adverse effects. Such action may well be justified. Alternatively, a patient may be responding well but not feeling any better. A suspected adverse effect may turn out to be an unrelated symptom requiring further investigation. Thus maintaining a dialogue with patients about their drug therapy is very important. If no specific indicator of drug efficacy or toxicity is being investigated such dialogue may be the only form of monitoring to take place. It also helps to sustain any established concordance (see p. 344) between patients and their pharmacist and/or doctor.

### Reviewing the care plan

Outcomes from the plan are evaluated against the aims which were specified at the formulation stage. Where the aims are achieved, assurance is provided of the resolution of medicine-related problems. Where specific aims are not achieved, the pharmaceutical care plan is reviewed. Either the outcome achieved is accepted as being the best achievable for the patient, or an alternative plan is proposed. Pharmaceutical care planning requires to respond continuously to changes in the clinical status and requirements of patients.

## Transferring care

In the course of a single acute care episode, a patient may interact with several professionals in different settings. Patients suffering from several chronic diseases are likely to be seen by a large number of health care professionals in both primary and secondary care. Transfer of the care of patients between professionals and between health care sectors may be planned or occur in an emergency. Whatever the circumstance, every effort should be made to maintain continuity of care. This requires effective communication between professionals within and between health care sectors.

### Reviewing the care plan

Whenever a patient is transferred to another care environment, or to the care of another pharmacist, the care plan should be reviewed. Proposals should be made to deal with any unresolved medication-related issues and with any new ones which are linked with the transfer of care. Consideration should be given to the change in environment, to the level of patient support and to any shared-care protocols. High priority should be given to ensuring that supplies of medicines are available. Sufficient information should be given to the patient, carers and other health care professionals to enable care to continue as planned.

### Counselling and advising the patient or carer

The pharmacist should ensure that the patient or the patient's carer understands about the medication and is able to administer it correctly. Where appropriate, compliance aids such as calendar cards should be considered. Special labelling should be requested for patients with visual impairment. Consideration should be given to the particular needs of ethnic groups. The patient should be advised on the disposal of discontinued medicines.

Self-medication schemes operate in some hospitals. This usually involves the pharmacist in counselling selected patients on their knowledge, understanding and use of medicines at an early stage during their admission. These patients are then given responsibility for administering their own medicines prior to discharge. This enables the patients' ability to manage their drug regimen to be monitored. Outwith these formal schemes, patient counselling seeks to ensure that all patients are able and prepared to take their medicines as prescribed.

The principle of applying objective measures to monitoring progress and outcomes applies also to the assessment of patients' knowledge and understanding of their medicines. It is all too easy to tell patients how to take their medicines. It is also important to check that they actually have the ability to use their medicines properly (see Chs 37 and 41). There is particular scope for confusion when patients are discharged or transferred. For example, on admission a patient is taking Largactil. In hospital she is changed to generic chlorpromazine and is issued with a supply on discharge. No explanation is given to the patient who subsequently takes both and over-doses. Similar problems can occur when a medicine is discontinued during a hospital stay. The patient may be unaware that the medicine has been stopped, and continue to take it on returning home.

## Communication between professionals

As patients transfer from one health care environment to another, continuity of care relies on the identification of, and effective communication with, those professionals to whom responsibility is transferred.

Where a pharmacist is providing care to a patient, it is his or her duty to ensure that the element of care is continued when the patient is transferred. This is equally so whether the patient is being transferred from the acute medical admissions ward to a general medical ward, from one hospital to another, or from hospital into the community. On hospital discharge, a pharmacy discharge summary can conveniently be transferred with the patient to the community pharmacist. The Royal Pharmaceutical Society of Great Britain has developed documentation to facilitate this two-way communication between hospital and community pharmacists. There are recommended formats for information to be provided on transfer of patients both into and out of hospital.

The confidentiality of information relating to a patient and the patient's family should be respected throughout the transfer process. This also applies to the personal wishes of the patient. For example, patients should be asked which community pharmacy they routinely use. It is important to explain to patients the advantages of using one community pharmacy. This is particularly the case for patients with complex medication needs. Such patients include those receiving parenteral nutrition, pain control or dialysis and those taking multiple medication for one or more chronic diseases (e.g. cystic fibrosis patients).

The community pharmacist's computerized patient medication record is a unique record of patient information. While the GP may be aware of what has been prescribed, some prescriptions are never dispensed. In addition, GPs are unlikely to have any record of the OTC medicines taken by patients. Most patients consistently have their prescriptions dispensed at the same pharmacy. The community pharmacist is therefore ideally placed to provide information to enable a complete medication history to be taken on admission of patients to hospital.

Computer data which are transferred between health care professionals at different sites should be registered with the Data Protections Registrar. All health care professionals involved should comply with the requirements of the Data Protection Act.

## Case study

### a. Poor transfer of care

Mr Brown, a regular customer in the pharmacy, asked to see the pharmacist. He was pale and quite upset. For several years he had taken antacids for indigestion. In the last 3 months he had little relief and during the last week had been feeling sick. On that morning he had been sick and the vomit was brown.

Mr Brown's medication record listed only the antacid which he had been buying and bendrofluazide, which was prescribed for control of blood pressure. The community pharmacist advised the patient to see his doctor immediately. The doctor admitted Mr Brown to hospital for urgent investigation of the problem.

On admission, no record was made of Mr Brown's bendrofluazide since he had forgotten to bring his supply with him. Although asked about medicines, he was confused and thought that the hospital doctor was only interested in medicines for indigestion. He was diagnosed as having a duodenal ulcer and discharged on ranitidine 300 mg daily.

He continued to smoke, had 'several pints with his mates' on Friday nights and drank milk whenever he was bothered with indigestion. 6 months later he was still taking the same dose of ranitidine and still complained of indigestion. He routinely took his ranitidine after breakfast. During a routine check his blood pressure was found to be high.

This example illustrates the potential for problems on transfer of care. Although each of the professionals involved dealt with his or her part of the problem, the overall quality of care was less than adequate.

Because the GP failed to inform the hospital doctor about bendrofluazide, this was missed in hospital and thus was not included on the discharge prescription. No mention was made on the discharge prescription of the duration of treatment with ranitidine. The receptionist amended the repeat prescription, deleting bendrofluazide and adding ranitidine. No one gave the patient health promotion advice and no one informed the community pharmacist about the continuing care of the patient. The scenario depicted in b. below indicates how Mr Brown might have fared in different circumstances.

### b. Effective transfer of care

Having recognized the potential seriousness of Mr Brown's condition, the pharmacist referred him to his family doctor. Mr Brown was given a copy of his patient medication record which he was advised to keep and show to his doctor. On referring Mr Brown to hospital, the GP included an up-to-date medication history in the referral letter. Consequently an accurate medication history was taken on admission and bendrofluazide was continued. Having been diagnosed as having a duodenal ulcer, he was discharged on ranitidine 300 mg at night. The family doctor was informed that treatment should be continued for 8 weeks and then reviewed. Since the patient was infected with *Helicobacter pylori*, a course of eradication therapy was recommended to be commenced once the ulcer had been healed.

Before discharge, the pharmacist gave Mr Brown a detailed explanation of his treatment. Advice was also given upon sensible eating and drinking and the need to stop smoking. A pharmacy discharge summary was sent to the community pharmacist. The treatment plan was described and reinforcement of health promotion advice was recommended.

6 months later Mr Brown's ulcer had healed and his blood pressure was well controlled. *Helicobacter pylori* had successfully been eradicated and he was symptom free. He had adopted sensible eating and drinking habits. With the assistance of nicotine patches suggested by the community pharmacist, he had also significantly reduced the number of cigarettes he smoked each day.

## ASSESSING CLINICAL PHARMACY PRACTICE

As members of the health care team and their own professional body, pharmacists are ethically and professionally accountable to patients and clients for the services which they provide. Assuring the quality of these services involves consulting the 'customers'. These may be the patients, carers, clients or other health care professionals. There is a need to involve each in continuous quality improvement (CQI) initiatives.

Quality may be described as a level of excellence which gives complete customer satisfaction. It also ensures that a product or service is fit for the purpose intended (Clinical Resource and Audit Group 1996). Quality assurance (QA) is achieved through a combination of all the activities and functions associated with achieving quality. Pharmacists have been familiar with this concept for some time, particularly in relation to the quality of medicines (see Ch. 29). More recently, QA has been concerned with assessing clinical pharmacy services.

Health care organizations are broadening the scope of their efforts to ensure quality, which involves a move towards CQI. This approach to quality considers systems within the organization as a whole. It focuses on process and the need to generate objective data on which the quality of services can be judged. The philosophy of CQI demands that all staff have a responsibility to strive for improvement in the services which they provide. Thus within the community pharmacy this might include the

manager/pharmacist, the dispenser/technician and the shop assistants. However, what patients might be equally concerned with is how well the community pharmacy service interacts with the other services involved in their care. CQI then concerns itself not only with intraprofessional processes, but also with interprofessional processes. As illustrated by the case study in the previous section of this chapter (p. 350), the latter can make or break the overall quality of patient care. When assessing clinical pharmacy practice, therefore, processes involving the pharmacist require to be examined in the context of total health care. In keeping with this has been the move within the NHS towards multidisciplinary audit (see Ch. 43).

### Defining the level of service

In hospital pharmacy practice, clinical pharmacy services may be based on written service specifications. These are produced in conjunction with management and other clinical care staff. Patient representatives should also be consulted to ensure that services are designed to meet patient needs. Specifications describe and define the level of service offered to various groups of patients. Clinical pharmacists' objectives should be based on these service specifications. The extent to which pharmacists meet these objectives can then be determined by various processes. These include performance appraisal, peer review, professional audit and clinical audit.

In community pharmacies, pharmacists produce a practice leaflet detailing the professional services offered by the pharmacy. This is part of the requirement for receiving a professional practice allowance. At the present time, the professional services offered by the majority of community pharmacists may be less well defined than those provided by hospital clinical pharmacists. However, community pharmacists are now required to participate in audit in order to qualify for their professional practice allowance.

The Royal Pharmaceutical Society's Statement of Principles and Standards of Good Practice for Hospital Pharmacy in the United Kingdom (1995) complements standards included in an Appendix to the Society's Code of Ethics. Pharmaceutical Officers in the NHS have also defined standards of practice for hospital pharmacists. These documents recognize the need to produce more detailed local clinical pharmacy standards.

### Generating objective data for performance appraisal, audit and peer review

A structured systematic approach to individual

patient care is recommended within this chapter. If properly documented, this approach is capable of generating data required for the assessment of clinical pharmacy practice. At best, the data would comprise fully documented pharmaceutical care plans and outcomes for every patient. This would be unrealistic at the present time. However, some hospital pharmacy services generate pharmaceutical care plans for selected priority groups of patients. A number of pharmacists working in primary care also document pharmaceutical care plans. In these cases it is possible to obtain a reasonable assessment of clinical pharmacy practice.

One of the most common methods of assessing clinical pharmacy practice has been the recording of interventions. These are usually actions by the pharmacist to clarify prescription or administration charts, to promote drug efficacy or economy in the use of medicines, or to prevent or reduce adverse effects. Whilst this may have done a great deal to demonstrate what pharmacists were capable of, it does not generate objective data on practice. In such a system, pharmacists record only what they observe and see fit to act upon. There are no records of patients for whom there was no pharmaceutical intervention. Pharmacists may also select to omit unsuccessful interventions or those in which they lacked confidence. Thus there is no opportunity to subject aspects of the pharmacist's performance to independent scrutiny. Another major deficiency of the system is that it is often based on a contribution made retrospectively by the pharmacist, that is in relation to the prescribing process. It could be argued that, if appropriate contributions are made prospectively, then the need for interventions would decrease. This would be good clinical pharmacy practice. However, practice has often been assessed on the basis of both the number and nature of pharmacists' interventions.

## Audit

Over recent years, audit has become an established component of the NHS. Professional audit is that carried out within a particular profession, usually by that profession. Clinical audit on the other hand is multidisciplinary in nature. It may be undertaken by health care professionals of any discipline. It should also involve the 'customers' of the services being audited, i.e. other health care professionals, clients, patients and their carers. Clinical audit often examines a clinical process which involves a number of different health care professions. Professional and clinical audit are described in more detail in Chapter 43.

## Peer review

Assessing the performance of clinical pharmacists involves issues of professional judgement. Peer review methods are appropriate for this purpose. They generate useful subjective measures of performance. This can complement the objective measures of performance achieved through audit.

Peer review is often used as part of a professional development programme rather than as part of a formal assessment of clinical pharmacy practice. It involves members of the same profession and should be non-threatening. The aim is to develop the clinical knowledge and skills of pharmacists to improve the quality of their practice.

---

### Key Points

- Clinical pharmacy aims to help maximize drug efficacy, minimize drug toxicity and promote cost-effectiveness.
- Pharmacists are accountable to patients for the services which they provide.
- Pharmacists are required to respect the confidentiality of information relating to a patient and the patient's family.
- Responding to symptoms, the effective use of patient medication records and the provision of counselling and advice on medicines are key functions of community pharmacists.
- Studies on medication errors in the 1960s led to the development of prescription and drug administration records and to ward pharmacy.
- The establishment of formal postgraduate courses in clinical pharmacy effected the transition from ward pharmacy to clinical pharmacy.
- The development of hospital-based clinical pharmacy practice facilitated the integration of the pharmacist into the health care team.
- Independent inquiry (Nuffield Foundation 1986) and government circulars ('The way forward for hospital pharmaceutical services' 1988) and a joint working party report (Royal Pharmaceutical Society 1992) provided valuable support for the further development of clinical pharmacy.
- The professional responsibility of pharmacists involves them in the development, implementation and monitoring of policies and methods designed to promote the rational use of medicines in particular patient groups.

- Irrespective of their location, patients have a right to have their pharmaceutical needs assessed and met.
- Appropriate skill mix should be deployed in pharmacy staff establishments and in the health care team such that best use is made of the pharmacist's time and clinical expertise.
- Prioritization of care can be achieved by adopting a systematic approach to practice in which patient groups at greatest risk of medicine-related problems are targeted.
- Screening and assessment of patients in targeted groups identifies those patients in active need of the pharmacist's attention.
- Maximum use should be made of all sources of information available to the pharmacist and medication histories should be taken where appropriate.
- Pharmacists should be mindful of the concept of concordance in their consultations with patients.
- Pharmacists should continuously address and document the changing pharmaceutical needs and medicine-related problems of patients.
- Formulation and documentation of a pharmaceutical care plan need to be achieved within the context of the overall clinical management of the patient.
- In planning care, pharmacists should be able to describe for each issue an aim, action(s) and a method of monitoring progress towards the aim.
- Where there are valid objective measures of the therapeutic or adverse effects of drugs, pharmacists can take responsibility for monitoring and taking action within protocols.
- Patients can play an important role in monitoring for toxicity provided that they are given a knowledge and understanding of the possible side effects of their medicines.
- Monitoring the patient's level of satisfaction with drug therapy is important.
- When patients are being transferred from one care environment to another, the care plan is reviewed to take account of relative priority on transfer. Due consideration should be given to the change in environment, the level of patient support, continuity of supply and existing shared care protocols.
- Patients (or their carers) should receive sufficient counselling and advice to enable their medicines to be used correctly.

- As patients are discharged or transferred, continuity of care relies on effective communication with those professionals (and/or carers) to whom responsibility is to be transferred.
- The philosophy of continuous quality improvement demands that all staff have a responsibility to strive for improvement in the services which they provide.
- 'Customers' of clinical pharmacy services should be involved both in specifying and assessing these services.
- More detailed local clinical pharmacy practice standards are required.
- Comprehensive documentation of clinical pharmacy practice would greatly facilitate its assessment.

## FURTHER READING

Baker J A 1967 Recent developments in the pharmaceutical service at Westminster Hospital. Journal of Hospital Pharmacy 24: 400–406

Calder G, Barnett J W 1967 The pharmacist in the ward. Pharmaceutical Journal 198: 584–586

Clinical Resource and Audit Group 1996 Clinical pharmacy in the hospital pharmaceutical service: a framework for practice. Report of a working group (Chairman, Cromarty J A). The Scottish Office, Edinburgh

Cotter S, Barber N, McKee M 1994 Survey of clinical pharmacy services in United Kingdom National Health Service hospitals. American Journal of Hospital Pharmacy 51: 2676–2684

Cromarty J A, Hudson S A, Young A B, Braddick L G, Davey P G, McMaster K U 1996 Clinical pharmacy services in NHS hospitals in Scotland. Pharmaceutical Journal 257, suppl: R9

Crooks J, Clark C G, Caie H B, Mawson W B 1965 Prescribing and administration of drugs in hospital. Lancet i: 373–378

Hepler C D, Strand L M 1990 Opportunities and responsibilities in pharmaceutical care. American Journal of Hospital Pharmacy 47: 533–543

Nuffield Foundation 1986 Pharmacy. A report to the Nuffield Foundation. The Nuffield Foundation, London

Rogers M L, Barrett C W 1972 The drug information centre at the London Hospital. Pharmaceutical Journal 209: 37–39

Royal Pharmaceutical Society of Great Britain 1992 Pharmaceutical care: the future for community pharmacy. Report of the joint working party on the future role of the community pharmaceutical services. The Royal Pharmaceutical Society, London

Royal Pharmaceutical Society of Great Britain 1995 Statement of principles and standards of good practice for hospital pharmacy in the United Kingdom. RPSGB, London

Royal Pharmaceutical Society of Great Britain 1996
Medicines, ethics and practice : a guide for pharmacists.
RPSGB, London, No 17, October 1996, p 89
Royal Pharmaceutical Society of Great Britain, Merck, Sharp
& Dohme 1997 From compliance to concordance:
achieving shared goals in medicine taking (Chairman,
Marinker M). Royal Pharmaceutical Society, London, and
Merck, Sharp & Dohme, Hoddesdon
Secretaries of State for Health, Wales, Northern Ireland and
Scotland 1989 Working for patients. CM 555. HMSO,
London
Secretaries of State for Social Services, Wales, Northern
Ireland and Scotland 1987 Promoting better health. CM
249. HMSO, London,
Vere D W 1965 Errors of complex prescribing. Lancet i:
370–373

# 32

# Adverse drug reactions

*G. Cunningham and J. Krska*

After studying this chapter you will know about:

**The classification of ADRs (adverse drug reactions)**
**Factors affecting the incidence of ADRs**
**Recognition and assessment of ADRs**
**Monitoring systems**
**Drug interactions**
**The role of the pharmacist in ADRs.**

## Introduction

Adverse reactions are a recognized hazard of drug therapy. However, since the problem was first addressed in the 1950s, the number of potent prescribed drugs in use has increased dramatically. In addition, the incidence of adverse drug reactions (ADRs) is known to rise with age. This, in combination with the proportionately increasing ageing population, signifies the growing importance of ADRs.

Patients themselves are becoming more aware of potential side effects of their drug therapy. The pharmacist, along with the prescriber, has a duty to ensure that patients are aware of side effects of their medicines and a suitable course of action should they occur. With their detailed knowledge of medicines, pharmacists have the ability to relate unexpected symptoms experienced by patients to possible adverse effects of their drug therapy.

The reporting of adverse reactions to drugs is certainly not new, and has taken place haphazardly throughout history. However, interest in ADRs and their monitoring has increased greatly since the association between thalidomide, a hypnotic, and limb deformities in babies was made in the early 1960s. Until then, thalidomide was thought to be a safe hypnotic, and was prescribed during pregnancy with disastrous results. ADR reporting systems were introduced in most developed countries following this tragedy. Although these systems encourage physicians to report suspected ADRs to all drugs, and to include details of self-medication by the patient, very often these details are unknown by the doctor. The result is that ADRs to non-prescription medicines are under-reported. In the UK more prescription medicines are being re-regulated as the Government extends the selected list of medicines available without prescription. Community pharmacists in particular, are in an ideal position to be involved in identifying ADRs to non-prescription medicines. This is essential if the safety of recently available over-the-counter (OTC) medicines is to be monitored effectively.

## INCIDENCE OF ADRS

Many studies have assessed the incidence of ADRs in the community, in hospital and as a cause of hospital admission. However, the absence of standardized criteria for identification and assessment of such problems means that estimates of incidence vary widely. It is therefore often difficult to compare such studies.

### Hospital inpatients

The risk of ADRs increases when a patient is hospitalized, owing to the high number of drugs prescribed per patient at any one time. Approximately 10–20% of hospitalized patients are thought to have experienced an ADR during their hospital stay.

### Community

Estimates of the incidence of ADRs in general practice vary widely, from 2% to over 40%, depending on the study methodology. More studies are required to assess the true incidence of the problem in the community.

## Hospital admissions

Approximately 5% of all hospital admissions are due to ADRs, although estimates of drug-related admissions range from 3% to 27% depending on the patient population studied. This represents a significant cost to the National Health Service in terms of bed occupancy and treatment of these adverse effects. A small number of studies have investigated drug-related hospital admissions in children, with admission rates for ADRs in the region of 2–3%.

## Drug-related deaths

Up to 3% of deaths in hospital inpatients are thought to be due to the adverse effects of drugs. Of those patients admitted to hospital due to ADRs, the death rate is approximately 5%. The Committee on Safety of Medicines receives reports of fatal suspected ADRs, and 476 such reports were received in 1995. The top three drugs most commonly associated with fatal suspected reactions in that year were clozapine, diclofenac and ethinyloestradiol.

A large proportion of these ADRs are considered to be preventable through good prescribing practice – mainly by individualizing dosage, and avoiding inappropriate and unnecessary drug therapy. In order that pharmacists can make a valuable contribution to the identification, monitoring, reporting and prevention of ADRs to both prescription and non-prescription drugs, they should have a thorough understanding of the aetiology and classification of ADRs.

## THE CLASSIFICATION OF ADRS

An ADR is defined by the World Health Organization (WHO) as 'a noxious, unintended effect of a drug that occurs in doses normally used in humans for the diagnosis, prophylaxis or treatment of disease'. ADRs can be classified into two types.

- Type A (augmented) reactions
- Type B (bizarre) reactions.

## Type A reactions

Type A reactions are due to known pharmacological actions of the drug. These may be:

- Excessive effects of the intended pharmacological action of a drug, e.g. haemorrhage with anticoagulants.

**Table 32.1    Some known teratogenic drugs which should be avoided in early pregnancy**

| Drug | Effect on fetus |
| --- | --- |
| Androgens | Masculinization of female fetus, congenital defects |
| Antiepileptics (*Note:* benefit of treatment outweighs risk to fetus) | Congenital malformation, increased risk of neural tube effects |
| Cytotoxic drugs | Multiple congenital defects |
| Diethylpropion | Congenital malformations |
| Diethylstilboestrol | Vaginal adenocarcinoma, urogenital abnormalities, and reduced fertility in daughters |
| Lithium | Neonatal goitre |
| Oral anticoagulants | Congenital malformation, fetal haemorrhage |
| Podophyllum resin | Neonatal death and teratogenesis |
| Radioactive iodine | Permanent hypothyroidism |
| Retinoids – acitretin, etretinate, isotretinoin | Congenital defects |

- Unwanted pharmacological actions of a drug, e.g. antimuscarinic effects of tricyclic antidepressants which can cause blurred vision, tachycardia, dry mouth and urinary retention.
- Withdrawal reactions, which may occur with abrupt withdrawal of some drugs after prolonged use, e.g. rebound hypertension with clonidine, acute adrenal insufficiency with glucocorticoids.
- Delayed adverse effects such as vaginal adenocarcinoma in the daughters of women who received diethylstilboestrol during pregnancy for the treatment of threatened abortion. Examples of other known teratogenic drugs which have a high risk of causing fetal abnormality and should therefore be avoided in early pregnancy are shown in Table 32.1. A full table of drugs which may have harmful effects in pregnancy can be found in Appendix 4 of the *British National Formulary* (BNF). The period of greatest risk for producing congenital abnormalities is considered to be from the 3rd to the 11th week of pregnancy. Since many women are unaware of their pregnancy at this stage, care should be taken in prescribing drugs to all women of child-bearing age. Pharmacists should also bear this in mind when recommending non-prescription medicines.

Some Type A reactions may be a result of failure to individualize dosage. Although the patient may be prescribed a dose which is within the normal recommended range, impaired renal or hepatic function affects clearance of the drug and may result in adverse effects. This type of ADR could be considered to be preventable. The predictability of these reactions is an important factor in selection of a drug for an individual patient. A knowledge of factors influencing the likelihood of any patient experiencing a predictable ADR is therefore important.

## Type B reactions

Type B reactions are unexpected effects which are unrelated to the known pharmacological actions of the drug. Many of these reactions have an immunological basis, for example anaphylaxis with penicillins. Others are due to genetic abnormalities such as drug-induced haemolysis in patients with glucose-6-phosphate dehydrogenase deficiency, when given oxidative drugs. For some Type B reactions, the cause is unknown. These allergic drug reactions are idiosyncratic, and normally unrelated to dosage. Management of such ADRs, therefore, usually requires stopping the offending drug. Type B reactions are often associated with serious illness and death, but are relatively rare. At other times, only mild urticaria or pyrexia may be experienced.

The differences between the two subgroups of ADRs are highlighted in Table 32.2. More detailed information on Type A and Type B reactions is given in Walker & Edwards (1994).

## FACTORS AFFECTING THE INCIDENCE OF ADRs

Pharmacists should be aware of the main factors which influence the occurrence of ADRs so that they can identify patients most at risk.

## Multiple drug therapy

An obvious association exists between the number of

drugs being taken and the risk of experiencing an ADR. Some studies have shown a sharp, disproportionate, rise in ADRs with increasing numbers of prescribed drugs. Drug interactions may contribute to this situation.

## Age

The incidence of ADRs is known to rise with age. Changes in pharmacokinetics and pharmacodynamics associated with age may be partly responsible. It is not clear, however, whether age itself is an independent risk factor. The increase seen with ageing may be partly due to the elderly taking a greater number of prescribed medicines than younger age groups. Multiple pathology in the elderly may also contribute.

Neonates also have reduced drug clearance, resulting in increased risk of ADRs. A well-known example is the 'grey baby' syndrome with chloramphenicol. Another common adverse reaction in neonates is respiratory depression due to opioids given to the mother during labour.

## Multiple disease states

Some disease states may alter a patient's response to drug therapy. This in turn may influence susceptibility to ADRs. Patients with particular disease states may be more likely to experience an ADR with certain drugs. Examples include patients with peptic ulcer disease being at increased risk of bleeding when prescribed non-steroidal anti-inflammatory drugs, and those with asthma who may suffer bronchospasm with beta-adrenoceptor blocking drugs. However, in severely ill patients, it is also possible that effects related to their disease states may be attributed in error to ADRs.

## Types of drugs prescribed

Some drugs are more likely to cause ADRs than others. ADRs may also be more likely to occur when the drug regimen includes medicines with a narrow therapeutic index. Examples of such drugs include digoxin, anticoagulants and insulin. Many commonly taken drugs have been implicated in ADRs serious enough to warrant hospital admission. Those most commonly involved are cardiac drugs, diuretics, non-steroidal anti-inflammatory drugs, corticosteroids, anticoagulants, antimicrobials and psychotropics.

## Dosage

Many Type A ADRs seem to be dose related, and

| Table 32.2 | Classification of adverse drug reactions | |
|---|---|
| Type A | Type B |
| Normal, augmented response | Abnormal, bizarre response |
| Predictable from pharmacology | Unpredictable from pharmacology |
| Dose related | Not dose related |
| Reasonably common | Uncommon |
| Seldom fatal | Often causes serious illness or death |

can be managed by a reduction in dose of the drug in question. Individualization of drug therapy is essential in avoiding these ADRs. Examples of dose-related adverse effects are drowsiness and ataxia with anticonvulsants such as phenytoin, phenobarbitone and carbamazepine, and bradycardia, hypotension and heart failure with beta-adrenoceptor blocking drugs.

## Route of administration

If drugs are given too quickly by the intravenous route, ADRs can arise especially with drugs which act on the heart. The problems can be reduced by giving intravenous injections slowly. For instance, rapid intravenous injection of digoxin may cause nausea and arrhythmias, and for this reason should be avoided. Rapid infusion of vancomycin may lead to anaphylactoid reactions such as severe hypotension, wheezing, dyspnoea, urticaria, pruritus and flushing of the upper body, known as 'red man' syndrome.

## Formulation

ADRs can be due to excipients in pharmaceutical formulations, for example colouring agents, sweeteners, preservatives. Changes in formulation affecting bioavailability led to toxicity in previously stabilized patients with digoxin because of changes in particle size. In the case of phenytoin capsules, a change in capsule filler from calcium sulphate to lactose increased bioavailability of phenytoin, again leading to toxicity.

## Sex

Some ADRs appear to occur more frequently in females. The reason for this is unknown.

## Race and genetic factors

Differences in susceptibility to ADRs have been demonstrated between races. This is probably due to differences in genetics and metabolism.

## Patient compliance

Non-compliance with drug therapy, which can be defined as the extent to which the patient follows a prescribed regimen, may also play a part in ADRs. Taking too much of the prescribed drug may lead to adverse effects or unexpected drug toxicity (see Ch. 42).

## RECOGNITION AND ASSESSMENT OF ADRS

Pharmacists and other health care professionals responsible for a patient's drug therapy should be vigilant for any new symptoms which may be drug related. Once a suspected ADR has been detected, a causal relationship between the drug and symptom should be established. Causality assessment is used to determine whether the adverse event is definitely, probably or possibly due to the drug. The following factors are important:

- temporal relationship with drug
- type of reaction
- nature of reaction
- exclusion of other possible causes
- dechallenge
- rechallenge
- diagnostic tests, e.g. plasma drug concentrations.

It is important to question the patient on the use of all other drugs, including non-prescription drugs. Several algorithms have been developed to standardize the assessment of the relationship between the suspected drug and the adverse event. Some are detailed and time-consuming, and have a limited application in practice. Ultimately, a degree of clinical judgement is needed to determine whether an adverse event is due to a drug. Table 32.3 shows the criteria used in assessing the relationship between drug and ADR. The classification of ADR depends on which criteria are satisfied. For example, for an ADR to be categorized as 'definite', all five criteria must be satisfied.

It should be noted, however, that it is sometimes difficult to apply these criteria in practice. It is seldom ethical to rechallenge a patient who may have had an ADR. In some cases, the adverse effect is not reversible, so is unlikely to disappear on dechallenge. Depending on the adverse event experienced, the time of onset may vary from minutes to years. Difficulties may arise in relating the symptoms to a drug years after it was first prescribed.

## DETECTION AND MONITORING SYSTEMS

Although all new drugs undergo clinical trials to demonstrate efficacy and detect adverse effects, only the most common ADRs will probably have been detected by the time the drug is marketed. At this

**Table 32.3  Criteria to determine a causal link between drug and symptoms**

| Criteria | Likelihood of ADR | | | |
| --- | --- | --- | --- | --- |
| | Definite | Probable | Possible | Unlikely |
| Known ADR | Yes | Yes | Yes | No |
| Time of administration related to onset of reaction | Yes | Yes | Yes | No |
| Disappears on dechallenge or dose reduction | Yes | Yes | Yes | No |
| Symptoms unexplained by clinical condition of patient | Yes | Yes | No | No |
| Symptoms reappear on rechallenge | Yes | No | No | No |

stage, only Type A reactions are likely to have been identified. In addition, clinical trials are unlikely to have been carried out on some groups of patients, such as the elderly or pregnant women. It is, therefore, important to monitor pharmaceutical products after marketing to identify any more unusual, serious, or delayed adverse effects.

## The yellow card system

As a result of the thalidomide disaster in the early 1960s, the Committee on Safety of Drugs was established in the UK in 1963. The chairman of this committee, Sir Derrick Dunlop, encouraged the reporting of suspected adverse effects of drugs by the medical profession. An assurance was given that the information would never be used for disciplinary purposes or for enquiries on prescribing costs. This assurance is probably the reason the scheme has been so successful. The Committee on Safety of Drugs was later superseded by the Committee on Safety of Medicines (CSM) after the Medicines Act in 1968. The CSM is responsible for the assessment of new drugs before clinical trials and marketing have taken place. They also manage the reporting system which monitors the occurrence of ADRs.

The CSM's spontaneous reporting scheme asks doctors to report all suspected reactions to new products which are marked with a black triangle in the BNF and the *Monthly Index of Medical Specialities* (MIMS). Doctors are also asked to report all serious suspected reactions to established drugs, even if it is considered that the adverse effect is well recognized. As well as drugs, the reporting scheme also applies to contact lens fluids, vaccines, intrauterine contraceptive devices, surgical or dental materials and absorbable sutures. Standard report forms or 'yellow cards' are conveniently located inside the back cover of the BNF, MIMS, ABPI data sheet compendium and on prescription pads. In addition to the voluntary reporting of ADRs by the medical profession,

pharmaceutical companies are responsible for reporting reactions to their licensed products.

Although the CSM advises doctors not to be put off reporting because some details are unknown, there is a minimum amount of data required for a report to be accepted. The following information is required:

- the identity of the patient
- the identity of the reporting doctor
- the suspected drug, dose, route of administration, and start and stop dates
- the nature, severity and outcome of the suspected ADR, and its start and stop dates.

The yellow cards also ask for additional information which may or may not be available. This includes:

- patient details – age, sex, weight
- other drugs taken in the last 3 months, including non-prescription drugs
- other relevant information including medical history, investigations, allergies.

The CSM receives over 20 000 ADR reports annually. To ease ADR monitoring, a system capable of capturing, retrieving and processing the yellow card data has been developed, known as ADROIT (adverse drug reaction on-line information tracking facility). The yellow card scheme has been successful in identifying both common and rare reactions, and can also provide early warnings of possible adverse drug reactions. Other methods can then be instituted to study these in more detail. Some drawbacks do exist:

1. The incidence of a particular ADR is unknown owing to a lack of information on the number of patients exposed to the drug. A rough estimate can be calculated from the number of prescriptions dispensed.

2. Considerable under-reporting takes place because of lack of time and the mistaken belief that

an adverse effect must definitely be due to a drug for a report to be made.

3. Some bias may be introduced if doctors tend to report ADRs which are well publicized or which they have just heard about.

4. ADRs which are as yet unknown are difficult to spot and so may be prone to under-reporting.

Before April 1997, all yellow cards had to be signed by a doctor, and could not be submitted by pharmacists alone.

Pharmacist reporting of ADRs already takes place in several countries, including the USA, Australia, Belgium, France, Germany, Ireland and New Zealand. Some countries (USA, Germany) even allow reporting of ADRs directly from patients, although this has provided little in the way of useful reports. The Committee on Safety of Medicines and the Medicines Control Agency agreed to extend the UK's official ADR reporting scheme to allow reporting of ADRs by hospital and community pharmacists from April 1997. ADR reporting by hospital pharmacists with direct involvement in patient care has been established nationally. After discussion with senior medical staff, a hospital pharmacist can complete and sign a yellow card report. A modified version of the yellow ADR reporting card is used, which has space for details of the reporting pharmacist and of the consultant or general practitioner. Demonstration schemes have initially been established for community pharmacists in the four CSM regional monitoring centres. Although these community pharmacists are able to submit reports on any suspected ADR, they have been asked to focus their reporting on areas where there is limited reporting by doctors, e.g. non-prescription medicines. The demonstration scheme will be evaluated over two years. The development has been welcomed by the pharmacy profession, which has been advocating pharmacist ADR reporting for many years. It is essential, therefore, that pharmacists are sufficiently educated on ADRs if they are to be competent and confident in their reporting.

As well as reporting ADRs to the CSM, pharmacists and prescribers should report ADRs to drug manufacturers. All manufacturers are interested to receive such information about their products. Many are also active in carrying out post-marketing surveillance on their products. Indeed the CSM expects this for many new products. If serious ADRs are suspected during any company-sponsored post-marketing surveillance, the company's medical department should be informed as well as the CSM.

## Other detection and monitoring systems

### Anecdotal reports (case reports)

Case reports from individual doctors are often published in the medical literature and may be important in detecting new ADRs. These single reports usually require further studies to confirm an ADR, but some serious adverse effects have been brought to light by this mechanism. Notable examples include the oculomucocutaneous syndrome due to practolol, and agranulocytosis caused by chloramphenicol.

### Cohort studies (prospective studies)

A 'cohort' of patients taking a specified drug is identified in this type of study. They are then monitored for adverse effects. Ideally, a control group is identified, who are drawn from the same population but are not taking the drug, in order to compare the incidence of adverse effects detected.

### Case control studies (retrospective studies)

These retrospective studies involve a group of patients with symptoms which may be due to an ADR. The patients are investigated to see if they have taken the drug in question. The prevalence of drug taking is compared to that of a control group who do not have the specified symptoms. These types of studies are useful for determining whether there is an association between a drug and an adverse effect, but only once the relationship has been suspected. They cannot detect new ADRs. Case control studies have been important in confirming associations between venous thromboembolism and oral contraceptives, phocomelia and thalidomide, and the adverse gastrointestinal effects of aspirin and NSAIDs.

### Record linkage studies

Patients' medical records are used to match drugs prescribed with adverse effects experienced in record linkage studies. Prescription event monitoring is an example of this type of study. Record linkage studies may be particularly useful for identifying long-term adverse effects of drugs.

### Hospital-based ADR reporting schemes

These are useful for determining the incidence of ADRs in hospitalized patients, or on admission to hospital. An example of this type of scheme is the Boston Collaborative Drug Surveillance Program, which involves selected hospitals in several countries.

### International ADR reporting

The World Health Organization Collaborating Centre for International Drug Monitoring was established in 1968. The centre collates spontaneous ADR reports from participating national centres, and aims to increase early recognition of new and unexpected ADRs. Very rare adverse reactions can be detected in this way.

### Feedback from CSM

Analysis of data collected by the CSM spontaneous reporting scheme takes place routinely. Recently discovered ADRs and other important points are communicated to doctors and pharmacists via the 'Current Problems in Pharmacovigilance' information sheet, which is produced by the CSM and the Medicines Control Agency (MCA).

### Pharmacy medication monitoring systems

Post-marketing surveillance of medicines can be carried out using patient medication records (PMRs) in community pharmacies as a database to identify patients taking particular medicines (see Ch. 39). These records can be more complete than medical records, so may be more likely to include the majority of patients. Patients can be issued with questionnaires when they collect prescriptions, or can be contacted on the telephone and asked a series of standard questions about their medication and the appearance of any potential ADRs. These systems have been piloted in Canada, the USA and Scotland and may provide a valuable method of detecting ADRs which complements other systems.

### Drug use evaluation studies

Pharmacists are usually involved in this type of study (described in Ch. 34), in which the actual use of drugs in a cohort of patients is evaluated in terms of appropriateness and outcomes, including ADRs.

## DRUG INTERACTIONS

Although not classified as ADRs, drug interactions are important contributors to adverse effects of medicines experienced by patients. Since they are preventable, it is important for the pharmacist to be able to identify and deal with common drug interactions. A recent example which illustrates this point is the low risk of arrhythmias known as torsades de pointes with terfenadine and astemizole. The risk of this serious adverse effect increases when the patient is prescribed drugs which interact with these antihistamines, such as ketoconazole or erythromycin. The pharmacist should be aware of this when recommending antihistamines over the counter, ensuring that the patient receives an alternative antihistamine.

Drug interactions occur when the effects of one drug are altered by the effects of another. The interaction may cause one drug to potentiate or antagonize the effect of the other. Adverse effects from drug interactions are well known, and the potential for drug interactions is great. However, not all are clinically significant. It is not possible to discuss all clinically significant interactions within this chapter. Recommended further reading is indicated at the end.

Some patients are at increased risk from drug interactions. These include those with impaired hepatic or renal function, and the elderly. The use of multiple medications also increases the risk of drug interactions. Also, the adverse effects due to drug interactions may be treated with an additional drug, resulting in increased polypharmacy. Drug interactions are normally divided into three types: pharmacodynamic, pharmacokinetic and pharmaceutical. The first two are the most common and are most likely to be potential contributing factors to ADRs.

Pharmacodynamic interactions occur when one drug alters the effect of another by acting at the same site of action, on the same pharmacological receptors or on the same physiological system. They are normally predictable from a knowledge of the pharmacology of the drugs involved. Common examples are increased anticoagulation when warfarin is given with corticosteroids, tetracyclines or oestrogens, alcohol taken with CNS depressant drugs resulting in CNS depression, and digoxin with beta-adrenoceptor blocking drugs resulting in bradycardia.

Pharmacokinetic interactions occur when one drug alters the absorption, distribution, metabolism or excretion of another drug. Those involving metabolism are the most frequent causes of ADRs. The rate of metabolism of a drug can be increased or decreased by another drug. This occurs through induction or inhibition of the hepatic microsomal enzyme system. Some common examples of drug

**Table 32.4    Common drug interactions involving enzyme inhibitors**

| Enzyme inhibitor | Affected drug(s) | Effect |
|---|---|---|
| Azapropazone | Warfarin | Inhibits metabolism → enhanced effect, haemorrhage |
| Phenylbutazone | Phenytoin | Increased plasma concentration |
| Cimetidine, selective serotonin reuptake inhibitors | Warfarin, theophylline antiarrhythmics, antiepileptics | Increased plasma concentrations |
| Isoniazid | Phenytoin, carbamazepine | Inhibits metabolism → enhanced effect |
| Metronidazole | Warfarin | Inhibits metabolism → enhanced effect, haemorrhage |
| Allopurinol | Azathioprine, mercaptopurine | Inhibits xanthine oxidase → reduced clearance, risk of bone marrow suppression, toxicity |

**Table 32.5    Common drug interactions involving enzyme inducers**

| Enzyme inducer | Affected drug(s) | Effect |
|---|---|---|
| Rifampicin | Warfarin, oral contraceptives, antiarrhythmics, anti-diabetics, phenytoin, corticosteroids, cyclosporin | Reduction in plasma concentration → reduced effect |
| Phenytoin, carbamazepine | Corticosteroids, warfarin | Metabolism of corticosteroids, warfarin accelerated (enhancement also reported with warfarin) |
| | Oral contraceptives | Reduced contraceptive effect |
| | Cyclosporin | Reduced plasma concentration |
| Griseofulvin | Warfarin, oral contraceptives | Metabolism accelerated → reduced anticoagulant or contraceptive effect |
| Barbiturates | Warfarin, antidepressants, corticosteroids, cyclosporin, oral contraceptives | Reduced effect |

interactions involving enzyme inhibitors or enzyme inducers are given in Tables 32.4 and 32.5 respectively. In addition, cigarette smoke may also induce hepatic microsomal enzymes. Examples of drugs whose metabolism is increased in smokers include theophylline, pentazocine and imipramine. This may be important in practice if, for example, a patient prescribed theophylline gives up cigarette smoking. Without a reduction in the dosage of theophylline, potentially life-threatening adverse effects may be experienced.

An example of an interaction involving excretion is the reduction in excretion of lithium by thiazide and loop diuretics, through an increase in proximal tubular reabsorption of lithium. This interaction can cause lithium toxicity, and lithium doses should therefore be reduced if these drugs are to be administered concurrently.

Clinically important drug interactions usually involve drugs with a small therapeutic ratio, or drugs which need careful dosage control. In both instances, small increases or decreases in their plasma concentrations may produce either toxicity or lack of effect. Careful monitoring is necessary to avoid these.

## THE ROLE OF THE PHARMACIST

Pharmacists have an important contribution to make in the prevention, identification, documentation and reporting of ADRs and drug interactions.

### Identification and documentation

ADRs may be drawn to community or hospital pharmacists' attention during the course of their work. In hospital, the pharmacist checks for ADRs on a daily basis when reviewing prescriptions. During this process a check is made on:

- whether the drug prescribed is most appropriate for that individual patient
- why the patient is receiving particular medicines
- whether the dose prescribed is appropriate for the indication
- whether any drug interactions are present
- whether any contraindications to therapy are present
- whether any medicines are being continued unnecessarily
- any excessive therapeutic effects of medicines
- any abnormal laboratory values which could be ADRs.

When screening prescriptions, pharmacists should be vigilant in noting whether patients are prescribed or have recently received any of the drugs that are often used to treat ADRs. Examples are antacids, laxatives, antimuscarinics, antihistamines, hydrocortisone and topical skin preparations. In seeking the indication for these drugs the presence of an ADR is often identified. The pharmacist is then in a position to prevent recurrence of the reaction. Documentation of confirmed and suspected ADRs is poor, both in hospital and in the community. ADRs should be recorded in medical notes, nursing notes and on prescriptions in hospital. In the community, they should be recorded in the medical notes, the practice computer and the pharmacist's patient medication record. The minimum information needed is the suspected medicine and the reaction which occurred. By being vigilant in recording this information themselves and in ensuring that others do so, pharmacists can play a major role in preventing patients from being unnecessarily exposed to the same or similar medicines again.

The accuracy of recorded information is equally important in preventing patients from having potentially useful medicines withheld because there is a suspicion of a previous reaction. A common example is the use of the term 'penicillin allergic', often recorded in medical notes of patients who may have experienced type A reactions of minor importance, such as diarrhoea or skin irritation. Penicillins of all types will not be available to this patient, which could have important consequences if a serious infection occurs.

Pharmacists can also be alert for any alterations to a patient's drug regimen while in hospital. A drug may be discontinued owing to adverse effects. If so,

this should be recorded. Patients are often more open about their experiences with medicines to pharmacists than to doctors. It is, therefore, important that hospital pharmacists have direct contact with patients and are able to obtain relevant details from them to allow assessment of potential ADRs. In community practice, pharmacists may see patients more frequently than GPs and they are often the health care professional most able to identify ADRs. As in hospital, suspicions may also be aroused by prescriptions or requests for certain medicines which could be used to treat ADRs, or by changes to prescribed medicines. This is an important reason for the pharmacist to be involved in the sale of non-prescription medicines.

Once an ADR is suspected, it should be recorded as such. If confirmed later, the record should be modified to include this. Suspected ADRs should be reported to the patient's medical practitioner and consideration given to whether a report to the CSM is appropriate.

## Monitoring and reporting

Reporting rates for ADRs to the CSM are low. It is estimated that a maximum of 10–15% of ADRs are reported. Pharmacists are now able to report directly to the CSM, but they can act as facilitators by encouraging physicians to report ADRs, and by filling out yellow cards. Hospital pharmacists are often involved in setting up and running ADR reporting schemes in hospitals. Pharmacists working in drug information centres may prepare information for distribution to GPs and pharmacists on the most common ADR problem areas. A pilot scheme, in which hospital pharmacists submitted ADR reports to the CSM after discussion with physicians, was successful in increasing reporting of serious reactions.

A trial scheme for community pharmacists to report ADRs to specific medicines showed that most community pharmacists were willing to participate in such a scheme. Most GPs also believe that community pharmacists should play an active part in ADR monitoring, and welcome assistance in reporting to the CSM.

Non-prescription medicines may be largely ignored in ADR reporting. The incidence of ADRs to these medicines may increase as more are re-regulated from POM to P or GSL status. Community pharmacists have a substantial contribution to make in the identification of ADRs due to non-prescription medicines. If comprehensive patient medication records are held, with information on prescribed and non-prescribed medicines, the community pharmacist is best placed to identify possible adverse effects of therapy and potential drug interactions. The patient can be referred to his or her GP if an ADR is suspected. The GP may not even be aware that the patient is self-medicating, and so be unlikely to attribute any adverse effect experienced by the patient to a non-prescription medicine.

Pharmacists are generally very interested in monitoring and reporting ADRs, and most community pharmacists feel that they should be involved in this area. Although a joint working party on the future role of community pharmaceutical services recommended that the ADR reporting system should be extended to community pharmacists, the demonstration schemes mentioned earlier are the only development so far. It has also been advocated that for non-prescription medicines, the pharmacist should directly report any adverse reactions of which he is aware. The future of the community pharmacist's role in ADR reporting will be clearer following the outcome of the demonstration schemes.

## Prevention

Since many ADRs are preventable, a major part of the pharmacist's role in ADRs should be to reduce the occurrence of the problem. Pharmacists in all branches of the profession are currently involved in improving the use of medicines in patients through:

- Identifying potential side effects of drug therapy.
- Avoiding unnecessary polypharmacy by encouraging and carrying out review of therapy already prescribed. Review enables the identification of medicines no longer required, those that have no clear indication, those prescribed for adverse effects which could be prevented by changes to therapy, and duplication of similar medicines. Medicines that may initially have been indicated but have become unnecessary may be highlighted in this way. For example, a patient taking a NSAID may have been prescribed concurrent therapy with ranitidine for prophylaxis of NSAID-induced duodenal ulcer. On stopping the NSAID, the ranitidine may be inadvertently continued.
- Choosing the least toxic drugs where possible.
- Careful consideration of the dosage requirements for individual patients.
- Ensuring that therapeutic drug monitoring or other appropriate laboratory tests are carried out.
- Checking for a history of allergy or previous reactions to a drug.

- Checking for drug interactions and advising on what action to take – increasing or decreasing the dose of one drug, monitoring the patient, replacing one drug with another. For example, the metabolism of theophylline may be reduced by cimetidine, leading to an increase in the serum level. If prescribed, advice should be given on the avoidance of adverse effects by either reducing the theophylline dose, or by careful monitoring of the serum theophylline concentration. A request for cimetidine in a patient taking theophylline should be met with an offer of an alternative $H_2$ antagonist. By also explaining the reason for this, future purchases of potentially interacting products may also be prevented
- Education of patients on their drug regimen, especially when new treatments are initiated. This should include specific details of any medicines available without prescription which should be avoided. In the above example, a patient prescribed theophylline should be educated about not purchasing cimetidine and cough remedies which contain theophylline.
- Encouraging patients to complete courses of medication and dispose of unused drugs to prevent hoarding and sharing of drugs.
- Encouraging patients to report any new symptoms.
- Questioning the patient on any new drug therapy, including non-prescription medicines.
- Advising the patient of expected side effects of therapy and a safe course of action should they occur.
- Taking drug histories, which may identify previous adverse effects or allergies to particular drugs.
- Drawing up formularies and prescribing protocols to ensure appropriate selection of medicines, and appropriate use in a given situation.
- Advising on simplifying dose and drug regimens to encourage good compliance.

Further developments which may help in the prevention of ADRs may include routine sharing of information between primary and secondary care, both on admission to hospital to prevent ADRs occurring during hospitalization, and on discharge from hospital, which should help minimize ADRs in the community. Information shared on discharge could include reasons for a drug being stopped or changed in hospital, dose changes, new drugs prescribed. Discharge planning schemes in hospitals should ensure that all patients are educated in their drug regimen, especially where new treatments have been initiated. Patients seeking treatment in community pharmacies should be questioned to establish whether any relationship exists between newly prescribed drugs and recently occurring symptoms. The use of one particular pharmacy should be encouraged. Patients having prescriptions dispensed at different pharmacies may be at greater risk of ADRs since the pharmacist will not have a complete picture of the patient's drug regimen.

Although ADRs are unwanted effects of drug therapy, for many drugs, the risk of adverse effects is small compared to the likely benefits of treatment. When adverse effects are experienced, however, the patient may be left in a worse condition than before he or she was prescribed the medicine. Pharmacists are ideally placed to play an active role in the prevention of ADRs. The benefits to patients in terms of reduced suffering, hospitalization and anxiety are considerable. Significant resource savings to the NHS could also be achieved through reduced hospitalization rates for ADRs, and reduced treatment costs.

---

### Key Points

- Adverse drug reactions (ADRs) are found in both hospital and community practice and may be 'augmented' (Type A) or 'bizarre' (Type B).
- Type A ADRs may be due to excessive or unwanted pharmacological effects, withdrawal reactions, delayed effects or failure to individualize dosage.
- Many Type B ADRs have an immunological or genetic basis and are normally unrelated to dosage.
- Factors influencing ADRs include multiple drug regimens, multiple disease states, type of drug, route, formulation and dosage, age, sex, race and level of compliance.
- Causality of an ADR can be categorized using set criteria.
- At the time of marketing a new drug, not all ADRs may be known.
- The 'yellow card' scheme is used by the CSM to help provide post-marketing surveillance.
- A wide range of methods are also used to complement the yellow card scheme.
- Drug interactions may contribute to ADRs and are preventable.
- Patients with impaired renal and hepatic function and the elderly are at increased risk of drug interactions.
- Prescription monitoring provides an opportunity for identifying some ADRs.

---

- Antacids, laxatives, antimuscarinics, antihistamines and hydrocortisone added to a prescription, or purchased by the patient, may indicate an ADR.
- Reporting rates for ADRs are very low.
- Pharmacists are in the best position to report non-prescribed medicine ADRs.
- Pharmacists can help prevent ADRs during their normal practice.

## FURTHER READING

British National Formulary, current edn. British Medical Association and Royal Pharmaceutical Society of Great Britain, London (Updated twice yearly)

D'Arcy P F, Griffin J P 1986 Iatrogenic diseases, 3rd edn. Oxford University Press, Oxford

Davies D M 1991 Textbook of adverse drug reactions, 4th edn. Oxford University Press, Oxford

Dukes M N G 1996 Meyler's side effects of drugs, 13th edn. Elsevier Science Publishers, Amsterdam

Lee A, Rawlins M D 1994 Adverse drug reactions. In: Walker R, Edwards C (eds) Clinical pharmacy and therapeutics. Churchill Livingston, Edinburgh, ch 3, p 31

Mann R D, Rawlins M D 1993 Spontaneous adverse drug reaction reporting systems. In: Mann R D, Rawlins M D, Auty R M (eds) A textbook of pharmaceutical medicine – current practice. Parthenon Publishing, Carnforth, ch 27, p 323

Roberts P I, Booth T G, Wolfson D J 1993 The community pharmacist and adverse drug reaction monitoring: (1) A historical and geographical perspective. Pharmaceutical Journal 250: 875–878

Stockley I H 1996 Drug interactions – a source book of adverse interactions, their mechanisms, clinical importance and management, 4th edn. Pharmaceutical Press, London

Wolfson D J, Booth T G, Roberts P I 1993 The community pharmacist and adverse drug reaction monitoring: (2) An examination of the potential role in the United Kingdom. Pharmaceutical Journal 251: 21–24

# 33
# Responding to symptoms

*E. J. Kennedy*

---

After studying this chapter you will know about:

**The skills required for effective responding to symptoms in the pharmacy, including observation, questioning and decision making**
**The use of protocols, mnemonics and treatment guidelines**
**How to distinguish between major and minor illness**
**Special considerations with children, the elderly, pregnant and breast-feeding women and patients with chronic conditions**
**Minor diseases which are suitable for OTC management; treatment, advice and outcomes**.

---

## Introduction

The community pharmacist has an important role in advising the general public on symptoms of minor illness. Many people buy medication to treat symptoms and may seek advice from the pharmacy, rather than seek attention from their family doctor. The term 'responding to symptoms' refers to the procedure that a pharmacist goes through when asked for advice by a customer in a community pharmacy, in response to the symptoms that they describe. The process involves a complex mix of knowledge and skills. The community pharmacist is able to distinguish between minor illness and major disease and recommend treatment or to refer the customer to an appropriate medical practitioner.

Self-care and self-medication make up a large and growing component of health care in the population of the UK. A study commissioned by the Proprietary Association of Great Britain, published in 1987, found that an average of five ailments each were reported by the British population in any 2 weeks.

The ailments most commonly experienced by adults in the sample were tiredness (35%), headache (29%) and muscular aches and pains (23%). Those most commonly reported by children were colds (27%), bruises (22%) and minor cuts and grazes (21%). Many of these ailments were simply tolerated and people drew on their own experiences and those of their family and friends to discriminate between minor ailments and those requiring advice (see Ch. 2). People generally exercised caution in the use of medicines and believed that it is important to have non-prescription medicines widely available. Pharmacists were recognized and used as an important expert source of advice on health and medicines.

Several options are available to people who suffer from symptoms. They may:

- take no action
- use a home remedy, for example a hot water bottle and lemon and honey drink for a cold
- use a prescription medicine already available at home
- use a non-prescription medicine
- see a doctor or dentist.

Medicines that are available over the counter fall into two categories; general sales list (GSL) medicines may be sold in many retail premises, Pharmacy category medicines (P) are restricted to sale by registered pharmacies. These latter sales should be supervised by a registered pharmacist, who should be ready to intervene in a sale whenever appropriate, for example if the patient is taking other medication or suffering from concurrent illnesses. Prescription-only medicines (POM) are increasingly being re-regulated and becoming available to buy over the counter (OTC). The role of the community pharmacist to ensure that these are sold for appropriate indications and used safely is becoming increasingly important. There are stringent safeguards when classifying medicines and there are various data requirements in order to facilitate the switch of a medicine from POM to P:

• Safety data are required to demonstrate safety in overdose, minimal interactive potential, a wide therapeutic index and low toxicity profile.

• Efficacy data should provide evidence that the indications and dosage are suitable for self-medication and the appropriateness of the indications is being recognized by customers and not confused with serious, treatable diseases.

• Product information that will lead to safe consumer use to include warnings and advice on duration of treatment and when medical advice should be sought.

Examples of medicines that have been switched from POM to P recently include beclomethasone for topical treatment of allergic rhinitis and topical piroxicam for relief of mild arthritic and rheumatic pains. An example of a recent change in a P licence is the use of topical hydrocortisone for treatment of mild to moderate eczema.

A pharmacy assistant is often the first person that the customer approaches in the community pharmacy. A written protocol covers the procedure to be followed by staff when medicines are sold or advice on treatment of a medical condition is sought from community pharmacies. The protocol should indicate the points at which direct involvement of a pharmacist is deemed necessary in that particular pharmacy. Examples may be, if specific requests for advice are made, or where there are requests for exceptional quantities of medicines. Protocols should also include a list of medicines for which requests should be referred directly to the pharmacist. This list would normally include medicines which have recently been re-regulated or which are liable to intentional misuse. All members of staff whose work will regularly involve the sale of medicines should also have completed an accredited course containing specified elements. These measures will ensure that all medicines are sold safely and appropriately from community pharmacies and ensure that pharmacists have more time to devote to transactions where their involvement is considered essential.

The duty of the pharmacist when responding to symptoms is to ensure that appropriate action is recommended when a person seeks advice on symptoms. This may be to advise non-drug treatment, treatment using a suitable non-prescription medicine or advice to visit a doctor or dentist. If non-prescription treatment is recommended the pharmacist needs to ensure that patients are advised on how to use the medicine safely and that suitable health care advice is given at the same time. This will help to diffuse fears from general medical practitioners (GPs) that the devolution of health care to self-treatment is preventing the patient from receiving appropriate health care advice. There are many advantages of self-medication. These include reduced workload for GPs and a decreased national drug budget. Increasingly drug costs are being borne by the patient. This may not be well received by patients who receive free NHS prescriptions. This partly explains the profile of self-medicators: relatively few elderly patients or children self-medicate. As the consulting role of the pharmacist becomes better established as an alternative to the GP for minor ailments, the status of the pharmacist in primary care will be enhanced.

The greater availability of medicines over the counter allows pharmacists and doctors the opportunity to cooperate and collaborate more effectively to advise patients and give better patient care. Pharmacists' recommendations for OTC medicines should be taken into account when producing practice prescribing policies, and vice versa.

## SKILLS INVOLVED IN RESPONDING TO SYMPTOMS

Skills required by the pharmacist to respond successfully to symptoms encompass a wide mix. These include knowledge of diseases and their treatment, astute observation, and excellent communication and questioning skills to obtain all the information required to make a decision about whether to treat or refer. Skills in selection of the most suitable treatment, explaining how to use the treatment, provision of advice on related health care and finally informing the patient of the action to take if symptoms do not improve within appropriate time scales are necessary.

General communication skills have been dealt with in Chapter 3. Other relevant skills are discussed here.

### Observation

A great deal of information can be gained by observing the patient. It is, of course, crucial that the pharmacist knows whether the person who is describing the symptoms is in fact the patient, or a representative of the sufferer. An evaluation of the appearance and demeanour of the patient will help when attempting to assess the seriousness of the symptoms reported. This is necessary because people's terms of reference will differ according to what they regard as normal. Non-verbal communication and body language will tell a lot about a patient. A migraine sufferer, for example, may be quiet and have screwed-up or red, heavy eyes, since bright lights can aggravate the headache. Pharmacists must also pay attention to their reactions, both verbal and nonverbal, to customers who are reporting symptoms and show sympathy and concern.

In the case of children, the parent or guardian will often give a detailed description of the symptoms. It is useful to actually observe the child as well. It enables the pharmacist to see how unwell the child appears and helps in the process of deciding whether to treat or refer.

Some conditions, such as skin diseases, are very difficult to advise on unless direct observation can be made. There are a large number of conditions which affect the skin and often only by examining the presenting signs can a reasonable assessment be made and a recommendation for treatment given. There are some symptoms which aid differential decisions on some conditions, for example, sites affected by the condition and progression. Eczema is a common condition which is intensely itchy. There is often inflammation present and small red spots or cracked, weepy skin. This is often made worse by scratching the skin. The distribution is often symmetrical, commonly occurring on the backs of knees, wrists, the neck, elbows and ankles.

Contact dermatitis appears as an eczematous-like rash and can be caused by various irritants such as chemicals, detergents or substances that come into contact with the skin. Details of job, hobbies and of any new agents handled by the sufferer will give clues about the cause of the rash. The site of the rash is often an important clue. Classic examples which will present are the appearance of a contact dermatitis on the wrist or round the neck resulting from new jewellery that contains nickel (which is a common allergen) or a rectangular rash under the area where a sticking plaster was placed, due to the resin colophony used in the adhesive. Nickel-free jewellery and hypoallergenic plasters are available to use to avoid these particular allergens. Occupational allergens that commonly cause contact dermatitis are perm solutions used by hairdressers, some plants (gardeners) and cement, used in the building trade. The rash often improves when away from work or on holiday and the use of gloves may be appropriate in some occupations to avoid contact with the rash-provoking substance.

## Questioning the patient

Effective questioning is essential in order to obtain all the relevant information. This enables pharmacists to decide whether to treat the symptoms or refer to a GP. Open questions should be used in preference to closed questions. This allows patients to tell the pharmacist about the symptoms. They are encouraged to open up and feel relaxed with the pharmacist, rather than feel that they are being interrogated as often happens if a barrage of closed questions is given. Points from a patient's account can be taken up by the pharmacist and specific, closed questions asked on these for clarification at a later stage.

## Identifying the patient

The patient should always be identified. Customers who are reporting symptoms may not always be the person suffering from them. It is important that assumptions are not made.

## Questioning on symptoms

The next stage in questioning should be to identify what the problem is. This involves obtaining detailed information on the presenting symptoms, any other symptoms and anything that makes the symptoms better or worse. For example, if a patient is reporting symptoms of indigestion and epigastric pain, it will be useful to know whether exertion makes the pain worse, as this could potentially be a sign of cardiac pain rather than dyspepsia. Information about the site or location, together with the intensity or severity, of any pain or symptoms may help in an initial diagnosis. Asking specifically about the spread or radiation of certain types of pain will be significant in certain conditions, for example, abdominal pain. A pain that starts centrally and spreads to the right side may be suggestive of appendicitis.

Patients often make a self-diagnosis before seeking professional help. Confirmation of their symptoms should always be sought. For example, a patient may present stating that she wants a remedy for cystitis, but the symptoms of cystitis can easily be mistaken for vaginal thrush and vice versa. Patients do not always volunteer all the important information about symptoms, therefore asking about any other unusual symptoms will be an important prompt. If somebody is complaining of a cough, it would be significant to know whether he is coughing up blood or coloured sputum, as these are both signs for referral to a doctor. It will be useful to know about changes in lifestyle, such as a recent holiday or change in job, as some symptoms could be attributed to this.

Anything that the patient reports which can be

linked with the onset of symptoms may give a clue as to the symptoms' cause. A bout of overeating of rich food may be linked to an episode of abdominal pain and dyspepsia, which can therefore be treated with simple antacids and advice not to repeat the overindulgence.

A history of the symptoms, including their duration and recurrence, is necessary. This will contribute to the assessment of the severity of the condition because most minor ailments are self-limiting and resolve within a few days. The information will also help distinguish between some types of condition. For example with headache, a tension headache will occur regularly, sometimes daily, whereas a classic migraine headache should not last longer than 2 days and will rarely occur twice in the same week. Some conditions are seasonal. Another example is hay fever when recurrence of symptoms is expected when pollen counts are high.

## Questioning on current medical conditions and medication

Questions on past medical history and detail of any current medication are required. This will allow the possibility of adverse drug reactions or possible drug interactions to be identified (see Ch. 32). Some symptoms may arise as a result of a current medical condition worsening. For example, coughing at night may be a sign that asthma is poorly controlled and requires referral for medical assessment.

Information on current medical conditions and medication taken will also be necessary. It allows the pharmacist to make an appropriate treatment recommendation that will not interact with existing medication or medical conditions. Information on any medicines that have been tried, successfully or otherwise, for the reported symptoms is also important. Many customers will have already tried something that is currently in their medicine cabinet, either a prescribed or an OTC medicine, or one that they have borrowed from a friend or relative. If the patient has used an apparently appropriate treatment already, then referral to the GP may be warranted.

## Questions to confirm a diagnosis

It is important not to jump to conclusions about what the person may be suffering from early in the consultation and thereby ask questions which could exclude other possibilities. Key questions are those which are particularly significant to be asked about the conditions or symptoms that are being reported by the patient. An example of a key question for headache would be: 'Is there a possible trigger factor?'. Some foods can trigger headaches, for example Chinese food (monosodium glutamate), cheese (cheese delays gastric emptying and decreases food absorption, which may trigger migraine), chocolate and red wine. Stopping excess coffee intake has been known to cause caffeine withdrawal headaches. Stress may precipitate tension headache, hypoglycaemic headaches can occur during dieting or fasting. Deteriorating eyesight may cause headaches in association with periods of close work, such as examination revision.

### Using mnemonics as a structured approach to questioning

There are various suggested structures for questioning, many using mnemonics as a prompt. Some of these are simple and act as a useful aide mémoire. Others are more complex and designed to facilitate detailed consideration of the patient's condition. The mnemonic approach is particularly suitable for training pharmacy assistants (and for pharmacy students!) to help them decide whether to refer the patient to a pharmacist or sell an appropriate product. As practice and experience are gained in responding to symptoms, and knowledge of particular conditions increases, a more intelligent and thoughtful approach to questioning is warranted. The use of mnemonics helps to minimize the risk of missing vital information, especially in a busy pharmacy where there are many potential distractions and interruptions. Care should be taken not to follow the checklists robotically and without thought as this will not give the customer confidence in your professional ability. Attention must be paid to the responses given by the customer, following up any additional aspects as necessary. Examples of several popular mnemonics, ASMETTHOD, WWHAM, SIT DOWN SIR and ENCORE are shown below.

A  Age and appearance of the patient?
S  Self or for someone else?
M  Medication the patient is taking?
E  Exactly what does the patient mean by the symptoms?
T  Time/duration of symptoms?
T  Taken anything for it or seen the doctor?
H  History of any disease or condition?
O  Other symptoms being experienced?
D  Doing anything to aggravate or alleviate the condition?

W  Who is the patient?
W  What are the symptoms?
H  How long have the symptoms been present?
A  Action already taken; what medicines have been tried?
M  Medication being taken for other problems?

S  Site or location?
I  Intensity or severity?
T  Type or nature?
D  Duration?
O  Onset?
W  With (other symptoms)?
N  annoyed or aggravated by?
S  Spread or radiation?
I  Incidence or frequency pattern?
R  Relieved by?

E  Explore
   N  Nature of symptoms
   O  Obtain identity of patient
   C  Concurrent medication or treatment
   E  Exclude possibility of serious disease
   O  Other associated symptoms.
N  No medication
   Remember that in many instances a medicine is not necessary and may indeed be contraindicated.
C  Care
   G  Geriatric patients
   P  Paediatric patients
   P  Pregnant women
   L  Lactating mothers.
O  Observe
   O  Other tell-tale signs
   D  Demeanour of patient
   D  Dramatization by patient.
R  Refer
   P  Potentially serious case
   P  Persistent symptoms
   P  Patients at increased risk.
E  Explain
   Discuss with patients why a particular course of action is suggested.

Worked examples of two of the mnemonics are illustrated in Case studies 33.1 and 33.2.

### Case study 33.1: Mr Johnstone

Mr Johnstone is a young man who asks you to recommend something for diarrhoea.

You question Mr Johnstone using the WWHAM structure:

Who is it for? It is for himself.

What are the symptoms? He is passing regular, watery stools.

How long have the symptoms persisted? Since late last night.

Action taken already? None, but he hasn't eaten anything today.

Medicines being taken for other problems? Occasional antacids for dyspepsia.

From this information, as a pharmacist, you would want to explore what may have triggered these symptoms and obtain more detail about severity of symptoms and any accompanying symptoms. Mr. Johnstone tells you that he had a pub meal in the early evening yesterday, and wonders whether this is what may have triggered the diarrhoea. When questioned about other symptoms, he tells you that he has also been sick, but there is no abdominal pain. He is passing stools less frequently now.

From this information, you conclude that it is likely that he has eaten food which has been microbiologically contaminated. (This could be confirmed by locating other people who ate the same food with Mr Johnstone at the pub last night, to find out if they are suffering from similar symptoms.) You recommend an oral rehydration sachet to Mr Johnstone and advise him to fast for the day, although if he does feel hungry he may eat, but to avoid milk and dairy products, as lactase is temporarily inactivated in the gut. He should drink plenty of fluids and the diarrhoea should subside completely in the next 2 days. If it does not, he should visit his GP. He should also be advised to avoid taking antacids that contain magnesium as they tend to have a laxative action which may aggravate his current condition.

### Case study 33.2: Miss Anderson

Miss Anderson asks to speak to the pharmacist in private. She looks rather embarrassed and worried. She tells you that she has had a vaginal discharge that is curdy and irritating for the last 2 days.

You question Miss Anderson using the ASMETTHOD mnemonic.

Age and appearance of the patient? She is a student, who looks healthy, but is embarrassed about this problem.

Self or for someone else? She is suffering from the symptoms herself.

Medication the patient is taking? She is taking the contraceptive pill and has recently had a course of antibiotics for a chest infection.

Exactly what does the patient mean by the symptoms? The discharge is curdy, thick and creamy, but not coloured or smelly and there is no bleeding.

Time/duration of the symptoms. She has already told you that she has noticed the symptoms for the last 2 days.

Taken anything for it or seen the doctor? No.

History of any disease or condition? No.

Other symptoms being experienced? The vulval area is itchy and it is quite painful when she passes water.

Doing anything to aggravate or alleviate the condition? She has been having hot baths to try to relieve the symptoms, but this hasn't helped much.

The pharmacist suspects that Miss Anderson is having an attack of the fungal infection, thrush, caused by the organism *Candida albicans*. This infection commonly follows a course of antibiotics, which kill the commensal bacteria of the vagina which normally keep the growth of *Candida* under control. The symptoms confirm this. There may also be a link between the use of the oral contraceptive and candidiasis, because the vaginal environment may be altered, making it more susceptible to overgrowth of the *Candida*. There is no suggestion that there is any other vaginal infection as there is no offensive smell or coloured discharge. There is no blood in the discharge which might indicate a more serious underlying cause.

The pharmacist asks Miss Anderson if she has ever suffered from vaginal thrush before. She has not, to her knowledge. As this is the first time she has suffered from the symptoms, she is advised to visit her GP for confirmation of the suspected diagnosis. An intravaginal imidazole treatment, such as a pessary or cream, is the most effective drug of choice, but must be prescribed by the GP in this case. Hot baths, especially if she has used perfumed bath additives, will probably aggravate and irritate the condition. Warm salt baths or showers may be more soothing. Miss Anderson can also be advised to avoid tight-fitting and synthetic clothing, such as tights, and to wear cotton underwear. Topical application of vinegar or yoghurt should be discouraged as this can reduce the effectiveness of the imidazoles.

## Decision making

After obtaining all the relevant information from the customer, the pharmacist must assess and interpret the situation. The most important task will be to distinguish between symptoms of minor ailments that can be reasonably treated and those that may indicate more serious illnesses. The latter require refer-

ral for further examination by the doctor or prescription-only medication. An initial diagnosis is made by the pharmacist which is based on the information obtained through detailed, structured questioning. The role of diagnosis is often claimed to be the doctor's domain only. However, there are various levels at which diagnoses may be made. Many patients perform self-medication after making a self-diagnosis based on limited knowledge. At the next level, the pharmacist can apply more knowledge and make a diagnosis aimed at excluding the presence of more serious disease. The doctor will be able to make a more sophisticated diagnosis based on past medical history of the patient, examination of the patient and more detailed knowledge of medical conditions. It should be remembered that the GP may refer the patient to a hospital specialist.

Guidelines to follow when responding to symptoms are available for many therapeutic areas and act as a useful aide mémoire for pharmacists and counter assistants. Development of local guidelines, from discussion between community pharmacists, general medical practitioners and hospital specialists in the field, may be of particular benefit, especially if discussion includes agreeing referral criteria between community pharmacists and GPs.

An example of published guidelines for treatment of lower GI tract symptoms is given in Figure 33.1. The guidelines consist of a flowchart which summarizes the counselling which should be followed. Additional notes are provided for pharmacists using the guidelines which detail the rationale behind the recommendations. The flow chart uses the WWHAM questions as a starting point.

It should be remembered that patient expectations may influence the pharmacist's course of action. For example, recommending a steam inhalation, with the addition of menthol crystals, will not be of any particular benefit, nor any harm, in a suspected case of sinusitis that you refer to the doctor. Often, however, patients feel happier if they feel that they have something that could give them symptomatic relief until they can obtain an appointment to see a doctor.

Assertiveness is often a vital skill in the process of decision making (see Ch. 3). Patients may not approve of the pharmacist's recommended course of action, such as referral to the doctor. Pointing out the reasons for the decision may help. Remaining professional and firm about the decision is important. There may also be times when sales of pharmacy medicines have to be refused for a range of reasons. An example is when the indication lies outwith the pharmacy medicine product licence, or if there is a suspicion that the medicine is likely to be

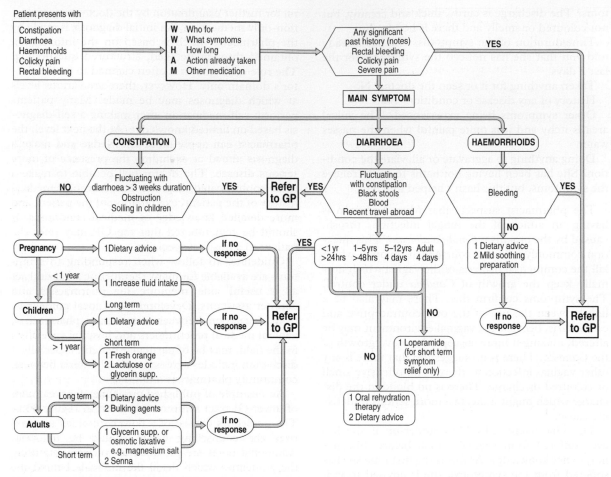

**Fig. 33.1** Guidelines used in responding to symptoms of the lower gastrointestinal tract (reproduced by permission of the Department of General Practice, University of Aberdeen).

abused. Again, there is a need to be assertive and remain professional, especially when the patient does not react well to the decision. The pharmacist is the person who is ultimately responsible for the safe and appropriate supply of over-the-counter medicines and will be liable if they are used incorrectly.

## Distinguishing between minor illness and major disease

Pharmacists should be able to screen the many cases that they see each day, through observation and intelligent questioning, and identify those symptoms for which there may be a potentially serious cause. These latter patients should then be referred to a doctor for treatment. It is difficult to define a minor illness, although criteria which have been applied are

that the condition should be of limited duration, self-limiting and something which is perceived as non-threatening. There are also conditions which are recurrent or persistent which can be managed by an individual following an initial consultation with a doctor, for example cold sores, eczema or allergies.

There are particular danger symptoms to be aware of which will always require referral of the patient to the doctor as they may be a sign of a more serious disease. These are listed in Table 33.1.

Failed medication will often require a referral to the GP, if the medication was apparently appropriate for the patient's condition. Further investigation may be necessary, or a more potent medicine may be required.

Pharmacists should be alert to suspected adverse drug reactions as a causative factor of symptoms (see Ch. 32). Information on medication that the patient

**Table 33.1    Danger symptoms which should be referred for medical investigation**

Ankle swelling
Blood in stools or vomit – may be associated with internal bleeding
Unexplained weight loss (anorexia) – may be associated with a malignancy
Difficulty in swallowing (obstructions)
History of severe and particularly penetrating injury
Increasing breathlessness
Menstrual abnormality
Pain in the chest, abdomen, head or ears
Persistent or recurrent pyrexia
Spontaneous bruising
Swelling or lumps of any size (malignancies)
Tenderness over the blood vessels
Urinary symptoms (possible infection)
Yellow or green discharge from the penis or vagina (underlying infection)
Yellow or green sputum (infected discharge)
Yellow skin colour (jaundice)

is currently, or has recently been, taking is essential. The timing of commencement of any new medicine regimens will also be important in linking it to a suspected adverse drug reaction. If adverse drug reactions are suspected, then a referral to the GP should be made so that the patient's medication may be reviewed.

## TREATMENT AND ADVICE

Once a full assessment of the symptoms has taken place, and a decision has been made that the patient does not need referral, appropriate recommendations should be made by the pharmacist.

Recommendation of a treatment often involves a diagnosis having been made. Selection of an appropriate treatment for a condition involves application of a knowledge of pharmacology, therapeutics and pharmaceutics. The first step will be to choose an appropriate therapeutic group to recommend. The next step would be to assist the customer in the choice of product within the therapeutic group. For many therapeutic groups there are a wide variety of products available, often supported by widespread advertising. The pharmacist should take into account the effectiveness of the product, potential side effects, interactions, cautions and contraindications. The patient's needs should be borne in mind when selecting a product. Factors such as the ease of use of a formulation and dosage regimens should be

considered. The customer will also be interested in value for money. There are many forms of OTC drugs available, from tablets, easy-to-swallow capsules and caplets to dispersible tablets and liquids. The form which will suit the patient's needs best should be chosen. For example, antacids are available in both tablets and liquid form. Tablets are more convenient to carry around for occasional use, but the liquid will work more quickly if immediate relief from symptoms is required. Previous experience by customers of some products may also have an influence on the selection of a particular OTC medicine. For example, if they have tried an analgesic and it worked well, customers will be more likely to want to purchase the same analgesic again.

Patients should be advised on how to use the treatment that has been recommended, including the recommended dose, when to take it and for how long. Any other important advice, such as how to use the preparation, should also be offered, for example how to use nasal sprays. Advice on storage is also important, for example informing the customer that eye drops and ointments should be disposed of 28 days after opening.

Non-drug treatment should also be offered where appropriate. There are often non-drug suggestions which will help to manage a condition in addition to the use of OTC medicines. For example, for prevention of motion sickness, in addition to the use of anticholinergics, visual mechanisms, such as looking out of the car, focusing on distant objects, or keeping eyes closed in a fixed position help to reduce symptoms (this helps to settle the brain's receipt of conflicting messages). Advice on increasing dietary fibre and fluids is an essential part of the management of conditions such as constipation and haemorrhoids. Advice on diet, alcohol and other health promotion activities is important so that the patient may learn how to attempt to avoid recurrence of the symptoms (see Ch 38). Occasions where pharmacists are being consulted by patients for advice on symptoms are ideal opportunities for health promotion and should be utilized. For example, if a customer is asking for advice on a cough mixture, part of the management of the condition will include asking him about his smoking habits, if any. Advice to stop or cut down is then an essential part of the management of the condition.

### Outcomes

It is important that the pharmacist is aware of the timescales for treatment of conditions with OTC medication. This will allow the patient to be given a reasonable time period over which to try the treatment before seeking further advice from a GP. Timescales will vary considerably from condition to condition. The status of the patient may also have an effect. For example, a toddler of 2 years suffering from diarrhoea will be referred to the GP in a shorter timescale than a teenager with the same symptoms. Customers should be encouraged to monitor outcomes of their therapy so that they can take further action if required. If there has been a long duration of symptoms, then the patient should be referred.

## Counselling areas

It is important that pharmacists are sensitive to the needs of their patients when giving advice. A patient's body language may indicate that he wishes to speak privately, or in a quiet area, away from other customers. Every effort should be made to provide a quiet area for conversation with the customer, so that others cannot overhear. A counselling area is ideal for this purpose. Many community pharmacies are now being designed to allow for the inclusion of such an area. A counselling area is usually screened off from the main pharmacy counter area, or may be a separate room, although studies have shown that patients may feel inhibited in an enclosed space. If this is not possible, the pharmacist should take the patient to a quieter area of the shop, so that other customers cannot overhear them. The pharmacist should always seek to create an atmosphere of privacy and confidentiality in these circumstances.

## Special considerations when responding to symptoms

### Children

Special care and consideration is needed when responding to children's symptoms. Children in their first months of life are particularly susceptible to complications from certain conditions. For example, dehydration will result very quickly in a 1-month-old baby compared to an older child or adult. If there is any doubt about symptoms, then referral to the GP is the safest and most sensible course of action. Parents of young children will often consult the pharmacist to obtain reassurance that this is the best course of action.

There are more restrictions on the medicines available to recommend for children's symptoms. Pharmacists should be alert and watch out for signs of common childhood infections, especially those which present with seemingly normal symptoms, for

example meningitis. Children of primary school age are particularly susceptible to viral infections and other contagious conditions that are currently prevalent in the local schools. Local knowledge, and communication with the local doctor's surgery, will be invaluable to the pharmacist in recommending treatment for these conditions.

When selecting treatments to recommend for children, it is important to bear in mind that medicine consumption in children is very high and that sugar in medicines can contribute to increased levels of dental decay, especially when medicines are to be given at bedtime. This is the worst time to consume anything containing sugar, because the saliva flow is greatly reduced whilst sleeping and cannot, therefore, buffer the acid attack from plaque. Sugar-free OTC medicines should always be offered to children in preference to equivalents that contain sugar.

### Elderly patients

Elderly patients are more likely to be taking other prescription medicines and therefore extra caution is required to check that there are no drug–drug or drug–disease interactions with the medication being recommended. The possibility of adverse effects from current drug regimens should also be considered to avoid the unnecessary addition of new medicines when a change in the existing regimen may lead to resolution of the symptoms. Treatment timescales may also be shorter compared to those for fit, healthy adults. Renal and hepatic function will also be affected by age, which may then alter the metabolism or excretion of drugs and subsequently require dosage alterations.

### Pregnant and breast-feeding mothers

Drugs may cause harmful effects to the fetus during pregnancy. The potential effect of OTC drugs should not be forgotten. The period of greatest risk of congenital malformations is from the 3rd to the 11th week of pregnancy. The effects of drugs during the second and third trimesters tend to be on growth and functional development. All drugs should be avoided if possible during the first trimester, although there is of course a risk–benefit situation with some conditions. There is a lack of information on the effects of OTC drugs in pregnancy and their use should be minimized. There are, however, some minor conditions which will be commonly suffered during pregnancy for which OTC medicine use is considered relatively safe, such as paracetamol for headaches, or low sodium content antacids for dyspepsia. Drugs which are known to cause definite adverse effects in pregnancy include aspirin, non-steroidal anti-inflammatory drugs, sympathomimetics and medicines with a high sodium content. These should, therefore, be avoided.

Some drugs may be excreted, in varying amounts, in the breast milk. This can potentially lead to toxicity in a baby who is being breast-fed. Those that are excreted in significant amounts and which could have an effect include aspirin, sedating antihistamines, caffeine, iodides, phenolphthalein and vit min A.

### Sufferers of chronic medical conditions

Patients who suffer from some chronic medical conditions, such as diabetes mellitus, will be more likely to suffer from specific minor illnesses and will be more likely to be taking other medication.

Care will need to be taken when recommending medicines to diabetics, because many pharmaceutical preparations contain sugar. A list of sugar-free medicines is available from the British Diabetic Association and the National Pharmaceutical Association. Sorbitol is often used as a sweetening agent in sugar-free medicines and excessive consumption of this agent can lead to an osmotic diarrhoea. Foot problems, particularly foot ulcers, may arise as one of the long-term complications of diabetes mellitus because of increased susceptibility to infection, neuropathy and vascular disease. Any lesions including corns and callouses in a diabetic patient should be treated by a chiropodist so that wound healing can be adequately monitored.

It is important to remember that some important drug–disease interactions will preclude certain medicines from being recommended. For example, cold remedies containing sympathomimetics, such as ephedrine and pseudoephedrine, should not be taken by patients with hypertension, hyperthyroidism, coronary heart disease and diabetics.

Some OTC medicines may provoke bronchospasm and should be avoided in asthmatics, such as alcoholic head lice lotions, e.g. Prioderm lotion. Asthmatics may also be sensitive to non-steroidal anti-inflammatory drugs, such as aspirin and ibuprofen, which should be avoided where sensitivity reactions have occurred, or if the asthmatic has not used these painkillers before.

## Drug interactions of OTC medicines and other drugs

Medicines that are available for sale to the public are relatively safe. However, there are some common drug–drug interactions to be aware of when recommending OTC medicines. Interactions may occur with prescribed medicines or other non-prescription medicines. Few are clinically significant, especially when associated with short-term use of OTC medicines. Those that may be clinically significant are listed in Table 33.2. A more detailed table may be found in the *OTC Directory* produced annually by the Proprietary Association of Great Britain.

## Misuse of non-prescription medicines

It is important to educate the general public that, although non-prescription medicines are perceived as being freely available and the pharmacist has been involved in their supply, there are still potential problems with their use. These will be minimized if the medicine is being used for its intended purpose and at the correct dose and dosage interval.

Overdosing has occurred with non-prescription medicines, particularly those that contain paracetamol. This most commonly occurs when patients take more than one paracetamol-containing product. Adverse reactions can also occur, but are rare. Non-prescription medicines may also be overused and lead to further problems. For example, liquid paraffin, which, if used on a habitual basis, can interfere with absorption of fat-soluble vitamins, amongst other problems. Medicines may also be used for indications which are not licensed when sold OTC, such as hydrocortisone cream used on the face. This may result in a delay in the patient seeking advice from a doctor. Inadequate storage of drugs in patients' homes can also lead to problems, especially if they are accessible to young children.

Pharmacists should therefore ensure that advice and information are available on the safe and effective use of medicines. There is also a vast array of information available to the consumer about health issues. This has led to members of the public being better informed, and wanting to know more about the medicines that they take.

Some products that are available for sale in community pharmacies may also be subject to intentional misuse by some people (see Ch. 42). It is important that pharmacists are aware of the products that have the potential for misuse, either through frequent use of the product over a long period of time or by taking substantially higher doses than are recommended. Pharmacists should be able to exercise professional judgement to prevent the sale or supply of any product that they suspect is not being used for a genuine medicinal purpose. Commonly abused products are listed in Table 33.3.

**Table 33.2  Common potential OTC drug–drug interactions**

| OTC drugs | Interacting drug | Nature of interaction |
|---|---|---|
| Paracetamol-containing products, e.g. Lemsip, Night Nurse, Sudafed cold and flu, Resolve, Solpadeine | Co-drugs containing paracetamol, e.g. co-proxamol, co-dyrdamol, co-codamol | Potential overdose of paracetamol, leading to hepatic damage |
| Non-steroidal anti-inflammatory drugs: ibuprofen, aspirin | Methotrexate | Reduced excretion of methotrexate leading to an increase in serum levels and potential toxicity |
| | Other NSAIDs and corticosteroids | Increased risk of GI bleeding |
| | Lithium | Reduced excretion of lithium with ibuprofen, leading to toxicity |
| | Anticoagulants | Antiplatelet action of aspirin increases prothrombin times and increased likelihood of GI bleeds |
| Sympathomimetics, e.g. ephedrine, pseudoephedrine, phenylpropanolamine | MAOIs | Concurrent administration can lead to severe hypertensive crisis |
| H$_2$ antagonist, e.g. cimetidine | Anticoagulants, phenytoin, theophylline, some calcium channel blockers | Inhibits microsomal liver enzymes, generally resulting in increased levels of affected drugs and possible toxicity |
| Antihistamines, e.g. astemizole | Imidazole antifungals such as ketoconazole and macrolide antibiotics such as erythromycin | Inhibited metabolism of antihistamines leading to increased levels and, rarely, hazardous arrhythmias |
| | Drugs with arrhythmogenic potential, e.g. antipsychotics, tricyclic antidepressants, diuretics | Increased risk of ventricular arrhythmias |
| Sedative antihistamines such as chlorpheniramine and promethazine | Alcohol, tricyclic antidepressants, benzodiazepines | Increased sedative effect |
| Dextromethorphan | MAOIs | Rare but severe reactions reported |
| Theophylline | Allopurinol, some antibacterials, calcium channel blockers | Raised theophylline levels |
| | Anticonvulsants and rifampicin | Reduced theophylline levels |
| Caffeine | Antihypertensives | Caffeine can lead to an increase in blood pressure |
| Iron | Tetracyclines | Chelation, resulting in poor absorption if taken at same time of day |
| Antacids | Ciprofloxacin, phenytoin, tetracyclines, iron, some antifungals (ketoconazole), some ACE inhibitors, chloroquine, anxiolytics | Chelation, resulting in poor absorption if taken at same time of day |
| Mebendazole | Carbamazepine and phenytoin | Lowers serum mebendazole |

## Minor ailments treatable in the pharmacy

There are a wide range of symptoms and ailments that can be treated using OTC medicines. Further reading will be required for details on symptoms, key questions, referral points and treatment and advice to give.

### Gastrointestinal system

Symptoms of the gastrointestinal system include dyspepsia, which is a term that covers a broad range of symptoms such as heartburn, epigastric discomfort and intestinal gas. Other conditions are infant colic, constipation, haemorrhoids and diarrhoea. Infestation of the gastrointestinal system with

| Table 33.3 Products liable to misuse which are available to buy |
| --- |
| All products containing solvents or propellants, e.g. Zoff, PR spray, methylated and surgical spirits, Ralgex spray<br>Chemicals, e.g. citric acid<br>Combinations of codeine, ephedrine, morphine, antihistamine, e.g. Gees linctus, kaolin and morphine mixture, Veganin<br>Antihistamines alone, e.g. Avomine, Nytol<br>Cyclizine preparations, e.g. Valoid, Femigraine<br>Laxatives, e.g. Nylax, Dulcolax<br>Sympathomimetics, e.g. Sudafed, Actifed<br>Ephedrine, pseudoephedrine and phenylpropanolamine, e.g. Mucron, Sinutab |

threadworm may occur. Ailments that may inflict the oropharynx are mouth ulcers, oral thrush, xerostomia (dry mouth) and halitosis.

## Central nervous system

Pain is an unpleasant sensory and emotional experience associated with actual, or potential, tissue damage, or which is described in terms of such damage. It is a complex syndrome which can often, but not always, be a symptom of an underlying condition. The cause of the pain should be ascertained so that the underlying condition can be treated and the source of the pain removed, if appropriate, rather than masking the symptoms. There are two categories of pain – which can be further subdivided according to the severity of pain. Acute pain is a symptom of injury, disease or disorder, e.g. dental, postoperative, obstetric or period pain, accidental strains and sprains. Chronic pain is persistent pain, e.g. cancer, osteoarthritis, rheumatoid arthritis.

A common CNS complaint is headache. There are many different types of headaches, for example vascular headaches resulting from dilatation or constriction of the blood vessels in and around the brain, traction headaches caused by inflammation (e.g. meningitis), migraine headaches, headache associated with sinusitis and tension headaches. It is important to question the patient about the site and the type of pain.

Other CNS complaints include sickness, motion sickness, teething and toothache. Sleep disturbance may arise as a result of many conditions, such as heartburn or coughing at night. Advice may be given to help establish a sleeping pattern.

## Respiratory system

Minor ailments of the respiratory tract include the common cold, productive or non-productive coughs and sore throat. Symptomatic relief can usually be offered as long as more serious causes have been eliminated. For example, a persistent dry cough in children, particularly at night, may be an early sign of asthma and the child should be referred to the doctor for further investigation. Nasal congestion may be due to a cold, sinusitis or hay fever.

## Eye and ear conditions

Many patients present in the pharmacy with minor eye complaints. These may be red eye, due to allergic or infective conjunctivitis, inflammation of the eyelids or a tear deficiency. Painful eyes or visual disturbances require referral.

Disorders of the ear that may be treated with OTC medicines include excessive build-up of ear wax, dermatitis of the outer ear, eustachian catarrh and barotrauma (pain due to mechanical pressure factors such as during the descent of an aeroplane). Ear pain, especially in children, or infective dermatitis should be referred.

## Skin conditions

The skin conditions which may present in community pharmacy are wide and varied. They include infestation by head lice and scabies, fungal infections such as athlete's foot, and cold sores. Other common conditions include acne, sunburn, insect bites, dermatitis and eczema, general rashes and pruritus, scalp conditions such as seborrhoeic dermatitis and cradle cap, nappy rash, verrucas and warts.

## Musculoskeletal disorders

The musculoskeletal system consists of the bony skeleton and associated soft tissues including ligaments, muscles and tendons. Disorders of the musculoskeletal systems include sprains, strains and bruises, often resulting in inflammation, swelling and pain. The pharmacist is often required to give advice for acute conditions that are associated with falls or sporting injuries, or for relief of pain associated with chronic conditions such as backache.

## Women's health

Specific conditions that women suffer from and which may be treated with OTC medicines include cystitis, vaginal thrush and premenstrual syndrome.

## Children's health

Mothers of young children are regular users of community pharmacies and may often seek the advice of the pharmacist for their children's ailments, particularly teething and feeding problems. The parent often wants reassurance from a health care professional that her child is not suffering from anything serious, or advice on whether to take the child to the doctor. Other children's ailments which commonly present in community pharmacies include skin conditions such as dermatitis, eczema and nappy rash, childhood infections such as measles, chickenpox and mumps, oral thrush, threadworm, vomiting and diarrhoea, infant colic and earache.

## Travellers' health

The pharmacist is in an ideal position to give advice on measures to take to avoid suffering from symptoms or to advise on a simple first aid kit to take to treat common ailments suffered when holidaying or travelling abroad. Advice on the recommended regimen for prophylaxis against malaria and other travel vaccinations can be given in the pharmacy. A change in climate and diet often leads to symptoms such as 'holiday tummy' and dyspepsia. Oral rehydration sachets are an ideal remedy to pack in a holiday first aid kit, as these replace lost fluid and salts which can rapidly occur in hotter climates through sweating as well as through diarrhoea. Sun protection creams, travel sickness remedies, insect repellents and bite treatments, dyspepsia remedies, antidiarrhoeals for convenience and analgesics are also useful items to have when travelling.

---

### Key Points

- Pharmacists are recognized and used as sources of advice on health and medicines.
- Drugs are increasingly being re-regulated to allow pharmacy sale.
- Protocols are required for use by pharmacy assistants in responding to requests from customers.
- There are both advantages and disadvantages in the move to self-medication.
- A wide mix of skills is required by the pharmacist to successfully respond to symptoms.
- Observation of the patient, particularly with skin conditions, can greatly assist advice giving.

---

- Open questions are best in the early stages of finding out about symptoms, using closed questions to seek clarification of specific aspects.
- It is important not to jump to premature conclusions about a diagnosis.
- Useful questioning mnemonics include 'ASMETTHOD', 'WWHAM', 'SIT DOWN SIR' and 'ENCORE'.
- Flowchart treatment guidelines are useful aids in the pharmacy.
- Assertiveness may be required if the patient does not agree with the pharmacist's decision.
- There are a range of symptoms, suspected adverse drug reactions and failed treatments, which should always lead to a referral to a GP.
- Patients will require recommendations on therapeutic groups, particular drug and dosage form.
- Non-drug treatment should be offered where appropriate, including health promotional advice.
- A quiet area where privacy and confidentiality can be provided should be available.
- Particular care is required when dealing with symptoms in young children.
- The elderly are more prone to adverse drug reactions.
- The use of drugs during pregnancy should be minimized.
- Diabetics should avoid sugar-containing medicines.
- Some OTC medicines may not be recommended for sufferers of some chronic diseases.
- There are a number of clinically significant drug interactions involving over-the-counter medicines.
- Pharmacists must be alert to the possibility of misuse of OTC medicines.

---

## FURTHER READING

Blenkinsopp A, Paxton P 1994 Symptoms in the pharmacy, 2nd edn. Blackwell Scientific Publications, Oxford

Bond C M 1994 Guidelines for dyspepsia treatment. Pharmaceutical Journal 252: 228–229

Edwards C, Stillman P 1995 Minor illness or major disease? Responding to symptoms in the pharmacy, 2nd edn. The Pharmaceutical Press, London

Harman R J 1990 Handbook of pharmacy health care: diseases and patient advice. The Pharmaceutical Press, London

Matheson C, Bond C 1995 Lower gastrointestinal symptoms. Pharmaceutical Journal 255: 656–658

OTC Directory. Treatments for common ailments, current edn. Proprietary Association of Great Britain, London (Updated annually)

Proprietary Association of Great Britain 1987 Everyday health care: a consumer study of self-medication in Great Britain. PAGB, London

# 34
# Formularies

*J. Krska*


After studying this chapter you will know about:

**The development and structure of formularies**
**The advantages and disadvantages of using a formulary**
**Factors involved in producing a formulary**
**The relationship of formularies to prescribing policies**
**Formulary management systems**
**The use of prescribing data in formulary development and management**.

## DEFINITIONS AND TYPES OF FORMULARIES

Formularies are not a new idea. For centuries there have been compilations of medicinal preparations, listed with the formulae for compounding them, which gave rise to the term formulary. The modern definition of a formulary is a list of drugs which are recommended or approved for use by a group of practitioners. It is compiled by members of the group and is regularly revised. Drugs are usually selected for inclusion on the basis of efficacy, safety, patient acceptability and cost. Drugs listed in a formulary should be available for use. Information on dosage, indications, side effects, contraindications, formulations and costs may also be included. An introduction, giving information on how the drugs were selected, by whom and how to use the formulary is usually provided.

Formularies, as lists of recommended drugs, have been widely used in hospitals in the USA for many years. The American Society of Hospital Pharmacists published guidelines on how they should be produced and used in 1978. Since 1977 the World Health Organization has published a list of 'essential drugs' which it recommends as necessary for basic health care in developing countries. The basis of these lists is that the drugs they contain are of proven therapeutic efficacy, acceptable safety and satisfy the health needs of the populations they serve.

The most common formulary in use in the UK is the *British National Formulary* (BNF), which is a compilation of all the drugs available. It is produced by the Joint Formulary Committee, whose members include doctors and pharmacists, as well as representatives from the Department of Health. It is revised every 6 months and is issued to all prescribers and registered pharmacies in both hospitals and the community. A formulary for dentists, the Dental Practitioners' Formulary, and one for nurse prescribers are also included in the BNF.

Local formularies are becoming widespread throughout the UK. These are compiled by pharmacists, hospital doctors, general practitioners and nurses who practise within a locality. Some are designed for small groups, such as one general medical practice, some are for all prescribers within a hospital, others may be intended for all prescribers within a large geographical area. They may be similar in appearance to the BNF or very different. Most acute general hospitals have a formulary, a quarter of all general medical practices use a formulary and there are examples of joint formularies between hospital and general practice. The Royal College of General Practitioners has adopted the Northern Ireland formulary, which is used by many general practices as a basis for their own formulary.

A formulary may be thought of as a prescribing policy, because it lists which drugs are recommended. Prescribing policies should, however, be much more detailed than a formulary, giving details of drugs which should be selected for use in specific medical conditions. Examples of prescribing policies in common use are antibiotic policies, head lice eradication policies and malarial prophylaxis policies.

## REASONS FOR COMPILING A FORMULARY

Drug costs are a major component of the total cost of the NHS and are constantly rising. As the resources of the NHS are finite, it becomes increasingly necessary to contain the escalation in drug costs. A lot of evidence has accumulated to show that drugs are not always prescribed appropriately. Therefore some of the expenditure on drugs could be reduced if prescribing were improved. Formularies, which recommend specific drugs and exclude others, are one means by which this can be achieved. Guidelines to assist prescribers in using the drugs in a formulary and specific treatment protocols make them even more useful. Thus the main reason for compiling a formulary is to promote rational and cost-effective prescribing.

The presentation and content of the BNF were radically changed in 1980 to its present form. The aim of this change was to encourage rational, effective and cost-conscious prescribing. It is now a very good means of providing relatively impartial information on drugs for prescribers in a user-friendly form. It gives some guidance on selection of drugs and provides price comparisons to help users to become cost-conscious. Cost-effective prescribing may in the long run reduce costs, which benefits all patients. Local formularies usually include only some of the drugs listed in the BNF. If prescribers only use the range of drugs included in a local formulary, the range stocked by pharmacies can decrease, which reduces costs further.

Most local formularies have been compiled for these reasons, but, because these formularies usually contain a restricted number of drugs, there is a further benefit. Prescribers who use a restricted range of drugs should know more about those drugs and their formulations. This also benefits the patient, as the increased knowledge should reduce the risk of inappropriate prescribing, which could have led to adverse effects, interactions or lack of efficacy.

There are even greater benefits if a local formulary has been put together by prescribers and pharmacists in both primary and secondary care. Prescribing from the same range of drugs whether patients are at home or in hospital, makes continuing drug treatment easier. This is the main reason for compiling a joint formulary, such as that in Grampian. As patient packs become increasingly available, patients may be more likely to use their own drugs during a hospital stay. A joint formulary helps this, as there is less chance of drug therapy having to change to comply with a different formulary on admission to hospital.

### Additional advantages

Local formularies have many additional advantages besides those already mentioned. Using a restricted range of drugs may allow pharmacists to buy in bulk those which are prescribed. This may reduce costs. If fewer products are stocked, monitoring of expiry dates becomes easier and cash flow may improve. Any money saved by using a formulary in hospital or on general practitioners' budgets may be used in other ways to benefit patients. Formularies encourage generic prescribing, which has educational benefit and may further reduce costs. As drugs included in a formulary are selected primarily on the basis of efficacy and safety, drugs which are less satisfactory can be avoided. This may reduce the incidence of drug-related problems in patients. Because formularies encourage rational prescribing, the extent of their use can be used as an indicator of the quality of prescribing. They can also stimulate audit. In the long term, the widespread use of formularies may encourage manufacturers to direct research towards therapeutic needs, rather than just considering commercial aspects. A further advantage is the improved relationships between prescribers and pharmacists which often result from their joint input into developing a local formulary.

### Disadvantages

There are relatively few disadvantages to using a formulary. Some prescribers dislike losing the freedom to prescribe as they choose and may reject the formulary and its concept. Often prescribers have developed personal drug preferences over the years and, even if they have no objection in principle to prescribing a different drug, may easily forget when actually writing prescriptions. Changing prescribing habits is difficult to achieve. Constant reminders may be necessary to maintain prescribing within the recommendations of a formulary or prescribing policy. Pharmacists are most often called upon to provide these reminders and it can be very time-consuming.

Formularies vary considerably in the number of drugs they contain. If they are too restrictive, there are likely to be more problems in their use. Conversely, a formulary containing a large number of drugs is less likely to achieve rational prescribing or to reduce drug costs.

When a formulary is introduced, some patients

will be receiving medicines which are not included and they, too, may be resistant to change. The doctors who prescribe for these patients may also be unhappy about changing individual patients' drugs. This is especially likely if the patient is well stabilized on a particular drug, with little adverse effect. As drugs included in a formulary will have been selected on a sound basis, the situation may arise that a formulary drug would be more suitable for a patient than his/her current drug. Change may therefore be of benefit. Education of prescribers and patients may be necessary to convince them of potential benefits. Again, pharmacists are often those most actively involved in educating and persuading prescribers to carry out changes. Even without changing individual patients' drug therapy, if the drugs recommended in a local formulary are used for all patients starting new therapy, most prescriptions will in time be for formulary medicines.

The main disadvantage of formularies is not in using one, but creating one. They take a very long time to produce; several years is not uncommon. Obtaining everyone's opinions and discussing the drugs to be included is the main reason for this prolonged time. A formulary then needs to be updated regularly if it is going to be useful, which is a further time commitment. All prescribers and pharmacists need to have access to the formulary, which means it may cost a substantial amount of money to produce.

## CONSIDERATIONS IN COMPILING A FORMULARY

The first consideration is who should compile a formulary. Clearly pharmacists should be involved, or the subject would not be included in this book! Hospital pharmacists help to compile hospital formularies and community pharmacists should help with general practice formularies. In the case of joint formularies between hospital and general practice, representatives of both branches of pharmacy should be involved. Prescribers must also be included. If a formulary is for one general medical practice, all the prescribers in that practice should help to produce the formulary. Those to be used by larger groups will need to have appropriate representatives actually doing the work, although the opinions of most should be sought. This is a very important point in formulary development. The people expected to use a formulary must have the opportunity to give their views on its content. If their opinions are not asked,

| Table 34.1   Examples of formularies | |
|---|---|
| Purpose | Example formulary |
| General use | British National Formulary |
| Hospital formulary | Dundee Teaching Hospitals Trust Drug Formulary and Antibiotic Policy |
| General practice | Lothian Formulary (Royal College of General Practitioners, South East Scotland Faculty, University of Edinburgh) |
| | Practice Formulary (Royal College of General Practitioners, Northern Ireland Faculty) |
| | A Basic Formulary for General Practice (Grant et al 1987) |
| Joint formulary | Grampian Joint Formulary (Grampian Medicines Committee, Drug Monitoring Unit, Aberdeen Royal Infirmary) |

they may feel that it does not apply to them and will be less likely to use it.

There are two basic ways of producing a new formulary; either start from scratch or modify an existing one. Adapting another formulary to suit local needs is much less time-consuming than starting from scratch. Whichever way is chosen, studying existing formularies is a good way to begin. A list of formularies which may be useful is given in Table 34.1.

Although much can be learned from looking at someone else's formulary, simply deciding to adopt it without any changes is not a good idea. Producing a formulary is an educational process, during which all concerned learn from each other's experience and update their clinical pharmacology and therapeutics along the way. Producing a formulary brings a sense of ownership, which encourages commitment to it and increases the chance of it being used. Local needs should also be addressed by a local formulary, so copying someone else's may not be satisfactory.

### Content

The formulary should start with an introduction, giving the names of those who have compiled it, stating who is expected to use it and explaining its format. It is important to state whether all the drugs included are recommended for all users and if not, how different recommendations can be distinguished. The BNF, for example, lists drugs the Committee considers less suitable for prescribing in small type. Local formularies may choose to place restrictions on some drugs, for use by specialists only, for certain indications or in certain locations only. These drugs should be easily distinguishable from the others in the formulary.

A list of contents should be included to make the formulary easier to use. An index may also be included, but is more difficult to compile.

Most formularies follow the lead of the BNF, listing their drugs in the same order and by therapeutic indication or pharmacological class. Reference to the relevant BNF section is helpful if a local formulary is designed to be used in conjunction with the BNF. Users can be directed to read the monographs there for information on dosage, indications, side effects, contraindications and precautions. Some formularies include all this information, but only for the recommended drugs. Other important information which may be given is drug costs and the reasons for selection of the drugs included.

Drug costs are one of the factors taken into account when compiling a formulary (see below). The price of a drug can be expressed in several different ways. The prices given in the BNF are the prices of different pack sizes or for 20 doses of generics at Drug Tariff prices. The cost of a period of treatment may be more useful if comparisons are being encouraged. A suitable period may be 1 day, 1 month (28 days) or a standard course of treatment (5 days for antibiotics, for example). Since the price of the drug usually varies with the pack size, this may not be as easy to calculate as it first appears. A further complicating factor is the differing prices in hospital and community. If a formulary is designed to be used in hospital only, the hospital price may seem most relevant. However, the price of the drug may be different in general practice and patients may take the drug while living in the community for much longer than they take it in hospital. Many hospital prescribers wish to take community prices into account when selecting drugs, so ideally both should be provided. A joint formulary should have both hospital and community drug prices. Hospital prices are of little relevance to a general practice formulary.

When large numbers of prescribers are to use a formulary, it is possible that not all of them will have been consulted about its content. If that is the case, providing explanations of how drugs have come to be included in a formulary is of particular importance. Many formularies state the general basis of drug selection as being efficacy, safety, patient acceptability and cost. Sometimes additional information is given about specific drugs. The BNF gives this type of information in introductory paragraphs to each section. An example is that most other thiazides have no advantages over bendrofluazide, but are more expensive. It may be desirable to reference

the formulary to give readers the opportunity to see the evidence on which statements such as these are based. It may also be useful to explain local preferences, particularly in the case of antibiotic selection, which should take local microbiological sensitivities into account.

Some or all of the formulary may be presented as prescribing policies. Again this is most likely for antibiotics, but may extend to any group of drugs. If this approach is taken, details of which drugs are to be used in specific medical conditions should be given. It may be necessary to include alternatives and the particular occasions when they should be used. In a prescribing policy, details of the recommended dosage, route and method of administration and duration of therapy should also be included.

A local formulary may have sections relating to prescribing in certain types of patients, such as the elderly, children, those with renal or hepatic impairment or in pregnancy and breast-feeding. As there is little point in reproducing the BNF, the content of these sections, if included, should be local recommendations, like the rest of the formulary.

## Presentation

The appearance of the formulary is an indicator of the importance attached to it by those who have produced it. If it is presented on a few tattered sheets of paper, those who are expected to use it are unlikely to have a great deal of respect for its content. This may lead to poor adherence to its recommendations. It is therefore worth creating a document which is attractive and looks professionally produced.

The size of the formulary document should also be considered. Ideally, it should be pocket-sized, perhaps compatible in size with the BNF, to make it easy to use the two together. A large document which cannot be carried around is much less likely to be available when needed. This again may result in its recommendations being ignored. Ensuring that the formulary is up to date is extremely important and its presentation must allow for this. Loose-leaf binding will enable easy updating, but relies on everyone modifying his or her own copy.

The formulary should be easy to use, to encourage prescribers to refer to it when necessary. This will be helped by a contents list, which means the pages have to be numbered. Arranging the drugs in the same order as the BNF will also help to make the formulary easier to use, as prescribers should be familiar with this order. Using different typefaces and print size can make a formulary easier to use. Highlighting the drug names in some way can be

# Chapter 1

# GASTRO-INTESTINAL SYSTEM

### 1.1 ANTACIDS

MAALOX/MUCOGEL
GAVISCON

**Maalox and Mucogel** *(sugar-free suspension)* are proprietary brands of the same generic preparation, co-magaldrox. This is an effective combination of aluminium hydroxide and magnesium hydroxide with a low sodium content (less than 1 mmol per 10mL dose).

**Gaviscon liquid** *(sodium alginate, sodium bicarbonate and calcium carbonate)* is recommended for the treatment of **gastric reflux only** as it is **less effective** as an antacid than co-magaldrox. It has a high sodium content (6 mmol per 10mL) and is sugar-free.

**Gaviscon tablets** *(alginic acid, aluminium hydroxide, magnesium trisilicate and sodium bicarbonate)* are indicated where a tablet formulation is required. Each tablet contains 2 mmol sodium.

#### SPECIAL INDICATIONS

**Mucaine** *(sugar-free suspension)* contains aluminium hydroxide, magnesium hydroxide, and the local anaesthetic, oxethazaine. It is recommended for use in procedures such as radiotherapy where the local anaesthetic ingredient may be helpful in relieving oesophageal pain. The suspension should not be washed down with water.

**Altacite Plus** *(sugar-free suspension containing activated dimethicone and hydrotalcite)* is used in the hospital for biliary gastritis only.

**Citrate antacid mixture** is used in patients undergoing elective caesarean section.

#### PRESCRIBING POINTS FOR ANTACIDS

● Liquid preparations are more effective than tablets.

● Antacids are best given when symptoms occur or are expected, usually between meals and at bedtime - four or more times daily.

● Antacids, taken at the same time as other drugs, may impair their absorption. They may also damage enteric coatings designed to prevent irritant drugs from dissolving in the stomach.

**Fig. 34.1**   Example of formulary recommendations, illustrating style of presentation (reproduced by permission from Grampian Joint Formulary 1995, copyright Grampian Medicines Committee).

useful, as often the name of the recommended drug may be all that someone is seeking (see Fig. 34.1). Colour can add to the appearance of the formulary, but also adds to the cost. The cover of the formulary must be durable enough to withstand regular use, so should be of card rather than paper.

## Selection of products for inclusion

It is important to decide at the outset the range of indications which the formulary should cover. Most hospital formularies do not attempt to include drugs to treat all possible conditions. Some deliberately exclude certain drugs, such as those used in cancer chemotherapy and anaesthetics. These areas are extremely specialized, so drugs in these groups are never likely to be used by most prescribers. A formulary for use in general practice should aim to include enough drugs to treat between 80% and 90% of all common conditions which present to a general practitioner. It is also useful to include emergency drugs, such as those which should be carried by GPs in their emergency bags. Clearly if a formulary includes all the available drugs, as does the BNF, it will not only be bulky, but will also not have many of the advantages that a local formulary can provide. It should be possible to cover most needs, either in hospital or general practice, with about 300–500 drugs.

## 1.2 ANTISPASMODICS AND OTHER DRUGS ALTERING GUT MOTILITY

### ANTISPASMODICS

**DICYCLOMINE
MEBEVERINE**

**Dicyclomine** *(tablets, syrup)* is an anti-muscarinic drug which also has direct muscle relaxant properties. It is used as an adjunct in the treatment of gastro-intestinal disorders such as irritable bowel syndrome and diverticular disease. It has less marked anti-muscarinic actions than atropine, but atropine-like side-effects are common. It is contra-indicated in patients with glaucoma and urinary retention. It should be avoided in patients with oesophageal reflux.

**Mebeverine** *(tablets, liquid)* is believed to act as a direct relaxant of intestinal smooth muscle and has no anti-muscarinic actions. It is well tolerated. It may be used with bulk forming agents in irritable bowel syndrome.

#### SPECIAL INDICATIONS

**Peppermint water** may be used to relieve wind pain after abdominal surgery.

**Peppermint oil** *(capsules, e/c capsules)* has a direct relaxant effect and may be useful for relief of abdominal colic and distention. It may cause heartburn. The capsules should be swallowed whole as peppermint oil can cause irritation of the mouth or oesophagus.

**Hyoscine butylbromide injection** is useful in endoscopy and radiology.

#### PRESCRIBING POINTS FOR ANTISPASMODICS

● All antispasmodics should be avoided in paralytic ileus.

● Absorption of other drugs may be affected by altering gut transit time.

● The elderly are particularly susceptible to anti-muscarinic side-effects.

**Fig. 34.1** *cont'd*

In selecting drugs for inclusion in a formulary, it is important to remember that recommendations are being made to treat the majority of the population. However, individual patients' needs and preferences should, where possible, be taken into account. This means that there may be individuals for whom the recommended formulary drug is not suitable, but the formulary should attempt to make provision for most commonly encountered situations. An example would be the inclusion of a histamine $H_2$ antagonist which does not inhibit cytochrome P450, to cover the situations when a patient is also taking a drug which is metabolized by this route.

As already stated, most formularies include drugs on the basis of efficacy, safety, patient acceptability and cost, but other factors are also usually considered. A list of factors which influence selection of drugs for inclusion is given in Table 34.2.

The most important factors are efficacy and toxicity. Drugs which are included in a formulary must be effective, for whatever indications they are to be used, with minimal toxicity. Evidence of efficacy should be based on well-conducted clinical trials, rather than anecdotal reports. Generally, prescribers' personal preferences are not a sound basis for selection of a particular drug or product. This is especially true when the formulary is to be used by many prescribers, as each may have his or her own preference. Occasionally there may be a range of similar drugs from which to select, but not all are licensed

---

**Table 34.2   Factors influencing selection of drugs for inclusion in a formulary**

- Efficacy for the indications to be included in the formulary
- Side effect profiles and contraindications of individual drugs
- Interaction profile of individual drugs
- Pharmacokinetic profiles of individual drugs
- Acceptability to patients – taste, appearance, ease of administration
- Formulations available
- General availability, including generic availability
- Cost
- Usage patterns

---

for all the indications the formulary is to cover. An example is calcium channel blockers, some of which are licensed for angina and hypertension, while others are only licensed for hypertension. In this situation, selection of the drug which covers most indications may be appropriate. Alternatively, separate drugs could be selected for different indications. This option is most difficult to monitor, as it is impossible to tell from looking only at prescribing data whether the drug is prescribed in line with the formulary recommendations. It therefore requires a lot of work to determine whether or not prescribers are adhering to the formulary.

If two drugs are equally efficacious, as is often the case within a group of pharmacologically similar drugs, the one which is least toxic is preferable. In this situation, any differences between the drugs in terms of their pharmacokinetics, contraindications, adverse effects and potential for interaction become important.

A knowledge of the pharmacokinetic profile of drugs is important to enable selection of a drug with an optimum half-life for its indications. It is also essential to know whether drugs undergo hepatic metabolism, to make recommendations for patients with hepatic dysfunction. Similarly it is important to know about the effect of renal impairment on a drug's elimination. It may be possible to select drugs which are minimally affected by either liver or renal impairment. Among the benzodiazepine group, for example, those with short half-lives and which have no active metabolites are preferred as hypnotics, as they have no hangover effect. Differences in drug handling in children and the elderly may require different drugs to be recommended for use with these patients. A knowledge of the passage of drugs into the placenta and secretion into breast milk will enable selection of drugs to be used in pregnancy and breast-feeding.

The range of contraindications, precautions and adverse effects may differ for drugs within a group from which a selection is being made. Often these are a drug class effect, but this is not always the case. Beta-adrenoceptor antagonists are a good example of a situation where there are differences between the individual drugs in the class. Differences are most often found in the frequency and severity of adverse effects between drugs in a class. Where possible, drugs should be selected which have the lowest frequency of and least severe adverse effects.

If drugs are similar in terms of efficacy and toxicity, but have different potential for interaction, this could be a deciding factor. Drugs with fewer possibilities of interaction mean fewer problems in use.

Patient acceptability is an important factor, which will be affected by efficacy and toxicity. If drugs do not work, or if they cause side effects, patients are less likely to accept the need to take them. For orally administered drugs, palatability and ease of swallowing will contribute to acceptability. Other considerations may also be important, such as the extent to which a dispersible preparation actually disperses, or not being able to break a modified-release tablet in half. Inhaled drugs are available in many different formulations and their selection will depend to a large extent on what patients will use properly, to achieve maximum efficacy. For topical products, such as creams and ointments, patient acceptability is particularly important.

A local formulary may simply list drugs which are recommended or it may specify particular dosage forms of those drugs. Patient acceptability is likely to influence the different formulations selected for inclusion in a formulary more than the drug entities. However, the range of formulations available, which will in turn affect patients' acceptance of drug therapy, may be a factor in deciding which drugs to include. If a drug is available in a wide range of formulations, it may be a better choice than one which has very few. It is simpler for the prescriber to remember one drug name when a particular class of drug is required, rather than to worry about which drug he should prescribe based on the formulation needed.

Many formularies exclude all combination products on classical clinical pharmacological grounds. A combination product includes two or more drugs in fixed ratio. It is impossible to increase the dose of one drug without also increasing the dose of the other(s). Some patients may receive higher doses of one of the constituents than they require as a result. However, combination products are particularly favoured in general practice, where they are considered to improve patient compliance. A further factor is the need for patients to pay only one prescription charge, for a condition for which they may be prescribed two drugs. Combination products are often used unnecessarily for these reasons. The products may be useful if the pharmacokinetic characteristics of the components are compatible. They can be used appropriately if the patient has been shown to require, and to obtain benefit from, all the components individually, in the same ratio as the combination product. Unfortunately, very few combination products are used in this way. Their inclusion in a formulary will depend very much on local preferences and appropriate use will subsequently depend on individual prescribers.

Cost considerations are also important, since the aim of a formulary is to encourage rational and cost-effective prescribing, not primarily to save money. Cost-effective prescribing involves the use of the drug with the lowest costs which is also effective, has minimal toxicity and is acceptable to patients. The cheapest drugs may not be the most acceptable, or of adequate efficacy. For some groups of drugs, prescribing costs may actually rise as a result of using a local formulary, since the optimum drugs may be the most expensive. However, where efficacy, toxicity and patient acceptability are equal, cost should be the deciding factor in drug selection. As described above, both hospital and community costs of drugs should be considered when selecting drugs for a hospital formulary, as the bulk of the cost is likely to be borne by general practitioners. The purchase price of a drug may not be the only factor to be taken into account when considering costs. Pharmacoeconomic evaluations which take account of the costs of the consequences of treatments may also be necessary.

Drugs to be included in a formulary should be easily available, so 'specials', drugs available in hospital only, or on a named patient basis, should be avoided. Generic availability is a bonus, since it usually means costs are lower than for drugs which are only available as branded formulations. Most formularies specify that prescribing should be generic, where appropriate. The use of computer systems for prescribing, which automatically change prescriptions to the appropriate generic name, increases the proportion of generic prescriptions considerably. This should also reduce costs.

## Use of prescribing data

All the factors mentioned so far are also applicable to

the selection of drugs for individual patients. A further factor which is often considered when selecting drugs to include in a formulary is current prescribing habits. The main reason for this is that it is much easier to encourage use of a formulary if it involves few changes of habit. However, if the drugs found to be commonly prescribed are not efficacious, or have a high incidence or severity of toxicity, it is better not to include them. Just because a drug is often prescribed, it is not necessarily an appropriate choice for a formulary. Information about the drugs currently prescribed is obtainable for either hospital or general practice prescribers. In hospital, these data may relate to wards or to directorates and can be obtained from computerized pharmacy supply systems. In UK general practice, data are available as Prescribing Analysis and CosT (PACT) in England and Wales, as Scottish Prescribing Analysis (SPA) in Scotland and as COMPASS (COMputerised on-line Prescribing Analysis for Science and Stewardship) in Northern Ireland. Prescribing data are generated by the Prescription Pricing Authority in England, the Health Common Services Agency in Wales, the Pharmacy Practice Division of the Common Services Agency in Scotland and the Central Services Agency in Northern Ireland. The data can identify prescribing by an individual general practitioner or by a practice. Prescribing is compared to the average for the health authority or health board. Detailed data which are useful in compiling a formulary are obtainable from the PACT catalogue in England and SPA Level 2 in Scotland. Examples of these types of data are shown in Figures 34.2 and 34.3. The raw data for practices in Northern Ireland are subjected to computer analysis by the Drug Utilization Research Unit at Queen's University, Belfast. This identifies medicines which may not have been prescribed as cost-effectively or as rationally as the latest evidence suggests. These items are highlighted, their rational use is described and potential cost savings calculated. An example is given in Figure 34.4. This makes it particularly helpful in compiling a formulary.

Prescribing data provide information about the frequency with which different drug products are prescribed. From this it is usually possible to identify one or two drugs within each group which account for the bulk of prescriptions for that class. These should usually be considered for inclusion in a formulary, as little change in prescribing habits will be needed if they are selected. As already stated, they should be efficacious and have minimal toxicity. It may be possible to include only these drugs in a formulary, or there may be a need for others to be

```
Request Ref:  GP                    Dispensing Month(s): MAR 1997 to MAY 1997   REF:GP /14-AUG-1997    PAGE

                                    No. times      Total              Total   Average Average
                                    prescribed     Quantity           cost    quantity cost

    1.      GASTRO-INTESTINAL SYSTEM
            This group represents of your prescribing costs:  18.62%
                              Scotland average:  18.38%

        CHAPTER TOTALS:                  292                          £5173.86
                                       =====                     ==============

    1.1    Antacids
        SECTION TOTALS:                   26                           £75.05
                                       -----                     --------------

        GAVISCON LIQ.........................................   10      5500 ml.      29.70     550    2.97
        GAVISCON PEPPERMINT TABS 500MG...................... .  4       240            9.00      60    2.25
        MUCAINE SUSP.........................................   1        400 ml.       1.52     400    1.52
        GASTROCOTE LIQ.......................................   2       1000 ml.       5.58     500    2.79
        INFACOL SUSP 40MG/ML.................................   3        150 ml.       5.28      50    1.76
        GASTROCOTE TABS......................................   5        600          22.02     120    4.40
        ASILONE SUSP.........................................   1        500 ml.       1.95     500    1.95
```

**Fig. 34.2**    Example of SPA data. (Reproduced with permission from the Pharmacy Practice Division.)

included on a more restricted basis. If the commonly prescribed drugs are inappropriate on therapeutic grounds, an alternative may be required. There are some classes of drugs for which none is considered appropriate by many clinical pharmacologists. An example is peripheral vasodilators. There is no established efficacy for any of these drugs in the conditions for which they are prescribed. None is recommended in the BNF. However, a review of prescribing data may well show a high frequency of prescribing. Here is an opportunity to encourage rational prescribing by not including drugs such as these.

A common finding on studying prescribing data is that different prescribers tend to favour different drugs. If a formulary is being developed for a group where this is found, extensive discussion will often be needed. Pharmacists have a key role to play in providing unbiased information about any differences in efficacy and toxicity between the different drugs. One useful source of such information is the National Prescribing Centre in Liverpool, England or the Scottish Medicines Resource Centre in Edinburgh. *Drug and Therapeutics Bulletin*, which is published monthly, also provides good short summaries of trials of new drugs and considers their place in relation to existing therapies. This information may be most effective when incorporated into routinely issued prescribing data, either individualized, as in Northern Ireland, or general, as in PACT.

## FORMULARY MANAGEMENT SYSTEMS

A formulary needs to be flexible and dynamic. A system must be devised which allows this. This is known as the formulary management system and it covers many different aspects of formularies which have not yet been mentioned.

## Production, distribution and revision

Producing a formulary is a very time-consuming task. Usually in hospital a drug and therapeutics committee will oversee this, but the work may be given to one or more small groups of individuals, possibly experts in particular fields. A pharmacist should be included in all groups. In a group general practice, all GPs should be involved, as well as local community pharmacists. The task of producing a formulary involves collecting together the data on which the drug selection will be based (published evidence, prescribing data and expert or all group members' opinions). Once the selection is made, the format of the material and the design of the final document must be considered. Thought is required as to who will need to have a copy, to help in deciding how best it should be produced. Photocopying is cheapest for small numbers and can still incorporate colour and be attractively bound for a professional appearance. However, if large numbers are required, printing becomes more economical.

| CATALOGUE OF PRESCRIBING (full) | | | | |
|---|---|---|---|---|
| **3. Respiratory System** | Quantity | No. of items | Quantity x items | Cost(£) |
| **3.10 Systemic Nasal Decongestants** | | | | |
| 3.10.0 Systemic Nasal Decongestants | | | | |
| Pseudoephed HCl Elix 30mg/5ml | 100 | 1 | 100 | 0.94 |
| | | 1 | 100 | 0.94 |
| Pseudoephed HCl Tab 60mg | 24 | 3 | 72 | 4.23 |
| | 24 | 1 | 24 | 1.41 |
| | | 4 | 96 | 5.64 |
| **Sub-total Pseudoephed HCl** | | 5 | | 6.58 |
| Sudafed®Tab (60mg) | 84 | 3 | 252 | 14.76 |
| | | 3 | 252 | 14.76 |
| **Sub-total Sudafed (Nsl Decongestant)** | | 3 | | 14.76 |
| Dimotane Plus®Elix S/F | 300 | 4 | 1200 | 8.32 |
| | | 4 | 1200 | 8.32 |
| **Sub-total Dimotane Plus** | | 4 | 1200 | 8.32 |
| **Sub-total Chem. Sub. Pseudoephedrine Hydrochloride** | | 12 | | 29.66 |
| **Sub-total 3.10.0** | | 12 | | 29.66 |
| **SUB-TOTAL 3.10** | | 12 | | 29.66 |
| **Total: Respiratory System** | | 405 | | 2,843.73 |

**This report covers prescribing attributed to Dr WORKLOAD's Practice**

**11**

APRIL 1995
BNF version number 24

© Copyright Prescription Pricing Authority 1996

**Fig. 34.3** Example of PACT data. (Reproduced with permission from the Prescription Pricing Authority.)

The method of distribution must also be considered if the formulary is to be used by large numbers of people. Mailing may be easiest and will require a covering letter, but hand delivery, with verbal explanation may help to encourage interest and therefore adherence to a formulary's recommendations. Launching of a new formulary (or indeed a revision) can usefully be accompanied by a meeting to explain its aims, describe how to use it and encourage discussion of its contents.

After all the effort which goes into producing a new formulary has resulted in the final document, the thought of revising it is likely to be far from popular. However, because of the time taken to produce a new formulary, it will soon go out of date. If this is allowed to happen, respect for its content will decline. Adherence to its recommendations may follow suit. Revision should therefore be considered even before the formulary is finished. The BNF is

revised every 6 months, but most local formularies cannot hope to achieve a similar frequency, because of the amount of work involved. Annual or biennial revision should be aimed at. This should be included as one of the aims when launching a new formulary. As new drugs are coming onto the market all the time, even 6-monthly revision will not be adequate to keep a formulary right up to date. Some system, therefore, needs to be devised to allow new drugs to be considered for inclusion.

## Responding to the needs of practice

Change is the norm in the world of drugs. New drugs are constantly becoming available, old drugs are removed from the market, new clinical trials provide evidence for efficacy of existing drugs in novel indications and post-marketing surveillance provides constantly changing data on adverse effect profiles.

| PRACTICE NAME: | | PRACTICE NUMBER: 345 | |
|---|---|---|---|
| MONTH SURVEYED: | March 1996 | | |
| | | | *% OF ALL COSTS* |
| PRESCRIBING COST(£) - ALL DRUGS: | | £103,916 | |
| PRESCRIBING COST(£) - COMPASS DRUGS: | | £41,757 | *40%* |
| **POTENTIAL SAVINGS (£) FOR COMPASS DRUGS:** | | **£28,876** | *28%* |
| POTENTIAL SAVINGS AS A PERCENTAGE OF COMPASS COSTS | | 69% | |

TO THE PRESCRIBER: Here is a record of your Practice's prescribing for : March 1996 showing where a substantial proportion of drug cost might be saved, without prejudice to the quality of treatment.

| | ACTUAL COST (£) | POSSIBLE SAVING (£) |
|---|---|---|
| Peripheral vasodilators have no effect on stenosed arteries. They dilate healthy arteries and arterioles, risking 'steal' syndrome. The Drug and Therapeutics Bulletin declares them "not worth giving". except in vasospastic conditions. They include Sturgeron,Hexopal, Ronicol, Trental, Opilon, Hydergine and Praxilene. Paroven is also of dubious efficacy (in treating venous insufficiency) - see BNF. | 925.1 | 925.1 |
| Persantin (dipyridamole) is no more effective than Dispersible Asprin BP 75 mg and costs 101 times more. (Persantin may be used in anti-coagulated patients, where gastic bleeding is a risk). | 79.06 | 78.03 |

**Fig. 34.4**  Extract from COMPASS data. (Supplied by Dr H. McGavock, Drug Utilization Research Unit, Queen's University, Belfast.)

An awareness of all the facts this generates is essential, so that the formulary does not go out of date and can respond to the changes. In implementing a formulary, patients must not be deprived of the benefits of new information and drugs. There will also inevitably be an occasional need for patients to receive treatment outwith a formulary's recommendations, since a formulary cannot be expected to cover all possible situations. Methods are therefore needed to allow drugs to be considered for inclusion in the formulary, to allow drugs to be removed from the formulary and to supply non-formulary drugs when these are appropriate.

A method for allowing drugs to be considered for inclusion in a formulary should not be restricted to newly available drugs. It must allow any user of the formulary to propose a drug for consideration and should be able to provide an evaluated response within a reasonable time. Evidence of any advantages the proposed drug has over drugs already included, in terms of efficacy, reduced toxicity or cost will be needed. This must be based on well-designed published clinical trials, the same basis as that used in the initial formulary development. Many hospital formulary management systems require a form to be completed; an example is given in Figure 34.5. The person making the request must be informed as to whether the drug will be included and, if so, whether any restrictions will be placed on its prescribing. One option is to have an appraisal period, during which prescribers can gain experience with a newly recommended drug, after which its continuing recommendation can be reviewed; 6 months would seem to be a suitable time for such an appraisal period.

If a drug is accepted onto an existing formulary between revisions, it is essential to inform all users of the change. One way of achieving this is to issue information bulletins. A similar method can be used to inform users of any changes in the indications or

---

**Request for an Inclusion of a New Drug in a Formulary**

Drug name _____

Formulation and strength(s) available _____

Indication(s) for which request is made _____

Usual duration of treatment _____


Type of inclusion       ☐   general recommendation

                         ☐   specialist use only

If so, which specialists? _____

                         ☐   restricted indication(s)

If so, which indication(s)? _____

Reason for request        ☐   novel therapeutic advance

                         ☐   benefits over existing drug

Will the new drug replace an existing drug? YES/NO

If so, which? _____

Estimated number of patients per year

likely to be treated _____

Estimated costs of treatment _____

Evidence in support of request (References required)

---

**Fig. 34.5** Example of a form which could be used to request new drugs to be considered for inclusion in a formulary.

doses of drugs which may also occur during the life of a formulary. Similarly, if drugs are to be withdrawn from the formulary, users must be kept informed.

Withdrawals may occur because of manufacturers ceasing production, product licences being withdrawn or changes in manufacturers' recommendations. However, it may also be useful to consider withdrawing drugs from the formulary if they have not been prescribed for a long time. Again, 6 months would be a suitable time to study the prescribing of most drugs, except those whose use is seasonal. This could be done on a regular basis between major revisions, but would require consultation with prescribers before the withdrawal were implemented. The advantage of a practice such as this is that it helps to keep the number of drugs in the formulary to a minimum.

As there will be situations when a non-formulary drug is requested for a patient, it is necessary to have a method of ensuring that the request is dealt with promptly. In general practice, there should be no problem in supplying a non-formulary drug, although there may be a delay if it is not stocked by local pharmacies owing to rare use. In hospital, however, pharmacies tend to stock only a limited range of drugs. Formulary drugs should always be easily available, but non-formulary drugs may need to be specially purchased. This will lead to delays in treatment. Some hospitals require completion of a form for every non-formulary drug which is prescribed. The purpose of this is twofold: it acts as a deterrent to prescribing non-formulary drugs and also allows monitoring to see whether any drugs are frequently requested. Consideration may be given to including frequently requested drugs in the formulary. Usually forms require a senior medical staff signature, but there is a possibility that this requirement may be abused. Once a form with the appropriate signature is received, pharmacists should not simply assume that the request should be complied with. If this occurs, all that has been achieved is an elaborate ordering system. For the formulary system to operate effectively, all prescribers requesting a non-formulary drug should be questioned to determine the reasons why a formulary drug is not suitable.

One of the most frequent reasons for requesting a non-formulary drug in hospital is that the patient was taking the drug prior to admission and prescribers are reluctant to change it. This can be viewed as an opportunity to review the medication, ensuring that it is appropriate for the individual patient. If it proves to be so, it may be possible to use the patient's own supply of the drug, if it has been brought into hospital. Further systems will then be necessary for ensuring that patients' medicines are those prescribed and are fit for use. It is possible to save money and prevent delays in treatment by using patients' own drugs.

If this is not an option, the decision must be made as to whether the requested drug will be supplied from the pharmacy. The systems in place must ensure that this is a rapid process, particularly if a special purchase is required.

In general practice too, the most common reason for using non-formulary drugs is that patients are already taking them and either they or their GPs are reluctant to change the prescription. If regular medication reviews are undertaken, this provides an opportunity to consider the appropriateness of any non-formulary drugs prescribed. An alternative time to look at this is during regular review of repeat prescribing, which takes place in many practices. Pharmacists may contribute to both activities.

The promotional activities of drug manufacturers' representatives will need to be controlled to prevent them from undermining the principles of the formulary. This is not to say that their role is unimportant, but the inclusion of a drug in a formulary must be evidence based and unbiased. Manufacturers can be an extremely useful source of information and many now specifically address the possibilities of placing their products in formularies.

Clearly a lot of effort goes into operating a formulary and there are many advantages of a good formulary management system. The measure of success of any formulary is in the extent to which it is used or adhered to and the demonstration that prescribing is more rational. It may be possible to show improvements in efficacy and reduced toxicity and also cost savings, but these may be more difficult to achieve and to demonstrate. The same type of prescribing data which were used to help develop the formulary can again be used to look for adherence to it.

## Feedback on performance

The simplest way to gauge whether a formulary is being used is to look at prescribing data. Computerized data, such as PACT and SPA or their hospital equivalent, can easily be studied to assess whether formulary drugs are being prescribed. However, this type of data provides no information about the patients for whom the drugs have been prescribed. It cannot, for example, identify why patients have received prescriptions for non-formulary drugs. Nor can it be used to determine whether the formulary drugs were prescribed appropriately. Despite these limitations, prescribing data are a valuable source of information which should be used to provide feedback to prescribers on the extent of their adherence to the formulary.

For data to be of any use, they must be easy to interpret, accurate and up to date. They must also be of direct relevance to the prescriber to whom they are given and may allow comparison either to earlier prescribing or to the prescribing of others. Comparing the prescribing of several GPs or hospital doctors to each other is known as peer review. Comparison to a 'norm' of prescribing practice, or to the practices of others in the same peer group, often increases the desire of prescribers to conform to the 'norm' or the peer group. However, it is important to ensure that the 'norm' is desirable. For example, reducing the cost of prescriptions for steroid inhalers to that of the lowest cost prescriber in a peer group may be considered to be a suitable target at which to aim. However, therapeutic guidelines suggest these products should be increasing in use, so costs should also be increasing.

Hospital data are often generated by the pharmacy computerized stock control system. As such they may refer to drugs issued to wards or directorates and care must be taken to determine whether this equates to drugs prescribed. Any drugs used on wards, which were not issued through the computer system, such as patients' own drugs, will not show up in these data. It is possible for drugs which are included in the formulary to be identified in the computer records, so that determination of formulary adherence is relatively simple. Care should, however, be taken to ensure that the quantities of the different drugs used are taken into account in some way.

For example, if a ward uses 180 tablets of a formulary drug and 20 tablets of a range of four other non-formulary drugs, adherence should be quantified as 90% (180 out of 200 tablets used in total). It could also be calculated that adherence was only 20%, if the range of drugs were used (one out of a range of five), but this would not be a reasonable representation of the overall prescribing on the ward.

Another source of data which can be valuable in hospital is the request forms for non-formulary drugs, if they are used. Review of these can indicate the extent of non-formulary prescribing. These also have the value of explaining the reasons why non-formulary drugs were used. Records of clinical pharmacists' interventions which have involved non-formulary prescribing can also be studied.

In general practice, PACT and SPA represent the number of prescriptions dispensed, so are a useful indicator of prescribing practices. Only prescriptions which have not been presented to pharmacies and dispensed are excluded. They cannot, however, distinguish between formulary and non-formulary drugs. This must be done manually and a figure for adherence can then be calculated, again taking the quantities of each drug into account. Another source of data in general practice is the practice computer. This can be programmed to identify formulary drugs, but not all practices use computers to create acute prescriptions. If these are excluded, the prescribing patterns obtained will not show the full picture.

Regular provision of information on performance is an essential part of formulary management. Any data which are presented to prescribers as a means of informing them of adherence to formulary recommendations will need to be attractive and easy to use, just like the formulary itself. Colour will add to their appearance, and a simple highlighter pen can be used to emphasize parts of a table or figure which may be particularly important. Computers can also generate graphics and this can be a useful way of presenting data. One simple way of showing adherence is to plot the percentage of formulary and non-formulary drugs prescribed in each therapeutic category as a bar chart, such as that shown in Figure 34.6. Finally, evidence of cost savings, if they are made, may help to encourage use of the formulary. This is best expressed as actual expenditure compared to expected expenditure had the formulary not been used.

Using feedback information such as this provides pharmacists with another opportunity to market the formulary, to promote relationships with prescribers and to discuss prescribing policies.

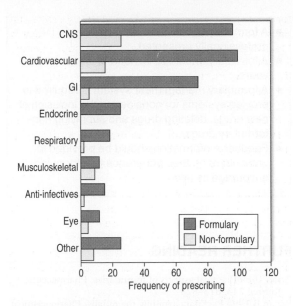

**Fig. 34.6** Example of graphic feedback on formulary and non-formulary prescribing.

One final point should be emphasized. It is important to remember that adherence to a prescribing policy cannot be ascertained from data such as these. If prescribing policies form a part of a formulary, drug utilization review will be needed to determine whether they are being followed.

## Key Points

- A formulary is a list of drugs which are recommended and available for prescribing.
- A formulary may contain prescribing policies, which detail the use of drugs in specific medical conditions.
- Local formularies are compiled to encourage rational and cost-effective prescribing.
- Compiling a formulary is a valuable educational exercise.
- Pharmacists and prescribers should work together on compiling a formulary.
- Drugs are selected for inclusion in a formulary on the basis of efficacy, toxicity, patient acceptability and cost.
- Use of a formulary containing a restricted number of drugs may reduce the incidence of adverse drug reactions, interactions and lack of efficacy.
- For a formulary to be accepted, there should be widespread consultation on its content.

- A formulary should be easy to use and professionally presented.
- A formulary should be revised at least every 2 years.
- A formulary management system is required to provide systems for considering the inclusion of new drugs, deleting drugs and supplying non-formulary drugs.
- Feedback information should be provided to prescribers on their adherence to a formulary to encourage its use.

## FURTHER READING

Anon 1989 Practical aspects of formularies. Pharmaceutical Journal 243: 813–820

Bevan B 1996 Pact data avoiding the pitfalls. Pharmaceutical Journal 257: 25–30

Clinical Resource and Audit Group 1993 Hospital drug formularies: an indicator of quality. Scottish Office, Edinburgh

Garvey G, Jappy B, Stewart D et al 1990 Grampian Health Board's joint drug formulary. British Medical Journal 301: 851–852

Grant G B, Gregory D A, Van Zwanenberg T D 1987 A basic formulary for general practice. Oxford University Press, Oxford

Jenkins A 1996 Formulary development by community pharmacists. Pharmaceutical Journal 256: 861–863

McGavock H, Wilson-Davis K, Rafferty T 1994 A 'compass' for general practitioner prescribers. Health Trends 26: 28–30

Waine C 1989 How to develop a practice formulary. Royal College of General Practitioners, London

# 35

# The evaluation of medicines

*J. A. Cromarty, J. Krska and J. Silcock*

After studying this chapter you will know about:

**Safety, efficacy and economy**
**Clinical trials**
**Post-marketing surveillance**
**Drug utilization review and evaluation**
**Pharmacoeconomic evaluation**.

## SAFETY, EFFICACY AND ECONOMY

The volume and complexity of modern medicines are increasing. Many new medicines are more potent than older medicines. The need to compare the therapeutic efficacy (i.e. benefits) of new medicines with their potential to cause harm (i.e. risks) remains of paramount importance. With the cost of medicines and related services increasing, economic evaluation is also important. Pharmacists are ideally placed to play a major role in the evaluation of the safety, efficacy and economy of medicines use. This opportunity exists before medicines are marketed through participation in clinical trial work. However, pharmacists may be even better placed to make significant contributions to post-marketing surveillance, drug utilization review and evaluation, and pharmacoeconomic evaluation.

At a macro level, the pharmaceutical industry decides which line of drug development would best serve its interests. Society and its health care systems are faced with difficult decisions on which specific patient populations to treat, or which expensive new drug therapy to approve for use. Increasingly, such decisions are likely to be based on economic evaluations. There is a need to calculate benefit : risk ratios for medicines for potential patient populations as a whole. However, at a micro level each clinician (doctor, pharmacist or nurse) requires to assess the relative risks and benefits of each medicine for individual patients.

Many factors can affect the disposition of the drug in individual patients. For certain drugs this results in wide interpatient variation in response. For example, differences in metabolizing capacity for phenytoin between patients can produce 10-fold differences in plasma concentrations achieved by the same dose. For other drugs variation in response between individuals can occur in the absence of significant differences in drug disposition. Concurrent disease states and/or drug therapy also contribute to variations in the safety and efficacy of medicines in individual patients (see Ch. 32).

Another important consideration in assessing benefit : risk ratios stems from the risk of the untreated disease itself. Thus there may be more justification for using an effective but toxic drug in a patient with a potentially fatal disease than an effective but similarly toxic drug in a patient with a non-fatal disease. Of course, what is justified or acceptable to one clinician or patient may not be to another. Equally, what is affordable to one health care system or individual patient may not be to another. Thus questions concerning the safety, efficacy and economy of medicines can be complex.

The pre- and post-marketing evaluation of medicines for safety, efficacy and economy takes several forms. These are summarized in Table 35.1, and described in a little more detail in the remaining sections of this chapter. Their overall purpose is to define in populations the safety, efficacy and economy of medicines. Where possible, they should also identify sub-populations or particular patients at risk of toxicity.

The results of these evaluations serve to inform clinicians of population-based benefit : risk ratios. This does not replace the need to consider carefully the potential for safety, efficacy and economy in their individual prescribing decisions (see Ch. 31 on

| Table 35.1 | Methods of evaluating medicines in humans | |
|---|---|---|
| **Method** | **Subjects** | **Outcome** |
| **Clinical trials** | | |
| Phase I | Usually healthy volunteers (≤60 adults) | • Pharmacokinetics of drug<br>• Tolerability and toxicity profile (SAFETY) |
| Phase II | Selected and limited target patient population | • Optimal dosage range (EFFICACY)<br>• Balance between safety and efficacy (THERAPEUTIC RATIO) |
| Phase III | Larger numbers of target patients (~1000–2000 patients) | • Comparative safety and efficacy of medicine<br>• Identification of common adverse drug reactions (<1 : 250 incidence) |
| **Post-marketing pharmacoepidemiological studies** | | |
| Post-marketing surveillance (Phase IV) | (Up to 10 000 patients) | • Less common and unpredictable ADRs<br>• Identification of patients at risk |
| Drug utilization studies or reviews | Variable numbers of patients using the medicine in routine clinical practice | • Quantitative studies → patterns of drug use<br>• Some qualitative studies → appropriateness of drug utilization |
| Drug utilization review programme or drug utilization evaluation or therapeutic audit | Variable numbers of patients using the medicine in routine clinical practice | Clinical, social and economic consequences of drug utilization |
| Pharmacoeconomic evaluations | Variable numbers of patients using the medicine in routine clinical practice | Comparative cost minimization, cost–effectiveness, cost–utility or cost–benefit |

Clinical pharmacy practice and Ch. 32 on Adverse drug reactions).

Medicines resource management aims to optimize the use of medicines to obtain maximum therapeutic benefit within available resources (Clinical Resource and Audit Group 1996). Pharmacists perform many functions in relation to this important multidisciplinary task. In promoting rational prescribing, pharmacists provide independently evaluated drug information (see Ch. 36), and manage formularies (see Ch. 34), clinical guidelines and treatment protocols (see Ch. 31). They also initiate and participate in studies on drug utilization review and evaluation (see p. 398).

## CLINICAL TRIALS

In most countries evidence of safety, efficacy and quality must be presented to government-appointed regulatory authorities before a new drug can be marketed. In the UK, the Committee on Safety of Medicines (CSM) requires to be satisfied with such evidence before it grants a product licence.

Prior to clinical trials in humans, the pharmacokinetics and pharmacodynamics of any new drug are studied during pre-clinical evaluation in animals. Such studies may indicate therapeutic and possible toxic effects in humans. However, there are often substantial inter-species differences in drug handling and in drug response. This usually results in the need for screening in more than one animal species. The often poor relationship between the effects of drugs in animals and humans necessitates cautious and step-wise trials in humans.

## Phase I trials

These first trials are normally carried out in healthy adult volunteers. Their main purpose is to determine the drug's toxicity profile and to assess tolerability. A dosage range is tested initially with a step-wise increase in drug dose being given to successive volunteers. Subjects in Phase I trials are intensively monitored to determine the nature and severity of any predictable dose-related adverse effects. Pharmacokinetic data are usually generated from both single- and multiple-dose studies.

The safety data obtained from Phase I studies suffer from a number of limitations. The subjects are healthy adults and unlikely to have compromised drug handling ability. Thus the potential risks of using the drug in patients at extremes of age, or in those with poor hepatic or renal function are not tested. There are also relatively few of them (e.g. 50–60), so only very common adverse effects are detected.

## Phase II trials

Phase II trials commence while Phase I studies are still running. They are carried out in relatively small groups of target patients and tend to be performed within hospital-based departments specializing in particular areas of medicine. Their main aims are to establish efficacy and to confirm an effective dose in closely monitored and controlled conditions. There is less emphasis on safety assessments during this phase. Phase II studies give the first indication of the likely value of the drug in patients. Double-blind randomized controlled trials use a control group with a matching placebo to assess the effectiveness of new drug therapies. Phase II studies also inform the design of Phase III studies which are more comprehensive. Phases II and III combined may study 1000–2000 patients. The regulatory authorities closely control Phase II and Phase III studies, for which clinical trial certificates or exemptions are required.

## Phase III trials

These are the better known trials of safety and efficacy. They are generally large-scale comparative trials with other treatments. Where appropriate, such trials should have a randomized controlled design which is generally accepted as the best method of conducting clinical research. Assigning each patient randomly to either the new treatment or the control helps to prevent bias in the interpretation of each patient's progress.

Phase III trials generate data equally between safety and efficacy. They are the main source of the information which appears ultimately in the product's data sheet.

Safety is assessed by close monitoring of clinical signs and symptoms during scheduled clinical examinations and consultations. This is complemented by

relevant laboratory investigations. Baseline pre-treatment data are compared with data obtained during periods of treatment with the study drugs. With the numbers of patients involved in Phases II and III, these trials are capable of identifying only Type A adverse drug reactions that affect 1 in ≤250 patients studied. Type B adverse drug reactions, which are neither pharmacologically predictable nor dose-related, tend to be rare (see Ch. 32). The larger number of patients involved in post-marketing surveillance studies are required, if they are to be detected.

## POST-MARKETING SURVEILLANCE

The most common type of post-marketing surveillance involves spontaneous reporting systems, e.g. the yellow card system, described in Chapter 32. Other forms of retrospective study (e.g. case-control studies) and of prospective study (e.g. cohort studies) are also outlined in Chapter 32.

Perhaps the main disadvantage of spontaneous reporting systems is the problem of under-reporting. This may reflect a number of factors including a lack of time, uncertainty about cause and effect, and failure to recognize a previously unreported effect. There may also be an element of a lack of incentive to report. A dramatic increase in the level of reporting was observed in one study following the experimental introduction of a financial incentive for doctors to report ADRs. Another factor in under-reporting in the UK stemmed from the fact that only doctors were allowed to report ADRs. After approximately 20 years of lobbying, the UK Medicines Control Agency have finally conceded in principle to permit pharmacists to report. This has been done successfully in other countries for many years. Another disadvantage of spontaneous reporting systems is that they fail to provide any reliable information on the incidence of ADRs. In spite of these disadvantages, the yellow card scheme has successfully identified many important, common and rare ADRs. The vigilance of pharmacists could serve to further enhance the usefulness of the scheme.

Cohort studies are like controlled clinical trials without the randomization. The incidence of ADRs is monitored in a group of patients exposed to the drug over a period of time. This is compared with the incidence of adverse events in a similar control group who have not been exposed to the drug. Unlike the yellow card system, cohort studies can generate information on the incidence of ADRs. They are also useful for monitoring drug safety where a wide range of side effects are associated with a single drug. They are less useful for studying rare suspected ADRs. This is because the large numbers of patients involved and the long duration of these studies (for long-term medication) make cohort studies very expensive. A particular disadvantage of the longer-term studies is the number of patients who are lost to follow-up.

Case-control studies retrospectively identify patients who have developed a particular ADR and determine their level of exposure to the suspected drug. This is then compared to a control group of patients without the ADR of interest.

Compared with cohort studies, case-control studies are smaller, much less expensive and generate results more quickly. However, case-control studies are not used to monitor ADRs, rather they are used to investigate suspected ADRs identified by other means, e.g. cohort studies or spontaneous reporting. They are capable of establishing attribution but do not generate information on the incidence of ADRs. Case-control drug surveillance is probably more effective for confirming Type B reactions to established drugs.

# DRUG UTILIZATION REVIEW AND EVALUATION

As well as evaluating new medicines, it is important to measure whether established medicines are being used appropriately. Their proper use increases the quality of patient care and promotes cost-effective health care.

Drug utilization review (DUR) is the assessment of patterns of drug use in a particular clinical context. Drug use evaluation (DUE) incorporates qualitative measures and emphasizes outcomes, including pharmacoeconomic assessment. Drug use evaluation can identify problems in drug use, reduce adverse drug reactions, optimize drug therapy and minimize drug-related expenditure.

It is usually necessary to be selective in the drugs chosen for study, as much of this work is time-consuming. Selection may be on the basis of high cost, wide usage or changes in usage, known or suspected inappropriate use or potential for improvements in patient care. Evaluations of the use of expensive drugs which are also widely prescribed, such as ulcer-healing drugs or antibiotics, are common. These are also examples of drugs for which DUR or DUE would be useful on the grounds of suspected inappropriate use. Studying the use of hypnotics and anxiolytics would also be valuable, because these drugs, although inexpensive, are widely used and often this use can be inappropriate. Changes in legislation can result in changes in the way medicines are used, for example alteration of the legal classification. Patterns of utilization often also change when a new product is marketed. Drug use review can provide information on what these changes are and drug use evaluation can determine whether they are beneficial.

## Drug utilization review

Initial drug utilization reviews were limited to the description of which drugs were being used and their costs. Hospital drug utilization review programmes developed in the USA in the 1970s initially focused on antibiotic use and involved the development of standards for the use of each drug or group of drugs. These were then used as criteria against which the actual use of the drugs could be measured. DUR is therefore a method of audit (see Ch. 43). Both DUR and audit are components of quality assurance programmes which, in this case, are designed to assure the quality of medicines usage.

## Drug use evaluation

Drug use evaluation programmes may relate the use of drugs to patient outcomes and often include interventions to ensure appropriate drug use. Such programmes are potentially of much greater benefit than drug utilization review. They can be retrospective, concurrent or prospective. Retrospective DUE requires, and may be compromised by a lack of, good documentation. It usually has little effect on the treatment of the patients included in the review. Concurrent or prospective DUE can be much more valuable as an aid to improving drug use, since changes in prescribing can be implemented after or even during the evaluation. In carrying out either DUR or DUE, prior agreement of the clinicians is essential, since the findings may be critical of their practice.

There are various levels at which the use of drugs can be studied. These range from very broad measures with little detail, usually obtained from routinely collected data to expensive methods, in which a great deal of useful information is obtained on individual patients.

## Methods

### Using drug purchase records

The simplest level of information about which drugs

are being used is obtained from drug purchase records. Both hospital and community pharmacies use computerized systems for purchase, which means these data are readily available. This type of information provides no clues as to how the drugs are being used, but can often point to potential areas which may need further investigation.

Various units can be used for the measurement of drug purchases, for example cost, number of containers, number of dosage units or number of defined daily doses (DDD). There is a DDD for every drug on the market, which is based on the average recommended daily maintenance dose for the drug when used for its most common indication in adults. It is expressed in g, mg, mcg, mmol or units or as the number of tablets for a combination product. The DDD for every drug is set by the Nordic Council on Medicines in conjunction with the World Health Organization. Its use as a measure of drug purchases allows comparison between pharmacies or over time.

### Using drug issue records

A more detailed record of drug use can be obtained from the drugs issued from pharmacies, either those dispensed from community pharmacies or those issued to wards in hospitals. Again, computerization allows these data to be obtained easily.

In the community, the data are captured when the prescriptions are priced by the Prescription Pricing Authorities in England, Wales and Northern Ireland or the Pharmacy Practice Division in Scotland. The data are then issued to prescribers as Prescribing Analysis and Cost (PACT) in England, Practice Audit Reports and Catalogues (PARC) in Wales or Scottish Prescribing Analysis (SPA). Data at this level are used to allow individuals to compare their drug use to that of a 'norm', such as the health authority (HA) (England) or health board (Wales, Scotland, Northern Ireland) equivalent. The type of data available is shown in Figure 35.1.

The units used for the measurement of drug issues are the same as those of drug purchase. An additional way of measuring drug use which is presented to prescribers is the average cost per prescription item. DDDs can also be used to make comparisons between prescribers from different areas. The quantity of a drug prescribed is usually expressed as the number of DDDs prescribed per 1000 people over a period of time. For example, the DDD of diazepam is 10 mg. It may be found that, in one area, diazepam is used with a DDD of 2000/1000/year. This means that for every 1000 people, 2000 doses of diazepam were prescribed in a year. This is equivalent to 2 doses per person per year. By using DDDs, not only are quantities prescribed accounted for, but an allowance is made for the frequency of administration. It is also possible to use the prescribed daily dose (PDD). This represents the average prescribed dose for a drug's main indication. The PDD may be the same as the DDD for some drugs, but the two measures may differ for drugs such as analgesics.

## PRESCRIBING BY BNF THERAPEUTIC GROUP IN YOUR PRACTICE

| | No. of items prescribed / HA equivalent | Comparison with HA (%) | Change from last year (%) Practice | HA | Dispensed generically (%) |
|---|---|---|---|---|---|
| Gastro-Intestinal System | 637 / 568 | 12 | 0 | 2 | 48 |
| Cardiovascular System | 1,768 / 1,268 | 39 | 2 | 5 | 72 |
| Respiratory System | 945 / 682 | 39 | 2 | -1 | 23 |
| Central Nervous System | 1,265 / 1,337 | -5 | -1 | 2 | 74 |
| Infections | 598 / 537 | 11 | -11 | -2 | 89 |
| Endocrine System | 471 / 389 | 21 | 8 | 7 | 61 |
| All other | 1,650 / 1,683 | -2 | -4 | -3 | 28 |

© Copyright Prescription Pricing Authority 1997

**Fig. 35.1** Prescribing analysis and cost (PACT) data: extract from page 3 of the standard PACT report (reproduced by permission of the Prescription Pricing Authority).

In some hospitals, it may be possible to link data from pharmacy issues to individual clinicians. This will increase with the development of on-line computer prescribing in hospitals. Often the data can only be applied at ward level, but this can still be helpful in developing and monitoring ward-based policies on drug use.

### Using prescription records

More detailed information from prescriptions, which includes the actual dose prescribed and the concurrent medication can be obtained in community pharmacies from patient medication records (see Ch. 39). However, without patient registration and the recording of non-prescription medicines purchased, these are incomplete. In hospitals, this level of data will only be easily obtainable with computer prescribing. Manual data collection from prescriptions is time-consuming, but provides information on the doses of drugs used, the extent of polypharmacy, prescribing errors and drug interactions.

These types of studies can not be used to determine the use of drugs in relation to indication and outcome. The information which they provide is incomplete and any suggestions of prescribing being inappropriate based solely on this type of data should be made cautiously.

### Using medical records and trained investigators

In order to obtain information about the decisions behind the use of particular drugs and their effectiveness, it is necessary to examine medical records. This requires expertise and time and can often be frustrated by the inadequacy of record keeping. Some hospital units and most general practices have computerized patient records, which allow links to be made to the drugs prescribed. In some hospitals links are also available to computerized laboratory data. Many systems, however, are either undeveloped or, as with pharmacy-based PMRs, the records are often inaccurate or incomplete. Clearly, it is not possible to compensate for either a lack of data or inaccurate data. However, small studies undertaken manually can still be of considerable value in determining whether drugs are being used appropriately and effectively. These studies usually involve the use of trained investigators reviewing medical records.

Prospective evaluation of drug use using trained investigators avoids the problem of inadequate records, by allowing data to be recorded and questions to be asked at the time of drug use. While this is likely to change prescribing behaviour, it may also help to improve the use of drugs. It can involve the patient, which thus provides a full picture of drug use, including outcomes and compliance. These latter methods are expensive, but both may be carried out by pharmacists, often as part of their normal activities.

### Using paper-based or computerized record systems designed for medicines use evaluation

A managerial requirement for better information on cost-effectiveness already points to the need for purpose-built systems for medicines use evaluation. Ideally, such systems should be computerized. This facilitates both multipoint, multidisciplinary data entry and information retrieval and analysis. Such systems require the use of standard terminology and data definitions. There are training implications for users. As with all computerized systems, the quality of the data obtained, in this case medicines use evaluation data, depends on the quality of data entry.

A paper-based system, based on the completion of full patient medication profiles by pharmacists, has been developed for use throughout the hospital pharmaceutical service in Scotland. This Clinical Pharmacy Information Project (CPIP) System has the potential to be computerized. It could also form the basis of a structured multidisciplinary record of drug therapy for inclusion in patients' medical records.

## The use of non-prescription medicines

Published information on the epidemiology of self-limiting minor illnesses is limited. Options available to those affected range from no treatment at all, through seeking advice from their pharmacist and/or purchasing an over-the-counter medicine, to visiting their general practitioner and having their medication prescribed. Similarly, data on the pharmacoepidemiology of the medicines used to treat these minor illnesses is either lacking or limited. The number of such medicines which can be bought from pharmacies or supermarkets is increasing. Many former prescription-only medicines have been deregulated to pharmacy medicines. Some former pharmacy medicines are now on the general sales list. These changes make medicines more available to the public. At the same time information on their use becomes less available.

There are as yet no methods developed for studying the use of non-prescription medicines. As increasing numbers of potent medicines become available directly to the public, the need for them to be included in DUE programmes increases.

# PHARMACOECONOMIC EVALUATION

Scarce resources within health care systems necessitate the promotion of cost-effective health care. This requires decisions to be made about whether to provide a particular health care programme and how to implement the chosen programmes. In making such choices, opportunities to provide some services will be lost. However, in order to ensure efficiency, health care has to be prioritized or rationed. This is essential if the health care obtained from the resources available is to be maximized. Medicines constitute a considerable resource and economic evaluation of medicines is needed to ensure that the best choices are made about which medicines should be used and how. This evaluation is termed pharmacoeconomic evaluation.

There are four main types of pharmacoeconomic evaluation. All have certain characteristics in common:

- at least two alternative methods of treatment are considered
- both the costs and the consequences of the alternatives are considered
- the evaluation has a clinical basis.

The four methods differ in the way they look at the consequences of treatments (outcomes), but not in the way they measure the resources (costs).

## Cost minimization analysis (CMA)

This is the simplest form of pharmacoeconomic evaluation. It is used to decide how to implement a particular health care programme or treatment method in situations where the outcome is known not to be dependent on the method of delivery. An example is the provision of domiciliary oxygen therapy. Oxygen can be provided using cylinders, delivered by community pharmacists, or by concentrators installed in the patient's home. Since the benefits are identical, the choice can be made on cost alone. All contributing factors to costs must, however, be included, such as the pharmacist's time. Concentrators have been found to be the cheaper option in most situations where long-term oxygen therapy is required.

Another example of CMA is the comparison of two different intravenous antibiotics to treat infec-

tions. The method can only be used where the efficacy of the two antibiotics is the same. In measuring the costs of these to help choose between them, it is necessary to include the purchase price, the administration costs (needles, syringes, swabs, nurses' time) and the costs of monitoring treatment, which could involve measurement of serum drug levels. A drug which is expensive to purchase but which can be given once daily and requires no special monitoring may work out to be cheaper than an inexpensive drug, given four times daily with a requirement for serum level measurements.

## Cost–effectiveness analysis (CEA)

This is a slightly more complex method, which is used to decide how to implement a health care programme, such as the best way to treat hypertension. In this type of study there may be differences in the outcomes when different methods of delivering care are used, so one method or drug may have a better effect than another. In CEA, the way in which outcome is measured must be the same. So for hypertension, it could be blood pressure in mmHg, life years gained or quality of life.

An incremental cost–effectiveness ratio is calculated, which shows by how much method 1 differs from method 2 in terms of costs and benefits. This is calculated using the equation:

$$\frac{\text{Cost of method 1} - \text{cost of method 2}}{\text{Benefits of method 1} - \text{benefits of method 2}}$$

Cost–effectiveness analysis has the disadvantage that it is restricted to one measure of the quantity or the quality of the life of the subjects studied. In reality, all aspects matter and so a cost–effectiveness analysis comparing two treatments may not show the whole picture.

## Cost–utility analysis (CUA)

Cost–utility analysis can be used to decide whether and/or how to implement a health care programme. It always incorporates measurement of patients' quality of life. This may be measured in various ways, usually by completion of questionnaires, such as the Nottingham Health Profile. In CUA, quality of life is multiplied by life expectancy to produce a parameter called the quality adjusted life year (QALY). This is therefore a measure of both the quality and quantity of life. Cost–utility analysis is often used by the pharmaceutical industry along with clinical evaluation in early stage clinical trials.

## Cost–benefit analysis (CBA)

Cost–benefit analysis can be used to help make many types of choices, even, for example, whether to build a hospital or a bypass. In CBA both costs and benefits are measured in monetary terms. This necessitates putting a cost on benefits such as quality and quantity of life. The commonest method of valuing life in health care research is the concept of willingness-to-pay (WTP). Questionnaires are designed to determine individuals' willingness-to-pay for various benefits or reductions in risks, which means that the public's preferences can be incorporated into health care decision making. It has been used, for example, in the study of the re-regulation of medicines from prescription-only to pharmacy medicines.

### Key Points

- Pharmacists have an important role to play in evaluating the safety, efficiency and economy of medicines' use.
- Medicine resource management aims to optimize the use of medicines.
- The Committee on Safety of Medicines (CSM) require evidence of safety, efficacy and quality before granting a product licence for a new drug.
- Clinical trials take place in three phases: Phase I determines the basic toxicity and tolerability, Phase II establishes efficacy and confirms the dosage, Phase III determines safety and efficacy on a larger sample.
- Post-marketing surveillance is required to establish many adverse reactions and involves spontaneous reporting.
- The yellow card system of reporting adverse reactions is being extended to pharmacists.
- Drug utilization review (DUR) assesses the patterns of drug use in particular clinical situations.
- Drug use evaluation (DUE) relates drug use to patient outcome.
- Methods for studying DUR and DUE include the use of drug purchase records, drug issue records, prescription records, medical records, specifically designed record systems.
- Pharmacoeconomic evaluation aims to promote cost-effective health care.
- Techniques for pharmacoeconomic evaluation include cost minimization analysis, cost–effectiveness analysis, cost–utility analysis and cost–benefit analysis.

## FURTHER READING

American Society of Hospital Pharmacists 1988 Guidelines on the pharmacist's role in drug use evaluation. American Journal of Hospital Pharmacy 45: 385–386

Clinical Resource and Audit Group 1996 Clinical pharmacy practice in the hospital pharmaceutical service: a framework for practice. Report of a working group (Chairman, Cromarty J A). The Scottish Office, Edinburgh

Drummond M F, Stoddart G L, Torrance G W 1987 Methods of economic evaluation of health care programmes. Oxford University Press, Oxford

Glaxo Group Research Ltd 1991 Drug safety: a shared responsibility. Churchill Livingstone, Edinburgh

Glenny H, Nelmes P (eds) 1986 Handbook of clinical drug research. The Association for Clinical Research in the Pharmaceutical Industry and Blackwell Scientific Publications, Oxford

Griffiths J 1989 Deciding priorities for drug usage review. Pharmaceutical Journal 242: HS38–HS40

Malek M 1996 Pharmacoeconomics (1) Introduction. Pharmaceutical Journal 256: 759–761

Malek M 1997 Pharmacoeconomics (2) Measuring quality of life impacts. Pharmaceutical Journal 258: 22–24

Malek M 1997 Pharmacoeconomics (3) Decision analysis and quality control. Pharmaceutical Journal 258: 99–101

Robinson R 1993 Economic evaluation and health care: what does it mean? British Medical Journal 307: 670–673

Strom B L (ed) 1994 Pharmacoepidemiology, 2nd edn. Wiley, Chichester

# 36

# Drug information*

*D. Stewart*

---

After studying this chapter you should know about:

**The types of drug information requests**
**Approaches to answering a drug information request**
**Nature of information sources**
**Evaluation of information**
**Drug information centres.**

---

## Introduction

The ability to provide up-to-date drug information is an important skill for all pharmacists. This is particularly true of those in hospital or community pharmacy who regularly provide drug information to patients and health care professionals. Increasingly, pharmacists are being employed within general practitioners' surgeries performing a variety of duties. These involve providing drug information to medical staff aimed at improving prescribing. Patients require information relating to medicines which they have been prescribed or have purchased over the counter. This topic is covered in depth in Chapters 33 and 37. Pharmacists also have a need for drug information in order to keep up to date with developments relevant to practice. Indeed there is a statement by the Royal Pharmaceutical Society of Great Britain that all pharmacists must participate in at least 30 hours of continuing education per year.

The need for up-to-date drug information has never been greater, mainly because of the increasing number and complexity of drugs. Doctors are also under increasing pressure to prescribe more cost-effectively, an area in which pharmacists are well placed to advise (see Ch. 34).

Drug information may be described as being reactive, that which is provided directly in response to a specific enquiry, or proactive, that provided other than in response to a specific enquiry. Examples of proactive drug information include:

- information and advice provided as part of patient counselling
- feedback to doctors on trends in prescribing
- production of information bulletins concerning recently marketed drugs.

Proactive drug information which is aimed at influencing prescribing is discussed further in Chapter 31.

This chapter concentrates mainly on reactive drug information in the following areas:

- types of drug information enquiries commonly encountered
- obtaining the background information to the enquiry
- sources of information
- the evaluation of clinical trials and promotional material
- specialist drug information centres.

---

## ENQUIRIES COMMONLY ENCOUNTERED

The range of topics on which information may be required is vast and extremely varied. Research has shown that health care professionals tend to require information in the following areas:

- drug choice, for example in pregnancy or breast-feeding
- dose
- dose interval
- route of administration
- adverse drug reactions

---

*Much of this chapter is based on the UK Drug Information Pharmacists' Group *Drug Information Procedures Manual* 1992, Leeds (with permission).

- drug–drug interactions
- drug–disease state interactions
- duration of therapy
- formulations
- storage
- cost.

Patients, however, are more likely to require information relating to either over-the-counter or prescribed drugs, in the following areas:

- what the drug is for and how it works
- how much to take
- when to take
- length of time until treatment begins to work and expected duration of therapy
- side effects
- over-the-counter drugs to avoid
- storage.

Whatever the nature of the enquiry, the same approach can always be used. This involves:

- identifying the enquirer, his or her status
- establishing the degree of urgency of the enquiry
- obtaining the full background information
- using the most appropriate source of information
- delivering the response.

## OBTAINING THE BACKGROUND INFORMATION

It is extremely important to obtain the full background information before attempting to answer any enquiry. The level of background information required will depend on the type of enquiry. For example, one of the most common types of enquiries from doctors is the most appropriate dose of a drug for an individual patient. Initially this may appear very straightforward but may become much more complex with the full background information which, in this case, will include:

- age of patient
- sex of patient
- other disease states
- levels of renal and hepatic function
- other drug therapy.

## SOURCES OF INFORMATION

Before starting to search the mass of literature avail-

able, it is important to know which sources have been checked by the enquirer. If this is not done, valuable time may be wasted simply repeating work that failed to provide a suitable answer. With this information in hand, the next stage is to determine the most appropriate sources of information. Rarely will an answer be obtained by consulting one source of information and often a variety of sources will be used. These sources of information can be classified into primary, secondary and tertiary.

Primary sources are those which provide new drug information mainly as research articles in journals. These articles are reviewed by one or more experts before being accepted for publication. There are many journals relevant to pharmacy, some of which are listed in Table 36.1. It would not be possible to read every journal of relevance to pharmacy. Instead it is much more sensible to become familiar with a smaller number of those of particular interest.

Secondary sources are those which provide reviews of the research articles that appear in primary sources. Examples of these are journals such as *Drug and Therapeutics Bulletin* and *Adverse Drug Reaction Bulletin*. Often those journals classed as primary sources may also contain review articles, as indicated in Table 36.1.

Abstracting systems are a useful secondary source of information. These systems regularly review selected journals and provide summaries of all research articles. One of the most useful abstracting systems for drug information is Medline, which reviews articles in journals relevant to medicine. These systems do, however, have limitations in that the summaries are short and do not always reflect the content of the original article. They are mainly used to help identify specific research articles. As articles are reviewed, important words or phrases known as keywords are highlighted. These can then be used to identify all research articles in a specific

| Table 36.1 Primary reference sources relevant to pharmacy |
|---|
| American Journal of Health-Systems Pharmacy* |
| British Journal of Clinical Pharmacy |
| British Journal of General Practice |
| British Medical Journal* |
| International Journal of Pharmacy Practice |
| Journal of Pharmacy and Pharmacology |
| Lancet* |
| New England Journal of Medicine* |
| Pharmaceutical Journal* |
| *Also contains review articles. |

**Table 36.2  Reference sources recommended for hospital and community pharmacies (adapted from UK Drug Information Pharmacists' Group 1992)**

British National Formulary
Association of British Pharmaceutical Industry (ABPI)
Compendium of Data Sheets
Diluent Directories (Internal and External)
Drug Tariff
Martindale: the Extra Pharmacopoeia (Reynolds 1996)
Medicines, Ethics and Practice – a Guide for Pharmacists

*Additional sources are also recommended for hospital pharmacies:*
Alder Hey Book of Children's Doses
Applied Therapeutics – the Clinical Use of Drugs (Young & Koda-Kimble 1995)
Basic Clinical Physiology (Green 1978; or equivalent text)
Clinical Pharmacology (Laurence & Bennett 1992; or equivalent text)
Davidson's Principles and Practice of Medicine (Edwards & Bouchier 1995; or equivalent text)
Dispensing for Pharmaceutical Students (Cooper et al 1975)
New Advanced First Aid (Gardner & Roylance 1977)
Paediatric Vade Mecum (Insley 1992)
Pocket Medical Dictionary

area. More information on these abstracting systems can be found in Appendix 7.

Tertiary sources are standard reference books which range from simple medical dictionaries to more specialized texts. The UK Drug Information Pharmacists Group has drawn up a list of textbooks recommended for all hospital and community pharmacies, as shown in Table 36.2. More detail on recommended sources can also be found in Appendix 7.

From the wealth of drug information available, it is important to be able to identify the most suitable sources of information for a particular enquiry.

Tertiary sources, which will provide a broad overview of a particular subject area, should be consulted first. Following these, secondary and then primary sources should be checked. However, not every community or hospital pharmacy will have access to a wide range of information sources and referral to a specialist drug information centre, as described later, may be necessary.

## Limitations of the literature

Every source of information has its limitations. With research articles there is a delay between writing the article and it being published. In the case of review articles and textbooks there will be an even greater delay due to gathering and reviewing the informa-

tion. As a result, the information provided may not be as up to date as it appears at first glance.

Journals vary enormously in quality and poorer journals may publish work that has been rejected by others. Simply because an article appears in print does not necessarily mean that its findings are valid. The area is fully discussed later in this chapter.

## DELIVERING THE RESPONSE

Once the appropriate sources of information have been checked and the response formulated, the next stage is to deliver the response. The form of response, whether verbal or written, should be agreed at the very beginning of the enquiry. Finally, the enquiry should be fully documented, including background information, sources of information used and response given. This may save a great deal of time if the same question is asked at a later date.

## EVALUATION OF CLINICAL TRIAL PAPERS

The efficacy and toxicity of drugs are assessed by carrying out clinical trials in which they are compared to standard treatment and/or placebo. Such studies may appear as clinical trial papers in primary reference sources, or form the basis of review articles in secondary reference sources. These studies are often used as sources of drug information and pharmacists must be able to critically analyse the data presented.

Research papers generally have the same format, as shown in Table 36.3.

The summary should provide a brief overview of the purpose of the study, methods, results obtained and main conclusions.

The introduction should briefly describe the full background to the study, including work previously

**Table 36.3  Standard format of clinical trial papers**

Title
Summary
Introduction
Methods
Results
Discussion and conclusion
References

published. The aims and objectives should also be detailed in this section.

Methods is probably the section that should be paid most attention; in reality, it may be quickly skimmed over by many readers. This section should describe methods which are appropriate to the aim of the study. If inappropriate methods are used, then misleading results and conclusions will be obtained. In particular, the methods section should fully describe the following:

• The types of patients included, how many were excluded from the study and why. Patient age, sex, whether they were selected from hospital or general practice, severity of disease, other disease states and drugs must also be described.

• The treatments given, including each treatment formulation, route of administration and how doses were selected. The method of assessing patient compliance with the treatment should also be described.

• The methods used to measure the effects of treatment. Where possible accepted and standardized methods should be used.

• The control group with which the drug under study was compared. Ideally comparison should be made with the standard treatment and placebo. This standard treatment should be the best available. In certain studies the use of a placebo would not be acceptable. Examples would be when studying the use of drugs in the treatment of cancers or pain control.

• The method of allocating treatments to patients. To prevent bias a random design should be used whereby each patient has an equal chance of receiving any of the available treatments. If this is not done, patients could be given treatments in the anticipation that they will respond in a certain way, thereby introducing bias into the study. Several methods of achieving a random design are available and the particular method used should be described.

• The method selected to ensure blindness. If the patient or investigator knows which treatment is being given, this may affect the response or measurement. To prevent this, a double-blind technique should be used, whereby neither the patient nor investigator knows the treatment being given. The method of achieving double-blindness in the study should be described.

• The number of patients included in the study. In the past the number of patients in a trial was often chosen depending on the amount of money or time available for the study. As a result many of these trials included too few patients to allow differences between treatments to be identified. The number of

patients to detect a clinically important difference between treatments can be calculated. These details must be included in this section.

Even if a trial is well designed, the way in which the results are presented may be inappropriate, leading to false claims of the effects of the drugs under study. When reviewing the results section, particular attention should be paid to the following:

• Graphs can be distorted to make the differences between drugs appear much greater than they actually are. This approach is sometimes used in promotional material and is described later in this chapter.

• All statistics included should be appropriate. Inexperienced readers can easily be misled by studies which analyse results using inappropriate statistical tests. If in doubt, it is best to consult a statistician for advice.

• Failure to account for all patients. Patients may withdraw from studies for many reasons, including side effects or worsening of the condition. The reasons for all withdrawals must be clearly described.

The discussion section should outline the importance of the findings, indicating any changes in practice which may occur as a result. Limitations of the study, such as problems in recruiting suitable patients, should also be highlighted at this point. The discussion should lead to the main conclusions of the study which should be justified from the study design and results.

The references section is the final section and must reflect the available relevant literature, not simply those studies agreeing with the views of the authors.

## EVALUATION OF PROMOTIONAL MATERIAL

Although not every pharmacist has access to a wide range of clinical trial papers, they do receive a steady stream of promotional material. These are basically advertisements making claims of superiority of one drug compared to others available. It is equally important to be able to critically analyse this type of material. The same basic approach can be used.

Graphics feature heavily in promotional material. Often bright colours and bold print are used to illustrate the results of the drug being promoted compared to the duller colours used for others. Figures 36.1 and 36.2 show just a few ways in which graphs can be used to exaggerate the effects of a drug.

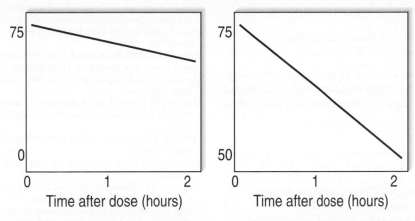

**Fig. 36.1** The response in the left-hand graph is identical to that in the right-hand graph, but at first sight appears to be much smaller.

Many claims are made in promotional material for the effects of a particular drug. However, more often than not, the data are not provided to justify these claims. Often data are listed as being 'on file' or 'to be published'. Such data should be viewed with caution, since they are not available for critical analysis by the reader.

## DRUG INFORMATION CENTRES

Drug information centres are situated within many hospital pharmacy departments in the UK. The first of these were established in 1969 at the London Hospital and Leeds General Infirmary. These centres, which are staffed by hospital pharmacists, are organized into local and regional levels. At present there are 22 regional centres, the addresses of which are listed in the *British National Formulary*. These information centres exist to serve health care professionals in both hospital and community. They have several functions, one of the most important being to provide an enquiry answering service. The regional centres work closely together, forming the National Drug Information Network. This network functions through two groups, the Drug Information Pharmacists Group and the Drug Information Sub-Committee. The main activities which have resulted from this network are:

- production of a manual covering all drug information procedures
- organization of national drug information training courses

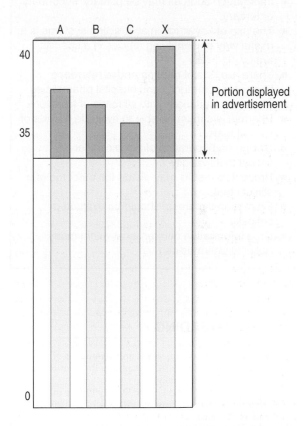

**Fig. 36.2** An 'amputated' bar chart gives the misleading impression that preparation X is superior in terms of response to a number of other competitors 'A', 'B', 'C' (reproduced by permission from UK Drug Information Pharmacists' Group 1992).

- development of Pharmline, an abstracting system
- production of new product evaluations
- production of information bulletins.

Drug information can also be obtained from other sources such as the drug industry and The Royal Pharmaceutical Society of Great Britain as described in Appendix 7.

---

### Key Points

- The RPSGB requires 30 hours of continuing education per year.
- Drug information can be reactive or proactive.
- There are differences between drug information needs of health care professionals and patients.
- Information sources may be primary, secondary or tertiary.
- The use of keywords in abstracting systems is a useful way of identifying articles in a specific area.
- There are lists of recommended reference books for community and hospital pharmacies.
- There are limitations with all forms of literature.
- Pharmacists must be able to evaluate reports of clinical trials.
- Design and operation of a clinical trial are critical to its validity.
- Presented results may distort the outcome of a clinical trial.
- Promotional material should be evaluated critically.
- Drug information centres exist within many hospital pharmacies.

---

Diluent Directories (Internal and External), current edn. National Pharmaceutical Association, St Albans

Drug Tariff, current edn. HMSO, London (Updated monthly)

Edwards C R W, Bouchier I A D 1995 Davidson's principles and practice of medicine. Churchill Livingstone, Edinburgh

Gardner A W, Roylance P J 1977 New advanced first aid. Pan, London

Gardner M J 1986 Use of checklists in assessing the statistical content of medical studies. British Medical Journal 292: 810–812

Green J H 1978 Basic clinical physiology. Oxford University Press, Oxford

Insley J 1986 Paediatric vade mecum, 12th edn. Lloyd-Luke, London

Laurence D R, Bennett N 1992 Clinical pharmacology. Churchill Livingstone, Edinburgh

Leach F 1986 A guide to evaluating drug advertisements. Pharmaceutical Journal 236: 172–173

McCabe J C, Richards R M E 1982 Drug information. In: Richards R M E, Lawson D H (eds) Clinical pharmacy and hospital drug management. Chapman & Hall, London, p 311

Medicines, Ethics and Practice – a guide for pharmacists, current edn. Royal Pharmaceutical Society of Great Britain, London (Updated twice yearly)

Pocock S J 1982 Clinical trials – a practical approach. Wiley, Chichester

Proudlove C R, Smith J C, Breckenridge A M 1988 Medical awareness and usage of a regional drug information centre. Pharmaceutical Journal 240: 394–396

Reynolds J E F (ed) 1996 Martindale: the extra pharmacopoeia, 31st edn. Pharmaceutical Press, London (Updated every 3 years)

Smith J C, McNulty H 1982 The national drug information network. Pharmaceutical Journal 228: 67–69

UK Drug Information Pharmacists' Group 1992 Drug information procedures manual. UK Drug Information Pharmacists' Group, Leeds

Young L Y, Koda-Kimble M A 1995 Applied therapeutics – the clinical use of drugs. Applied Therapeutics, Vancouver

## FURTHER READING

ABPI Compendium of data sheets and summaries of product characteristics, current edn. Datapharm Publications, London (Updated annually)

Adams P R, Woods F J, Luscombe D K 1990 Use of drug information services by hospital pharmacists. British Journal of Pharmaceutical Practice 12: 282–285

Alder Hey Book of Children's Doses 1994 6th edn. Liverpool Area Health Authority, Liverpool

Anon 1985 Reading between the lines of clinical trials. Drug and Therapeutics Bulletin 23: 1–8

British National Formulary, current edn. British Medical Association and Royal Pharmaceutical Society of Great Britain, London (Updated twice yearly)

Cooper J W, Gunn C, Carter S J 1975 Dispensing for pharmaceutical students. Pitman Medical, Tunbridge Wells

# 37
# Counselling

*M. M. Moody*

After studying this chapter you will know about:

**The rationale and need for counselling**
**Opportunities for counselling in hospital and community practice**
**Assessing the need for counselling**
**How to decide on the content and method of counselling**
**Aids to counselling**.

## Introduction

Pharmacies have always been places where the general public could obtain and were given advice on the use of medicines. In the days before the National Health Service, pharmacists were frequently used as an alternative and less expensive source of medical care. As the number of more effective drugs grew the number of prescriptions being dispensed increased. In many pharmacies this increased volume and pressure of work drove the pharmacist into the dispensary, hidden from the view of the general public. A 'good' pharmacy began to be perceived as one where prescriptions were dispensed quickly and the time pharmacists spent in discussion with customers declined. Various studies have shown that, because of lack of knowledge and information, many people take and use their medication or appliance incorrectly or inappropriately. This in turn leads to loss of efficacy and is an inefficient use of the considerable resources which are spent annually on drugs and appliances.

The pharmacist is often the last health care professional whom a patient sees, before starting drug therapy. It is well documented that well-informed patients are more likely to use their medication correctly. There is, therefore, a need for pharmacists to be actively involved in ensuring that patients are adequately informed. This has been recognized both by the Government and the Royal Pharmaceutical Society of Great Britain. In Scotland, one of the criteria which have to be satisfied for payment of pharmacists' professional allowance is the provision of advice on medicines and appliances. The Code of Ethics sets the standard of professional conduct for all pharmacists. The section entitled 'Standards of Good Professional Practice' states 'A pharmacist must seek to ensure that the patient or his agent understands sufficient information and advice to enable safe and effective use of the medicine'. This chapter explores the counselling role of the pharmacist.

## COMMUNITY PHARMACY

Working as a community pharmacist is a highly pressurized job. A huge variety of tasks need to be undertaken, with a high level of competence. Invariably, they all have to be done with limited time available. Unfortunately this often includes counselling patients on medication. Lack of expectation by customers for counselling and advice can also be a barrier. Many do not see the necessity of spending additional time in the pharmacy being given verbal information about their medication. However, the public's demand for information on a variety of issues, including drug therapy, is increasing and there is growing awareness of the advice-giving role of the pharmacist. Counselling on medication is not an optional extra, but is an integral part of the dispensing of a prescription. Pharmacists must ensure that they are visible and accessible in community pharmacies to provide it.

## COUNSELLING AND ADVICE GIVING IN HOSPITALS

There are many opportunities for patient counselling in hospital:

- on admission
- needs assessment
- on discharge
- at outpatient clinics
- rehabilitation groups.

In hospital, pharmacists have the advantage of access to a considerable amount of information about the patient. This can include details of disease states, current therapy and home circumstances, all of which can be useful in providing appropriate counselling. Unlike the community setting, where no formal screening takes place and the process is random, counselling in hospital can be approached in a more formalized way. However, the hospital pharmacist is also subject to pressure and considerable time constraints. Financial pressures in hospitals affect manpower levels and, because the benefits of counselling patients on drug therapy are difficult to quantify, staffing levels may be reduced. Not all wards have access to a pharmacist and, therefore, essential counselling may not occur. Patients in hospital often have their medication changed and they should be made fully aware of any alterations. Unfortunately patients may be discharged from hospital without the knowledge of the pharmacist. This can result in the patient going home with a variety of medicines but little guidance on their use. In some cases, because of limited resources, patients are screened to prioritize who is counselled. While this means that the most needy cases are dealt with, some other cases, where counselling would be beneficial, are missed.

## THE NEED FOR COUNSELLING

The purpose of counselling is to:

- ensure that patients are adequately informed about their medication
- pre-empt any problems which might cause loss of efficacy of the drug or be detrimental to the health of the patient
- identify any problems which might cause loss of efficacy of the drug or be detrimental to the health of the patient.

It has been suggested that patients need to ask their prescriber 20 questions in order to be well informed about their prescribed medication. The writing of a prescription is often seen as a symbolic act, signifying that the consultation is at an end. Patients may feel uncomfortable about prolonging the time and many leave the consulting room with many questions unasked. In many cases the prescriber will give excellent and comprehensive information but, because of the stressfulness of the situation, the patient may not take in all the information or retain it.

## HOW TO GO ABOUT IT

Wherever it occurs, in a community pharmacy, a hospital ward or a hospital outpatient department, counselling should take place in a thoughtful, structured way. The pharmacist must possess not only a sound knowledge of the drugs and appliances being dispensed, but also excellent communication skills. Pharmacists must have the ability to explain information clearly and unambiguously and in language the recipient can understand. They must know the right questions and how to ask them and, most importantly, they must know how to listen. For counselling and advice giving to be successful, it must be a two-way process. Rapport is built up between the pharmacist and the patient and a much more meaningful dialogue can take place. The communication skills needed have been discussed in detail in Chapter 3.

Each situation and each patient will have different information needs but as a general summary no patient who has been given medication should leave a pharmacy or hospital without knowing:

- how and when to take or use the medicine
- how much to take or use
- how long to continue
- what to do if something goes wrong, e.g. if a dose is missed
- how to recognize side effects and minimize their incidence
- lifestyle or dietary changes which need to be made.

One of the arguments used to defend why counselling has not taken place is that there was insufficient time. In many instances this is not true. Good counselling does not always need to take a large amount of time. If approached in a structured manner, time will be used efficiently and the counselling has a greater likelihood of success. The guidelines on Counselling and Advice on Medicines and Appliances in Community Pharmacy Practice produced in 1996 by the Scottish Office Clinical Research and Audit Group suggest the following plan:

- *Recognizing the need.* It is important to ensure that all patients who require counselling receive it.
- *Assessing and prioritizing the needs.* Different patients and different medication and appliances need different types and levels of counselling and advice.
- *Specifying assessment methods.* It cannot be assumed that because counselling and advice have been given, the patient understands the advice or is able to adhere to it. It is therefore important that, before embarking on any counselling and advice process, the pharmacist has an idea of how the success of the process can be measured.
- *Implementation.* This involves giving the necessary information to the patient in an appropriate manner.
- *Assessment.* Having given the information it is then of major importance to check how successful the interview has been. What does the patient understand, can he use his device, does he have any problems? The ideal, where possible, is to assess compliance through follow-up.

## Recognizing the need

Not every patient will require counselling and advice but it is important that pharmacists can correctly identify those who do. The most common error is to assume that a person is well informed. Use the following criteria to ensure that all the people who need advice get it.

### The prescription

*Is it for a medicine which the patient has not had before?* This is where a patient medication record (PMR) can be very useful (see Ch. 39). If the PMR cannot provide the answer and the patient is unknown, it is important to find out this information.

*Are there several items on the prescription?* This could cause the patient problems with compliance. Studies have shown that compliance decreases as the number of drugs increases (see Ch. 41).

*Are the instructions clear?* It is the pharmacist's responsibility to make sure that patients know what instructions such as 'p.r.n' or 'm.d.u.' mean. An open question should be used here, e.g. 'Tell me how you take this medicine'. If the patient does not know, then the necessary information can be provided. In some cases patients may be taking the medication incorrectly. The pharmacist is then in a position to rectify any misconceptions. Checking on imprecise dosage instructions can also pre-empt possible errors, as in the following example.

---

**EXAMPLE 37.1**

A prescription for 60 Nitrazepam tablets 5 mg was received. The instructions read 'm.d.u.'.

The prescription was dispensed as written and handed over to the patient with no dialogue taking place. Approximately 2 hours later the patient returned saying that the tablets had a different name and appearance from the ones he had previously been prescribed. On checking with the surgery the pharmacist found out that an error in entering the drug details into the surgery computer had occurred. The patient should have been prescribed Nutrizym capsules. The dose to be taken was 'three capsules with every meal and two with intervening snacks'. If the pharmacist had asked the patient how he was taking his medication she would have realized something was wrong, the normal dose for nitrazepam being 'two tablets at bedtime'. Fortunately in this instance no harm was done to the patient, but it illustrates very clearly how important the pharmacist's involvement is.

---

*Is the prescription for drugs which have a complicated or unusual regimen?* In some instances, with a little thought the pharmacist can simplify matters. The following example is an illustration.

---

**EXAMPLE 37.2**

A prescription for Questran sachets, 1 t.i.d., penicillin tablets 250 mg, 2 q.i.d. and captopril tablets, 25 mg b.i.d. was received.

Because Questran interferes with the absorption of drugs it must be given either 1 hour before, or 4–6 hours after other drugs. A considerable amount of organization is needed to get this regimen right. Trying to fit three doses of Questran around the other drug therapy could cause the patient considerable problems. Fortunately, Questran can be given as a single dose, instead of divided doses. This would considerably simplify the regimen.

---

### Prescribed medicines

If the drugs have a narrow therapeutic index the need for strict adherence to dosing should be emphasized. Drugs such as lithium or theophylline are common examples.

Drugs which have a potential for interaction should be identified and guidance given on their use. One of the commonest is warfarin. Appendix 1 in the BNF gives useful information.

Some drugs require additional, precautionary labels. The information on these labels should always be reinforced. As mentioned in Chapter 8, some precautionary labels may need further explanation. Appendix 9 in the BNF should be consulted.

Some drugs are presented in complex dosage forms such as transdermal patches or inhalers. The patient must have a clear understanding of how these should be used.

Certain drugs are more likely to cause side effects. In these instances the patient should be told, not only how to recognize the side effects, but also how to reduce the incidence or severity of them. For example tamoxifen has been known to cause nausea in some patients. To minimize the upset to the patient the dose can be taken at night. There are many drugs which can cause problems, e.g. non-steroidal anti-inflammatory drugs (NSAIDs) may cause GI irritation, and antihistamines cause drowsiness. Many pharmacists are unsure how much information about side effects should be given to patients. There is concern that the patient may be put off taking the medication because of the risk of suffering these unwanted effects. No two situations or patients are alike and it is difficult to make a definite statement about this. However, it has been shown that if patients are informed of commonly occurring side effects, how to recognize them and how to deal with them, they are less likely to be anxious. Select the side effects which are most likely to occur and advise on them.

### The patient

In general all patients who are elderly should be offered counselling and advice. If the prescription is for a child, the parent or guardian should be given advice.

The patient may be known at the pharmacy and have been previously identified as having problems with drug therapy. This could be due to a variety of factors such as:

- physical disability causing problems in opening containers
- confusion or forgetfulness
- anxiety
- known poor compliance.

Other instances which should alert the pharmacist to the need for counselling would be if the patient asks to purchase an OTC product which is incompatible with the prescribed medication, if the patient asks for an item not to be dispensed or if the patient asks to buy an OTC medicine which is to relieve the side effects of a prescribed medicine. Examples of these would be:

- A patient who is being prescribed atenolol to treat hypertension is heard asking for a packet of Sinutabs for his nasal congestion. Sinutabs contain a sympathomimetic, phenylpropanolamine. Sympathomimetics are contraindicated in cardiovascular disease. The pharmacist should investigate further, finding out how severe the congestion is. If medication is considered necessary a more suitable product can be recommended.

- If a patient asks for an item not to be dispensed this can be for a number of reasons including inadequate compliance. Whatever the reason the pharmacist should find out more information to ensure that any problems the patient is having with his medication are rectified.

- A patient who is being prescribed NSAIDs asks for an indigestion remedy. This should be investigated. The pharmacist will want to make sure that the stomach problem is not due to inappropriate use of the NSAID.

## Assessing and prioritizing the needs

Although a need for counselling has been recognized, the level and type of information given and how it is given will depend on a variety of factors.

- What counselling has the patient previously received?
- What are the patient's comprehension levels?
- What level of support does the patient need or have?
- Does the patient have sight or hearing problems. A patient with neither of these problems may require minimal advice to be given but a different approach needs to be adopted where these physical disabilities are present. A sight-impaired patient may not benefit from a patient information leaflet, while this may be the best way of providing information for someone who is hearing impaired.
- Is the patient pregnant or breast-feeding? These patients will need additional advice, specific to their condition. In patients such as these, only essential drug therapy should be given. This will have been checked by the prescriber but the patient may still require reassurance that the therapy is safe to take. A pharmacist who does identify a situation where a drug has been prescribed, which is contraindicated,

should always check with the prescriber. An example of extra advice which may be needed is for a breast-feeding mother who has been prescribed an antihistamine. In this situation a short-acting preparation such as chlorpheniramine is preferred. The mother should be told to take the medication immediately after feeding the baby and by the time the next feed is due the blood levels and consequently the level of drug in the milk will be low.

• Does a large amount of information need to be given? The average number of facts which can be retained at any one time is three. If several pieces of information have to be given it may be necessary to select what is considered to be the most important.

---

**EXAMPLE 37.3**

A prescription for metronidazole tablets is received.

Metronidazole tablets have five additional cautionary labels which should be added to the instructions. These are:

'Avoid alcoholic drink'. This is because, when combined with alcohol, a disulfiram-like reaction occurs and the patient may suffer nausea and vomiting. Patients who are not aware of this interaction may think, incorrectly, that the drug does not agree with them and stop taking it.

'Take at regular intervals. Complete the prescribed course unless otherwise directed'. Because of the antimicrobial effect of metronidazole, blood levels must be maintained and therapy must be continued for a minimum time period to prevent bacterial resistance developing.

'Take with or after food'. Metronidazole can cause GI irritation and the presence of food in the stomach will reduce the likelihood of this.

'To be swallowed whole, not chewed'. Metronidazole tablets are film coated which gives a degree of protection to the GI tract. If the preparation is chewed the coating will be destroyed, the drug will come into contact with the stomach lining and GI irritation will occur.

'Take with plenty of water'. The film coating on the tablets may become sticky and if not taken with a reasonable draught of water can stick in the oesophagus. The drug will be released and could cause irritation to this, least protected, area of the GI tract.

Counselling on cautionary labels should always include the reason why the precaution should be taken. Obviously, in this instance, to go into a

detailed explanation for each caution could take a considerable amount of time. The large amount of information required might confuse the patient and the whole process becomes self-defeating. In instances like this the most important points should be selected for emphasis. Any other points may have to be left to another counselling session. If only two points could be selected for this prescription they would differ for different patients. In a patient who never drinks alcohol but is known to have a sensitive GI tract, the alcohol warning is less important than the warning about food intake and swallowing whole.

---

## Check assessment methods

This could consist of checking that the patient can read the label, use an inhaler device or open a container with a child-resistant cap. Checking on understanding may require follow-up, such as an enquiry, the next time the patient visits the pharmacy, to ensure that no problems have occurred and the response to the therapy is as expected.

## Implementation

### Environment

The appearance of the pharmacy is an important factor. The environment should have a professional appearance and it should be apparent that counselling and advice is offered as a professional service. The service can be advertised in practice leaflets and within the pharmacy. Trying to give patients advice about their medication in a busy pharmacy can be difficult. Some pharmacies have a room or a special area set aside for counselling. This is the ideal. If neither of these is available the pharmacist must try to take the patient to an area in the pharmacy where they will not be overheard and a private discussion can be carried on. Constant interruptions and customers milling around nearby are a major distraction and are barriers to good communication.

### Time

Time, or rather the lack of it, is a major barrier to good counselling. Patients should be given an indication of why you wish to speak to them and you should always check that they have the time to listen. A patient who is worried about missing a bus or concerned that the car is parked on double yellow lines is unlikely to give undivided attention.

### Professional appearance

How the pharmacist appears is also of importance. An organized, calm persona is more likely to instill confidence in the patient than a pharmacist who appears distracted, harassed and unsure of himself.

### Patient expectations

Over the last decade or so, through the National Pharmaceutical Association's 'Ask Your Pharmacist' campaign, the public have been made more aware of the pharmacist's role in the provision of health care advice. However, there are still many people who see pharmacies as merely collection points for their medicines. They are not expecting to be given advice, nor are they aware that they may need information about their medication. It is important that patients are made aware that pharmacies are sources of information about drug therapy and that information is available. If patients expect to be given information about their drug therapy then they will become more receptive to it.

### Patient

If the patient is unknown to the pharmacist, it is important at the beginning of the conversation to try to gauge, not just the amount of information that is needed, but also the patient's level of comprehension. The type of language used is very important, particularly guarding against being patronizing, by oversimplification. However, the use of medical terminology must be considered carefully.

The counselling process must not be a monologue by the pharmacist, giving a long list of information points. There should be ample opportunity for the patient to ask questions. The pharmacist should introduce aids to comprehension, if this is felt necessary, e.g. an explanatory leaflet or diagram, a placebo device.

## Assessing the success of the process

During the counselling process the pharmacist should be checking if the information is being understood by the patient. Watching the patient's body language and maintaining eye contact can give useful clues as to whether the message is being understood and whether it is likely to be complied with.

## AIDS TO COUNSELLING

Patient information leaflets, warning cards and placebo devices are all useful aids when giving advice to patients. Many products are now provided with information leaflets. These should be used where appropriate and important points highlighted. Placebo devices can be used to demonstrate a particular technique and also to check a patient's ability to use a device. The NPA is a useful source of information leaflets and warning cards. Leaflets on how to use ear drops, eye drops, eye ointment, pessaries, suppositories, a nebulizer, malaria tablets and head louse lotions are available. These, along with warning cards for anticoagulant therapy, lithium, MAOI and steroids should be available in all pharmacies, hospitals and any other areas where counselling patients on drug therapy takes place. Whether commercially produced or prepared by individual pharmacists, ensure that the quality of any information leaflet is of the highest standard and is comprehensible to the patient.

## SOME EXAMPLES

In the following examples details of a prescription and some biographical details of the patient are given. Various counselling points are identified and information which could be given to the patient, detailed. These examples illustrate the wide variety of issues which have to be dealt with in the counselling process. They are not intended to be comprehensive, as different situations and different patients will produce a variety of problems and issues.

---

### EXAMPLE 37.4

Mrs Gordon, an elderly lady of about 70 years, presents a prescription for ibuprofen tablets 400 mg. She has lived alone since the death of her husband, 2 years ago. When she is signing the back of her prescription she has difficulty holding the pen and complains that her hands and fingers are rather sore and stiff and hopes that the prescription will help. This is the first time she has had these tablets.

**Recognize the need for counselling**
Mrs Gordon has never been prescribed the tablets before, therefore basic information about the drug name and dose timings need to be given.

NSAIDs can cause GI irritation if not taken with or after food. The warning label which indicates this will need to be reinforced.

---

Mrs Gordon appears to have problems with her hands. Will she be able to open a bottle with a child-resistant cap? She lives alone so does not have anyone to help her.

She has not been to the doctor previously for a prescription for her hands but has she been buying anything OTC to try to alleviate the pain? Many of the OTC products available for relief of arthritic pain contain ibuprofen.

The tablets are quite large. Will she have any problems swallowing them?

There are a variety of issues here which will need to be checked.

### Assessing and prioritizing the counselling and advice needs

*Compliance problems.* It is important to ensure that Mrs Gordon can open the container and that she will have no difficulty swallowing the tablets.

*Side effects.* It is vitally important to alert Mrs Gordon to the fact that the tablets may irritate her stomach and how she can avoid this.

*OTC purchases.* To avoid any duplication of drug therapy it is very important to find out if Mrs Gordon is taking any OTC medicines, what they are and make sure they are not going to cause any problems.

*Timing of doses and duration of treatment.* Mrs Gordon should be told that the tablets are not simply painkillers, to be taken infrequently. NSAIDs should give pain relief within 1 week and successful anti-inflammatory action should be seen within 3 weeks. To achieve these benefits the drug must be taken at regular intervals. This should be explained to Mrs Gordon.

There is obviously a considerable amount of information which needs to be given to Mrs Gordon. However, none of it is too complex so it should be possible to deal with all of it.

A simple demonstration with a CRC will identify if she needs a container with a plain cap fitted. Showing her the tablets will also provide a clue as to whether she will be able to swallow them. Patients with swallowing difficulties can rarely conceal a look of horror when presented with tablets they know they cannot cope with. If swallowing is identified as a problem she can be reassured that alternative therapy is available in liquid or granular form. It may then be necessary to contact the prescriber to alert him to this.

Any potential OTC problems can be dealt with by simple questioning.

It is preferable to give the patient all the drug details, if possible. However, if it is felt this will be counterproductive, dosing in relation to food is one that should have high priority.

Mrs Gordon should be invited to let you know how she is getting on with her tablets and to contact you if she has any queries.

---

> **EXAMPLE 37.5**

You receive the following prescription:

Pulmicort LS inhaler
Mitte 1
Sig. 2 puffs m. et n.

Bricanyl turbohaler
Mitte 1
Sig. Use m.d.u.

The patient, Mr Christopher Ferguson is a patient of long standing. He has been on the steroid inhaler for several months and was also prescribed terbutaline as a metered-dose inhaler. He seemed to be well controlled and did not need to use his bronchodilator very frequently. He tells you that recently he has had one or two frightening wheezing attacks where his ability to inhale was severely impaired. For that reason, the doctor has given him a new type of inhaler.

### The need for counselling
Mr Ferguson has not had the turbohaler before. The different method of use will need to be explained. Because of the lack of propellant some patients are not aware they have inhaled the drug, when using this device.

He will need to be told that the turbohaler is the same drug as his terbutaline metered-dose inhaler and that he must not use them both.

The maximum dose of one puff four times daily will need to reinforced, as this is different from the metered-dose inhaler dose.

During the counselling session it is probably worth checking Mr Ferguson's inhaler technique. The deterioration in his condition may be caused by insufficient steroid being inhaled. This could lead to ineffective prophylaxis.

Although asthmatic patients are normally on long-term treatment, it is dangerous to assume that they have good inhaler technique or are knowledgeable about their drug therapy. There should be regular checking of how devices are used and how frequently they are inhaled. Further information on this is found in Chapter 18.

## EXAMPLE 37.6

The following prescription is received:

Atenolol tablets 50 mg
Hypromellose eye drops
Trimethoprim tablets 200 mg

You notice from your PMR that, other than the atenolol tablets, which had previously been prescribed as the proprietary brand, Tenormin, the other two items are new to the patient. A considerable number of issues need to be dealt with here.

An explanation needs to be given that, although the appearance and name have changed, atenolol and Tenormin are the same drug. If the patient has any left at home they should be finished and the generic then started. Unfortunately, cases are reported of patients who end up taking double doses of drugs owing to a generic being prescribed in place of the branded preparation.

Information about shelf life and storage of the eye drops should be given, i.e. the eye drops must be discarded 4 weeks after being opened and should preferably be stored in a fridge.

Compliance with eye drops should be checked and the need for a compliance aid ascertained.

The trimethoprim is for the treatment of a urinary tract infection. Advice on the duration of the therapy must be given. An indication of when an improvement in the condition can be expected should be given. If no decrease in the severity of the symptoms is seen within 48 hours it is possible that the organism is resistant to the antibiotic and alternative therapy may be needed. Basic advice on maintaining fluid intake should be given as an adjunct to drug therapy.

## CONCLUSION

Develop the habit of thinking about prescriptions from the patients' point of view. What do they need to know? Identifying counselling points from the information at your disposal is fundamental to good pharmacy practice. It is important to remember, however, that asking questions and listening carefully to the information provided by patients or in many cases, carers, is critical to the success of the process. The incidence of dispensing errors is relatively low, but approximately 16% of hospital admissions are directly due to adverse drug reactions. How many of these could have been avoided if the patient had received appropriate counselling and advice from the pharmacist?

### Key Points

- Evidence shows that well-informed patients are more likely to use their medicines correctly.
- Counselling in hospital is more formalized than in community practice.
- There are a number of factors which may reduce the opportunity for counselling in hospitals.
- Counselling must be structured and deal with the key information in an easily understood form.
- The prescription is a useful guide to possible counselling needs.
- The extent to which patients should be told about side effects will vary from one patient to another.
- Counselling should be used to reinforce adherence, potential for interactions and warning labels.
- Some groups can be identified as requiring special counselling – the elderly, where there have been previous problems, parents of children.
- It may be necessary to limit the amount of information given during counselling to avoid confusion and meet patients' needs.
- Checking is important in ensuring the effectiveness of counselling.
- A busy setting is a barrier to effective communication.
- Patients are becoming more aware that pharmacists can give valuable advice.
- Counselling is not a lecture – patients must be given the opportunity to ask questions.
- There are many aids to help counselling, including information leaflets, placebos and warning cards.

### FURTHER READING

ABPI Compendium of data sheets and summaries of product characteristics, current edn. Datapharm Publications, London (Updated annually)
ABPI Compendium of patient information leaflets, current edn. Datapharm Publications, London (Updated annually)

British National Formulary, current edn. British Medical Association and Royal Pharmaceutical Society of Great Britain, London (Updated twice yearly)

British Pharmaceutical Conference 1986 Communication, counselling and co-operation. Pharmaceutical Journal 238: 449–456

Clinical Research and Audit Group 1996 Counselling and advice on medicines and appliances in community pharmacy practice. HMSO, Scotland

Ley P 1988 Communicating with patients. Croom and Helm, London

Medicines, Ethics and Practice – a guide for pharmacists, current edn. Royal Pharmaceutical Society of Great Britain, London (Updated twice yearly)

Pharmaceutical Society 1988 Information leaflets. Pharmaceutical Journal 240: 98

# 38
# Health promotion and health education

*M. M. Moody*

After studying this chapter you will know about:

**The meaning of the terms 'health promotion' and 'health education'**
**Government health targets**
**Ways in which pharmacists can help meet government targets for health**
**Opportunities for health promotion and health education in the pharmacy**
**Health screening in the pharmacy**.

## Introduction

Before embarking on a discussion of the pharmacist's role in health promotion and health education it is important to understand what is meant by these two terms. Health promotion encompasses the whole situation and includes control of the environment, e.g. control of air pollution, which could be simply the creation of a no smoking area, or more complex, such as the control of emissions from a chemical plant. The creation of suitable housing and recreational facilities for a community must be considered. In short any factor is relevant if it will directly affect the maintenance of good health or help to improve the existing health state. These issues are the subject of social policy and the necessary changes are dealt with by government, pressure groups, economic measures and societal influences.

Health education is a component of health promotion and is much more specific. It aims to make individuals more aware of the factors which help to maintain good health and prevent ill health.

The cost of health care in the UK has been steadily increasing in real terms for many years. There are several diverse reasons for this, e.g. more sophisticated treatments which rely heavily on expensive technical equipment or require highly trained personnel to operate them and have expensive running costs.

In addition, the proportion of the population aged 60 years or over is increasing which in turn leads to greater demands for the provision of health care.

In order to utilize the finite resources which are available to operate the health care system of the nation, increasing emphasis has been placed on the maintenance of good health. In recent years the Government has highlighted several areas where the state of health of many of the population is a cause for concern. Five key areas where the need for improvements is greatest have been identified. These are:

- coronary heart disease and stroke
- cancers
- mental illness
- accidents
- HIV/AIDS and sexual health.

## Targets

Within these areas specific targets have been set (DoH 1992).

### Coronary heart disease (CHD) and stroke

- To reduce death rates for both CHD and stroke, in people under 65, by at least 40% by the year 2000.
- To reduce the death rate for CHD in people aged 65–74 by at least 30% by the year 2000.
- To reduce the death rate for stroke in people aged 65–74 by at least 40% by the year 2000.
- To reduce the prevalence of cigarette smoking in men and women aged 16 and over to no more than 20% by the year 2000.
- To reduce mean systolic blood pressure in the adult population by at least 5 mmHg by 2005.
- To reduce the percentages of men and women aged 16–64 who are obese, by at least 25% for men and at least 33% for women by 2005.

- To reduce the average percentage of food energy derived by the population from saturated fatty acids by at least 35% by 2005.
- To reduce the average percentage of food energy derived by the population from total fat by at least 12% by 2005.
- To reduce the proportion of men drinking more than 21 units of alcohol per week from 28% in 1990 to 18% in 2005 and the proportion of women drinking more than 14 units of alcohol per week from 11% in 1990 to 7% by 2005.

### Cancers

- To reduce the death rate for breast cancer in the population invited for screening by at least 25% by the year 2000.
- To reduce the incidence of invasive cervical cancer by at least 20% by the year 2000.
- To halve the year-on-year increase of skin cancer by 2005.
- To reduce the death rate for lung cancer by at least 30% in men under 75 and 15% in women under 75 by 2010.
- In addition to the overall reduction in prevalence of smoking (see CHD targets), at least a third of women smokers to stop smoking at the start of their pregnancy by the year 2000.
- To reduce the consumption of cigarettes by at least 40% by the year 2000.
- To reduce the prevalence of smoking amongst 11- to 15-year-olds by at least 33%.

### Mental illness

- To improve significantly the health and social functioning of mentally ill people.

### HIV/AIDS and sexual health

- To reduce the percentage of injecting drug misusers who report sharing injecting equipment in the previous 4 weeks by at least 50% by 1997 and by a further 50% by the year 2000.
- To reduce the rate of conceptions amongst the under-16s by at least 50% by the year 2000.

In all, 25 targets were set, with the option of altering or adding to the list with time. Since the publication of the targets in 1992, some progress has been made, but in three areas, obesity, smoking in the 11- to 15-year-old group and suicide, there have been increases.

In many areas throughout the country health promotion and health education departments have been created. The pharmacist's role in health education was formally recognized in 1986 with the launch of the 'Health Care in the High Street' scheme. Now entitled 'Pharmacy Healthcare', the scheme, which is supported by The Royal Pharmaceutical Society of Great Britain, the Family Planning Association, the Health Education Authority, the Health Education Board for Scotland, the National Pharmaceutical Association and Boots the Chemists Ltd, highlights the importance of pharmacists as a source of information on health education issues. Leaflets, produced by the various participating groups, are distributed through pharmacies. New topics are dealt with, usually every 4–6 weeks, often linking in with ongoing national campaigns. Prior to the release of the leaflets, pharmacists are given information on the leaflet contents.

## THE PHARMACIST'S ROLE

Where do pharmacists fit into the health education picture and how can they assist in helping to achieve the Government's targets?

### Appearance of the pharmacy

The perceptions and expectations which the general public have of pharmacy will have a major impact on the use they make of pharmacies. We live in an image-conscious culture and the appearance of an environment can have considerable influence. Pharmacies are readily identified by the general public as sources of prescription and over-the-counter medicines. In recent years, thanks to campaigns such as 'Ask Your Pharmacist', initiated by the NPA, pharmacies are increasingly being seen as places where advice and information on drug therapy can be obtained. For many people, the pharmacy is the first place to call for this type of advice. The area of health education is slightly more problematic. Many pharmacies have taken the initiative and are operating very successfully as specific 'health-promoting' pharmacies but the role of the community pharmacist as a health educator is still being developed.

### Provision of leaflets

The provision of information on health education can be done by having suitable leaflets available. Indeed some pharmacists find that owing to time constraints this is as far as they can become involved in health education. However, leaflet provision should be dealt with in a positive way. Selection of appropriate leaflets is as important as ensuring that they are situated in a suitable place. Pharmacists should be familiar with the content of the leaflets they have available, and up-to-date material should be used. They should always try to ensure that, if a national or local health education campaign is currently being promoted, information about the chosen topic is available. As already mentioned all pharmacies are sent the latest Pharmacy Healthcare leaflets. These are of excellent quality but there are many others to choose from, on an enormous range of subjects. The local health education officer should be able to give advice on where to obtain them. However, beware, the quality and suitability of leaflets are variable and any material should be critically evaluated before use. Several factors should be considered, one of the most important being the target audience. Space is always at a premium and therefore only the most useful leaflets should be given room. The following points may help in the selection of material best suited for a particular situation and clientele.

- *Page size*. This is an important consideration especially when storage facilities and a display stand are considered.
- *Layout*. The important areas to be considered here are clear type, uncluttered pages, clear illustrations which have plenty of space round them. Illustrations should relate directly to the text; if used purely for decoration they can cause confusion. There should be an appropriate use of colour. Studies have found that black print on a white or yellow background is best. Coloured prints and backgrounds can be difficult to read. Short paragraphs are less daunting than long ones, which can give the appearance of solid blocks. Logical organization of the material is essential and allows the reader to assimilate the information more easily.
- *Type*. As well as being of high quality, the style of print is of paramount importance. The use of capital letters should be kept to a minimum, as should the use of ornate styles which are often difficult to read. Underlining can be useful to emphasize particular points, but should be used sparingly as overuse can be counterproductive.
- *Text*. This should be kept simple and should be appropriate for the target audience. Short words, simple sentences and positive statements are more easily understood. Studies have found that personalizing the material by the use of 'you' rather than the impersonal 'he', 'she', or 'they' improves the reader's acceptance of the material. It is very easy when producing health-related material to fall into the trap of using medical terms or jargon which may not be understood by many of the readers. If used, these terms should be clearly defined in understandable language (see also Ch. 3).

Much work has been carried out to develop readability tests. Common ones in use are Flesch, FOG and SMOG tests. When these tests are applied to a piece of text, an average readability can be calculated which, theoretically, will give an indication of whether the material is suitable for the intended audience. However, a readability test used alone, without consideration of the points mentioned above, will not give an indication of the suitability of a particular piece of text. The reasons for this are:

- No account is taken of the reader's knowledge of the subject matter.
- No allowance is made for scientific or medical terms which may not be understood by the lay person.
- No allowance is made for the level of motivation a reader may have.

Having leaflets available in pharmacies is a useful method of disseminating information but needs to be approached thoughtfully and intelligently. Next time you pick up an information leaflet look at it with a critical eye and try to evaluate how useful it is.

## Opportunistic health education

There are many occasions during the working day in a community pharmacy on which health education can take place. However, each requires the pharmacist to be available, motivated, proactive and knowledgeable. It does take time but done well can greatly benefit the recipient and can increase the pharmacist's job satisfaction. The chapter on counselling (Ch. 37) deals with the information requirements of patients receiving medication. Information on appropriate drug use is an important facet of health education. However, there are many other occasions when opportunistic health education can be undertaken. Unfortunately in many pharmacies these are missed.

The following are some examples.

- Unless the pharmacist knows there is a specific medical reason for a request to purchase a laxative this can be an ideal opportunity to discuss a patient's eating habits. Advice on exercise and fluid and fibre intake could be offered. Although some pharmacists feel that this may be seen as interfering in people's lifestyles it can improve their health and quality of life.

- Purchasers of antacids could be questioned on their eating habits. Information can be given on foods to avoid and the types of lifestyle which can predispose people to stomach problems.
- Customers wishing to purchase so called 'slimming preparations' can be given information on an appropriate weight-reducing diet and advice on how retraining of eating habits can be undertaken.

Obviously for any of the above if the pharmacist suspects a serious health problem exists, referral to an appropriate practitioner such as GP or a dietitian should take place.

## SPECIFIC HEALTH CARE ISSUES

### Dental health

Many of the articles which are available for sale in pharmacies give ideal opportunities to become involved in health education. One of the most obvious areas, but which is often overlooked, is that of dental health. Most pharmacies sell toothpaste, toothbrushes, mouthwashes, fluoride drops and tablets, and varieties of dental floss. Currently there is considerable concern over the very poor state of dental health in the UK. For this reason dental health has been highlighted and added to the Government's health strategies for the year 2000. The following targets have been set:

- 60% of 5-year-old school entrants should have no cavities, fillings or extractions
- less than 10% of 45- to 54-year-olds should be without their own teeth.

Dental health is an area where pharmacists can make a major contribution. For this reason it is helpful if teeth-related products are positioned in a part of the pharmacy where the pharmacist, or suitably trained staff, can readily be on hand to offer advice and assistance. As always, a sound knowledge base is essential. This should be combined with an awareness of what is the most appropriate advice.

The most effective way of preventing the development of dental disease is in controlling the production of dental plaque. Plaque is a soft thin layer which deposits on teeth, gums and all appliances fitted in the mouth. It is formed by microbial action. Dietary sugars, in particular sucrose, contribute to the formation of plaque and their presence increases the rate of formation and thickness of plaque. The removal of plaque from the teeth and related areas is essential for the maintenance of a healthy mouth. However, because plaque adheres to the various surfaces on which it forms, removal must be of a physical nature; hence the requirement for efficient and regular brushing of the teeth. Brushing should be done at least twice daily and preferably after meals.

### Toothbrushes

The range of toothbrushes is enormous and is potentially bewildering. A few simple rules can help in the selection of an appropriate brush.

- A small- to medium-sized head is the best choice as this is more manoeuvrable and reaches into the back of the mouth more easily.
- Nylon bristles are better than natural which soften more quickly and are more inclined to harbour bacteria.
- Brushes which have multitufted, small bristles are better than those with fewer and larger bristles.
- Soft bristles are not as efficient at removing plaque. Medium bristles are therefore preferred. Soft bristles may be of benefit for people who have sensitive teeth or who suffer from gum disorders. Hard bristles should not be recommended as they can cause gum damage.
- A toothbrush should be replaced as soon as the bristles become bent as they are no longer able to remove plaque efficiently.
- Interproximal toothbrushes are specialized brushes which only have one tuft. These are extremely useful for people who have malaligned teeth or large spaces between their teeth.

### Toothpaste

The main agent in the tooth-cleaning process is the toothbrush. The purpose of toothpaste is to leave the mouth with a pleasant, fresh taste and also to act as a carrier for various active ingredients. These latter include fluoride, chlorhexidine, formaldehyde and strontium chloride which all have differing, but beneficial, effects on oral health.

- Fluoride has a topical effect which appears to increase the resistance of tooth enamel to attack by acid. This makes it an extremely useful agent in the prevention of tooth decay. Unless specifically contraindicated, fluoride toothpaste should be used.
- Chlorhexidine is active against the bacteria in dental plaque and helps to prevent plaque building up.
- Formaldehyde or strontium chloride is present

in so-called 'desensitizing' toothpastes. They reduce the sensitivity of dentine to painful stimuli.

Important advice regarding toothpaste use relates to quantity. An amount the size of a pea is all that is required. Large quantities cause excessive foaming which in turn produces the desire to spit. The mouth is then usually rinsed out and toothbrushing is stopped before a thorough cleansing of the mouth has been carried out.

### Dental floss

This is of great value in cleaning between the teeth and removing material which is resistant to brushing. Regular flossing should be carried out to ensure efficient teeth cleaning and thereby reduce the risk of tooth decay. However, for a variety of reasons, which include the amount of time that flossing takes, it is not undertaken as often as it should be. Pharmacists can encourage customers to use dental floss and inform them of the most appropriate method of use. It can be pointed out that flossing once per day has been shown to be effective when time is a problem. Dental floss is available as waxed or unwaxed. Pharmacists may be asked which is the more effective product. There appears to be little difference and choice comes down to personal preference. Some users find the waxed variety easier to use as it is less likely to fray than unwaxed. However unwaxed floss is often easier to pass through spaces where teeth are very close together and generally leads to more efficient cleaning. Floss must be used carefully as highly energetic flossing may cause the gums to bleed and can cause gum damage.

### Diet

As dietary sugars are the main contributor to the development of plaque, control of their intake should be encouraged. One of the main issues in health education is to try to achieve a change in lifestyle where current lifestyle is compromising health. However, it has been recognized that to attempt to eliminate sugars, especially sucrose, from the diet is neither realistic nor desirable. Dietary advice to help improve oral health is to reduce the quantity of dietary sugar, but perhaps more importantly, to reduce the frequency of the intake. A quantity of sugary items consumed at specific but infrequent times during the day is much less damaging than constant snacking throughout the day. This may not be the ideal, but because it is more realistic is likely to be a more achievable goal. If snacks must be consumed, savoury ones such as crisps are to be preferred, as are 'diet' varieties of soft drinks.

The commonly held belief that eating an apple is useful in keeping teeth clean and healthy should be corrected. The acidic nature of the fruit lowers the pH of the mouth and the enamel of the teeth is subjected to acid attack.

## Children and oral health

The oral health of children in the UK is amongst the worst in the western world. Recent reports indicate that improvements are being achieved in England and Wales but not in Scotland. This is a major area of concern and one where pharmacists should take a proactive role.

### Fluoride

Fluoride plays a major part in preventing dental caries or decay by increasing the resistance of tooth enamel to acid attack. It is effective both topically and systemically. Studies have shown that in areas where the fluoride concentration in the local water supply is at least 1 p.p.m. (1 mg/litre) the incidence of dental caries in children is much lower than in other areas. There has been considerable pressure for fluoridation of water supplies in the UK but a very strong lobby against this has developed. Consequently, other than in areas where it occurs naturally, water supplies in the UK are not artificially fluoridated.

Many children, particularly those with poor diet, poor tooth development, malaligned teeth or from a socially deprived background, will benefit from dietary fluoride supplements. These supplements should be started no later than 6 months old. The recommended doses are given in Table 38.1.

Opinion among members of the dental profession is divided about how long to continue fluoride supplements, but they should be continued at least until all the milk teeth have been replaced.

Low fluoride toothpaste does not need to be used with children and standard fluoride toothpaste is appropriate. However, as children are more prone to

**Table 38.1 Recommended doses of fluoride for children**

| | |
|---|---|
| Up to 2 years | 0.25 mg daily |
| 2–4 years | 0.5 mg daily |
| Over 4 years | 1 mg daily |

ingesting toothpaste, only a pea-sized quantity should be used. Overdose of fluoride can cause fluorosis. This gives the teeth a mottled appearance which is reversible and can be removed by a dentist.

### Toothbrushing in children

Brushing should start in children before the first tooth erupts. This allows the baby to become accustomed to the sensation of brushing. Toothbrushing should be supervised until the child is at least 6 years old.

### Sugar-free medicines

Wherever possible pharmacists should recommend sugar-free medicines, particularly for children.

## Advice on diet

Many pharmacies have weighing machines. Information on current guidelines on healthy eating and dietary advice should be available in the pharmacy, both orally from the pharmacist and in the form of leaflets. The adage 'we are what we eat' is of great significance today with considerable resources being used in an attempt to improve the diet of the population in the UK. Major initiatives involving food manufacturers, food producers, retailers and health professionals are being used to raise the awareness of the general public to the importance of healthy eating. Weight control is obviously an important factor in the maintenance of good health and pharmacists will frequently be asked for advice on how to lose weight. However many people who are not overweight have a very unhealthy diet and so advice on what constitutes a healthy diet should be available.

Recent government recommendations on what should be included in a healthy diet are:

- Fruit and vegetable intake to be at least 400 g daily
- Bread intake to be about 150 g and mainly wholemeal and brown
- Breakfast cereal intake to average 35 g
- Fat:
  - total fat to comprise no more than 35% of food energy
  - saturated fatty acids to be no more than 11% of total food energy
- Salt – average daily intake to be decreased from the UK average of 160 mmol (10 g) to not more than 100 mmol (approx. 6 g)
- Sugar intake in children to be less than 10% of total energy

- Fish:
  - white fish to be eaten at least once weekly
  - oily fish intake to be 88 g per week.

Healthy eating is central to the maintenance of good health. Research in this area is ongoing and recommendations may be changed in the light of new findings. It is important that pharmacists offering advice on diet ensure that they are up to date with current recommendations.

## THE ROLE OF THE PHARMACIST IN HEALTH SCREENING

Coronary heart disease (CHD) is a major cause of morbidity and mortality in the UK. A number of risk factors associated with an increased incidence of CHD can be identified. Opinion is divided as to the benefits of mass screening of the population for risk factors. However the Family Heart Association is committed to the view that risk factor screening in the population is fully justified.

The main risk factors which have been identified are:

- age
- gender
- genetic or inherited tendencies
- obesity
- smoking
- hypertension
- raised cholesterol
- diabetes.

The presence of one risk factor greatly increases the chance of developing heart disease and the presence of two or more increases the risk disproportionately. It is therefore important that a pharmacist who wishes to become involved in CHD prevention should offer a screening programme which will identify the presence or absence of all the major risk factors listed above. A blood pressure or a cholesterol measuring service offered in isolation does not provide the level of screening required.

To operate a comprehensive heart attack risk factor (HARF) screening programme clearly defined protocols must be adhered to. Important points to be considered are:

- What tests are being carried out?
- What equipment is required?
- What facilities are necessary?
- How much time will be allotted to each interview?
- What are the points of referral to the client's GP?

- What advice will be required by the patient?
- How the advice should be given, e.g. verbal, leaflets, etc?
- What support services need to be available for clients, e.g. smoking cessation?

## The information required

### Age and gender

In order to assess the number of risk factors present, the age and gender of the patient should be noted. Mortality due to CHD in 35- to 44-year-old men is five to six times higher than in women of the same age. This difference decreases with increasing age until at age 85 the mortality rate for men is only slightly higher than that of women.

### Genetic or inherited tendencies

The presence of heart disease in first degree relatives should be elicited.

### Obesity

Body mass index (BMI) should be calculated. This is done by measuring height and weight. BMI is expressed as weight/height$^2$ (kg/m$^2$). From the BMI figure an assessment of the degree to which the patient is overweight can be made. The relationship between BMI and obesity is given in Table 38.2.

### Hypertension

Because hypertension is asymptomatic, blood pressure must be measured in order to check whether this risk factor is present. Suitable apparatus must be used and the operator should be experienced in its use. A standard sphygmomanometer can be used, but electronic devices may be easier to use. As long as they are properly maintained they are an effective method of measuring blood pressure. The Royal Pharmaceutical Society of Great Britain Guidelines

for blood pressure monitoring in community pharmacies should be strictly adhered to (RPSGB Guidelines are contained in *Medicines, Ethics and Practice*).

*Taking a reading.* The patient should be seated and relaxed for approximately 10 minutes before the blood pressure is measured. If a high reading is obtained a subsequent reading should be taken at an interval of 15 minutes. If the reading is still above the recommended range a further reading should be taken on a different day. It should be explained to the patient that one, or even two, high readings do not necessarily indicate hypertension. Where the reading is high or borderline the patient should be referred to his GP. The general recommendation is that a diastolic pressure above 90 mmHg should be investigated, as should a systolic pressure above 160 mmHg. However, pharmacists who offer blood pressure measurement as a service should liaise with local GPs to determine what levels they consider appropriate for referral.

### Raised cholesterol

Cholesterol must be measured by a pharmacist who is not only highly competent in operating the equipment, but has an extensive knowledge base to answer any questions which the patient may have. The Royal Pharmaceutical Society Guidelines on testing body fluids should be strictly adhered to. A useful table on the interpretation of cholesterol test results is included in the Guidelines and is reproduced in Table 38.3.

The cholesterol which enters the bloodstream is carried by two proteins, HDL (high density lipoprotein) and LDL (low density lipoprotein). LDL transports cholesterol from the liver throughout the body. When cholesterol levels are raised it can be deposited onto the walls of blood vessels which can eventually lead to blocked arteries. HDL carries cholesterol back to the liver where it is broken down and excreted. The ratio of HDL to LDL is of importance. Some races, such as Greenland Eskimos, have a naturally high HDL:LDL ratio and very rarely suffer from heart disease. Unfortunately in western society the ratio is much lower, which means the balance of cholesterol is in favour of deposition. This can be improved by careful diet and, if necessary, by drug treatment.

It is not necessary for patients to fast before providing a blood sample for an initial cholesterol test. However, if a level above 6.5 mmol/l is measured it may be necessary for a second, more precise, measurement to be made. In this instance the patient

| Table 38.2 Body mass index and obesity | |
|---|---|
| | BMI |
| Underweight | 20 or less |
| Average | Over 20 to 25 |
| Overweight | Over 25 to 30 |
| Obese | Over 30 |

**Table 38.3  Interpretation of cholesterol test results (reproduced from *Medicines, Ethics and Practice* 1996)**

| Cholesterol levels (mmol/l) | Other risk factors | Degree of risk | Action |
|---|---|---|---|
| 5.2 or less | Minor or absent | Very low | None, although general lifestyle advice may be given |
| 5.2–6.5 | Minor or absent | Low | Advice on low fat diet and healthy lifestyle and reduction of risk factors where appropriate |
| 5.2–6.5 | Major or numerous | Moderate | Refer to GP for investigation. Advise on diet, lifestyle and reduction of risk factors where appropriate |
| 6.5–7.8 | Minor or absent | Moderate | Refer to GP for investigation. Advise on diet, lifestyle and reduction of risk factors where appropriate |
| 6.5–7.8 | Major or numerous | High | Refer to GP for investigation |
| 7.8 and over | Major or numerous | High | Refer to GP for investigation |

should fast for 14 hours prior to the sample being taken.

Cholesterol levels in the UK are quoted as mmol/l, however, some countries quote them as mg/dl. A conversion chart is given in Table 38.4.

Home cholesterol testing kits are available. Customers wishing to purchase these should be informed that raised cholesterol is only one risk factor and should not be viewed in isolation.

### Smoking

Smoking causes a variety of problems related to heart disease. These include damage to blood vessel endothelium caused by nicotine, vasoconstriction, a reduction of HDL cholesterol and an increase in platelet stickiness leading to a tendency to aggregate. Studies have shown the rate of CHD in smokers to be two to three times that of non-smokers. The level of risk also increases with an increase in the number of cigarettes smoked. Stopping smoking will decrease the risk. Recent studies have shown that while there are considerable benefits in stopping

smoking, they are neither immediate nor complete. The most important message is to persuade people not to start smoking. Many people have great difficulty stopping smoking and a smoking cessation programme, as described later (p. 427) could be run in conjunction with a HARF screening programme.

### Diabetes

The presence of diabetes has been shown to be linked with a twofold increase in CHD mortality. Patients should therefore be asked if they suffer from diabetes. A blood glucose test should also be carried out to check for the presence of undiagnosed diabetes.

### Other factors

Information on exercise patterns should be sought. Physically active people appear to have a lower risk of developing CHD than those who follow a more sedentary lifestyle. However, it should be noted that a good physical lifestyle will not counteract the risks brought about by raised cholesterol, hypertension or cigarette smoking. It could be argued that people who are aware of the importance of physical exercise are more likely to have a positive attitude to weight control, smoking and diet. Advice on regular, moderate exercise should be given. In his book *Coronary Heart Disease, Risks and Reasons*, A. G. Shaper states: 'It is probably better to sustain light or moderate activity on a regular basis than to have a glorious history of past vigorous exercise'. Exercise which slight-

**Table 38.4  Conversion of cholesterol concentrations between mmol/l and mg/dl**

Serum cholesterol conversion: mmol/l × 38.7 = mg/dl

| mg/dl | 77 | 116 | 155 | 194 | 232 | 271 | 310 | 348 |
|---|---|---|---|---|---|---|---|---|
| mmol/l | 2.0 | 3.0 | 4.0 | 5.0 | 6.0 | 7.0 | 8.0 | 9.0 |

**Table 38.5    Guidelines for low cholesterol eating**

| Advisable | In moderation | Not advised |
|---|---|---|
| Wholemeal flour, oatmeal, wholemeal bread, wholegrain cereals, porridge oats, crispbreads, wholegrain rice and pasta, sweetcorn | White flour, white bread, sugar-coated cereals, white rice, pasta | Fancy breads, e.g. croissants, Aberdeen rolls, savoury cheese biscuits, cream crackers |
| All fresh and frozen vegetables, e.g. peas, broad beans, sweetcorn. Dried beans and lentils are particularly high in fibre. Baked potatoes – eat skins wherever possible | Chips if cooked in suitable oil or fat, avocado pears, olives | Potato crisps cooked in unsuitable oil or fat |
| Fresh fruit, dried fruit | | |
| Walnuts | Almonds, brazil nuts, chestnuts, hazelnuts, peanuts | Coconut |
| All white fish, oily fish, e.g. herring, tuna | Shellfish occasionally | Fish roe |
| Chicken, turkey, veal, rabbit, game | Ham, beef, pork, lamb, bacon, lean mince. Liver and kidney occasionally | Visible fat on meat (including crackling), sausages, pâté, duck, goose, streaky bacon, meat pies, meat pasties |
| Skimmed milk, skimmed milk cheese, e.g. cottage and curd cheese, egg white (maximum of three egg yolks per week) | Edam, camembert and parmesan cheese | Whole milk, cream, hard stilton cheese, cream cheese, excess egg yolks |
| All fats should be limited | Margarine labelled 'high in polyunsaturates', corn oil, sunflower oil, soya oil, safflower oil | Butter, dripping, suet, lard, margarine not 'high in polyunsaturates', cooking vegetable oils of unknown origin |
| Skimmed milk puddings, low fat puddings, e.g. jelly, sorbet. Skimmed milk sauces. Pastry puddings, cakes and biscuits made with suitable margarine or oil and wholemeal flour | Pastry puddings, cakes and biscuits made with suitable margarine or oil and white flour. Ice-cream (low fat) | Tinned or whole-milk puddings, dairy ice cream, pastry puddings, cakes, biscuits and sauces made with whole milk, eggs, or unsuitable fat or oil. All proprietary puddings and sauces, mayonnaise |
| Bovril, Oxo, Marmite | Meat and fish pastes, boiled sweets, fruit pastilles, peppermints, etc., jam, marmalade, honey, sugar | Peanut butter, chocolate, toffees, fudge, butterscotch, lemon curd, mincemeat |
| Tea, coffee, mineral water, unsweetened fruit juices, clear soups, homemade soups, e.g. vegetable, lentil | Packet soups Alcohol | Cream soups |

ly raises the pulse rate should be taken for 20 minutes, three times each week.

*Diet.* Areas which should be checked are the intake of saturated fat, fibre and salt. Salt intake is often very difficult to measure because of the large quantities of salt which food manufacturers add to their products. Improved labelling should help in calculating a more accurate figure. Information on appropriate foodstuffs is given in Tables 38.5 and 38.6.

*Alcohol.* Several studies have reported that regular moderate drinking is 'good for the heart'. While it is true that alcohol increases the level of HDL the quantity of alcohol which has to be consumed to achieve this would cause considerable damage to the

| Table 38.6 How much fat? | |
|---|---|
| | Amount of fat |
| **Meat** | |
| Fried streaky bacon | 45% |
| Grilled streaky bacon | 36% |
| Grilled lamb chops | 29% |
| Pork pie | 27% |
| Luncheon meat | 27% |
| Liver sausage | 27% |
| Roast lamb (shoulder) | 26% |
| Fried pork sausages | 25% |
| Roast leg of pork | 20% |
| Fried beefburgers | 17% |
| Grilled rump steak | 12% |
| Casseroled pig's liver | 8% |
| Stewed steak | 7% |
| Casseroled chicken | 7% |
| Fried lambs' kidneys | 6% |
| Tinned ham | 5% |
| **Fish** | |
| Smoked mackerel | 16% |
| Fried fish fingers | 13% |
| Grilled kippers | 12% |
| Cod fried in batter | 10% |
| Steamed plaice | 2% |
| Steamed haddock | 1% |
| **Cheese** | |
| Cream cheeses | 50% |
| Stilton | 40% |
| Cheddar | 34% |
| Parmesan | 30% |
| Processed cheese | 25% |
| Camembert | 23% |
| Edam | 23% |
| Cheese spread | 23% |
| Cottage cheese | 4% |
| **Milk, butter and oils** | |
| Oil (all kinds) | 100% |
| Lard | 99% |
| Butter | 82% |
| Margarine (all kinds) | 80% |
| Double cream | 50% |
| Dairy ice-cream | 7% |
| Gold top milk | 5% |
| Silver top milk | 4% |
| Yoghurt | 1% |
| Skimmed milk | < 1% |

liver and kidneys. Advice on alcohol consumption should follow government guidelines which indicate a maximum weekly consumption of 8 units for men and 21 for women.

*Current disease states and medication.* Some disease states or medication may predispose patients to CHD; thus information about any drugs which the patient is taking should be sought.

Providing a HARF screening service is one way in which pharmacists can make a very major contribution to health promotion and health education. It must, however, be carried out by pharmacists who have carefully researched the area and have the necessary knowledge base to deal with the many and varied questions which they will be asked.

## PHARMACISTS AND SMOKING CESSATION

Smoking is a major cause of morbidity and death. It increases the risk of the development of CHD and is a common cause of lung cancer and other diseases of the respiratory tract. A decrease in smoking amongst pregnant women is one of the government health targets. Smoking in pregnancy leads to several obstetric problems and effects on the fetus. The likelihood of premature deliveries is increased and there is a higher incidence of low birth weight babies in mothers who smoke. There is an increased awareness of the problems caused by smoking and passive smoking has also been identified as a risk. Smoking is now banned in many public places including transport.

As well as being harmful to health, smoking also has an effect on certain drugs and in many instances there is evidence of an inadequate therapeutic response (Table 38.7).

### Withdrawal symptoms

Nicotine is an addictive drug and withdrawal symptoms can often cause problems for someone trying to give up smoking. In fact, concern about withdrawal symptoms may prevent many smokers from even trying to give up. Pharmacists can give help and advice on how to cope with these symptoms, emphasizing the positive aspect that the symptoms are an indication that the body is recovering from the effects of tobacco. The common withdrawal symptoms are as follows:

• *Craving.* This intense desire to smoke can occur only a few hours after the last cigarette. It is usually at its worst on day three, when all the nicotine has been eliminated from the body. It only lasts for 2–3 minutes and knowledge that the duration is short is often the key to helping the smoker to cope.

• *Coughing.* This is caused by reactivation of the cilia in the respiratory tract which have become paralysed during smoking. Accumulated mucus is

**Table 38.7    Pharmacists' guide to smoking and drug interactions (modified from Anon 1989)***

| Drug interactions with smoking | Management |
|---|---|
| Tricyclic antidepressants: Smokers tend to have lower plasma levels of tricyclic antidepressants than non-smokers. These lower levels would be expected to reduce the therapeutic response to the antidepressants in some patients | Watch for evidence of inadequate response to tricyclic antidepressants in smokers. They may require larger doses than non-smokers |
| Benzodiazepines: The sedative effects of diazepam and chlordiazepoxide may be lower in smokers than in non-smokers | Smokers may require larger doses than non-smokers for an equivalent sedative effect |
| Dextropropoxyphene: This drug may be less effective in smokers than in non-smokers | Heavy smokers (20+ cigarettes per day) may obtain better relief with an analgesic other than dextropropoxyphene |
| Heparin: Smokers tend to eliminate heparin more rapidly than non-smokers | Smokers may require larger doses of heparin than non-smokers |
| Oral contraceptives: The risk of serious cardiovascular adverse reactions from oral contraceptive use is increased in patients who smoke, especially those who are over 35 years of age and smoke 15 or more cigarettes per day | Women who smoke and take oral contraceptives should be informed of the increased risk of stroke, myocardial infarction or thromboembolism and urged to stop smoking |
| Pentazocine: Dose requirements for pentazocine tend to be higher in smokers than in non-smokers | Watch for evidence of inadequate response to pentazocine. Smokers may require larger doses of pentazocine than non-smokers |
| Phenothiazines: Chlorpromazine tends to produce less drowsiness and hypotension in smokers than in non-smokers | Watch for evidence of inadequate therapeutic response to chlorpromazine (and possible other phenothiazines) in smokers |
| Propranolol: Smokers tend to have lower serum propranolol concentrations. Smoking also inhibits the therapeutic effect of propranolol in the treatment of angina | Watch for evidence of inadequate response to propranolol. If propranolol is being used to treat angina, patients, should be informed that smoking will inhibit the therapeutic response to propranolol |
| Theophylline: Smokers metabolize theophylline more rapidly than non-smokers and may require larger doses | Watch for evidence of inadequate response to theophylline and inform patients that they may be at risk of inadequate plasma levels |

*The original table was published in the USA by the National Cancer Institute and the American Pharmaceutical Association.

cleared from the lungs. The cough is self-limiting and an explanation of the cause should be all that is necessary.

• *Hunger.* Many smokers are concerned that they will put on large amounts of weight when they stop smoking. Although hunger can be intense, careful control of diet minimizes any weight gain. It is worth mentioning that the average weight gain on quitting is only 4–8 lb.

• *Bowel disturbance.* Constipation or diarrhoea occasionally occur. Again this is of short duration and a high fibre diet can alleviate the constipation.

• *Dizziness and tingling.* This is caused by improved oxygenation of the tissues. It should be explained that this is a positive sign.

• *CNS disturbance.* On giving up smoking some people suffer irritability, mood swings or lack of concentration. This can be very difficult to deal with particularly for family, friends or work colleagues. Smokers should tell all these people they are trying to give up and allowances should be made and support given for the few weeks that the symptoms last.

## Anti-smoking aids

Smokers who want to give up must be self-motivated and will-power is the greatest factor in success (see Ch. 2 for information about the cycle of change). However, there are occasions when support in the form of an anti-smoking aid gives additional help.

Anti-smoking aids fall into two categories:

- nicotine replacements
- nicotine substitutes.

These replace or substitute nicotine in the bloodstream thereby reducing the feeling of craving and help reduce the withdrawal symptoms.

### Nicotine replacements

**Nicotine chewing gum.** The intranasal absorption of nicotine which occurs in smoking takes about 10 minutes. On chewing nicotine gum, absorption takes place through the buccal mucosa and takes about 30 minutes to achieve peak blood levels. This slower build-up eliminates the 'kick' given by the intranasal route. However, the presence of nicotine reduces the withdrawal symptoms of craving, irritability and lack of concentration.

*Method of use.* Nicotine gum comes in two strengths, 2 mg and 4 mg. Patients would normally start on the lower dose increasing to 4 mg later, if needed. The 4 mg gum should be used if 15 pieces of the 2 mg gum are being chewed per day. Patients should also start on the 4 mg strength if they fall into the '20/20 rule' category. This applies to smokers who smoke at least 20 cigarettes daily and also smoke within 20 minutes of getting up in the morning.

The gum must be chewed slowly to aid steady and maximum buccal absorption. If chewed quickly, saliva is increased, the nicotine is swallowed and becomes deactivated in the GI tract. Hiccups and indigestion may occur. The chewing process should be continued for 30 minutes. The gum should be used regularly for 3 months then gradually reduced.

**Nicotine patches.** These are transdermal delivery systems which are applied on a daily basis. The nicotine is absorbed through the skin into the systemic circulation providing a dose lower than that achieved by smoking, but sufficient to prevent or reduce the incidence of withdrawal symptoms.

*Method of use.* Patches are available in a variety of strengths which relate to the rate of release of nicotine. The rates range from 5 mg per 16 hours, through 7 mg per 24 hours to a maximum of 22 mg per 24 hours. Smokers of more than 20 cigarettes a day should start with the highest strength and those smoking fewer than 20 start with an intermediate strength. The dose should be reduced after approximately 4 weeks. Treatment should be reviewed if success has not been achieved by 3 months. The patch should be applied to a clean hairless area on the trunk or arm and removed after 24 hours (16 hours for Nicorette). A different area should be used each day.

**Nicotine spray.** The nasal spray produces a peak nicotine level in about 10 minutes. This more closely mimics the effect of smoking with the quicker absorption giving more of a 'kick'.

*Method of use.* The spray is available in one strength of 500 µg/metered dose. One dose is sprayed into each nostril a maximum of twice per hour up to a maximum of 64 per day. After 8 weeks the dose should be reduced and not continued beyond 3 months' treatment.

**Lozenges.** There are two proprietary lozenges marketed which are purported to be 'pure tobacco' and therefore contain nicotine. Little research has been done to assess blood nicotine levels and therefore comparisons with the other nicotine products are difficult.

### Nicotine substitutes

These contain substances which help to alleviate withdrawal symptoms.

## Smoking cessation initiatives

Giving up smoking is successfully achieved by many people, but there are many more who have great difficulty in breaking the habit. Many programmes like Weight Watchers and Alcoholics Anonymous are successful because of the support which they provide. Smokers are more likely to succeed in giving up smoking if they receive regular counselling and support. This support for smokers wishing to give up can be provided from pharmacies. Two examples of schemes operated by pharmacists to provide this support are discussed below.

### Smoking cessation monitoring system

This consists of a progress card and a profile sheet which are given to a smoker who wants to give up with the help of a pharmacist. The pharmacist records the date of contact with the customer, what advice was given, the number of tobacco-free weeks and information on any anti-smoking products used. Pharmacists also maintain a client profile sheet which contains similar information to the progress card, but also includes relevant medical information. This type of system formalizes the already helpful contribution many pharmacists give to smokers who wish to stop.

## Model cessation service

This model is based on work done by community pharmacist, Terry Maguire (1993). In research into smoking cessation he found that pharmacist support improved 'stop smoking rates' from 16% to 56% in 3 months and from 6% to 46% at 6 months. The need to stop smoking was discussed with patients presenting with smoking-related symptoms and also smokers. Clients who enrolled onto the programme had 10 one-to-one interviews with the pharmacist. This highly structured scheme includes window displays, literature and visual aids. In addition to the interviews, carbon monoxide monitoring is carried out on smokers who have claimed to stop.

Both of these schemes are supported by the NPA and are useful ways in which pharmacists can become actively involved in health promotion and education.

## SKIN CANCER

The sale of sun-protection products from pharmacies gives pharmacists an ideal opportunity to provide advice on reducing the risks of developing skin cancer.

Knowledge of skin types, warning signs and sun-protection factors is needed. Sunscreens marketed in the UK are all awarded a sun-protection factor (SPF). This is an indication of the level of protection provided against UVB radiation. An SPF of 6 or under should be considered as giving low protection, SPF 8–12 gives medium protection and greater than 12, high protection. Sunscreen products are additionally star rated to indicate the level of protection they provide against UVA radiation. One star (*) indicates low protection and four stars (****) high protection. This rating is independent of the SPF scale and some products can have a high SPF but a low star rating. Selection of the most appropriate sunscreen should be done on the basis of SPF. The greater the tendency for a person's skin to burn in the sun, the higher the SPF which should be recommended. Tables relating skin type to required SPF are available from several sources.

Pharmacists who become actively involved in health promotion and education have increased job satisfaction. The increased contact with customers raises the profile of pharmacy and raises the awareness of the general public to the level of advice and support which is available from a pharmacy. Pharmacists are more clearly seen as members of the primary health care team. Pharmacies are busy places and pharmacists are busy people who have many demands on their time. Involvement in health education is not a passive process and requires considerable commitment from the pharmacist in time and resources. However, as in many areas where considerable effort is required, the benefits frequently outweigh the effort.

## Key Points

- Health promotion is anything which positively affects health.
- Health education involves making people aware of factors which promote good health.
- The UK Government has set 25 health targets.
- The pharmacist's role in health promotion and health education is formally recognized.
- Many pharmacists operate 'health promotion pharmacies'.
- Leaflets can be useful for health education providing they are of a suitable quality.
- Important features of leaflet design include page size, layout, type and readability of the text.
- Pharmacists have many opportunities for health promotion if they choose to use them.
- Dental health has been added to the health targets and presents pharmacists with further opportunities for health education and health promotion.
- Diet and eating advice should be available from the pharmacist.
- Pharmacists are able to offer heart attack risk factor (HARF) screening.
- Measuring blood pressure or cholesterol alone is not helpful.
- Two types of product are available to help people stop smoking – nicotine replacement and nicotine substitutes.
- Pharmacists may recommend appropriate sun protection to help reduce the increase in skin cancer.
- Involvement with health education and health promotion increases pharmacists' job satisfaction.

## SELF-ASSESSMENT QUESTIONS

1. The terms 'health education' and 'health promotion' are synonymous. True or false?

2. What is the concentration of fluoride in the water supply below which fluoride supplements should be given to children?

3. What are the symptoms of fluorosis?

4. Fluorosis is irreversible. True or false?

5. What is the concentration of fluoride in the water supply in your area?

6. What is the current recommendation for maximum weekly intake of alcohol for adult males and females?

7. When is a person described as overweight and when is a person described as obese?

8. What does BMI stand for and how is it calculated?

9. List *five* heart attack risk factors.

10. If people suffer from two risk factors their chances of developing CHD double. True or false?

11. What strength of nicotine chewing gum should be used by a smoker who wishes to give up and smokes 15 cigarettes daily?

12. What effect does smoking have on theophylline levels?

13. The best dietary advice to reduce the incidence of dental caries is to eliminate sucrose from the diet. True or false?

14. List *three* reasons why readability tests alone are inappropriate for assessing the suitability of information leaflets.

15. What is the government target for smoking in the 11- to 15-year-old age group?

16. Describe why a smoker has an increased risk of developing a blood clot.

17. Pregnant women who smoke are more likely to give birth to undersized babies. True or false?

18. What is being measured in the Flesch readability index?

19. List *three* foodstuffs which should be avoided in a cholesterol-reducing diet, *three* where consumption should be limited and *three* which are advised.

20. List *three* benefits to community pharmacists from becoming more involved and proactive in health education.

## ANSWERS TO SELF-ASSESSMENT QUESTIONS

1. False. Health education is a component of health promotion and deals with specific information aimed at improving an individual's knowledge about preventing ill health and maintaining good health.

2. Less than 1 p.p.m.

3. Mottling of the teeth

4. False. It can be removed by a dentist.

5. This information can be obtained from the local water authority.

6. Adult males 21 units of alcohol

   Adult females 14 units of alcohol.

7. If BMI is over 25 and less than 30 – overweight

   If BMI is over 30 – obese.

8. Weight in kg divided by height in metres squared.

9. Genetic tendencies, obesity, smoking, hypertension, raised cholesterol.

10. False. Suffering from one risk factor increases the chances of developing CHD but suffering from two or more increases the risk disproportionately.

11. The 2 mg strength is appropriate for initiating therapy.

12. Theophylline levels are lowered.

13. False. Although this may be the ideal it is not realistic advice and so is not likely to be adhered to. Advice to reduce the frequency of intake is more likely to be accepted.

14. Readability tests do not take account of medical jargon and scientific terms, the motivation of the reader or the reader's knowledge base.

15. To reduce the prevalence of smoking in this age group by 33%.

16. Smoking causes a reduction in HDL cholesterol, the lipoprotein which transports cholesterol back to the liver. There is also an increase in platelet stickiness which in turn increases the tendency for the platelets to aggregate.

17. True. Intrauterine growth is retarded in pregnant women and there is an increased risk of premature birth.

18. The number of syllables in each word and the number of words in a sentence.

19. Any three from the relevant columns in Table 38.5.

20. Increased job satisfaction, increased customer contact, increased professional standing plus many more.

## FURTHER READING

Anon 1989 Smoking and drug interactions. Pharmaceutical Journal 242: 237

Blenkinsopp A, Panton R 1992 Health promotion for pharmacists. Oxford University Press, Oxford

Department of Health 1992 The health of the nation: a strategy for health in England. Cm 1986. HMSO, London

Kendle K E, Bell J H, Maitland J M, Moody M M 1991 Heart attack risk factor screening: an evaluation of a procedure suitable for application by community pharmacists. Pharmaceutical Journal 247: 734–738

Maguire T A 1993 A study of the feasibility of a smoking cessation service in a community pharmacy. Pharmaceutical Journal 251: R26

Martin J (ed) 1991 Handbook of pharmacy health education. Pharmaceutical Press, London

Medicines, Ethics and Practice – a guide for pharmacists, current edn. Royal Pharmaceutical Society of Great Britain, London (Updated twice yearly)

National Pharmaceutical Association 1994 Health promotion and the community pharmacist. The Health Education Authority, London

News Feature 1994 New initiatives for pharmacy smoking cessation. Pharmaceutical Journal 252: 289–290

Scottish Office Department of Health 1992 Scotland's health – a challenge to us all. Scottish Office Department of Health, Edinburgh

Scottish Office Department of Health 1996 Scotland's health – a challenge to us all. Eating for health. Scottish Office Department of Health, Edinburgh

Shaper A G 1988 Coronary heart disease risks and reasons. Current Medical Literature, London

# 39

# Patient medication records

*A. J. Winfield*

---

After studying this chapter you will know about:

**The types of patient medication records (PMRs)**
**The nature of the information which can and should be stored and how PMRs operate**
**The practical uses of PMRs**
**Legal aspects of keeping PMRs on computer.**

## Introduction

There has been a tradition of pharmacists keeping records on certain types of medication. Often this was keeping notes about types of insulin or the supply of oxygen cylinders. There has also been the legal requirement to record certain types of prescription and classes of drugs.

Over recent years there has been a marked increase in the use of records to include a wide range of patient groups and medicines. It has been claimed (Rogers & Rees 1996) that 95% of pharmacists now keep records, many on all patients. They are commonly called patient medication records (PMRs). The value of these records has been recognized by the UK Government who currently pay pharmacists, who must have completed appropriate training, a fee for keeping records. At present there should be a PMR for 100 patients over age 60 (50 patients in an essential small pharmacy). This fee is likely to become part of the professional allowance in the future.

## TYPES OF RECORD

There are three types of patient medication record in use, namely cards, computer-based systems and 'smart cards'. Each has its advantages and disadvantages.

Card systems rely on handwriting. The NPA has produced a card that enables most of the information to be recorded easily. Cards are stored in a box file, usually in alphabetical order.

Computer-based systems are commercially available as 'add-ons' to labelling programs, having been refined since their introduction in the early 1980s. They cost more to purchase and update, but give greater flexibility.

'Smart cards' are still experimental. They use a chip to record patient data on a card which the patient carries with him. Technology is developing rapidly in this area, so that large amounts of data can now be stored on a credit-card-sized card. However, there is as yet no standardization and they are only being used in local trials. This method has the potential to carry a lot of medical information about the patient and could have all medicines included in the record, irrespective of where dispensed. However, because it has not been developed sufficiently to make generalizations, it will not be discussed further.

A comparison of the advantages and disadvantages of the two main types of patient medication record is given in Table 39.1. The advantages of computer-based systems have resulted in the card-based systems being largely abandoned.

## Computer-based systems

The Royal Pharmaceutical Society of Great Britain (RPSGB) includes guidelines on pharmacy computer systems in *Medicines, Ethics and Practice*. This gives valuable guidance about the hardware and software aspects of installing a system, as well as addressing issues such as supplier support, multi-user systems, data standards, compatibility and the maintenance of databases. The types of data which the program should be capable of storing are summarized in Table 39.2.

Modern systems will also allow the addition of a range of other information. This could include preg-

**Table 39.1 Comparison of advantages and disadvantages of card and computer-based patient medication records**

|  | Advantages | Disadvantages |
|---|---|---|
| Card | Cheap, easy to set up, unlimited capacity, not prone to system failure | Takes time to update, slow, inflexible retrieval, no multiple access, identification of problems relies on vigilance |
| Computer | Quick to update, retrieval is fast and flexible, problems identified automatically | Software (and updates) costly, limited capacity (auto-delete on some systems), can have system failure |

**Table 39.2 Types of data to record on a patient medication system (based on RPSGB Guidelines 1996)**

| Should record | Patient | Name<br>Address and postcode<br>Telephone number<br>Sex<br>Age and date of birth<br>NHS number<br>General practitioner<br>Details of medicines |
|---|---|---|
|  | GP data | Name<br>Identification number<br>Practice name and telephone |
|  | Medicine | Name<br>Strength<br>Form<br>Quantity<br>Quantity unit<br>Dosage regimen<br>Date dispensed |
| Useful | Patient | Exempt prescription charges<br>Child-resistant closures unacceptable<br>Drug sensitivity<br>Drug allergy<br>Chronic illness |
|  | Medicine | Product licence (for generics)<br>Batch number |

The programs are structured as a number of separate files. These are normally a patient file, a prescription file, a drug file, a dosage instruction file (for labelling) and a doctor file. In operation, the computer links two files by a common set of data, called the linking field. Thus, for example, when a new prescription is entered, the computer would access a number of files. It would go to the patient file to check name and address and any special notes. The drug file would be checked for the drug strength and dosage. Both the patient file and drug file would be used to check for drug interactions and the instruction file would be used if the same label is required. On completion of dispensing the information is stored in the appropriate file and can be accessed in a very flexible way. Thus, for example, it would be possible to produce lists of all patients on a particular drug, all residents in a residential home, or all patients recorded as having a particular medical condition.

It is essential that any entry can be corrected if it is found to be incorrect. It must also be recognized that each entry takes up space on the computer disk. On older machines the hard disk memory may be quite restricted, and so it is necessary to either store on floppy disks or delete records. Some programs will carry out deletion automatically against predetermined criteria, such as after 6 months for most patients, but after 2 years for patients aged over 60 years. It is good practice with any computer system to make regular back-up copies of the data. When data are archived, the Consumer Protection Act requires that they are kept for 10 years. The Department of Health specify that data be stored for at least 1 year and preferably 2. It is essential that there is easy access to any archived data.

The ease of use of computer-based PMRs has led to a widespread use. However, some pharmacists may wish to limit the records to certain groups of patients, particularly when setting up a new system. In such a process, it is advisable to have clear priorities. The NHS contract only requires records for patients over the age of 60 years. Apart from this group, other priority groups could include children under 12, patients in receipt of domiciliary services or living in a residential or nursing home, some disease groups (asthmatics, epileptics), patients with special needs (penicillin sensitivity, regular multiple therapy, confusion, needing compliance aids), or patients on certain groups of drugs ($H_2$ antagonists, anticoagulants, oral contraceptives, steroids, antihypertensives). The ideal is to include all patients.

nancy, breast-feeding, smoking status, other characteristics or risks. They also have a facility to flag the patient the next time the record is accessed.

## *Data Protection Act*

In the UK the Data Protection Act 1984 must be complied with when using a computer-based PMR system. The user of the computer system must register with the Data Protection Registrar. The data stored can only be used for the purpose(s) for which they are registered, although they can be used for research providing that an individual cannot be identified. The Act is designed to protect an individual's right to confidentiality and the accuracy of the data. Thus, before a PMR can be created, patients must give their permission and they have a right to either see the whole record or receive a complete print-out. Programs allow for this and so in practice this is normally straightforward. However, there can be some ethical and legal problems. An example is whether the parents, the child or both have the right to see the record of a teenage child. In this example, there are detailed differences in the law across the UK. The Act also requires that the system is secure to prevent unauthorized access to the data.

## USE OF PMRS IN DISPENSING

The major use of a PMR is during dispensing a prescription. Computer-based systems have the capability of confirming the prescriber and that the name and address on the prescription and PMR match. The computer can be used to check for the safety and appropriateness of each item against the data on file, including drug interactions and any recorded contraindications and allergies. Doses may be checked, particularly for consistency with previous occasions of dispensing. Any notes on the patient's record, such as a need to avoid child-resistant closures, can be seen to optimize efficiency. When the item to be dispensed is a simple repeat of a previous prescription, most systems allow automatic label preparation. Finally, a single key stroke will update the record. Thus it provides a very efficient way of checking the safety of the prescription for the patient. In doing so, the ideal is that the record should be checked over a period of at least 2 years for any patient over 65 years and for 3 months for other patients.

In addition, the computer record can improve the efficiency of service provided in a number of ways. For example, the frequency of counselling or checking inhaler technique can be noted and a reminder flashed on the screen. Where generics are being dispensed, the source can be recorded in order to provide the same one where possible and so avoid anxiety in the patient if the appearance is different. These facilities are useful for a regular pharmacist but are invaluable for a locum pharmacist. The record can also help if errors are made or if information is missing from a repeat prescription, because drug name, dose, strength, quantity and instructions will all be recorded. However, the intention of the prescriber must always be confirmed.

## Drug interactions

The use of the PMR in recognizing a drug interaction is often given as one of the most important facilities. However, there are a number of possible problems with these programs. In order to operate effectively the program must be able to recognize drugs that are entered either by proprietary or generic name. The database used by the computer must be compiled from a reliable source and be updated regularly. Interactions vary in their severity and potential to cause harm, as recognized by the *British National Formulary* (BNF) in Appendix 1. Not only do the interactions vary, so do individual patients' susceptibility to them. This is recognized by most of the interaction programs, although the extent of discrimination varies between programs. Studies have demonstrated that different programs will produce different information about the same combination of drugs (Rogers et al 1993). In extreme examples this can range from major interaction to no interaction. The RPSGB guideline indicates that any interactions program should alert to every interaction listed in the current edition of the BNF and must be able to highlight any potentially hazardous interactions. There is a danger that people will come to rely on the computer, but the guidelines make it clear that the pharmacist still has personal responsibility for verifying the safety of any combination of drugs prescribed for a patient.

Increasingly, electronic point of sale (EPOS) systems are being used in pharmacies which can be linked into the PMR system. As a result, the records will include OTC medicines as well as dispensed medicines. This is important from a safety point of view, especially as more drugs are deregulated. However, information on OTC interactions is less well developed and the public still have to be convinced about its use when they wish to purchase a medicine.

## Other uses of PMRs

The other uses of PMRs derive from either the ease

and flexibility of access to the information or from the nature of the information which is stored.

There are a number of reasons why a pharmacist may not be able to dispense all the medicine requested on a prescription. This is usually due to the quantity ordered exceeding the amount in stock, especially when there has been a deliberate decision to keep stock low because of the high cost or short expiry date of the medicine. It could also arise because of a supply problem or a heavy demand leading to a need to 'ration' the supply. However the shortfall arises, the balance of product for the patient is usually called an 'owing'. Most PMR programs have a facility for recording this, producing a note for the patient and the label for the balance when it is available. This has a clear management advantage. It can be used, if thought necessary, to review the optimum stock levels of particular products. Decisions about stock levels can be difficult to make, because many factors influence them, including time to resupply and cost of items. The usage patterns of drugs can be analysed using the data in the PMR. Whilst this will not be the only information needed in order to reach a decision, it is important and can readily show the normal level of demand and any seasonal fluctuations.

In the chapter on residential homes, the need to be able to produce information on medicines is mentioned (Ch. 40). The computer is able to put together the records of all the patients in a given home, both for general information and as a prelude to a visit to that home by the pharmacist.

Another facility which may be useful for residents of homes, or for other patients, is that of producing medicine administration records. These are used with monitored dosage systems to provide the name, strength, form, quantity and administration times for each medicine.

Compliance charts are not dissimilar in that they also record the same information on paper for a patient or carer. They are used to act as a reminder or to record that the administration has taken place.

Invoices may be required for supplies made to surgeries and other similar places. These can be generated easily by the computer.

Patient information leaflets (PILs) can be produced by some programs. As with drug interactions, it is the responsibility of the pharmacist to ensure the accuracy of the information. Whilst the text could be typed in by the pharmacist the RPSGB guidelines advise against this.

It is likely that pharmacists will become part of the adverse drug reaction reporting scheme. In order to be in a position to make such a report, the pharmacist will need to be aware of the occurrence of adverse reactions. It is difficult to notice a pattern in isolated events, but by keeping a record of them on the computer, it will be much easier to recognize a problem.

From time to time a product recall is necessary. When this occurs, it is important to trace all the medicines that have been supplied. Most systems have the facility for recording product source and batch number. In the event of a recall, this information will allow the pharmacist to know exactly to whom the medicine has been dispensed, together with their addresses and the dates of dispensing. This makes recovering the product much more efficient.

Pharmacists may find it useful to keep health-related data which they have determined should be part of their service. Thus, for example, a diary-like record could be made of smoking cessation, blood pressure monitoring, peak flow measurement, blood cholesterol measurement.

Most systems also have a facility for stock ordering to ease the business management aspects of community pharmacy.

More advanced uses of PMRs have been suggested which make direct use of the information, or draw upon it together with other related information. Two examples are mentioned below.

As discussed in Chapter 41, compliance by patients with the prescribed medicines can be a problem. The PMR contains information about the quantity of medicines dispensed over a period of time and the frequency of dosage intended. Thus it is possible to see if this pattern corresponds with what would be expected from the prescription. This does not prove or disprove compliance, but may give a pointer to a problem and lead the pharmacist to ask further questions. A related use is when the method of administration requires a special technique, such as with a pressurized aerosol. It is advisable to check on the patient's technique regularly, but not necessarily every time a prescription is dispensed. A 'flag' can be placed in the PMR reminding the pharmacist to speak to the patient after a set number of prescriptions.

Some facets of health promotion require the identification of patients who are 'at risk'. The main difficulty of this is making contact with them. One way of doing this may be by using the PMR. It can work by using the drugs which are being prescribed, together with the other information which is stored on the PMR. Thus, as an example, influenza vaccination is recommended for elderly people and certain other groups. The PMR can easily identify elderly people. It can also identify people who have respiratory disease, either by using the notes, or by deduction from the drugs being prescribed. Whichever way they are recognized, a flag on the PMR means that the next these these patients have a prescription dispensed, they can be asked whether they have had the vaccination.

## PROBLEMS WITH PMRs

A number of problems with PMR systems have been mentioned already, such as variable information about drug interactions. There are a number of other problems, both technical and practical.

Most systems at present are designed for use by one operator at a time. This may be inadequate. For example in a busy pharmacy, where there is more than one pharmacist, multiple access is required. This need also arises where EPOS is being used, or where the pharmacist wants to have the PMR available at the position in the pharmacy where patient counselling is taking place as well as in the dispensary. The hardware and software are now being developed to allow these additional facilities.

The greatest problem with PMRs in pharmacies is that they are probably incomplete. Patients are not required to use the same pharmacy every time and they may purchase GSL medicines from non-pharmacy outlets. As a result, several different pharmacies may have incomplete records on the same person. In the UK, one multiple outlet company has developed a system which interlinks all its stores. Apart from this, at present there have been no initiatives towards interlinking records to produce a more complete record. Likewise, there has been no move towards a scheme in which a patient must register with one pharmacy. The smart-card form of patient medication record has the potential to overcome this serious limitation, if the technical aspects can be standardized. However, even that may not be the complete answer, because the card is ultimately dependent on patients carrying it with them at all times. The evidence from the limited trials suggests that patients do not do this.

- Most records are now kept on computer.
- Modern computer-based PMRs store a wide range of information and offer great flexibility in use.
- The RPSGB has guidelines on the capabilities of computer-based PMR systems.
- Priority groups for keeping records can be identified and may be useful when developing a system, but the ideal is to include all patients.
- The Data Protection Act controls the use of computer-based PMRs and all its requirements must be complied with.
- The PMR can give prompts during the dispensing process and provide safety checks.
- Recognition of drug interactions is useful, but can give rise to some problems.
- The records can be used for 'owings', stock control, to help service residential homes, for compliance charts, information for patients and in product recalls.
- PMRs have the potential to assist compliance monitoring and targeting health promotion.
- Without patient registration, PMRs are likely to be incomplete.

## FURTHER READING

British National Formulary, current edn. British Medical Association and Royal Pharmaceutical Society of Great Britain, London

Medicines, Ethics and Practice – a guide for pharmacists, current edn. Royal Pharmaceutical Society of Great Britain, London (Updated twice yearly)

Morris G 1989 Patient medication records: a personal view. Pharmaceutical Journal 242: 351–352

Rogers P J, Carroll J, Rees J E 1993 Problems associated with the use of drug interaction monitoring software. Pharmaceutical Journal 251: R23

Rogers P J, Rees J E 1996 Comparison of the use of PMRs in community pharmacy 1991 and 1995: (1) PMR use and recording of product details. Pharmaceutical Journal 256: 161–166

## Key Points

- There has been a tradition of pharmacists keeping records.
- Pharmacists are now paid for keeping PMRs.
- Records can be kept on cards, computer or on 'smart cards'.

# 40
# Residential care

*A. J. Winfield*

After studying this chapter you will know about:

**Development of residential care**
**Medicine management problems in residential homes**
**Arrangements for provision of pharmaceutical services to residential homes**
**Possible involvement of pharmacist with residents, staff training and clinical review**.

## BACKGROUND

Over recent years there has been a move towards caring for patients in the community. The process was given impetus by the White Paper 'Caring for People' (1989) and the National Health Service and Community Care Act 1990. There has also been a progressive reduction in the number of long-term hospital beds. To meet the resulting need, private, local authority and voluntary residential care facilities have been developed. These homes may be thought of as being in three groups. Sheltered accommodation is designed for those who still manage with a high level of independence, including their medicine administration. Residential homes are for elderly residents whose needs are higher, but who have a wide spectrum of independence. Nursing homes meet the needs of people with specific medical requirements. In practice they tend to overlap in the services they provide. There are legislative differences between residential and nursing homes. The aim of providing pharmaceutical care is the same for both.

Not only have the elderly moved into the community, so too have their pharmaceutical needs. The physiological changes which occur with age mean that medicine consumption is likely to be high and the possibility of complications will increase proportionately. Community pharmacists have a role in ensuring the safe and effective handling of these medicines whilst allowing residents maximum independence. Thus they have been presented with the new challenge of providing clinical services in addition to their normal supply function. This contribution to patient care in residential homes has been recognized by the Government who have authorized payment to pharmacists who have had suitable training and who have signed an agreement to provide services to such a home.

It should also be noted that there are homes caring for others with needs, including children, the mentally ill and those with physical and learning difficulties. Whilst this chapter considers residential homes for the elderly, the principles are applicable to other situations.

### Medicine administration in homes

There are a wide variety of ways in which residents may receive their medicines. The home may be flexible enough to allow for variation with the resident's ability to manage or otherwise. Where possible residents should have complete control of all their medicines, both prescribed and bought over the counter (OTC). In such situations, the pharmacist should be alert to the potential need for assistance with maintaining compliance (see Ch. 41). However, it is more usual for there to be some form of centralized control over prescribed medicines. Where this is used, there are two basic approaches to medicine administration. In direct administration, residents are given their medicine directly from the original pack by a suitably qualified member of staff. In redispensing, the dose is placed in a suitable container for the resident to take, often at a meal table. There are advantages and disadvantages of both methods, which are summarized in Table 40.1. Whichever method is

**Table 40.1 Comparison of the redispensing and direct administration methods of medicine administration in residential homes**

| Redispensing | Direct administration |
|---|---|
| Two-stage process | Single-stage process |
| Higher risk of error | Lower risk of error |
| Lower staff time | Higher staff time |
| Can be prepared in advance | Prepared with resident |
| Resident has to remember to take medicine | Resident told to take medicine |
| Consumption not seen | Consumption seen |
| Distribution is rapid | Distribution is slow |
| Little help available to resident | Help available to resident |

used, pharmacists should be prepared to give advice to ensure that, as far as possible, errors or omissions do not arise. Apart from the actual methods of administration to be used, this will require that adequate records are kept. In addition, it will also need to link with wider issues such as delivery, storage and disposal of medicines and the methods of stock control.

# PHARMACY SERVICE TO RESIDENTIAL HOMES

A number of issues arise, which will be dealt with individually, although they are interlinked.

## Documentation and recording

It is necessary to have some form of formal recording of medicines in a home for a number of reasons. These include the problems created by a large number of staff, often on shift work, use of relief staff and the large quantities of medicines that will be handled at any one time. In addition, the use of records will facilitate the smooth and effective operation of medicine administration. It is generally accepted that at least three types of record should be used. These are:

• A medicines record, which is used as a central record of ordering and receiving medicines. Its main function is in effective stock control to ensure that patients do not run out of medicines.
• The medication profile is a record for each patient. The information required will be the same as that on the patient's PMR (see Ch. 39) and may be computer generated. It will, therefore, include information such as allergies, in addition to details of current and past medicines.

• The administration record is used to record the giving of a medicine to a resident. Ideally this should be on the same sheet as the medication profile, so that checking the actual administration with the prescriber's instructions is facilitated. Many computer systems can produce these sheets. The time and nature of each dose administered are recorded and signed by the member of staff. Over time a complete profile is built up. This indicates the giving of the medicine, but can only guarantee its use where the member of staff gives it directly to the resident and sees that it is taken or used. Stories abound of dining room floors covered with assorted tablets after meals!

## Storage and control of medicines

Unless residents look after their own medicines, there will be a need to keep large quantities of medicines centrally. This must be in a manner which will avoid confusion, be secure and provide appropriate conditions for the storage of the medicines.

Two main types of storage are used – cupboards and medicine trolleys. Ideally a cupboard should be specially designed and lockable, although in some situations use of an existing cupboard may be appropriate. It is best if the key is kept by the person in charge. A cupboard should be large enough to allow good separation between different residents' medicines in order to avoid the risk of mixing them, but not large enough to encourage hoarding. Medicine trolleys should be stored in a room not normally accessible to residents and fastened to a fixed object when not in use. The storage conditions required for the medicine must also be considered (see Ch. 7). In particular there may be the need for refrigerator storage. It is not necessary to have a refrigerator dedicated to medicine storage in residential homes, but it must be lockable and medicines should be kept separate from other items in a mixed-use refrigerator. The temperature inside storage cupboards should be checked and the trolley storage point should not be near to a radiator. There is no need for special storage of controlled drugs, except in nursing homes which must comply with the Misuse of Drugs Act.

## Procedures for administering medicines

Ideally any procedures should apply to both prescribed and OTC medicines. It is important in designing them to minimize the possibility of errors being made. Key stages are summarized in Table 40.2. The method of administration chosen by a particular home will affect the ease with which some of these

**Table 40.2    Stages involved in the preparation of a medicine for administration to a patient**

1. Check the identity of the patient
2. Check the resident's medication record, especially ensuring that the dose has not already been given and noting any changes made by the doctor
3. Identify the medicine and check that the label has the resident's name and corresponds with the medication record
4. Administer the medicine, or place it in receptacle for giving to resident
5. Endorse the medication record immediately
6. Record any reason why a dose is not taken

can be carried out. The giving of medicines at meals is open to many problems. These include identification if residents sit in a different position, the person not being present, taking the medicines intended for a neighbour, not noticing or forgetting to take the medicine. More significantly, the times when a medicine is required to be administered may not correspond with meal times, for example when it is required half an hour before food. Such practical issues will need to be discussed by the pharmacist and resolved with the home administrators.

## Ordering and delivery of medicines

Apart from short-term treatments, most medicines used by residents in homes are supplied from repeat prescriptions. It is generally accepted that a 1-month supply is adequate. Ideally, home staff know when to order a repeat prescription from the medication profile of the patient and the stock level. This can be reinforced by agreement about the minimum stock level to allow adequate time for prescription preparation, collection, dispensing and delivery. Once agreed, a time for reordering can be marked on the administration record.

Occasionally awkward situations may arise, such as when there is an urgent need for a medicine, or where a delay means that a repeat medicine is required before a prescription is received. In the former situation the aim of the pharmacist must be to provide the medicine as quickly as possible – the same as for any patient. One way of speeding the process is for a responsible member of staff in the home to read the prescription over the telephone. The actual prescription can then be collected and checked by the pharmacist before the medicine is handed over. A speedy service in such situations is often quoted as one of the main benefits of a home being registered with a particular pharmacy.

When a request is received for a repeat medicine without a prescription a number of courses of action are open to the pharmacist. It could be that the staff are using the pharmacist as a 'first call', whereas a telephone call to the surgery could produce the prescription. A second option, after contacting the doctor, is to treat the request as a normal 'emergency supply'. Where the doctor cannot be contacted, the request would have to come from the resident and the pharmacist would need to be satisfied of the need. Finally, the pharmacist could refuse to supply the medicine if not satisfied as to the validity or accuracy of the request. Adequate records, such as the PMR (Ch. 39), will make reaching a decision easier.

## Disposal of unwanted medicines

Remaining medicine should be destroyed when a treatment is completed or discontinued, when it has passed its expiry date and when a resident has died. In the latter case, disposal should be left for 1 week in case the medicine is required by the coroner. Special attention must be paid to short expiry date medicines, such as eye drops. For these medicines a start of use date is also useful. The overall responsibility for the disposal of unwanted medicines should lie with the pharmacist and arrangements with the home must ensure that this occurs. Medicines must not be flushed down the toilet or put in the dustbin. The medicines record can be initialled by both pharmacist and responsible person in the home. In no situation should medicines be kept by the home for use by other residents.

## Regular visits by the pharmacist

Clearly, the putting in place of protocols for recording, administration, storage and disposal of medicines will require time being spent between the pharmacist and home administrators. How much time will be required will vary with the size, nature and needs of a particular home. However, the need for meetings is not over when this process is complete. Indeed, there is a requirement for regular visits, with appropriate records, as part of the remuneration package. At the simplest these visits are important to develop trust and goodwill. However, there are more important aspects to these visits, some of which have been mentioned already.

The pharmacist needs to check the records in the home on a regular basis, perhaps every 3 months. This helps ensure that residents are receiving the medication profile intended by their doctor, that the stock levels correspond with the entries in the medicines record and that any changes in treatment have been correctly introduced. At the same time, checks should be made of the expiry date of all medicines in stock and that all medicines in stock are in current use. This will enable the establishment of an awareness by the staff of the home of the importance of safe disposal of medicines when they are no longer needed and reduce the risk of errors in administration. It also helps to avoid the use of medicines for other residents. All these are routine matters but can be used as a focal point for discussion between the pharmacist and home staff about the safe and effective use of medicines and how to deal with any problems which may arise on a day-by-day basis. Using such an approach, any errors, or less than ideal practices, can be corrected in a relaxed and informal manner.

In addition, the pharmacist can use regular visits to develop other aspects of the service to the home. The pharmacist could assume a more clinical role by reviewing the medication profiles of patients. This can be particularly useful when a new resident enters a home. The process helps to identify problems arising with combinations of medicines, dosage form or selection of drug. Issues surrounding this are discussed in Chapters 31 and 32. Where problems are identified and corrected, the care of the resident is improved.

## Contact with residents

As with any patient receiving a dispensed medicine, residents are entitled to expect any questions about their medicines to be answered by a pharmacist. They should not be denied this because of the surroundings in which they live. Thus direct contact with residents can be made part of regular visits and could be especially useful when a person first takes up residence. It allows informal discussion, probably with more time available than in the normal community pharmacy situation. During this time it will be possible to answer questions and ask about any problems which the person is experiencing. The ideal is that a resident is counselled by the pharmacist each time there is a change of medication. As with any similar situation, the pharmacist can also make an assessment as to whether the patient might benefit from the use of a compliance aid (see Ch. 41). Likewise, the pharmacist can find out whether the patient is having other difficulties with the medicine, for example with swallowing a tablet, which might lead to a suggested change in dosage form or regimen. In homes where residents are allowed to use their own OTC medicines, the pharmacist can use this time to discuss the needs of the patient, respond to any symptoms and offer general advice.

## Staff training

In the preceding discussion, contact with staff in the home has, by implication, been limited to the senior, responsible personnel. These people may have qualifications and experience which enable them to appreciate easily what is being discussed. However, on a daily basis it is usually the less qualified or experienced carers who come in contact with the residents and who may have to operate the procedures for the administration of medicines. Thus it is important that all levels of staff in a home have an adequate level of knowledge and understanding about medicines and how to operate the agreed procedures. Thus there is a need for training which brings the staff up to a suitable level of proficiency by instruction or practice. This training is needed at the start and should then be maintained on an ongoing basis. Technically, this is the responsibility of the District Pharmaceutical Officer or Chief Administrative Pharmaceutical Officer. In practice, general training may be provided by the health authority or board, or be left to the community pharmacist to provide. Ongoing training is likely to be the responsibility of the pharmacist responding to the expressed needs of the staff as the relationship develops. There are a number of potential topics which are summarized in Table 40.3. The level at which the training takes place should match the ability and need of the staff to comprehend it. In general this means using language which would be suitable for the general public.

| Table 40.3 Summary of topics suitable for training sessions with staff of residential homes |
| --- |
| Administration procedures for medicines |
| Record keeping |
| Acquisition of medicines |
| Disposal of medicines |
| Storage of medicines |
| Types of pharmaceutical formulation |
| Handling of different types of medicine |
| Fate of drugs in the body |
| Side effects of drugs |
| Sources of information and the meaning of some technical words |
| Use of over-the-counter and household medicines |
| Differences in legal classification |
| Safe use of medicines |

## Operation of procedures

All staff who are going to give medicines to residents must understand the record-keeping system; why it is there, how to use it, how to check the medicine and dosage, and how to record that a dose has been given. Failure to appreciate the operation of the system and its importance will result in meaningless records and potential danger to the residents as the risks of confusion and error increase.

## The nature of medicines

Staff in homes should be aware of the different types of formulation used. This should then be developed to include an awareness of what should and should not be done with them. Thus, for example, with tablets staff need to be aware which tablets can be split or crushed and which cannot. With liquids, they need to know how to shake a bottle effectively and how to measure a dose accurately. With more specialized dosage forms, such as eye drops and inhalers, staff will need to know how to use them. Practical sessions spent handling products, or placebos, which are in current use in the home will be beneficial.

## Information sources

Some form of reference work should be available in each home. The BNF is a useful source, but the language is technical and may not be helpful to untrained staff. Thus, sessions in which terms are explained may be a useful way of increasing knowledge and encouraging their use.

## Drugs and their effects

It is useful that staff have an awareness of the basic concepts of pharmacokinetcs. This should not be advanced, but rather establish the concepts of absorption, metabolism and excretion. This can then be developed to give an appreciation of why different dosage regimens are used and why it is important to adhere to them. A further development of these ideas can be used to give an appreciation of side effects, why they arise and how they can be minimized. Both the kinetics and side effects can be taught using drugs which are used regularly in homes as examples.

## Other aspects of training

Home staff need to be aware of the legal restrictions on the supply of medicines, especially that they should not be given to residents other than the one for whom it was prescribed. It can also be useful in establishing that all prescription-only medicines, irrespective of their dosage form, must be treated with the same respect. The use of OTC medicines for trivial complaints can be discussed, together with advice on what to use and when to seek further advice. Also the use of household remedies and other related products can be addressed.

It should be remembered that training is best given on a little-and-often basis. Large blocks of information are unlikely to produce the desired effect.

# ADVICE FOR PHARMACISTS

The ultimate responsibility for the provision of pharmaceutical services to residential homes lies with the District Pharmaceutical Officer or Chief Administrative Pharmaceutical Officer. Depending on the local situation, the Community Services Pharmacist or equivalent may undertake the day-by-day management. This involves an inspection role. It may also include pharmacist training, draft protocols for pharmacists to use with homes and the provision of centrally organized training for home staff. In addition pharmacists can gain other guidance from various sources such as the Royal Pharmaceutical Society of Great Britain, the National Pharmaceutical Association and the Centres for Postgraduate or Postqualification Pharmaceutical Education (Distance Learning).

> ## Key Points
>
> - There has been a move of patients and their pharmaceutical needs into the community.
> - Pharmacies can contract to provide services to residential homes.
> - An aim should be to allow residents control of their medicines whenever possible.
> - Actually giving the medicine to the patient and supervising its correct use is one of the greatest problems in residential homes.
> - Direct administration is made by a qualified member of staff from the original pack to the patient.
> - Redispensing involves placing the medicine in a container for the resident to take.

- It is necessary to have adequate records of medicines in residential homes.
- Records which are normally kept are a medicines record, a medication profile and an administration record.
- Storage of medicines must be secure and well organized.
- Arrangements for ordering and delivery of medicines need to be agreed by pharmacist and home.
- Adequate pharmacy records will assist in responding to requests for emergency supply.
- Pharmacists must be responsible for safe disposal of all unwanted medicines.
- Regular visits by the pharmacist are required as part of a contract.
- Visits can be used to check medicine stocks and records, and discuss issues of concern.
- Pharmacists have an obligation to treat residents in the same way they would any other patient.
- There is a need to provide training for all levels of staff on topics such as procedures, the nature of medicines and their use.

## FURTHER READING

Anon 1990 Administration of drugs in residential homes. The Rivington Press, London

Pharmaceutical Society Working Party Report 1986 Administration and control of medicines in residential homes. Pharmaceutical Journal 236: 631–636

Royal Pharmaceutical Society of Great Britain and Age Concern 1989 Joint guidelines for the use of medicines in residential homes. RPSGB and Age Concern, London

Royal Pharmaceutical Society of Great Britain 1990 Pharmaceutical services to nursing homes. RPSGB, London

Secretary of State for Health, Social Security, Wales and Scotland 1989 Caring for people: community care in the next decade and beyond. HMSO, London

# 41
# Compliance

*A. J. Winfield*

> After studying this chapter you should know about:
>
> **Definitions of compliance and non-compliance**
> **The methods used to measure compliance**
> **Some of the causes of non-compliance**
> **Techniques for improving compliance.**

## Introduction

A dictionary definition of compliance is 'an action in accordance with a request or command'. In the context of medicines, the request comes from the doctor in prescribing a treatment regimen. Thus, patient compliance is the extent to which a patient takes or uses his medicine in accordance with the directions or follows the general health advice given by his doctor. The word 'compliance' has an implication of authority of the doctor over the patient. To avoid this 'adherence' or 'concordance' are used as an alternative.

Patients do not comply for a variety of reasons which will be discussed later. When this occurs it is called non-compliance or non-adherence and may be accidental or deliberate. Non-compliance is usually thought of as not taking a dose, but it could be taking it at the wrong time, or taking too much. It is also necessary to decide the level of deviation from the instructions that will be called non-compliance. There is no clear answer, although many who study the problem regard three out of four doses taken correctly as being compliance.

An ethical question is whether the patient should comply. In the late 20th century, the attitude is that it is for the patient to decide. In order to reach a rational decision, the patient requires sufficient knowledge and understanding. Thus, the pharmacist has an important role in ensuring that the patient has enough information in an understandable form. It must also be recognized that unused medicines represent a waste of NHS resources. One estimate suggests that, in the UK, more than 25% of medicines are not used at an annual cost of about £500 million.

Non-compliance is not a new phenomenon. Hippocrates, around 400 BC, warned of patients who 'lie about taking their medicines and refuse to confess when things go wrong'. Such secrecy means that there are no reliable methods for measuring compliance. Nevertheless, studies indicate a wide spread in the levels of compliance with an average in the range of 40–60% compliance. The factors which affect it will be discussed in more detail, along with methods which may be used to improve compliance.

## MEASUREMENT OF COMPLIANCE

A number of different methods for measuring compliance have been devised (see Table 41.1), but none is accurate. Some rely on the honesty of patients in reporting their own compliance, whilst others are intrusive and thereby alter the level of compliance which is being measured. Some of the methods are briefly discussed.

### Patient reports

The method relies on asking patients about their compliance. It is important that the question is asked in a non-judgemental way. Despite care with the use of words, there is a tendency for patients to exaggerate their compliance. However, some patients will deliberately indicate a poor level of compliance. This is called social non-compliance and can arise with, for example, lonely people in receipt of home visits. The patient report method assumes that the patients know how to take their medicine. Thus, they may think they are complying, but actually be misusing their medicine. A way of finding out about this is to

**Table 41.1  Methods of measuring compliance by patients with their prescribed medicines**

| Method | Comments |
| --- | --- |
| Patient reports | No observation, relies on patient. As reliable as any other method |
| Pill and bottle counts | No proof of consumption or timing |
| Body fluid tests | Only indicate short-term compliance, individual kinetics varies. Very invasive |
| Mechanical devices | Do not indicate taking of medicine. Indicate timing |
| Direct observation | Useful for checking technique. Impractical for routine use |
| Outcome measurement | Insensitive and makes assumptions. Clinical judgement is not reliable |
| Discussion | Talking to patients – may be best |

ask people to keep a diary of their medicine taking. This reduces any implied criticism and enables an assessment of compliance to the regimen to be made. It is, however, difficult to sustain diary keeping for long periods of time.

## Pill and bottle counts

The principle here is that a spot check is made to count the number of doses which have been removed from the container since the last check. Visits usually have to be prearranged, so alert patients can ensure that the correct number of doses are missing. No information about the timing of doses, or whether the dose was actually taken is obtained. It is invasive of a patient's privacy and time-consuming.

## Blood and urine tests

Concentrations of drug in blood or urine can be measured. With a knowledge of drug kinetics, an estimate of dosing can be made. There are a number of problems with this approach, not least being the invasion needed to obtain the samples for analysis. Usually samples are obtained on visits to clinics. However, it is well recognized that patients tend to become more compliant just prior to such visits. A second problem is that the half-life of drugs means that drug-taking behaviour can only be assessed over the last 48 hours at best. The one exception at present is the measurement of haemoglobin A1c (glycosylated haemoglobin) which gives a 5- to 6-week

history of insulin compliance. There is also interest in the possibility that drug laid down in hair could provide a record over a longer time span once analytical techniques are sufficiently sensitive. A third problem is that, because individual kinetics vary, answers can only be approximate.

## Mechanical devices

These were first used with eye drops. A device was built into the cap that recorded each inversion of the bottle, which was taken to indicate use. However, the bottle could have been deliberately inverted, accidentally inverted or a genuine attempt made to instill a drop which failed. Similar technology can be adapted to show the opening of bottle tops, but with similar reservations about interpretation.

## Direct observation

Medicine administration in residential homes (Ch. 40) and in hospitals could involve observing that the patient actually takes the medicine. In the domiciliary situation, this is impractical. It has been argued that in the care situation, the patient is being coerced into taking the medicine, rather than being allowed freedom of choice. However, direct observation is a useful tool when a level of skill is required in order to use a medicine successfully. This will arise with, for example, eye drops, various inhaler devices, use of buccal tablets. Here the method is being used to help give patients the skill to comply, rather than to measure their level of compliance.

## Outcome measurement and clinical judgement

In theory, if an effective drug is being taken correctly, there should be an observable improvement in the condition, which would not occur if there were poor compliance. There are a number of objections to this hypothesis. Firstly, the diagnosis may not be correct, secondly the drug may not be effective, thirdly the outcome may not be sensitive to small changes in compliance, and fourthly there may be other factors involved, such as socioeconomic pressures. Likewise, reliance on the clinical judgement of a doctor is unreliable. Studies have shown that, whilst doctors thought their patients had no problems with compliance, up to 70% of the same patients admitted non-compliance.

Apart from these formal methods, an impression of compliance may be formed from comments made by patients and from the frequency with which they present repeat prescriptions.

**Table 41.2   A summary of the main factors contributing to patient non-compliance**

| | |
|---|---|
| Understanding | Inability to read |
| | Intellectual ability |
| | Poor instructions |
| | Misunderstanding |
| | Confusion |
| Medicine management | Number of medicines |
| | Times of day to be taken |
| | Lifestyle issues |
| | Forgetfulness and confusion |
| Disease-related factors | Physical effects |
| | Vomiting and diarrhoea |
| | Progress of disease |
| | Asymptomatic diseases |
| | Prophylaxis |
| | Mental state |
| | Health beliefs |
| Physical limitations | Obtaining medicines |
| | Physical dexterity |
| | Dysphagia |
| Drug-related factors | Organoleptic properties |
| | Side effects |
| | Generic variations |
| | Religious factors |
| Other factors | Social and psychological |
| | Cost of prescriptions |
| | Confidence in the doctor and medicine |
| | Religious observances |
| | Help seeking |

## CAUSES OF NON-COMPLIANCE

There is an almost endless list of reasons why patients fail to comply. Table 41.2 lists the main groups of reasons. However, under each heading there are many complex reasons. Where an individual fails to comply, there may be several simultaneous factors. Some of the main reasons for non-compliance will be discussed in more detail.

## Understanding and comprehension

It appears that this is one of the most important reasons for non-compliance, but there are many aspects to it.

The patient may be unable to understand the instructions. Some people cannot read, others have poor eyesight, the writing may be too small, or the ink too faint. Understanding is impaired by the choice of language. If it is vague, confusion may arise. Instructions may be ambiguous, such as 'two tablets a day'. When patients are counselled, they may not be listening, may have a hearing difficulty, may have a problem with their educational level or their level of consciousness. They could also be suffering from mental confusion. With frail elderly patients, it may be a carer who collects the prescription, so that the pharmacist does not see the patient. Another difficulty is a failure to appreciate the need for, or use of, particular medicines. Such situations are common with asthma sufferers who are prescribed inhalers for both prophylaxis and relief.

## Medicine management

Some people are well organized. Such people will probably be able to manage their medicines. However, those who are less well organized may have difficulties with their medicines. The more different medicines the patient has, the more the problems increase. Likewise, the more complex the regimen, the worse will be compliance. Thus if all medicines are to be taken at the same time of day, compliance will be higher than if several different times throughout the day are used. Confusion can also arise over which medicine is which. These problems are increased where the patient is either confused or forgetful, both of which tend to increase with age. Since, in general, it is the elderly who require most medication, the incidence of non-compliance is higher in this group. However, problems are not confined to the elderly. Those in work may also have problems, for instance where tablets are expected to be taken regularly through the day with food, but the patient has very irregular meal times, or with dose administration in a working environment. Another problem is remembering whether a dose has been taken. Calendar packs are designed to help this process. However, they too can be confusing, depending on their layout, how they label the doses and how they accommodate differing starting days.

## Disease-related problems

Various aspects of a patient's state of health can influence compliance. The disease may simply interfere with the patient's ability to comply. Thus an arthritic may have problems opening a container, a skin condition may require application of a cream to a part of the body which the person cannot reach. A patient may be suffering from vomiting or diarrhoea, so that, despite taking a tablet, he may only gain a small benefit from it. A patient in pain is more likely to comply with analgesia because of the relief which it brings.

The attitude of the patient to the disease is also important. The more 'serious' and life threatening the patient regards it, the more likely he is to comply with its treatment. This is not universal. Some recent studies have shown, for example, that a high proportion of transplant patients fail to take the drugs used to prevent tissue rejection. Compliance is more critical in conditions such as diabetes and epilepsy, where small fluctuations in drug plasma concentration are required for effective control.

The reaction of patients to the progress of their disease is also important. A common example is of patients prescribed a 1-week or 10-day course of antibiotics who stop taking their medicine after a few days because they are better. Patients may also stop because they do not perceive any improvement in their condition. This is a particular problem with asymptomatic conditions such as glaucoma and high blood pressure. The patient does not feel unwell at the start and so sees no improvement, and may even feel worse. A similar situation arises with prophylactic medication, for example with anti-malarials, where the individual may see no advantage in taking a medicine with its associated risks. Some patients may overuse a medicine to 'complete' a cure, such as using topical corticosteroids in some skin conditions.

The state of mind of the patient will also have an impact on compliance. The psychological state of an individual can markedly affect his or her compliance, although the effect is not necessarily predictable. Depression, distress, tension and aggression can reduce people's motivation towards taking their medicines. However, the effect may be reversed, with the patient coming to rely on medicines, almost as a ritual. Some of the factors which affect patients' reactions to disease and treatment have been discussed in Chapter 2 and are relevant here. Anything about their beliefs or perceptions which supports medicine taking, will improve compliance. On the contrary, factors which undermine people's confidence or belief in the medical service in general, will increase their non-compliance. Thus attitudes to the 'sick role' and health beliefs are going to be important in compliance.

## Physical limitations

A number of factors are important under this heading. One aspect is how easy the patient finds it to either obtain a repeat prescription or have it dispensed. Distance, particularly where the patient has limited access to transport or lives in a rural area, can be a major problem. Hills can also be difficult for some elderly people. Access to surgeries and pharmacies may be a problem for people working long hours or difficult shift patterns.

Physical dexterity is required for administering some medicines. Eye drops are the most obvious, where the patient requires to tilt the head, squeeze on a small bottle and aim accurately a short distance from the eye in order to successfully instill a drop. Many find this very difficult or impossible. Inhaler devices, especially pressurized aerosols, require coordination between fingers and breathing which many either find difficult or require training in order to achieve. Other dosage forms may also present some problems, including injections, ointments and creams, suppositories and pessaries, skin 'patches', buccal tablets. Very small tablets can present handling problems for people with arthritic fingers, because they do not have the fineness of movement required to pick them up.

Dysphagia, a difficulty in swallowing, is often overlooked, but is a problem for many, not just in certain medical conditions (such as stroke and parkinsonism) where it is recognized. Many people will indicate a problem in swallowing large tablets. There also appears to be a minimum size of tablet, below which swallowing also becomes difficult. In severe dysphagia, swallowing thin liquids will be a problem, often leading to aspiration of the liquid.

## Drug-related problems

The medicines themselves can also create compliance problems. Side effects of a drug, particularly if unpleasant, may deter the patient, although the effect is minor if the patient believes that the medicine is helping him. Some have argued that non-compliance is an advantage in that it protects the patient from adverse effects. In the past, taste, smell and colour were problems which could reduce compliance. With improved technology, most medicines can be flavoured and coloured to avoid the problems. However, a related problem arises with colour, size and shape, where generic products are being used. Since there is no standardization on colour, size and shape, patients may get tablets which are different in appearance each time a prescription is dispensed. This can produce uncertainty, confusion, even a rejection of the tablets, with a consequent effect on compliance.

Religious beliefs can also affect compliance because of materials used in medicines. Examples include the use of alcohol in medicines for Muslims, porcine insulin for Jews and gelatin for Hindus. In addition people of some cultures may associate disease with spiritual causes and not see the relevance of physical treatments.

## Other factors

Because of their complexity, there are many other factors which may affect a particular individual. One of the most often quoted over recent years, has been the impact of prescription charges. Since each item incurs a substantial charge, there are many reports of patients asking the pharmacist which is the more important item. A less obvious consequence of this is that patients may try to make a medicine last longer by 'rationing' their doses, say to one or two per day instead of the three prescribed.

Social and psychological influences on patients will be important (see Ch. 2). Of particular importance is the level of confidence which patients have in the doctor. If confidence is low, they are less likely to comply, because they will also doubt the effectiveness of the treatment. Conversely, if they have a very high level of confidence, they may tend to over-comply if there is no improvement. Related to this is the confidence of patients in the drug which has been prescribed. From their own experience, or, more commonly from neighbours or publicity, they form an impression of the efficacy of a drug. In some situations, doctors can come under extreme pressure to prescribe particular drugs because of magazine articles or the neighbourhood 'grapevine'. If these influences are positive, compliance will be enhanced. If they are unfavourable, it can become a self-fulfilling prophecy, where the patient 'knows' it will not work, has poor compliance and so does not improve.

People have different beliefs about medicines. Many see them as beneficial and helpful. Others regard them as poisons to be used as a last resort. This attitude has led, amongst other influences, to the present interest in alternative therapies such as homoeopathy (see Appendix 6). People with such attitudes will take medicines reluctantly, often with poor compliance.

Some patients feel that they are being used as guinea pigs when they are prescribed a medicine. They are, therefore, sceptical about the medicine and its potential benefit to them. As a result, compliance is reduced, particularly if there is no immediate improvement.

There can be situations when people quite deliberately do not comply because of the effect non-compliance will have. One example was mentioned earlier, where people living on their own come to rely on a visit by a member of the health care team for their only social contact. An improvement in their condition could result in their loss of that visit. Another example can arise with mentally ill people who prefer to live in a hospital rather than the community. If they do not comply, their condition will be assessed as being unsuitable for community living.

Finally under this heading, the impact of religious observance must be remembered. Perhaps the most significant is the Muslim observation of Ramadan, where medicine should not be taken between dawn and dusk throughout the month. Less significant in its impact may be short-term fasting or an unwillingness to take any food in a morning before a ritual has been completed.

## IMPROVING COMPLIANCE

The foregoing section has reviewed briefly some of the main factors which influence the compliance of an individual patient. The point has already been made that, ultimately, the patient has the right not to comply. However, it may be regarded as a professional responsibility to try to persuade the patient of the benefit of compliance, before accepting the situation. The following section considers some of the many techniques which the pharmacist can use to achieve this.

### Understanding and comprehension

The aim is to ensure as a high a level of understanding by the patient as possible. This means that optimum communication skills must be used. Orally, this will come from counselling patients (see Chs 3 and 37). This may simply involve passing on relevant information to the patient. However, the pharmacist needs to be alert to indications of the patient's health beliefs. If these are at variance with fact, an attempt may be required to correct the error.

Apart from routine counselling, it may be necessary to give additional information to fill in gaps in understanding following the patient's consultation with the doctor. Alternatively, it could be providing information about the disease, the drug, lifestyle advice or giving training in using the medicine. Where a patient relies on a carer, it is advisable to involve the carer in any counselling or other advice which is being given.

Along with verbal communication, written information is supplied. Labels must be clear, easy to read and unambiguous. Where necessary, large-print labels can be produced by some computers, and Braille labels are available for a limited range of instructions. Other written information must be in non-technical language to make it readily understood.

Compliance charts may also be useful and are discussed below.

## Medicine management

When compliance aids are discussed, it is usually those designed to assist medicine management which are thought of first. The aim of any actions taken is to assist patients to manage their medicine taking. There are three main approaches which can be tried. A diary of the day, indicating on it the times at which each medicine should be taken is the simplest form of compliance chart. Colour coding may be used to link the medicine bottle and chart. Computers can assist in producing these charts. Marking the chart as each dose is taken assists in preventing readministration.

Compliance aids can be used. There is a wide range of different designs of memory aid devices. Monitored dosage systems can be used as an alternative. The principle on which they all operate is that compartments are used to hold doses, each compartment corresponding to a time of day. The patient works through the device as the day progresses, removal of the medicine indicating that it has been remembered. Audible devices are available, but are more expensive. There can be some problems. Errors may be made in filling the aid, there are questions about the stability of some medicines in these devices and some patients may have difficulty getting the tablets or capsules out of the compartments. Liquids are much more difficult to handle using these aids. Table 41.3 lists some of the main compliance aids and monitored dosage systems available.

The third possibility is to review the medicines to see if the regimen can be simplified to make it easier to manage. Thus the use of sustained-release dosage forms reduces dosage frequency and combination dosage forms reduce the total number to be taken.

## Disease-related problems

Careful counselling can answer many of the problems which arise from a lack of understanding about the disease and its treatment. This can be particularly important with asymptomatic conditions or prophylactic treatments. Where the disease has reduced the manipulative ability of the patient, some compliance aids or other simple measures may be useful.

**Table 41.3** Compliance aids and monitored dosage systems which will assist patients to remember to take their medicines

| | |
|---|---|
| Compliance aids | Beehive |
| | Daily Pillminder |
| | Dispensatab |
| | Dosett |
| | Medidos |
| | Mediset Mini |
| | Mediwheel (and week pack) |
| | Medsystems (and week pack) |
| | Pico |
| | PillMill |
| | Redidos |
| | Weighand-Bulach |
| Monitored dosage systems | Compliapack |
| | MDS |
| | Nomad |
| | Park-Pak |
| | Ventalink |
| | W+W |

The simplest is to suggest non-child-resistant closures for some elderly patients. Larger bottles can be used to make handling easier. Devices are available to get tablets from blister packs, which many arthritics find particularly difficult. A long-armed roller is available to assist applying ointments and creams to parts of the skin which are difficult to reach.

## Physical limitations

Many compliance aids have been developed to assist people use their medicines. The main groups are shown in Table 41.4. Different aids can contribute in different ways, so selection needs to be made to meet the specific needs of the patient. For example, there are different types of aids to help with eye drops. Some help with aim only, others with aim and squeezing. For pressurized inhalers the 'Haleraid' helps squeeze and various spacer devices are available, or it may be more appropriate to change to a breath-activated delivery device. Small tablets are a problem for those with limited movement in their fingers, but the Tiltab tablet shape can help.

Where dysphagia is a problem, an alternative dosage form or route of administration may be the best option. When tablets must be used, they may need to be crushed and suspended in liquid or semisolid. Care is needed to ensure that the tablet is not designed to give any type of modified release. In all cases, very thin liquids are best avoided to reduce the danger of aspiration. Adopting an upright position is

**Table 41.4 Compliance aids available to help patients overcome specific problems of medicine use or administration**

| | |
|---|---|
| External preparations | Mediderm applicator |
| Eye drops | Autodrop and Autosqueeze<br>Easidrop<br>Opticare-2 |
| General | Medicine bottle opener<br>MedTime Minder (audible) |
| Inhalers | Haleraid<br>Spacers |
| Liquids | Ezydose and other non-spill spoons<br>Oral syringes<br>Rotadose (liquid dispenser) |
| Tablets | Pill-out (foil and blister pack tablet remover)<br>Tablet crushers<br>Tablet splitters |

advisable and small changes in head and neck position can be of considerable help.

## Drug-related problems

Many community pharmacists find it difficult to obtain generics for dispensing which are always consistent in appearance. Thus it may not be possible to reduce the problems which arise from changes of colour, shape and size, other than by reassuring the patient. Where some control is possible, the use of the PMR to record the source of tablets dispensed for an individual will reduce these variations to a minimum (see Ch. 39). Control of side effects may require a change in prescription. However, it is sometimes possible to modify the method of taking a medicine to reduce the problems such as avoiding tablets on an empty stomach to reduce the incidence of nausea. Where ingredients would be unacceptable to some patients, it is necessary for the pharmacist to be aware of the problem and to be in a position to suggest alternative products where possible.

## Other problems

Pharmacists cannot alter the cost of NHS prescriptions. However, they can ensure that all those exempt charges are claiming exemption, and they should be alert to situations where it is cheaper to purchase a non-POM medicine. Where patients are not having all their medicines dispensed, a discussion with the doctor might be useful to see if rational priorities can be established.

There are no simple answers to many of the other sociological and psychological factors which affect compliance. Depending on their nature, effective counselling by the pharmacist may assist with improving compliance. In other situations it may require a concerted effort by the whole health care team to help patients understand their treatment and the personal value of compliance for them.

Compliance can be a very difficult problem which may go undetected. When non-compliance is recognized, the pharmacist is in a good position to offer support to the patient. The approach should be to attempt to remove obvious barriers to compliance first, for example by suggesting compliance aids, drawing up compliance charts or instructing in the method of administration. For many, this will be adequate. Others will have remaining problems, where a range of techniques may be required. Some patients will always be poor compliers, but many can be helped towards effective use of their medicines.

---

**Key Points**

- Non-compliance may be accidental or deliberate.
- Untaken medicine costs the NHS a lot of money each year.
- No method for measuring compliance is accurate, although many have been devised.
- There is an almost limitless list of reasons for non-compliance, reflecting a complex interplay of factors.
- One of the main reasons for non-compliance is a lack of understanding or comprehension about the medicine and how to use it.
- Poor medicine management is a problem with many, especially when they are on complex regimens.
- Compliance levels may be affected by the disease.
- Physical limitations can have a marked effect on compliance in some situations.
- Increasing understanding and comprehension can increase compliance.
- It may be necessary to counsel a carer rather than the patients about medicine taking.
- Compliance charts and aids may help some patients who are trying but failing to comply.

- Whilst useful for some, compliance aids must be selected to meet the specific needs of the patient.
- Pharmacists must be alert to problems which may arise from the cost of medicine and take appropriate action.
- Some patients will always be poor compliers.

## FURTHER READING

Clepper I 1992 Noncompliance: the invisible epidemic. Drug Topics (Aug 17): 44,45,49,50,56,59,60,62,65
Ley P 1988 Communicating with patients. Croom Helm, London
Rivers P H 1992 Compliance aids – do they work? Drug Therapy 2: 103–111
Roberts K 1987 Compliance. Pharmacy Update (March): 90,92,94–96,98–100

# 42

# Substance misuse and harm reduction

*A. J. Winfield and E. J. Kennedy*

---

After studying this chapter you will know about:

**The potential for harm in drug use**
**Substances which are deliberately misused, including**:
    Over-the-counter medicines
    Prescription-only medicines
    Materials derived from plants and other chemicals
    Everyday consumables
**The particular dangers of misuse of drug by injection**
**The concept of harm reduction**
**The pharmacist's role in harm reduction, in particular with**:
    Nicotine-replacement therapy
    Syringe and needle exchange
    Methadone.

---

## Introduction

There is a potential danger in the use of any drug. These dangers come from many possible sources. The main sources are:

- *Incorrect diagnosis*. If the wrong diagnosis has been made, then the drug prescribed may do more harm than good.
- *Incorrect choice of drug*. Even if the diagnosis is correct, the choice of a particular drug for a particular patient is important, for example care is required for an asthmatic patient receiving a beta-blocker. Other examples of the issues involved are discussed in Chapters 31, 32 and 34 and in Walker & Edwards (1994).
- *Side effects*. These are possible with all drugs. The more severe they are, the more the potential harm. However, their incidence may also be idiosyncratic and unpredictable and so be unavoidable.
- *Over-compliance*. If the patient takes too much

of the medicine, whether by accident or on purpose there is the potential for harm. This is discussed in Chapter 41.

- *Inappropriate use*. Patients may misunderstand the purpose or effect of a drug, or they may pass their medicine on to other people in the mistaken belief that it will help other conditions.
- *Deliberate misuse*. Unfortunately, because of the effects which some drugs produce, there are individuals who choose to use drugs to give pleasurable sensations. Some of these drugs are habit forming, others are addictive. Both can cause very real problems for the people using them.

The inadvertent harm resulting from the legitimate use of drugs is a clinical problem and is outside the scope of this book. The unnecessary or inappropriate use of drugs, as for example the excessive consumption of analgesics or vitamins, will not be considered in detail. The deliberate misuse of drugs is the subject of this chapter. It will review some of the substances which are misused, consider the problems which result and address the ways in which the pharmacist can be involved in minimizing harm.

---

## SUBSTANCES WHICH ARE MISUSED

There have been many reviews on the subject in the literature and a series of articles in *The Pharmaceutical Journal* in 1993 and 1994 by Wills is a useful introduction. It should also be remembered that, apart from producing a 'high' or 'buzz' or 'fix', misuse may occur for a number of other reasons. The drugs used will generally have an effect on the central nervous system, producing either a stimulation ('upper') or depression ('downer'). They may be used by some people to complement each other. Thus, for example, a 'downer' may be used to help a person return to 'normal' after using 'uppers'. For convenience, the materials misused will be considered under a number of different headings.

## Over-the-counter medicines

There are a surprising number of 'safe' over-the-counter medicines which can be misused. Pharmacists must be aware of what these are and the reasons for misuse, so that they can intervene if necessary.

Aspirin has been reported to produce some intoxicating effects at very high doses. Paracetamol has been used, also at high dose, to induce vomiting in people with eating disorders. A number of opioid drugs are available in over-the-counter (OTC) medicines. Abuse of codeine linctus is well known. Other medicines which contain opioids are shown in Table 42.1 together with the drug concerned.

Dextromethorphan is chemically similar to the opioids, but has a different mechanism of action producing different effects. As a cough suppressant it is used in a range of medicines, but has been subject to abuse. A wide range of antihistamines is available over the counter, but only two are documented as open to abuse. These are cyclizine and dimenhydrinate. Cyclizine, available as Valoid and also in some prescription-only medicines (POM) such as Migril and Diconal, appears to enhance the effects of opioids. Given intravenously it produces exhilaration and hallucinations. Dimenhydrinate, in Dramamine, is most often abused by anorexic patients wanting to produce vomiting. Ephedrine, pseudoephedrine, phenylephrine and phenylpropanolamine are all sympathomimetics widely used in cold treatments. They produce amphetamine-like responses if taken in large doses.

Laxatives are most often abused by patients with eating disorders or bowel obsession. Bulimic and anorexic patients use laxatives to prevent weight gain.

Bowel obsession is a condition, often amongst older people, in which they wish to defecate regularly at the same time, or to produce a stool of a particular consistency. Long-term use of laxatives produces a reliance on them and the use of ever-increasing doses. As a consequence, there can be severe damage of the colon, constipation and faecal impaction.

## Prescription medicines

A number of prescription-only medicines are subject to deliberate misuse. These include not only the obvious amphetamines, opioids, benzodiazepines and anabolic steroids, but also antimuscarinic agents, barbiturates and anaesthetics.

The opioids are the most widely known drugs of abuse and also carry the greatest consequences for the person using them. Heroin is the most widely used and has various names such as 'junk', 'H', 'smack'. Most is made for the illicit market and is diluted ('cut') with many different powders. Other common opioids are dipipanone (as Diconal, which also includes cyclizine), buprenorphine and methadone. Most opioids are still taken orally, but because of the slow onset and reduced effect due to metabolism, some people prefer to use other routes. Heroin can also be inhaled ('snorted'), heated and the vapour inhaled ('chasing the dragon') or smoked ('reefers'). All give a more rapid and intense sensation than the oral route. The intravenous (i.v.) route is said to produce a rapid sense of euphoria. The use of tablets or cut powders, which may contain insoluble material, to prepare non-sterile injections can have serious consequences for the user. These include damage to blood vessels, abscess formation and severe infection.

Apart from the dangers arising from potential overdose, adverse reactions to the drug, or injection site damage, the main problem is dependence. This has two clear elements, receptor tolerance leading to increasing dosage, and physical dependence. The latter gives rise to withdrawal symptoms. The pharmacist's possible input with opioid misusers is discussed later in the chapter.

Cocaine misuse is on the increase. Crystalline cocaine hydrochloride has been extracted from coca leaves as abuse has spread. On the street it is known as 'coke', 'snow' or 'blow'. It is usually taken by inhaling it through a small tube into the nose – called 'snorting'. 'Crack' is the alkaloid base. This has a greater chemical stability and so can be smoked or heated to produce a vapour which is inhaled. Injection is less common. The effects of cocaine are relatively short-lasting (up to an hour orally), so

| Table 42.1 Some of the over-the-counter medicines which contain opioids | |
|---|---|
| Medicine | Drug |
| Codeine linctus | Codeine phosphate |
| Gee's linctus | Camphorated opium tincture |
| Kaolin and morphine mixture | Morphine tincture |
| Collis Browne's mixture | Opium liquid extract |
| Dimotane Co (and paediatric) | Codeine phosphate |
| Terpoin | Codeine phosphate |
| Codis, Panadeine, Solpadeine | Codeine phosphate |
| Paramol | Dihydrocodeine |

**Table 42.2 Amphetamines which are commonly misused, together with street names**

| Drug name | Street name(s) |
|---|---|
| Amphetamine | Speed, whizz, Uppers |
| Methylamphetamine | Ice |
| 3,4-methylenedioxymethamphetamine | Ecstacy |
| Diethylpropion | |
| Phenteramine | |
| Methylphenidate | |
| Pemoline | |

repeated use of the drug often occurs. Cocaine taken as the base appears to have a very high addiction rate, although there is debate as to whether this is a true addiction.

Amphetamine and its derivatives, some of which are not now used therapeutically, are abused. The drugs, with their common names, are listed in Table 42.2. As with the opioids, they may be taken orally, by nasal inhalation, smoking or by injection.

The hallucinogenic drug LSD (lysergic acid diethylamide – street name 'acid' or 'trips') has never been established as a therapeutic agent although it was studied as a possible psychotherapeutic agent. When abused it is taken orally as tablets or on pieces of blotting paper, gelatin or sugar cubes to produce euphoria and psychedelic effects. Phencyclidine, which has similar, though shorter-lasting, effects has not been as widely abused.

The benzodiazepines are the most widely abused of the regularly prescribed drugs. This abuse takes different forms. They are abused by inappropriate and overprescribing, which has resulted in many patients becoming dependent on them. There are now guidelines designed to reduce the prescribing of these agents and assist in the withdrawal of patients who have become dependent. The second form of abuse is on the street, where intravenous administration is often used. Temazepam is the most commonly abused of these drugs. It was available as a liquid-filled soft gelatin capsule, the contents of which were easily removed and injected. In 1990, the liquid was replaced with a gel in an attempt to reduce this practice. However, they were still used and the macrogol gelling agent caused many serious clinical problems in those misusing the capsules. In 1996 they were withdrawn.

Anabolic steroids have been subject to increasing abuse in recent years. Originally used by athletes, abusers now include body builders, weight trainers and those who feel that they produce a more desir-able physical appearance. Both oral dosage and intramuscular injections are used. 'Pyramid' and 'stacking' regimens are used to minimize the side effects of use.

The abuse of barbiturates has declined markedly in recent years. Other occasional misuse may be found with antimuscarinic agents, such as benzhexol and orphenadrine. It is a matter of history that many volatile anaesthetics were abused. Nitrous oxide is recognized as being addictive, ketamine has been used orally, halothane, cyclopropane and enflurane have been reported as being misused.

## Plants

Drugs already mentioned such as cocaine and morphine are derived from plants. However, some plants are used without extraction of the active ingredient. This is known to have happened for at least 10 000 years. Perhaps the plant which is at the centre of most debate is cannabis. The active constituents are within the resin, although different forms of the plant are used. 'Marijuana' is the dried and crushed flowers and leaves. 'Hashish' is the resin separated from the plant, whilst 'hash oil' is concentrated resin. It is usually taken by smoking marijuana or by mixing the resin with tobacco. The resulting cigarettes are called 'reefers' or 'joints'. A pipe may be used or it may be taken orally. Stopping cannabis after regular high-dose use can produce withdrawal symptoms, although psychological rather than physical dependence is more common.

In the UK there are about 12 species of wild mushrooms which contain psychoactive compounds. They are often referred to as 'magic mushrooms' although the name is also used for *Psilocybe semilanceata* in particular. The alkaloids in this mushroom produce effects ranging from relaxation and euphoria to hallucinations depending on the quantity taken. One of the main dangers in the use of mushrooms is incorrect identification. There are many toxic mushrooms that look very similar to both edible ones and those which contain psychoactive alkaloids.

A number of other plants are reported as being abused occasionally. Nutmeg contains amphetamine-like ethers. When eaten, smoked, inhaled or vapourized, nutmeg can produce similar reactions. Also related to amphetamine is mescaline, in the peyote cactus and cathine in *Catha edulis*. Morning glory seeds contain D-lysergic acid amide, which is closely related to LSD. Weaker effects may be found with betel ('nut' or 'leaf'), ginseng and members of the Solanaceae family such as mandrake, henbane, datura and deadly nightshade.

## Other chemicals

This heading is used to describe volatile substance abuse and the so-called 'smart drugs'. In 'glue sniffing' or 'solvent misuse' volatile solvents are inhaled. This practice is often associated with children and teenagers from the lower socioeconomic groups. A wide range of materials may be used. These include glues, paints and thinners, correction fluids, cleaning fluids, stain removers, nail varnish remover, lighter fuel, bottled gases, aerosol propellants, petrol, butyl nitrite, marker pens. The fumes are inhaled from a closed or confined space, such as a polythene bag, often by rebreathing in order to increase the effect. Occasionally, and dangerously, the solvent may be sprayed directly down the throat.

The so-called 'smart drugs' are generally described as being able to increase learning ability and enhance other higher functions such as memory and concentration. Some would argue that they are not drugs of abuse, and it is certainly a difficult ethical area. Many of these materials started as diet supplements, but now some POMs are also used. The review by Wills (1994b) gives a good introduction to some of the materials and the issues involved.

## Everyday consumables

These are caffeine, tobacco and alcohol. Tobacco is the dried leaf of the plant *Nicotiana tabacum* which contains nicotine. Smoking is the usual way of using tobacco, although it can be chewed or the powder inhaled. Smoking often begins in teenage years and the reasons for starting to smoke are many and varied. The effects of nicotine can be very rapid – within about 7 seconds of inhaling it reaches the brain – producing a sense of relaxation and relief of tension. Although tobacco has been used in Europe for about 400 years, it is only in the past few decades that the harm which it can cause has been recognized. Lung cancer is the best known, but cancers of the mouth, pharynx, larynx, oesophagus, bladder and pancreas are also caused by tobacco, and it is implicated in stomach, liver and cervical cancers and adult leukaemia. It also affects airways, cardiovascular and digestive system morbidity. Nicotine causes physical dependence which, together with a negative reinforcement arising from a fear of withdrawal symptoms, makes stopping smoking very difficult.

Alcohol, which has been available for a long time is, of course, consumed orally in a variety of different drinks. In the UK the actual alcohol concentrations of these are controlled within set limits which can be as high as 55% for some spirits. Intoxication with alcohol is implicated in many accidents (road, pedestrian, at work and home) and violent crime. Long-term damage can include cirrhosis, hepatitis, liver cancer, pancreatitis, neuropathy and cardiac disease. Death can result from concentrations in the blood of 3–4 g/l. Alcohol can induce physical dependence. Withdrawal symptoms may be severe, often leading to relapse.

Caffeine is present in tea, coffee, cocoa, chocolate and cola-drinks at concentrations of up to 2.5%. A number of medicines, herbal products and stimulants also contain caffeine. It is, therefore, probably the most widely used psychoactive material. After drinking, caffeine reaches a peak concentration in the blood after 15–45 minutes. In the brain it acts as a stimulant. As the dose increases, so do the side effects of headache, anxiety, tremor and insomnia. There are no diseases clearly linked to the use of caffeine, but a dose of 5–10 g is usually fatal. Physical dependence on caffeine is shown by tolerance to its effects, especially diuresis, and specific withdrawal symptoms including headache, anxiety, restlessness, lethargy, poor concentration and antisocial behaviour. In addition there is a social dependence. Unlike some other forms of dependence, there does not appear to be a tendency to increase the amount consumed. However, it is generally advised that caffeine consumption should be kept to moderate levels.

## DANGER OF MISUSE BY INJECTING

The spread of HIV has been linked to the sharing of needles used for intravenous drug administration. The virus is sufficiently robust to survive on contaminated needles. Injecting drugs is often a social event where sharing equipment may be part of the ritual of preparing the injection. Thus the danger of spreading the disease is increased, especially when needles and syringes are difficult to obtain. The practice of sharing is decreasing as a result of information campaigns and supplies being made available. The role of pharmacists in this is discussed on page 457. However, this is not the only danger associated with i.v. drug use. There is a far higher risk of transmission of hepatitis B than there is of HIV. More recently, hepatitis C has been highlighted as being a greater danger because it can be transmitted by sharing crockery, cutlery and other equipment used in preparing the injections. Street drugs are seldom pure. Dealers 'cut' them with diluents which may be soluble and inert, or insoluble and toxic. Where tablets and capsules are used as the source of the drug, excipients in the formulation may be included in the injection. In both situations, solid matter may be injected intravenously in a non-sterile solution. Particles can block capillaries and small veins. Infections can arise leading to abscess formation. There are many reports of severe damage to limbs, amputation, even death, from such practices. Some steps which can be taken to minimize the harm are discussed later in the chapter.

## HARM REDUCTION

Whilst ideally there should be no drug misuse, it has to be acknowledged that there will be persons who will misuse drugs. There are many reasons for this, some of which have been mentioned in the earlier description of the drugs. Physical and psychological addiction or dependence are major factors. There are also social and psychological factors that can be very strong. Because of the illicit nature of much drug misuse, those who participate tend to live in a separate social environment. Their friends are around them, they may be involved in criminal activities to support the habit, and may be under peer pressure not to change. Ritual becomes an important part of their life, making it more difficult to move away from what they see as secure and known. Thus to stop misusing a drug, especially where there is a physical dependence, will be very difficult. It will probably require external help. Before this is sought, and in order to see it through, the user will require a 'change of mind' to give the psychological determination to change lifestyle and all that goes with it. Even when that happens, the process will take time, and many will relapse and have to start again. The so-called 'cycle of change', described by Prochaska & DiClemente, has been discussed in Chapter 2.

There was a policy that no drug misuse should be tolerated – the so-called 'zero tolerance' approach. However, it is clear from the short discussion above, that this is a simplistic approach. The misuser may be unable to stop even if he or she wishes to do so. As a consequence, the idea of 'harm reduction' developed. The principle behind harm reduction is to provide help to reduce as far as possible the adverse effects of drug misuse until the user has decided, or is able, to stop using the drug. Thus it is a practical rather than theoretical approach to the problem. Some people, for good ethical reasons, have reservations about this approach because it could be seen as sanctioning drug misuse.

One of the difficulties with the term 'harm reduc-

tion' is that it can mean different things to different people. Thus it could mean:

- reducing the harmful effects without reducing the consumption of the drug
- taking any steps necessary to reduce harm, including a reduction in consumption
- taking stringent steps to eliminate all illicit drugs.

It is the first of these which is gaining in acceptance. In 1993 the World Health Organization adopted such an approach, citing examples of needle exchange and nicotine patches. The United Nations International Drug Control Programs, in 1994, concluded that 'While ridding the world of drug abuse remains a central objective, it is a long-term goal. Therefore, the most useful short-term outlook should aim to contain the immediate threat to society'.

From this it is suggested that there are three aspects to harm reduction:

- The user's decision to use drugs is accepted, but not necessarily approved of.
- The user is treated as a normal human being, providing he or she behaves responsibly
- Harm reduction is neutral regarding longer-term goals.

### The pharmacist's role in harm reduction

Pharmacists have become increasingly involved in a number of measures, some introduced by government, which attempt to reduce harm to drug misusers. These have usually been concerned with opioid drugs and intravenous use. In addition, there are other measures which may be helpful, but which are not at present encouraged. The main schemes – syringe and needle exchange and methadone prescribing – which most closely involve pharmacists are considered below after nicotine-replacement therapy has been briefly discussed.

### Nicotine-replacement therapy

Stopping smoking can be very difficult owing to both the social and behavioural contexts of smoking and the physical dependence on the nicotine. The latter can be relieved by using some form of nicotine-replacement therapy. Different forms are available, including gums and patches. These may be prescribed on private prescription or they can be purchased over the counter. They are capable of providing nicotine in a reasonably controlled way to replace that which is not being obtained from cigarettes. However, many smokers who try to stop still fail, perhaps because of social and behavioural factors. Pharmacists and counter assistants have a role to play in supporting their clients and giving encouragement. It has been shown that just keeping records of the sales on the patient medication record encourages the client. If this is extended by giving continued counselling, there are demonstrable improvements in the success rate of smoking cessation. A more detailed coverage of this topic is given in Chapter 38.

## Syringe and needle exchange

Intravenous drug misusers require syringes and needles, called 'works'. Until 1982, community pharmacists were able to sell needles and syringes on request. Whilst these were expected to be for diabetics needing them for their insulin injections, drug misusers were not prevented from buying them. Because of the ethical concerns that this raised, in 1982 the Royal Pharmaceutical Society of Great Britain (RPSGB) recommended that needles and syringes should only be sold to known diabetics. As a result intravenous misusers found it very difficult to obtain the necessary equipment. This led to misusers sharing what equipment was available, and also intensified the social and cultural context of the misuse. During this time it also emerged that sharing needles increased the transmission of HIV and contributed to the increase in cases of AIDS. In 1986, the RPSGB withdrew its recommendation. In the same year, the first needle exchange scheme in the UK was set up. Government-sponsored pilot studies were undertaken to evaluate whether such schemes could reduce the transmission of HIV. The positive conclusion led to the setting up of a large number of such schemes. Pharmacists were also allowed to sell needles and syringes to misusers. Most needle exchange schemes were operated from specialized centres dealing with drug misusers. In 1992, the UK Government introduced a needle exchange scheme operated through contracted community pharmacists, which was free to the misusers. Pharmacists would receive payment for their participation.

The stated aims of the move were given as follows:

*1. To provide access to sterile injecting equipment to determined or potential injecting substance misusers with anonymity, dignity, and professional responsibility.*
*2. To remove contaminated sharp waste from the environment at approximately the same rate as it is generated.*
*3. To provide appropriate educational material,*

| Table 42.3 Practical aspects of needle and syringe exchange schemes |
| --- |
| • Supply of hypodermic needles, syringes and equipment free of charge |
| • Receive from misusers, normally in exchange for the new needles and syringes, the used needles and syringes |
| • Used equipment would be disposed of safely |
| • Display a logo indicating that the scheme is operated |
| • Participating pharmacists should attend a training course within the first year of operation of the scheme |
| • Following further training, a counselling service could be offered to drug misusers |

*health aids, and health advice in keeping with harm reduction and alteration of life style.*

The essential practical aspects of the schemes are shown in Table 42.3.

Pharmacists were required to keep records of the number of individual clients, of the number of needles and syringes issued and estimate the number returned for disposal. These were to be submitted monthly to the health authority or board. Guidance to pharmacists indicated that a maximum of 10 needles should be given per visit, provided that needles and syringes were returned. When there were no returns, the number should be reduced to a maximum of five.

Some of the practical and ethical issues involved are presented in the RPSGB guidelines (which can be found in *Medicines, Ethics and Practice*). This makes it clear that it is the responsibility of the pharmacist to carry out the exchange. The pack that is given out contains needles and syringes, condoms, educational literature and useful contact names and telephone numbers. Local variations are allowed for, with some schemes also including small disposal units ('cin bins') for example. Water for injections cannot be supplied, although it would reduce the risk of infection arising from injecting non-sterile solutions. It is illegal to supply needles and syringes for intramuscular injection of steroids under this scheme, although they are available through some other agencies.

The most difficult practical problem for the pharmacist is what to do when no 'works' are returned in an exchange. This could imply that they are being used by others, or that they have been discarded creating a risk to the general public. The return rate appears to vary with the level of insistence by the pharmacist. However, it is a difficult decision, which can only be based on knowledge of the local situation.

## Methadone prescribing

Opioid withdrawal has a relapse rate of up to 70%. Methadone can be used to replace heroin and reduce the withdrawal symptoms. With a fairly rapid reduction in the dose of methadone, the aim is to achieve a drug-free state within about 10 days. Such a strict regimen would need to be carried out under supervision in hospital. In the community a much slower programme is used, with a reduction of methadone dose of about 10% per week being normal. The rationale for methadone use is that it has a long half-life of 35 hours ($\pm$ 12 hours), allowing once-daily dosing. It also means that it will take about a week to reach a steady state plasma level initially and following a reduction in dose (estimated from 5 half-lives). Methadone is available as a mixture 1 mg/ml and as a concentrate 10 mg/ml. An initial dose in the range 10–40 mg is quite normal.

An alternative is to use methadone as a maintenance drug. Here the target is to replace the illegal opioid with the legal methadone. Such practice is more controversial, although there is growing evidence of both improved behaviour and health when people are stabilized on methadone. The aims of maintenance with methadone are to:

- reduce the danger of injecting drugs
- decriminalize the drug misuser
- stabilize misusers until they are ready for further change
- allow misusers to contribute to society.

Maintenance programmes are based in the community, so community pharmacists are involved. Methadone has the same abuse potential as morphine and is subject to the Misuse of Drugs Regulations 1985. Because of this, the trend is for supervised consumption on the premises in order to avoid the methadone being sold to others illegally. Later, when the user can be trusted, he may gradually be allowed twice-weekly, then weekly 'take home' supply privileges as part of his rehabilitation. Practical aspects of this supervised consumption will now be considered.

It is important that the treatment of the methadone user should always be the same. Thus a written protocol available to all those working in the pharmacy, including locums, is advisable. This should cover the main processes involved as shown in Table 42.4.

### Starting a new patient

When a doctor starts a patient on methadone, the

| Table 42.4 Stages involved in operating methadone dispensing |
|---|
| Starting a new patient |
| Procedures for daily dose administration |
| Contract between patient and pharmacist |
| Counselling the patient |

| Table 42.5 Items for inclusion in a contract between pharmacist and methadone user |
|---|
| • Explanation of procedure for administration |
| • What to do if the pharmacy is closed |
| • Time when the dose may be collected (if restricted) |
| • What to do if a dose is missed |
| • Acceptable and unacceptable behaviour (where to wait, abuse, under influence of drugs or alcohol) |
| • Statement of the consequences of breaking the contract (no further dispensing and the doctor will be informed) |

patient is asked to nominate a pharmacy. The pharmacist is asked to agree. It is important that pharmacists are not pressurized and that they do not have to deal with more patients than they can reasonably cope with. If a patient presents a prescription without prior arrangement, the pharmacist must check with the prescriber to ensure that it is genuine.

A new patient should be asked to agree to a contract, which will explain the procedures followed in that pharmacy (see Table 42.5). It may also be necessary to include some means of formal identification, particularly where there are a large number of patients. A patient medication record should be created to cover the methadone, including a note that it is supervised consumption.

### Daily dose administration

Each day, the patient should make themselves known to a member of staff. The pharmacist should then deal with them as soon as possible, because delays can lead to tensions. Supervision of the dosing should ideally take place in a quiet area. It must be remembered that the patient has the same right to confidentiality as any other patient. In order to comply with the Medicines Act requirements for labelling of dispensed medicines, the methadone should be supplied in a labelled bottle. This may be prepared in advance (and stored in the controlled drug (CD) cabinet). However, in practice, a label would be produced from the PMR, the volume would be measured and poured into a cup from which the patient can consume the dose. The pharmacist must ensure that the dose is swallowed. Offering a drink of water serves two functions – it helps remove the taste and ensure that the dose has been swallowed. Getting the patient to speak also confirms that swallowing has taken place.

Records must be made. A GP10 prescription must have an instalment dispensing sticker on the back, and it should be initialled and dated each time a dose is given. An FP10 (MDA) or FP10 (MP) Ad should be similarly endorsed on the section provided. All doses supplied must be entered in the Controlled Drugs Register within 24 hours. Many pharmacists carry out the entries at the same time on a regular daily basis, for example, at night time.

### Contract

Many pharmacists have found it beneficial to draw up a contract between themselves and the patient. Its purpose is to inform patients what will happen on their daily visits and also to allow the pharmacist some control over the time of visits and the patients' behaviour during the visits. Possible items in a contract are given in Table 42.5.

When the patient has agreed, the contract should be signed by both pharmacist and patient and the patient given a copy.

### Counselling

The pharmacist will have very regular contact with the patients and so may be able to contribute to their overall management by the health care team. In particular the pharmacist will be able to comment on compliance, general state of health and any suspicions about continued drug misuse. Patients on methadone may have generally poor health, particularly if they have been injecting. General advice about diet, oral hygiene and exercise can be usefully offered. The pharmacist should be alert to side effects. Several are common, particularly at first, including insomnia, sweating, constipation, dry mouth, disrupted menstruation and reduced libido.

## Other issues surrounding illicit drug misuse

It is advisable to offer to all staff who may come into contact with drug misusers the opportunity to have a hepatitis B vaccination.

The drugs used for intravenous use are more soluble in acidic solutions. Many misusers try to use acids to help in the solution process. Citric acid is the most common, but others such as ascorbic acid and vinegar are also used. Pharmacists are currently advised not to supply these materials if they suspect that they will be used for this purpose. With or without the use of acids, many tablets have water-insoluble ingredients. Drug misusers have devised a number of filters, including toilet paper, cotton wool and cigarette filters. Some drug user support centres supply more efficient filters but these are not yet available through pharmacies.

There are many ethical issues surrounding the care of people who choose to abuse themselves by abusing drugs. No doubt these will develop and change over the years. At present, the consensus is that drug misusers' health should be preserved as far as possible until such time as they decide that they wish to stop misusing drugs.

---

### Key Points

- Many types of material may be misused including OTC medicines, prescription medicines, plant products, solvents and everyday consumables.
- Injecting drugs increases the danger, especially if there are insoluble solids present.
- Sharing injecting equipment increases the risk of infection with HIV, hepatitis B and hepatitis C.
- Harm minimization tries to reduce the harmful effects of misuse without necessarily reducing consumption.
- The pharmacist has a role in supply of nicotine-replacement therapy, syringe and needle exchange schemes and methadone dispensing.
- Exchange schemes aim to provide clean syringes and needles in exchange for used equipment.
- Methadone is taken once daily and must be observed by the pharmacist.
- Procedures which will operate in methadone dispensing in a pharmacy must be drawn up.
- Methadone-taking patients should sign a contract with the pharmacy.
- The pharmacist, when dealing with substance misusers, is in a good position to offer general health advice.

---

## FURTHER READING

Erikson P G 1995 Harm reduction: what it is and is not. Drug and Alcohol Review 14: 283–285

Lunec S 1992 Practice update: needle and syringe exchange schemes. Pharmaceutical Journal (Dec 12): i–iv

Medicines, Ethics and Practice – a guide for pharmacists, current edn. Royal Pharmaceutical Society of Great Britain, London (Updated twice yearly)

Single S 1995 Defining harm reduction. Drug and Alcohol Review 14: 287–290

Walker R, Edwards C 1994 Clinical pharmacy and therapeutics. Churchill Livingstone, London

Wills S 1993a Volatile substance abuse. Pharmaceutical Journal 250: 381–383

Wills S 1993b Abuse of prescription drugs. Pharmaceutical Journal 250: 537–540

Wills S 1993c Amphetamines and hallucinogens. Pharmaceutical Journal 250: 871–874

Wills S 1993d Plants. Pharmaceutical Journal 251: 227–229

Wills S 1993e Cannabis and cocaine. Pharmaceutical Journal 251: 483–485

Wills S 1993f Over-the-counter products. Pharmaceutical Journal 251: 807–810

Wills S 1994a Opioids. Pharmaceutical Journal 252:157–160

Wills S 1994b Smart drugs – do they work? Pharmaceutical Journal 252: 673–675

Wills S 1994c Caffeine. Pharmaceutical Journal 252: 822–824

Wills S 1994d Tobacco and alcohol. Pharmaceutical Journal 253: 158–160

Wodak A, Saunders B 1995 Harm reduction means what I choose it to mean. Drug and Alcohol Review 14: 269–271

# 43

# Professional and clinical audit

*J. Krska*

---

After studying this chapter you will know about:

**Meaning and significance of audit**
**The relationship between audit, quality assurance and practice research**
**Types of audit**
**Structures, processes and outcomes which may be audited**
**The audit cycle**:
  Standard setting
  Data collection
  Comparison with standards
  Identifying problems
  Implementing change
  Re-audit.

---

## DEFINITIONS

The word 'audit' is derived from the Latin *audio*, meaning 'I hear'. It originates from the verbal delivery of accounts by stewards, which were heard by their landowners. It has therefore long been associated with financial accounts or with the question of whether one is getting value for money. Recently the term audit has been used to mean the comparison of actual practice with best practice and it is in this sense that pharmacists need to understand audit and to undertake it.

As a profession, pharmacists are involved in the creation of standards, for example registration procedures and standards of professional practice. The hallmark of a professional is the maintenance of these standards, which exist to protect the public from poor-quality services. Audit is also about quality – the quality of professional activities and services. Those who carry out audit seek to determine whether best practice is being delivered and, equally importantly, to improve practice. A most useful definition of audit is thus 'the process of reviewing the delivery of health care to identify deficiencies so that they may be remedied'.

Any of the health care professions may carry out audit of services provided by their own peer group. This is professional audit. Some aspects of pharmacy are concerned with professionalism per se, such as continuing education and the standard of pharmacy premises. Audit of these aspects may, therefore, be termed pharmaceutical audit.

Most of the activities of health professionals, however, have an impact on patients, either directly or indirectly. Any service which has an effect on the outcome of a patient's care may be deemed to be a clinical service. An audit of these services may be called clinical audit. Clinical audit is defined by the Government as the systematic and critical appraisal of the quality of clinical care.

At first, it may appear relatively easy to identify who provides specific services. However, there are actually few instances where pharmacists provide a service to patients in isolation from other health care professionals. The provision of advice and sale of non-prescription medicines may be one such area. Even in this area, many patients will need referral to the GP or a GP may have advised patients to seek help from a pharmacist. The dispensing of prescriptions always involves some sort of review of prescribing by another professional. Additionally counselling by a pharmacist does not stand alone as a service, since the patient will usually have had some instruction from others as well. Thus clinical services are in the main multidisciplinary and the audit of these clinical services must also be multidisciplinary.

Since audit is about standards of service, it provides a method of accountability, both to the public and to government. In the prevailing atmosphere of purchasers and providers of health services, it is also essential that managers have information about the quality of the services they are purchasing or which their staff are providing. Although this may seem to be a somewhat threatening situation, ultimately the aim of audit is to improve the efficiency and effectiveness of services, to promote higher standards and, in the case of clinical audit, to improve the outcome for patients. It also allows changes in practice to be evaluated. Therefore it is an essential component of any professional's work and should be seen as an integral part of day-to-day practice.

## RELATIONSHIP BETWEEN AUDIT, QUALITY ASSURANCE AND PRACTICE RESEARCH

Audit techniques are very similar to quality assurance techniques in that both are concerned with standards and the continuous measurement of parameters selected to ensure that these standards are met. Both look at resources, procedures and outcomes or end products. Quality assurance also requires that action is taken if deficiencies are discovered. It has tended to be applied to non-clinical services and is at present separated from multidisciplinary clinical audit.

Research has a very different purpose, but is a necessary basis for much audit, because research is designed to establish what is best practice. The findings of research are therefore used in setting standards for audit.

There are many similarities in the methods used to obtain data for research and for audit, such as questionnaires and interviews. Many of the parameters measured may be the same, particularly when considering measures of outcome in clinical audit. In research, it is important to have controlled studies, to be able to extrapolate the results and to have large enough samples to demonstrate statistical significance of any differences between groups. None of these applies to audit. Audit compares actual practice to a predetermined level of best practice, not to a control. The results of audit apply to a particular situation and should not be extrapolated. Audit can be applied to a single case; large numbers are not required.

## TYPES OF AUDIT

Audit may be of three types, classified according to who undertakes it. These are:

- self audit
- peer or group audit
- external audit.

Self audit is undertaken by individuals and may be seen as the development of a professional attitude to work, in which critical appraisal of actions taken and of their results is constantly being made. It is most commonly undertaken by pharmacists who work in isolation from other pharmacists, such as in single-handed community pharmacies.

Peer audit is undertaken by people within the same peer group, which usually means the same profession. This means that there is joint setting of standards and the activities of everyone in the group are assessed by the other members of the group. For example, pharmacists from several hospitals could get together and audit a service which is provided by each hospital. Pharmacists from one hospital would look at the services provided from other hospitals, while their own service would be open to the scrutiny of pharmacists from these hospitals.

Multidisciplinary group audit is the most common type of group audit. It is usually required for clinical services audits. In this type of audit, it is essential to ensure that one subgroup is not auditing the activities of another subgroup. This would lead to tensions and be counterproductive. An example of how this could occur is an audit of prescribing errors detected by pharmacists. The pharmacists may consider there are too many errors, without the prescribers being involved in deciding what constitutes an error or what is an acceptable frequency of errors. If the prescribers are not part of the team responsible for designing the audit, there is also little chance of any improvement.

External audit is carried out by people other than those actually providing the service and because of this, is perceived as threatening by those whose services are being audited. It may be more objective in its criticisms than self or peer audit, but there may be less enthusiasm for corrective action to improve services.

Externally organized audits may be particularly suitable for services which are difficult for individuals to audit, such as responding to symptoms in community pharmacies. However, it is still possible to involve those whose services are to be audited in deciding what best practice should be and in making improvements. This is not the same as external audit in which the standard of best practice is imposed and where there is a perceived threat if an individual's performance is not of the standard required.

## WHAT IS MEASURED IN AUDIT

There are three aspects of any professional activity which may be audited. These are:

- the structures or resources involved
- the processes used
- the outcomes of the activity.

Structures are the resources available to help deliver services or carry out activities. Examples are staff, their expertise and knowledge, books, learning materials or training courses, drug stocks, equipment, layout of premises.

Processes are the systems and procedures which take place when carrying out an activity and may include quality assurance procedures and policies and protocols of all types. An example of this could be a hospital pharmacy which has a written procedure to be followed when patients bring their own medicines into hospital. Another is the protocol that all community pharmacies should have which should be followed when a request is made for advice.

Outcomes are the results of the activity and are arguably the most important aspect of any activity. In clinical audit, where the outcomes involve patients,

they may be very difficult to measure, since a change in health status or attitude or behaviour will be involved. Changes in the behaviour of other health professionals may be another outcome measure, for example changes in prescribing. In pharmaceutical audits which look, for example, at drug procurement or distribution, continuing education or standards of premises, outcomes will be much easier to measure.

## THE AUDIT CYCLE

The audit of any activity is a continuous process, which follows a cycle of measurement, evaluation and improvement. This cycle is shown in Figure 43.1. It incorporates:

- the setting of standards for practice
- measuring actual practice
- comparing the two
- finding out any reasons why best practice is not being achieved
- changing what is done to improve this.

Although the process is continuous, it is not practicable to audit all activities or services all the time. It

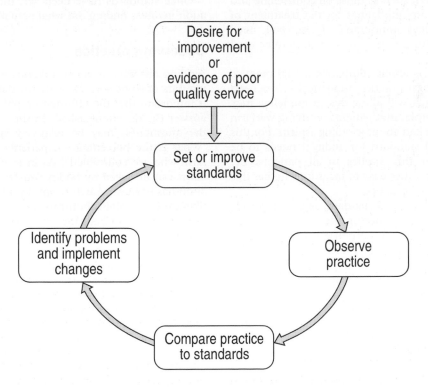

**Fig. 43.1**　The audit cycle.

is often appropriate to have intervals between periods when actual practice is measured, to allow for changes to take effect. It is also important to select topics for audit carefully, because of the time involved in doing the audit. In choosing which activities should be audited, two of the main criteria to be considered are whether or not there is a problem and whether there is a realistic possibility of improvement. If this is the case and an audit is planned, then the first stage is to set standards, against which practice will be measured.

## Setting standards

All audit should be based on standards which are widely accepted in terms of what should be done (i.e. best practice). There are many standards provided by the Royal Pharmaceutical Society of Great Britain for individual aspects of pharmacy practice. These are published 6-monthly in *Medicines, Ethics and Practice*. In addition, other organizations may have produced standards. There are, for example, Regional Pharmaceutical Officers' standards for hospital pharmacy services or the CAPOs' equivalent in Scotland; often individual pharmacies or companies have standards. Other guidelines may be available which can be used, such as those on counselling and advice or the many guidelines for the treatment of individual medical conditions. These will need modification to form criteria or standards to be used for audit.

Because audit is about comparing actual practice to standards of best practice, numerical values need to be added which will allow this. A guideline may suggest, for example, that patients receiving warfarin should be counselled about avoiding aspirin. For this to form a useful standard for audit, it needs to be clarified whether this applies to all patients, i.e. 100%. It then becomes easy to measure whether this is the case in actual practice.

This is termed an ideal standard, since it is ideally what should happen. However, the level of standard set may need to be a compromise between what is desirable and what is possible, since resources may be limited. In this case, an optimal standard may be set. Using the previous example, it may be considered that there were insufficient staff to ensure that 100% of patients receiving warfarin could be counselled about avoiding aspirin. A useful compromise could be that 100% of patients prescribed warfarin for the first time are counselled. Another type of standard is the minimal standard, which, as its name implies, is the minimum level of service which is acceptable. This type of standard is often that used in external audits.

For some of the services or activities which are to be audited, there may be no published guidelines or standards to help, in which case it will be necessary to devise them. This may involve searching the literature, for example recent journals, standard textbooks or perhaps educational material. Whether devising standards from scratch or making guidelines into standards, it is important that everybody involved in providing the service is also involved in deciding what the standard will be. For much of clinical audit, this will include other health professionals and is most likely to involve at least medical practitioners. However, nurses, health visitors, technical staff and non-medical staff, such as receptionists or porters, may also need to be involved. It may also be appropriate to include patients or their carers as recipients of services.

By involving everyone who plays a part in a health care service in deciding standards, the audit is clearly a peer or group audit. This avoids the potential feeling of threat which may be created by excluding individuals. To anyone excluded at this stage, it appears that the audit is external. This could result in the whole exercise being a waste of time, since these individuals may refuse to help in raising performance later.

Once standards have been set, the next stage of audit involves finding out what actually happens.

## Observing practice

Finding out what is actual practice involves collecting data of some sort. As with any data collection, it is important that the information obtained is able to answer the questions asked. In the case of an audit the question(s) may be relatively simple, such as 'What is the percentage of patients receiving warfarin who are counselled?' As in research, time and effort can be saved by finding out whether a similar audit has been done before and by adapting or modifying the data collection procedures used. If a new procedure is required, the same basic requirements as for any data collection must be considered (see Table 43.1).

In addition, because audit is about improvement of services, it is often necessary to find out why best practice is not followed. Again using the warfarin counselling as an example, the data may show that only 75% of patients were counselled. If no reasons have been found to explain why the remainder were not counselled, it may not be clear what needs to be done to improve practice. After all, maybe the 25% who were not counselled already knew about avoiding aspirin. On the other hand it may be that these

**Table 43.1   Requirements for data collection procedures**

- Provide information required
- Validity
- Reliability
- Controlled for bias
- Adequate sampling technique
- Feasible
- Quantitative or qualitative
- Retrospective or prospective
- Routinely or specially collected
- Pilot study

prescriptions were all handed out by one particular member of staff, who felt unhappy about counselling. Another cause could be that the prescriptions were all given out when the pharmacy was particularly busy and staff felt that they had no time for counselling. Each of these different reasons for best practice not being delivered would need different solutions, so it is essential to determine the reasons as part of the audit. This shows that the data collection procedures need to anticipate, to some extent at least, potential causes of failing to provide best practice.

The method of data collection must be valid and reliable. If sampling procedures are used, they too must be appropriate, avoiding bias and equally importantly, it must be feasible to carry them out.

Validity is the extent to which what is measured is actually what is supposed to be measured. To use the warfarin counselling example again, the standard was about advice concerning aspirin. If the only data collected were the number of patients who were counselled and not what advice they were given about aspirin, these data would be invalid, since they did not measure what they set out to measure.

Reliability is a measure of the consistency or reproducibility of the data collection procedure. Good reliability can be difficult to achieve when trying to measure outcomes in health care. It is therefore important to use recognized measures wherever possible. Reliability may also vary among individuals collecting data, despite their using the same data collection tool. It is important to check this and ensure that they agree before they start to collect data which will be used for audit.

Sampling is important in collecting data for audit, because the data should be unbiased or representative of actual practice. It may be that the numbers and time involved are small enough that all examples of the activity are included in data collection procedures. In the case of large numbers, it may be easier

to include just a proportion in the audit. If so, a plan is needed which ensures that those selected are representative. A range of different sampling methods have been devised. A combination of random number tables and systematic sampling can be used where, for example, the counselling given to every tenth patient presenting a prescription for warfarin is to be audited. Another way is to decide in advance that a certain percentage of the total population will be sampled, usually ensuring that they will be typical of the population. These techniques require that the total population size within the audit period is known. If large, the population may need to be stratified into subgroups first before using these techniques.

Sampling, or even large numbers, may not always be necessary. Since audit is about a particular service or activity, carried out by one or more particular individual professionals, an audit can be carried out on a service provided to one patient. It is still the determination of whether actual practice equates to best practice.

Feasibility of data collection is very important. It must be possible to collect the data which are required to answer the question. It is often necessary to incorporate data collection for audit into routine work, so the time taken is an important consideration.

Some of the data which will answer audit questions may already be collected on a routine basis. Data kept on computerized patient medication records or on patient profiles may be useful for some types of audit. Some pharmacies routinely log the time when prescriptions are handed in and given out, so an audit of turnaround time could easily be carried out using these data. Hospitals routinely collect data on length of stay and number of admissions, discharges and deaths, which may be useful outcome measures. Often data have to be specially collected for the audit, which needs a specifically designed data collection tool. This may be simply a form, onto which data from other sources are transferred. Methods of collecting data for audit include all those employed in practice research, such as interviews, questionnaires and surveys.

Data for audit can be either quantitative or qualitative in nature. Qualitative data are often useful in obtaining opinions about services or for measuring outcomes in patients. Large numbers are not required for producing qualitative data. It may be useful to undertake qualitative work which can then be used to help design a good data collection tool to be used in a quantitative way, using larger numbers. Quantitative audit almost always generates large amounts of data, which require subsequent analysis, usually using statistics. These may be purely descriptive or simple comparative statistics.

Whether the data collected are retrospective or prospective depends to a large extent on the topic of the audit and the data available. Retrospective audit can only be undertaken if good records of activities have been kept. Prospective audits should ensure that the data required are recorded, even if only for the audit period. The possibility of practice changing during the audit period simply because the audit is being undertaken is a real one. This may not always be a problem if practice is better than usual and if audit is continuous, since the ultimate aim is to improve services, after all. It is more important to be aware of this effect if practice is measured periodically, although it is very difficult to control for.

In large audits, as in most practice research, piloting the data collection tool which will be used is a valuable way of finding out if it is suitable. It is always worth spending time undertaking a small pilot study, using a sample similar to those to be included in the audit. This should avoid the discovery that there were difficulties in interpretation or

that vital information has not been recorded after acquiring large amounts of data.

## Comparing practice to standards

This is the evaluation stage of audit, in which actual practice is compared to best practice. This involves the analysis and presentation of the data obtained. Most audit data require only descriptive analysis, such as percentages, means or medians, along with ranges and standard deviations to show the spread of the data. Comparative statistical tests are useful for looking at one or more subgroups of quantitative data. This could be for different data collection periods (audit cycles) or for subgroups within one audit. Examples where comparison may be useful are three different pharmacies' prescription turnaround times or the counselling frequencies for patients presenting prescriptions for warfarin for the first time compared to those who have taken it before. The statistical test must be appropriate for the type of data. Chi-square is used for nonparametric data, such as frequencies. For parametric data which are normally distributed, $t$-tests can be

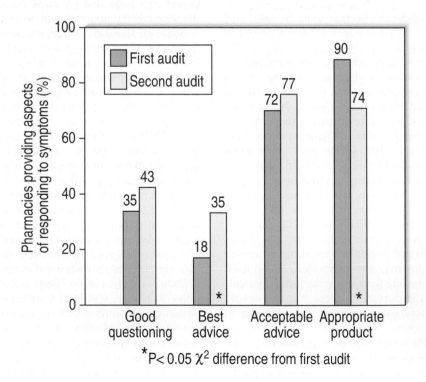

*$P < 0.05$ $\chi^2$ difference from first audit

**Fig. 43.2**   Performance of pharmacies in an audit of responding to symptoms.

used. An example of comparative data from an audit is given in Figure 43.2.

In audit, as in any use of statistics, it is important to consider the practical significance of the data. An improvement which is statistically significant may not always be of practical significance and vice versa.

Data collected for audit purposes relate to the activities of individual professionals and to their effects on patients. It is therefore essential to maintain confidentiality. Permission is required before any information about one individual's practice is given to other members of the audit team. Managers who may need this sort of information should be part of the audit team anyway. The general results of an audit should, however, be made available to others, after ensuring that no individual practitioner or patient can be identified. This is essential if the audit is to improve services, as it will help others to learn and allow comparisons to be made.

When comparing the results of audits between centres, there will most probably be differences, perhaps in staffing levels, population served, case mix and so on, which could account for differences in apparent performance. The results of any audit should not be extrapolated beyond the sample audited. Audit applies to a particular activity, carried out by particular individuals and involving particular patients.

In presenting data collected during audit, as with any other data, graphics can be particularly useful, as tables can be discouraging to many people. This is particularly important in a group audit, where everyone needs to see the results. Simple graphics should be adequate, such as pie charts or bar charts.

Providing the standards for the audit have been set appropriately, it should be relatively easy to determine whether they have been achieved. Often the most difficult part of audit is finding out why best practice is not being delivered and ensuring that improvement occurs.

## Identifying problems

It is important in any audit to find out not only what is wrong with a service, but why it is wrong. The underlying causes of failure need to be established. Thus the data collected during measurement of practice should have attempted to identify them. Sub-optimal practice can arise b1ecause of inadequate skills or knowledge, poor systems of work or patient attitudes and behaviour. Each should be examined as a possible contributory factor to disap-

pointing results of an audit. In most audits, health care professionals' lack of knowledge is not a problem, although lack of awareness about, for example, guidelines for disease management can contribute to their lack of use. Lack of skill may be related to infrequency of carrying out a particular activity. Both are relatively easily remedied. Both behaviour and the way in which work is organized are more difficult to change. The strategies adopted for effecting change will need to differ depending on which of these underlying causes is present.

## Implementing changes

Achieving an improvement in practice requires a change in behaviour. Change can be threatening simply because of its novelty. It may also involve increased work and is often resisted. For this reason all those whose work pattern may need to change should be active members of the audit team from the start. Change must be seen as leading to improvement in performance and ultimately benefits to the patient. The changes proposed to improve practice must be closely tailored to the underlying cause of the sub-optimal results. They should be specific to the situation which has been audited, rather than general. They should be non-threatening and may need to be introduced gradually. Change may require resources, including time. It may also have other knock-on effects which need to be anticipated. The effect of changes must be monitored, to see whether they have been successful. This can be done by re-audit.

## Re-audit

In some audits it may be appropriate to reconsider the standards before undertaking a further period of data collection. Standards which were set too high may always be unattainable, although this may not have been apparent before practice was measured. It is equally possible to have used low standards and to have found they were surpassed. In this case it may be appropriate to raise them, which is a good way of improving practice. Whether or not the standards remain the same, a second period of measuring practice is needed if changes have been implemented, so that the effectiveness of these changes can be determined.

It is always difficult to change behaviour and improvements in practice may be short-lived. It may therefore be necessary to repeat audits at regular intervals to reinforce the desired practice and maintain the improvement in service.

## Key Points

- Pharmacists are involved in setting standards of practice and need to be able to show that they meet them.
- Audit may be of professional activity or clinical service.
- Audit may be seen as a form of accountability by a profession.
- The main aim of audit must be to improve standards of service and outcome for patients.
- There are similarities and differences between audit, quality assurance and practice research.
- The three main types of audit are self, peer and external audit.
- Audit may measure structures, processes or outcomes.
- The time taken to carry out audit restricts what can be audited.
- Actual practice should be compared to best practice using a numerical basis.
- Standards may be ideal, optimal or minimal.
- Standard setting should involve at least all those involved in delivering the service being audited.
- Data collection must answer the audit question and have the potential to give reasons for failure to meet the standard.
- Sampling has to ensure that the data are representative of the total activity.
- Piloting the data collection ensures that it is suitable and comprehensive.
- Comparison with standards will normally involve very simple descriptive or statistical analysis.
- Confidentiality must be respected, but outcomes should be shared with all the audit team.
- Implementing change may feel threatening to an individual.
- Re-audit is a way of testing whether changes have achieved their objective.

Regional Pharmaceutical Officers' Special Interest Group 1991 Standards for pharmaceutical services in health authorities in England.

Medicines, Ethics and Practice – a guide for pharmacists, current edn. The Royal Pharmaceutical Society of Great Britain, London (Updated twice yearly)

## FURTHER READING

Centre for Medical Education 1993 Moving to audit. Ninewells Hospital and Medical School, Dundee

College of Pharmacy Practice 1993 Introducing audit: a pharmacist's guide. College of Pharmacy Practice, Coventry

Crombie I K, Davies H T O 1996 The audit handbook: improving healthcare through clinical audit, 2nd edn. John Wiley, Chichester

# PART 5

# APPENDICES

# Appendix 1
## Current UK pharmaceutical legislation

*M. M. Moody*

## Introduction

When dealing with the supply of medicines, poisons and related substances, pharmacists must comply with a wide range of legal requirements. It is not the purpose of this appendix to reiterate many of these legal requirements but rather, to give some reasoning to the various legal procedures. Additionally, it is hoped that some commonly held misconceptions may be clarified. The legal procedures referred to are found in a variety of comprehensive reference sources, e.g. *Medicines, Ethics and Practice* (RPSGB, current edn), *Pharmacy Law and Ethics* (Appelbe & Wingfield 1993), *Pharmacy Law and Practice* (Merrills & Fisher 1997). All practising pharmacists, pre-registration students and pharmacy undergraduates should consult these volumes extensively. Only the most recent editions should be consulted as pharmaceutical law is constantly being updated to deal with the ever-changing requirements of medicines and medication. In addition, the Law and Ethics Department of the Royal Pharmaceutical Society of Great Britain (RPSGB) should be consulted regarding matters too recent to appear in any of the aforementioned publications. Changes in pharmaceutical law are published in *The Pharmaceutical Journal* and again it is every practising pharmacist's professional responsibility to keep up to date.

## CONSUMER PROTECTION ACT

Although this Act does not immediately appear to have a direct link with drug therapy it is of considerable relevance to pharmacists. It deals with products the quality of which is lower than the consumer should expect. Prior to this Act it was the consumer's responsibility to prove that the producer of a particular product was guilty of negligence. The emphasis has now shifted and it is the producer's responsibility to prove that negligence has not occurred. This obviously makes it a more realistic option for the average consumer to bring a genuine complaint against a producer who may be a multinational company with considerable resources and legal expertise at their disposal.

Why should this have a bearing on practising pharmacists? When community pharmacists supply medicines against prescriptions they are identified as the supplier because the medicine will have attached to it a label bearing the name and address of the issuing pharmacy. This in itself does not indicate that the pharmacist is the producer of the medication, but it does put the onus on the pharmacist to be able to identify who the producer is. There are four main areas which have direct relevance to pharmacists.

## 1. Generic prescribing

Pharmacists should always be able to provide evidence of their source of supply for generic drugs. It is advisable to use only a very limited number of generic suppliers and preferably use manufacturers who produce a product which bears a means of identification, e.g. a company trademark. A pharmacist who is unable to identify the source of a preparation will be held liable for any problems caused by the preparation.

## 2. Extemporaneous dispensing

When preparing an extemporaneous preparation, full records of the ingredients used, their batch numbers and who supplied them should be kept by the pharmacist. If a fault is identified, e.g. an ingredient used in good faith but supplied incorrectly labelled by the manufacturer, the pharmacist must be able to identify the supplier or manufacturer or he will be held liable for any problems caused by the product.

### 3. 'Own label' products

A pharmacist who has 'own label' products manufactured by an outside agency must ensure that full records and details of all supplies are available. This ensures that the manufacturer is liable for any product defects, not the pharmacist.

### 4. The provision of advice

The Consumer Protection Act requires the supplier of goods to ensure that the consumer is provided with comprehensive instructions on the safe use of the goods. This has obvious implications when supplying medicines. Although this requirement may be satisfied by the provision of a patient information leaflet, a patient may not receive one on every occasion. It is therefore essential that products are clearly labelled with instructions regarding safe use and pharmacists should satisfy themselves that appropriate information has been provided.

## THE MEDICINES ACT

This is the major piece of legislation which governs the professional activities of pharmacists and in particular, community pharmacists. The major thrust of this Act is to ensure the protection of the general public in respect of medicines. It ensures the quality, safety and efficacy of medicines and controls the level of access which the general public have to them.

The Act classifies medicinal products into three groups.

### 1. General sales list (GSL)

The products in this category have been deemed to be relatively safe and can be sold without any pharmaceutical or medical input.

### 2. Pharmacy medicines (P)

These preparations require some control and apart from a few exceptions, are only allowed to be sold from a registered retail pharmacy. The sale must be supervised by a pharmacist. This ensures that the sale of any inappropriate medicine should be avoided. The reality of this situation is less clear cut. In many instances, after questioning the purchaser, pharmacists will refuse a sale. It can often be very difficult to persuade customers that a particular product is not suitable for their needs. In some instances the customer may merely go to another pharmacy where the pharmacist and staff are less vigilant and the purchase is made. The introduction of protocols for the sale of medicines in pharmacies has helped to make the general public more aware that a degree of control is required on the sale of medicines.

### 3. Prescription-only medicines (POM)

These are medicines which can only be obtained by the general public if they are in possession of a valid prescription. All the preparations in this category have been identified as drugs which are to be used for conditions where appropriate diagnosis and treatment should be carried out by a properly qualified practitioner. Medical practitioners, dentists and vets may all prescribe POM drugs. Recently, a limited number of suitably qualified and trained nurses have been allowed to write prescriptions for a limited number of POM classified preparations.

## Emergency supply procedures

There are certain situations when a pharmacist may supply a POM to a member of the public who is not in possession of a prescription. This is known as an emergency supply.

Prior to this being made legal, community pharmacists often found themselves facing major moral dilemmas. A customer would present himself at the pharmacy in desperate need of a POM but with no prescription. No doctor was available to write one and the pharmacist knew that without appropriate medication the customer's state of health would be compromised. However, if the POM was supplied the pharmacist was in breach of the law. To overcome these very difficult situations the procedures for emergency supply of a POM were devised and became part of the Act. Used in appropriate situations they are a welcome addition to the Act. However, there are still some pharmacists who have difficulty interpreting this piece of legislation and for that reason details of correct procedures are given.

1. The person requiring the POM must be present and be interviewed by the pharmacist.

2. The pharmacist must satisfy himself that a genuine emergency exists, i.e. there is no possibility of obtaining a prescription (for this reason the majority of emergency supplies occur at the weekend and on public holidays). The emergency supply procedure

should not be used just because a patient cannot be bothered to visit the surgery.

3. The pharmacist should consider the consequences of not making the supply. For instance, how seriously will the patient's health suffer if the required medication is not available?

4. The pharmacist must ensure that the medicine being requested has previously been prescribed for the patient. The emergency supply procedure is not a situation where new drug therapy can be initiated by the pharmacist. The normal requirement is that the drug should have been prescribed within the last 6 months; however, this requirement is waived when the condition being treated occurs intermittently, e.g. hay fever or urinary tract infection. Many emergency supplies are given for medication which the patient is currently taking, e.g. antihypertensive therapy. This has led to a misconception among some pharmacists that only medication being currently taken by the patient is allowed on an emergency supply. This is incorrect. As long as it has previously been prescribed and the pharmacist considers it appropriate, it can be supplied.

5. Unless the medication requested is supplied in a complete container such as a tube of ointment, an aerosol or a course of contraceptive tablets, a maximum of 5 days' supply only may be given. During the interview with the patient the pharmacist must find out when a prescription can be obtained. Some patients may have adequate supplies of medication but have forgotten to bring them with them. Information on when they are going home should be sought. In many cases the maximum 5-day supply will not be required to be issued.

6. Drugs which are either Schedule 2 or Schedule 3 of the Misuse of Drugs Act may not be supplied as an emergency supply. The only exception to this rule is when phenobarbitone or its salts are required for the treatment of epilepsy.

For further details of Medicine Act legislation and the procedures to be followed to comply with the Act, the current edition of *Medicines, Ethics and Practice* should be consulted.

## THE MISUSE OF DRUGS ACT

This Act deals with all the drugs which have been identified as drugs of dependence or have the potential for dependence. The drugs are classified into five schedules, each schedule having varying degrees of control.

As far as pharmacists are concerned, prescriptions for drugs which are categorized in Schedules 2 or 3 require the greatest degree of scrutiny and highest level of vigilance.

One of the aims of the Misuse of Drugs Act is to control the supply of many of the drugs controlled by the Act. For this reason, with one or two exceptions, all prescriptions for Schedule 2 and 3 drugs must be written in the prescriber's own hand (handwriting requirements) and satisfy certain prescription requirements, e.g. the form of the drug must be stated, the quantity prescribed must be stated in words and figures and the dose to taken, indicated. The frequency of dose does not need to be stated but the dose taken at any one time does. Therefore, 'as directed' is not acceptable but 'one as directed' is.

## Private prescriptions for Schedule 2 and Schedule 3 drugs

Private prescriptions for POM drugs can be repeated if this is indicated on the prescription by the prescriber. However, this facility is not allowed if the prescription is for a Schedule 2 or 3 drug. If a prescription is received which has a repeat indication on it the pharmacist may have two courses of action.

1. If the prescription has not previously been dispensed and is in date, i.e. not older than 13 weeks, it may be legally dispensed. The repeat indication however must not be complied with. The pharmacist should explain to the patient that the prescription must be retained and a courtesy call made to the prescriber explaining the situation.

2. If the prescription has previously been dispensed and the patient has returned for a repeat supply, this may not be given. Another prescription must be obtained from the prescriber. In these situations it is more appropriate for the pharmacist to contact the prescriber and explain the situation. The prescription should be retained if the previous dispensing was carried out in that pharmacy. If the dispensing was carried out in different premises, it should theoretically be returned to those premises.

The situation above may arise if a drug is reclassified into a schedule with a greater number of controls. Recent examples are the reclassification of Equagesic from POM to POM Schedule 3 and temazepam from POM Schedule 4 to POM Schedule 3. Prescriptions were legal at the time of writing but immediately the reclassification comes into force the appropriate controls are applied and the repeat facility is disallowed.

## Record keeping for Schedule 2 drugs

It is a legal requirement that both receipts and supplies of Schedule 2 drugs are recorded in a Controlled Drug Register. Full information of the details to be kept are found in *Medicines, Ethics and Practice*. The law states that, if possible, the records should be entered at the time of receipt or supply but in any case within 24 hours of the transaction. However, pharmacists should make every effort to make entries at the time of the transaction as it is all too easy, in a busy pharmacy, to forget. The Register will then be incomplete and give the appearance of discrepancies in the stock held.

## Destruction of Schedule 2 drugs

### Drugs returned to the pharmacy by a patient or the patient's representative

Schedule 2 drugs which have been dispensed for a patient and are returned because they are no longer required may be destroyed by the pharmacist. A controlled drug denaturing kit can be used. No record of the destruction need be made nor does the destruction need to be witnessed. A pharmacist accepts returned drugs from a patient on the legal understanding that they are destroyed. On no account must these preparations be put back into stock.

### Destruction of stocks of Schedule 2 drugs held in the pharmacy

Out-of-date stocks or drugs which are no longer required can be destroyed but their destruction must be witnessed and an entry regarding the destruction must be made in the Controlled Drug Register.

*Witnesses.* The witness can be a police officer. Some pharmacies have regular visits from police officers who are chemist liaison officers. If there is no regular visit then a phone call to the local police station should be made to arrange for an officer to witness the destruction. In addition, a RPSGB inspector or a Home Office inspector can also witness controlled drug destruction.

*Records.* A record of the destruction should be made in the Controlled Drug Register. Details should be entered in the appropriate 'supplied' section of the Register and should include:

- the date of the destruction
- the name and quantity of the drug destroyed
- the signature of the witness.

Because of stricter waste disposal legislation which does not allow medicines to be disposed of into the water or sewage system, pharmacists may use a denaturing kit, which can then be put with other waste for disposal. If destruction does not need to be witnessed, the drugs can be handed to an authorized waste disposal carrier who is authorized to handle controlled drugs.

## Dispensing for drug addicts

With the rise in the number of registered drug addicts in the UK there has been a proportionate increase in the number of prescriptions issued for drug addicts. There are certain procedures which should be adhered to when dispensing prescriptions for controlled drugs for addicts.

- Ideally, the addict should be introduced to the pharmacy by drug addiction clinic staff or the prescriber issuing the prescriptions. Pharmacists have the right to refuse to take on a drug addict. Some pharmacists feel that they can only cope with a certain number of addicts while others have concerns about the effect the presence of addicts in the pharmacy may have on their other customers. Many pharmacists operate a written contract system with the addicts under their care. The addicts are required to sign a contract in which they guarantee to abide by certain rules, usually involving their behaviour and demeanour within the pharmacy. If an addict breaches the terms of the contract the pharmacist reserves the right to withdraw dispensing services.
- Only the registered addict may collect the dispensed items. If, for any reason, this is not possible, the pharmacist must receive a written instruction from the addict naming the representative who will collect the drugs.
- If the prescription has to be dispensed in instalments, the instalment must be collected at the appropriate time or the supply is forfeited.

### Dispensing by instalments

Where a drug is to be dispensed in instalments the prescription must satisfy certain criteria. The number of instalments, the intervals between the instalments and the quantity in each instalment must be stated. These three criteria may be written in a variety of ways but must be present for the prescription to be legal. Some prescribers may indicate a starting date. If present, this must be complied with. If no starting date is indicated then the prescription may be started any time within the legal time limits of the prescription, e.g. 13 weeks for a Schedule 2 or 3 drug. The timing of the instalments must be strictly adhered to. They may not be dispensed ahead of time and if a patient is late in coming to collect a supply it is forfeited.

The prescription must be endorsed with the date of dispensing and the quantity dispensed, each time an instalment is dispensed. If an instalment is not collected the prescription should be dated and the words 'not dispensed' added.

### Records for instalment dispensing

When the prescription is for a Schedule 2 drug a record of each instalment must be made in the Controlled Drug Register. This should not be done prior to the instalment being collected. If for some reason the instalment is not uplifted an incorrect entry would then have been made in the Register.

## POISONS ACT AND POISONS RULES

Substances which are legally classified as poisons are subject to a variety of controls. These controls are dependent on the classification of the poison.

## Classification of poisons

Poisons are either classified as Part 1 or Part 2 poisons.

*Part 1 poisons*, in general, may only be sold by retail from a registered retail pharmacy under the supervision of a pharmacist.

*Part 2 poisons* can be sold from either registered retail pharmacies or from a listed seller, i.e. a person whose name appears in a list of sellers maintained by a local authority.

The classification of a substance into Part 1 or Part 2 has nothing to do with the level of toxicity of the poison but is governed by the extent to which the substance is required for use by the general public.

## Poisons Rules

The Poisons Rules either cause additional restrictions to be applied to the poison or cause the regulations to be relaxed. The Rules classify certain, but not all, poisons into schedules. The two which pharmacists are most likely to have to deal with are Schedule 1 and Schedule 12.

### Schedule 1

Sales of Schedule 1 poisons are strictly controlled. The person purchasing the poison must be personally known to the seller as a person fit to be in possession of the poison. If the purchaser is not known to the seller he must provide documentation before the sale can be made. Full details of the documents required are found in *Medicines, Ethics and Practice*.

A record of the sale must be made in the Poisons Register by the seller. The details required are:

- the date of the sale
- the name and address of the purchaser
- details of any documentation required
- the name and quantity of the poison
- the purpose for which the poison is to be used
- the signature of the purchaser or, if appropriate, details of a signed order.

*Point to note.* Unlike entries for controlled drugs, the Poisons Register must be completed before the poison is handed over to the purchaser.

### Schedule 12

This schedule indicates the restrictions which apply to the supply of strychnine and other substances which are used to eliminate certain verminous animals. Full details of all the requirements are found in *Medicines, Ethics and Practice*.

## Labelling of poisons

All substances classified as poisons are subject to Chemicals (Hazard Information and Packaging) Regulations (CHIP).

### CHIP Regulations

These regulations are a major piece of Health and Safety legislation. They ensure that all chemicals which have potentially damaging or dangerous properties are clearly labelled.

The basic labelling requirements are:

- the name of the substance
- the name, address and telephone number of the supplier
- an indication of the general nature of the risk, e.g. toxic, corrosive, teratogenic
- the symbols specified for the above risks, e.g. skull and crossbones
- risk phrases – these are general statements of the properties of the substance, e.g. 'Causes severe burns'

- safety phrases – these contain advice on what to do to avoid problems, e.g. 'Wear suitable protective clothing', 'Do not breathe vapour'.

Because of the complex nature of these labelling requirements it is generally recommended that pharmacists should supply substances which are controlled by the CHIP regulations in the original container. The pharmacist must, of course, ensure that the labelling on the container complies with current legislation.

Further information in the form of a safety data sheet should also be supplied to the purchaser. This applies when the chemical is being used for business use, but is not a requirement when being used for domestic purposes. As long as the domestic purchaser is supplied with 'sufficient information' for the safe use of the chemical the regulations are satisfied. This does however put additional responsibility on the pharmacist. It is unlikely that the label alone will provide sufficient detailed information. It may therefore be appropriate, although not required by law, to provide all purchasers with a safety data sheet. Pharmacists should ensure that domestic users, in particular, understand the procedures required for the safe use of the substance.

## METHYLATED SPIRITS LEGISLATION

The Alcoholic Liquor Duties Act 1979 gives the power to Customs and Excise to make regulations regarding the sale and supply of methylated spirits.

There are several forms of methylated spirits but the two of main interest to the pharmacist are Mineralised Methylated Spirits (MMS) used for household purposes such as cleaning and lighting and Industrial Methylated Spirits (IMS) which is used for medical purposes. Substances containing IMS such as surgical spirit are also controlled by the legislation.

### Industrial Methylated Spirits

Pharmacists who wish to use or supply IMS must first apply to Customs and Excise for authority to receive IMS. On receipt of this authority a statement to that effect must be issued to the wholesaler from whom the pharmacist wishes to purchase the IMS. The statement must be renewed annually. Full details of the content and format of these two documents are found in *Medicines, Ethics and Practice*.

### Supply of IMS from a community pharmacy

IMS can be supplied:

- on receipt of a legally written prescription or order from a medical practitioner.
- on receipt of a signed order addressed to the pharmacist and signed by a medical practitioner, the quantity not to exceed 3 litres.

*Note* that the definition of 'medical practitioner' in this legislation differs from the definition in the Medicines Act. In the Methylated Spirits Regulations the definition is 'any doctor, dentist, nurse, chiropodist, veterinary surgeon or any other person entitled by law to provide medical or veterinary services in the UK'.

## Mineralised Methylated Spirits

Authority to purchase MMS is not required by pharmacists and it can be sold, subject to certain conditions, to the general public. There are, however, differences in procedures to be followed in England and Wales, Scotland, and Northern Ireland.

### England and Wales

No sales may be made between 10 p.m. on Saturday and 8 a.m. on the following Monday.

### Scotland

The same time restrictions which apply in England and Wales also apply. In addition a record of the sale of either MMS or surgical spirit must be made. Details required to be kept are:

- date of the sale
- name and address of the purchaser
- name of substance and quantity supplied
- purpose for use
- signature of purchaser or details of any signed order.

The maximum quantity which can be sold, if not for resale, is 4 gallons. The purchaser must be over the age of 14 years.

### Northern Ireland

Similar time restrictions apply, no records need to be kept but the minimum age of the purchaser must be 18 years.

For further information on the legislation governing methylated spirits consult *Medicines, Ethics and Practice*.

## DATA PROTECTION ACT

This Act is of relevance to pharmacists because it deals with the storage of information on computers. Any pharmacist who uses a computer for the maintenance of patient medication records must ensure that they are registered with the Data Protection Registrar. It is an offence to keep such records otherwise.

To comply with the Data Protection Act pharmacists should ensure that only essential information is held on computer, the information is kept up to date, security systems are in place to prevent unauthorized access and the pharmacy has a procedure for dealing with a request for computer-held data.

### Unauthorized access

- All systems should be protected by a password.
- Computer screens should not be on view to the general public.
- Computers should not be left running in an unattended dispensary.
- Staff should be informed of the necessity for total confidentiality.

### Requests for information

Pharmacists may receive requests from members of the general public for details of information held about them on computer. Except in instances where the physical or mental health of the person could suffer, the information must be supplied. The pharmacist must supply the information, in an understandable form, within 40 days of the request. Any pharmacist receiving such a request should not, however, immediately access the information. Details of who is requesting the information and the date on which the request was made should be taken. The pharmacist should then check on what information is held, consult with the patient's doctor if necessary, and then if it is deemed appropriate, send a copy of the information to the patient.

## FURTHER READING

Appelbe G E, Wingfield J 1997 Dale and Appelbe's pharmacy law and ethics, 6th edn. Pharmaceutical Press, London

Medicines, Ethics and Practice – a guide for pharmacists, current edn. Royal Pharmaceutical Society of Great Britain, London (Updated twice yearly)

Merrills J, Fisher J 1997 Pharmacy law and practice, 2nd edn. Blackwell Science, Oxford

# Appendix 2
## National Health Service dispensing

*M. M. Moody*

## Introduction

The provision of medicines ordered on National Health Service (NHS) prescriptions is the major activity in most community pharmacies in the UK. The NHS is administered separately in England and Wales from Scotland and Northern Ireland. This means that there are variations both in the requirements of the contract which community pharmacies have with the Government and in the levels of remuneration.

In England and Wales each pharmacy should have a contract with their local health authority. The terms of the contract are negotiated annually with the Department of Health. The negotiating body, on behalf of the chemist contractors in England and Wales, is the Pharmaceutical Services Negotiating Committee (PSNC). In Scotland the contract is with the local Health Board, is negotiated with the Scottish Office Health Department and the negotiating body is the Scottish Pharmaceutical General Council (SPGC). In Northern Ireland the Department of Health and Social Services is responsible for providing an integrated health service. There are four health and social services boards who are in contract with the contractors in their particular area.

Because the contracts are negotiated separately and there are differences in some of the terms and conditions it is important that pharmacists working in community pharmacy who move from one country in the UK to another, are aware of the different requirements and procedures. The terms and conditions of the contract are printed in the current edition of the Drug Tariff, which is published monthly in England and Wales and quarterly in Scotland. The Northern Ireland Drug Tariff is presented in a loose-leaf format and is updated quarterly.

## THE DRUG TARIFF

This publication contains details of all the requirements which have to be met when providing an NHS dispensing service. It includes information on allowances paid to contractors, medicines and appliances permitted to be prescribed on an NHS prescription form, prescription endorsement requirements, amounts payable, exempt categories of patients and details of charges made for prescriptions.

## PRESCRIPTION FORMS

The type of prescription forms issued in the various countries of the UK differ. Information about these prescription forms is found in Tables A2.1, A2.2, A2.3 and A2.4.

NHS prescription forms are issued by GPs and dentists in Jersey and by GPs in Guernsey. These forms are not valid for dispensing in England, Wales, Scotland, Northern Ireland or the Isle of Man.

## PAYMENT FOR PRESCRIPTIONS

On presentation of a valid NHS prescription at a pharmacy, pharmacists, under the terms of their contract, are required to dispense the prescription without undue delay. The prescription is then submitted to the Prescription Pricing Authority (PPA) in England, the Prescription Pricing Division in Wales or the Pharmacy Practice Division (PPD) in Scotland, where it is priced. The contractor is then reimbursed for the cost of the drugs or appliances

### Table A2.1   NHS prescription forms issued in England and Wales (E & W)

| Prescription code | Colour | Issued by | Reason issued | Valid to be dispensed in E, W, S, NI and IOM |
|---|---|---|---|---|
| FP10 | White | GPs and dispensing doctors | General practice patients | Yes |
| FP10 (HP) | Peach | Doctors from clinics or hospitals | Hospital outpatients | Yes |
| FP10 (HP) (ad) | Pink | Doctors from drug addiction clinics | Drug addicts | Yes |
| FP10 (MDA) | Light blue | GPs and dispensing doctors | Drug addicts | Yes |
| FP10 (D) | Green-blue | Dispensing doctors | Dispensing doctors' patients for drugs not in stock | Yes |
| FP10 (CN) | Green | Community nurses with nurse prescriber qualifications | General practice patients | Yes |
| FP10 (PN) | Lilac | Practice nurses with nurse prescriber qualifications | General practice patients | Yes |
| FP10 (DTS) | White | Sampling officers of Drug Testing Scheme | Drug Testing Scheme | E & W only |
| FP14 | Yellow | Dentists | Dental patients | Yes; only valid if written generically |

### Table A2.2   NHS prescription forms issued in Scotland (S)

| Prescription code | Colour | Issued by | Reason issued | Valid to be dispensed in E, W, S, NI and IOM |
|---|---|---|---|---|
| GP10 | White | GPs | General practice patients | Yes |
| GP10AW | White | GPs | Doctors' stock orders | S only |
| GP10 (CN) | Green | Community nurses with nurse prescriber qualifications | General practice patients | Yes |
| GP10 (PN) | Lilac | Practice nurses with nurse prescriber qualifications | General practice patients | Yes |
| GP10DTS | Pink | Sampling officers of Drug Testing Scheme | Drug Testing Scheme | S only |
| GP14 | Yellow | Dentists | Dental patients | Yes; must be written generically |
| HBP | Blue | Hospital doctors | Hospital outpatients | Yes |
| HBP(A) | Pink | Drug addiction clinics | Drug addicts | Yes |

### Table A2.3   NHS prescription forms issued in Northern Ireland (NI)

| Prescription code | Colour | Issued by | Reason issued | Valid to be dispensed in E, W, S, NI and IOM |
|---|---|---|---|---|
| HS21 | White | GPs | General practice patients | Yes |
| HS21 (C) | White | GPs (preprinted computer forms) | General practice patients | Yes |
| HS47 | Yellow | Dentists | Dental patients | Yes |

| Table A2.4  NHS forms issued in the Isle of Man (IOM) | | | | |
|---|---|---|---|---|
| Prescription code | Colour | Issued by | Reason issued | Valid to be dispensed in E, W, S, NI and IOM |
| HS10 | White | GPs and dentists | General practice patients<br>Dental patients<br>Hospital outpatients | Yes |

and paid the appropriate dispensing fee. Details of appropriate costs and fees are published in the Drug Tariff.

Currently, submission of prescriptions for payment is a paper-based, time-consuming exercise. Trials are presently being carried out on the electronic transfer of prescription information. This will provide a quicker and less labour-intensive method of submitting prescriptions for pricing.

## Prescription endorsement

To ensure accurate pricing of the prescriptions they must be endorsed before submission. If omissions or errors occur in the endorsing process, the prescription is returned to the pharmacy for clarification, thereby causing a delay in the pharmacist's remuneration. Endorsement requirements are clearly stated in the Drug Tariff which should be consulted. The National Pharmaceutical Association (NPA) publishes a guide to the Drug Tariff and NHS dispensing which also provides much useful information.

In general, the prescription should state, clearly and unambiguously, a description of the drugs dispensed, the strength and the quantity. If these are present the need for further endorsement is unlikely. Some common reasons why prescriptions are referred back to the submitting pharmacy are:

- Failure to endorse 'illegible' prescriptions
- Failure to endorse the prescription with details of the manufacturer or supplier, when required to do so
- Failure to endorse the prescription with pack size details, when required to do so
- Failure to endorse prescriptions which have vital details omitted by the prescriber, e.g. strength, when there is more than one
- Dispensing a prescription which has not been signed or dated by the prescriber.

## Disallowed payments

In addition, certain prescriptions will be disallowed for payment. There are a variety of reasons for this and the following list gives some examples.

- The item dispensed is blacklisted, i.e. an item which is not available on the NHS.
- The prescription is either a dental or a nurse's form and the item is not allowed to be prescribed by these practitioners.
- The prescribed item is a chemical reagent or appliance which is not allowed to be prescribed on an NHS form.

Neither of these lists is comprehensive and further information can be obtained from the PPA or PPD.

## PRESCRIPTION CHARGES

The Government currently levies a flat rate prescription charge on each prescription item. This must be collected by community pharmacists as part of their contractual agreement. There are several categories of people who are exempt from charges and a declaration to that effect and an indication of why they are claiming exemption must be completed on the reverse of the prescription form. A full list of exemption categories can be found in the Drug Tariff and includes groups such as men and women over 60 years old, children under 16 years and women who are pregnant. Some categories are automatically exempt while others must apply for exemption. Figures vary from area to area but approximately 70% of prescription items dispensed are for people who are exempt from prescription charges.

Pharmacists must ensure that the declaration on the reverse of the prescription form is accurately completed. Failure to do this could lead to contractors having prescription charges incorrectly deducted from their remuneration.

## Charges payable

One area where confusion can occur is when patients are charged incorrectly for prescription items. This can cause financial loss to the contractor and also confusion to the patient. A complete list of criteria on how many prescription charges should be made is found in the Drug Tariff. The following is a list of commonly occurring situations, with examples.

Unless the patient is exempt, one charge is payable if:

- Different strengths of the same drug, in the same formulation, are prescribed at the same time, e.g. warfarin tablets 1 mg and 5 mg.
- One appliance of the same type (other than hosiery) is supplied at the same time, e.g. six open-wove bandages 2.5 cm and six open-wove bandages 5 cm. Although the bandages are two different sizes and more than one of each is supplied only one charge should be made for this prescription.
- A drug is supplied with a throat brush, dropper or vaginal applicator, e.g. Ortho Dienoestrol cream with applicator.
- Different flavours of the same preparation are prescribed at the same time, e.g. 60 Fybogel sachets (plain) and 60 Fybogel sachets (orange).

Unless the patient is exempt, multiple prescription charges are made if:

- The same drug, in different formulations, is prescribed at the same time, e.g. Voltarol tablets 25 mg and Voltarol 75 mg SR. This is the area where probably the greatest number of errors occur. Combination packs cause problems. Patients think they are only receiving one item but in fact the pack may contain two or more. Examples of these are Canesten Combi which includes a pessary and a tube of cream. Two charges must therefore be made. A pack of Menophase tablets consists of six different types of tablet. Strictly speaking, six charges should be made but in this instance the Government has chosen to levy only two.
- More than one item of elastic hosiery, e.g. a pair of elastic stockings is counted as two items and two charges are made.

More examples of single and multiple charges are found in the Drug Tariff. In cases of uncertainty the PPA or the PPD is an extremely helpful and useful source of advice.

## THE BLACK LIST

In 1985 the Government issued a list of preparations which would no longer be prescribable on NHS pre-

scriptions. Various criteria were used in selecting which items would be 'blacklisted'. These included products which were deemed to be of limited therapeutic value, e.g. certain cough preparations, products which were too expensive and products where there was considerable duplication. The Black List may, therefore, contain a particular brand of a drug but the generic equivalent is allowable, e.g. generic diazepam may be prescribed on an NHS prescription but may not be written as the branded form, Valium, which is disallowed. A patient who wishes the proprietary brand must obtain a private prescription. The Black List is continuously updated with products being added or removed from the list. Practising pharmacists should ensure that they keep up to date with any alterations.

When presented with a prescription for a blacklisted item the pharmacist always has one option and the possibility of another three, if appropriate.

- The patient can always be referred back to the prescriber to obtain a private prescription for the blacklisted item.
- If the preparation is available in an allowable generic form, an NHS prescription for the generic could be requested, if this is acceptable to the patient and the prescriber.
- If the item can be legally purchased without a prescription, i.e. is not a POM, then this option can be offered to the patient.
- In exceptional circumstances, e.g. where it is impossible to contact the prescriber, it may be possible to use the emergency supply procedures, if requested by the patient.

## PRIVATE PRESCRIPTIONS

NHS prescription forms may not be used or treated as private prescriptions. The form is considered to be the property of the Secretary of State for Health and, as such, may only be used for the provision of drugs and appliances on the NHS. The two situations when problems might arise are:

- A blacklisted item, which is a POM, is written on an NHS prescription. If the patient wants this particular item he or she must return to the prescriber and obtain a private prescription. The pharmacist must not treat the NHS form as a private prescription, i.e. charge the patient for the item and retain the prescription in the pharmacy.
- The cost of the item prescribed is less than the prescription charge. It is against the NHS terms of

service to dispense NHS prescriptions as private prescriptions in order to save patients money.

## OTHER PROFESSIONAL SERVICES

Over and above the provision of dispensing services the terms of service require pharmacists to provide a range of professional services. These are the subject of negotiation with government and requirements change from one period of negotiation to another. Additions which have occurred in the last few years are:

- ensuring the availability in the pharmacy of appropriate health education leaflets
- the provision of a practice leaflet indicating the services provided by the pharmacy
- the provision, where appropriate, of counselling and advice on prescription medicines and appliances (currently Scotland only)
- maintaining patient medication records.

Pharmacists should consult a current edition of the Drug Tariff for information on the conditions which apply and the allowances payable.

## FURTHER READING

Chemist and Druggist Directory 1996 128th edn. Miller Freeman, Tonbridge (Use current edition)

National Health Service England and Wales Drug Tariff. HMSO (Published monthly – use current edn)

National Health Service in Scotland Drug Tariff. Scottish Office Home and Health Department (Published quarterly – use current edn)

NPA Guide to the Drug Tariff and NHS Dispensing. National Pharmaceutical Association, St Albans (Use current edition)

# Appendix 3
## Medical abbreviations

*D. M. Collett*

## Introduction

In order to practise the clinical aspects of pharmacy the student must become familiar with the terminology of the physician. It is beyond the scope of this book to include definitions of medical terms; the reader is referred to one of the excellent medical dictionaries published. However, the following list of the more commonly used medical abbreviations is included as a guide to the physician's shorthand. It is not intended to be comprehensive and users should be aware of local variations in the use of terms and their abbreviations.

## Some commonly used abbreviations for medical terms

| Abbreviation | Term |
| --- | --- |
| Ab | abortion |
| Abd | abdomen |
| ADH | antidiuretic hormone |
| ADR | adverse drug reaction |
| A & E | accident and emergency |
| AFB | acid-fast bacillus |
| A/G | albumin/globulin ratio |
| Ag | antigen |
| ALL | acute lymphocytic leukaemia |
| AMI | acute myocardial infarction |
| AML | acute myelogenous leukaemia |
| A-R | apical-radial pulse |
| ASCVD | arteriosclerotic cardiovascular disease |
| AV | arteriovenous, atrioventricular |
| BaE | barium enema |
| BBB | bundle branch block, blood–brain barrier |
| BM | bowel movement |
| BMR | basal metabolic rate |
| BNO | bowels not open |
| BOR | bowels open regularly |

| Abbreviation | Term |
| --- | --- |
| BS | bowel sounds, breath sounds, blood sugar |
| BUN | blood urea nitrogen |
| Bx | biopsy |
| c̄ | with |
| CA | cancer, carcinoma |
| CAPD | continuous ambulatory peritoneal dialysis |
| CAT | computer assisted tomogram |
| CC | chief complaint |
| CCF | congestive cardiac failure |
| CCU | coronary care unit |
| CHD | coronary heart disease |
| CHF | congestive heart failure |
| CNS | central nervous system |
| CO | cardiac output |
| C/O | complains of |
| COAD | chronic obstructive airway disease |
| COLD | chronic obstructive lung disease |
| COPD | chronic obstructive pulmonary disease |
| C & S | culture and sensitivity |
| CSF | cerebrospinal fluid |
| CSU | catheter specimen of urine |
| CVA | cerebrovascular accident |
| CVP | central venous pressure |
| Cx | cervical, cervix |
| CXR | chest X-ray |
| D | diagnosis |
| D & C | dilatation and curettage |
| DD | differential diagnosis |
| DH | drug history |
| DM | diabetes mellitus |
| DNA | did not attend (outpatient) |
| DOA | dead on arrival |
| DOB | date of birth |
| DOE | dyspnoea on exertion |
| DTs | delirium tremens |
| DU | duodenal ulcer |

| Abbreviation | Term | Abbreviation | Term |
|---|---|---|---|
| D & V | diarrhoea and vomiting | LVH | left ventricular hypertrophy |
| DVT | deep vein thrombosis | MCH | mean corpuscular haemoglobin |
| ECG | electrocardiogram | MCHC | mean corpuscular haemoglobin |
| ECT | electroconvulsive therapy | | concentration |
| EEG | electroencephalogram | MCV | mean corpuscular volume |
| EMS | early morning specimen | MI | mitral incompetence or |
| ENT | ear, nose and throat | | insufficiency |
| ESR | erythrocyte sedimentation rate | MI | myocardial infarction |
| EUA | examination under anaesthetic | MIC | minimum inhibitory concentration |
| FB | finger breadths, foreign body | MS | mitral stenosis, multiple sclerosis |
| FBC | full blood count | MSU | mid-stream urine specimen |
| FBS | fasting blood sugar | N | normal |
| FEV$_1$ | forced expiratory volume in | NAD | nothing abnormal detected |
| | 1 second | NBM | nil by mouth |
| FFA | free fatty acids | NG | nasogastric |
| FH | family history | NPN | non-protein nitrogen |
| FROM | full range of movement | NPO | nothing by mouth (non-peroral) |
| FUO | fever of unknown origin | NS | nervous system |
| FVC | forced vital capacity | NSR | normal sinus rhythm |
| Fx | fracture | N & V | nausea and vomiting |
| GFR | glomerular filtration rate | $^0$BS | absence of bowel sounds |
| GI | gastrointestinal | o | absent |
| GIT | gastrointestinal tract | O | oedema |
| GTT | glucose tolerance test | O/A | on admission |
| GU | genitourinary | Obs-Gyn | obstetrics and gynaecology |
| gyn | gynaecology | O/E | on examination |
| Hb, Hgb | haemoglobin | OOB | out of bed |
| Hct | haematocrit | OP | outpatient |
| HCVD | hypertensive cardiovascular disease | OPD | outpatients department |
| H & P | history and physical | Para | number of pregnancies |
| HPI | history of present illness | PBI | protein-bound iodine |
| HTVD | hypertensive vascular disease | PCV | packed cell volume |
| ICM | intracostal margin | PDQ | at once |
| ICS | intercostal space | PE | physical examination, pulmonary |
| ICU | intensive care unit | | embolism |
| ID | intradermal, initial dose | PERRLA | pupils equal, round, reactive to light |
| Ig | immunoglobulin | | and accommodation |
| IHD | ischaemic heart disease | PF(R) | peak flow (rate) |
| IM | intramuscular | PKU | phenylketonuria |
| INR | International Normalized Ratio | PM | postmortem |
| | (prothrombin time) | PMH | past medical history |
| IP | intraperitoneal, inpatient | PMT | premenstrual tension |
| IPPB | intermittent positive pressure | PND | paroxysmal nocturnal dyspnoea |
| | breathing | PO | oral (peroral) |
| IUD | intrauterine device | PR | rectal (per rectum) |
| IV | intravenous | Pt | patient |
| IVP | intravenous pyelogram | PT | prothrombin time |
| J | jaundice | PTA | prior to admission |
| JVP | jugular venous pulse | PUO | pyrexia of unknown origin |
| LA | local anaesthetic | PV | per vagina |
| LD | lethal dose | PVC | premature ventricular contraction |
| LE | lupus erythematosus | (R) | right |
| LVF | left ventricular failure | RA | right atrium, rheumatoid arthritis |

| Abbreviation | Term |
|---|---|
| RBC | red blood cells |
| RBS | random blood sugar |
| RCC | red cell count |
| RF | rheumatoid factor |
| RHD | rheumatic heart disease |
| Rh | rhesus factor |
| ROS | review of symptoms |
| RS | respiratory system |
| s̄ | without |
| S1 | first heart sound |
| S2 | second heart sound |
| SA | sino-atrial |
| SB | seen by, short of breath |
| SBE | shortage of breath on exertion |
| SBE | subacute bacterial endocarditis |
| SC | subcutaneous |
| SGOT | serum glutamic oxaloacetic transaminase |
| SGPT | serum glutamic pyruvic transaminase |
| SH | social history, serum hepatitis |
| SL | sublingual |
| SLE | systemic lupus erythematosus |
| SOA | swelling of ankles |
| SOB | shortness of breath |
| SOS | swelling of sacrum |
| STD | sexually transmitted disease |
| Sx | symptoms |
| T | temperature |
| T3 | tri-iodothyronine |
| T4 | thyroxine |
| T & A | tonsillectomy and adenoidectomy |
| TB | tuberculosis |
| TBA | to be arranged or to be administered |
| TIA | transient ischaemic attack |
| TIBC | total iron binding capacity |
| TKVO | to keep vein open |
| TLC | total lung capacity |
| TPN | total parenteral nutrition |
| TPR | temperature, pulse, respiration |
| TTO | to take out (home) |
| Tx | treatment |
| UA | uric acid, urinalysis |
| UC | ulcerative colitis |
| U & E | urea and electrolytes |
| UTI | urinary tract infection |
| UR(T)I | upper respiratory (tract) infection |
| VD | venereal disease |
| VP | venous pressure |
| VS | vital signs |
| VT | ventricular tachycardia |
| WBC | white blood cell |
| WBS | whole body scan |

| Abbreviation | Term |
|---|---|
| WNL | within normal limits |
| WR | Wassermann reaction |
| XR | X-ray |

## BIBLIOGRAPHY

Roper N 1987 Pocket medical dictionary, 15th edn. Churchill Livingstone, Edinburgh
Steen E B 1984 Abbreviations used in medicine, 5th edn. Baillière Tindall, London

# Appendix 4
## Latin terms and abbreviations

*D. M. Collett*

## Introduction

Prescriptions written in the UK should be written in English and the use of Latin is strongly discouraged. However, the use of some Latin terms persists and abbreviations are often used, especially to indicate the frequency of dosing.

The following lists include terms which may be encountered in current practice. For more comprehensive lists see previous editions of this book (Carter 1975) and the *Pharmaceutical Handbook* (Wade 1980).

## Dosage forms

| Latin name | Abbreviation | English name |
|---|---|---|
| Auristillae | aurist. | ear drops |
| Capsula | caps. | capsule |
| Cataplasma | cataplasm. | poultice |
| Collunarium | collun. | nosewash |
| Collutorium | collut. | mouthwash |
| Collyrium | collyr. | eye lotion |
| Cremor | crem. | cream |
| Guttae | gtt. | drops |
| Haustus | ht. | draught |
| Liquor | liq. | solution |
| Lotio | lot. | lotion |
| Mistura | mist. | mixture |
| Naristillae | narist. | nose drops |
| Nebula | neb. | spray solution |
| Oculentum | oculent. | eye ointment |
| Pasta | past. | paste |
| Pigmentum | pig. | paint |
| Pulvis | pulv. | powder |
| Pulvis conspersus | pulv. consp. | dusting powder |
| Trochiscus | troch. | lozenge |
| Unguentum | ung. | ointment |
| Vapor | vap. | inhalation |
| Vitrella | vitrell. | glass capsule (crushable) |

## Terms used in prescriptions

| Latin | Abbreviation | English |
|---|---|---|
| ante cibum | a.c. | before food |
| ante meridiem | a.m. | before noon |
| ana | aa. | of each |
| ad | ad | to |
| ad libitum | ad lib. | as much as desired |
| alternus | alt. | alternate |
| ante | ante | before |
| applicandus | applic. | to be applied |
| aqua | aq. | water |
| bis | b. | twice |
| bis die | b.d. | twice daily |
| bis in die | b.i.d. | twice daily |
| calidus | calid. | warm |
| cibus | cib. | food |
| compositus | co. | compound |
| concentratus | conc. | concentrated |
| cum | c. | with |
| dies | d. | a day |
| destillatus | dest. | distilled |
| dilutus | dil. | diluted |
| duplex | dup. | double |
| ex aqua | ex aq. | in water |
| fiat | ft. | let it be made |
| fortis | fort. | strong |
| hora | h. | at the hour of |
| hora somni | h.s. | at bedtime |
| inter cibos | i.c. | between meals |
| inter | int. | between |
| mane | m. | in the morning |
| more dicto | m.d. | as directed |
| more dicto utendus | m.d.u. | to be used as directed |
| mitte | mitt. | send |
| nocte | n. | at night |
| nocte et mane | n. et m. | night and morning |
| nocte maneque | n.m. | night and morning |

485

| Latin | Abbreviation | English |
|---|---|---|
| nomen proprium | n.p. | the proper name |
| nocte | noct. | at night |
| omnibus alternis horis | o.alt.hor | every other hour |
| omni die | o.d. | every day |
| omni mane | o.m. | every morning |
| omni nocte | o.n. | every night |
| parti affectae | p.a. | to the affected part |
| parti affectae applicandus | part. affect. | to be applied to the affected part |
| partes aequales | p.aeq. | equal parts |
| post cibum | p.c. | after food |
| post meridiem | p.m. | afternoon |
| partes | pp. | parts |
| pro re nata | p.r.n. | when required |
| parti dolenti | part. dolent. | to the painful part |
| quarter die | q.d. | four times daily |
| quater die sumendus | q.d.s. | to be take four times daily |
| quarter in die | q.i.d. | four times daily |
| quaque | qq. | every |
| quaque hora | qq.h. | every hour |
| quarta quaque hora | q.qq.h. | every fourth hour |
| | q.q.h. | every fourth hour |
| quantum sufficiat | q.s. | sufficient |
| recipe | ℞ | take |
| secundum artem | sec. art. | with pharmaceutical skill |
| semisse | ss. | half |

| Latin | Abbreviation | English |
|---|---|---|
| si opus sit | s.o.s. | if necessary |
| signa | sig. | label |
| statim | stat. | immediately |
| sumendus ter | sum. t. | to be taken thrice thrice |
| ter de die | t.d.d. | three times daily |
| ter die sumendus | t.d.s. | to be taken three times daily |
| ter in die | t.i.d. | three times daily |
| tussis | tuss. | a cough |
| tussi urgente | tuss. urg. | when the cough troubles |
| ut antea | u.a. | as before |
| ut dictum | ut. dict. | as directed |
| ut directum | ut. direct. | as directed |
| utendus | utend. | to be used |

## Numerals

The *cardinals* in Table A4.1 refer to number and thus are translated, one, two, three, etc.

The *ordinals* refer to position and thus are translated first, second, third, etc.

The *adverbs* qualify verbs and thus are translated once, twice, three times, etc.

## BIBLIOGRAPHY

Carter S 1975 Dispensing for pharmaceutical students, 13th edn. Pitman Medical, London

Wade A 1980 Pharmaceutical handbook, 19th edn. Pharmaceutical Press, London

**Table A4.1** Roman numerals: Roman symbol and corresponding Latin names for the cardinal and ordinal numbers and their adverbs

| Arabic number | Roman symbol | Cardinals | Ordinals | Adverbs |
|---|---|---|---|---|
| 1 | I | unus | primus, -a, -um | semel (once) |
| 2 | II | duo | secundus or alter | bis (twice) |
| 3 | III | tres, tria(n.) | tertius | ter (three times) |
| 4 | IV | quattuor | quartus | quater (four times) |
| 5 | V | quinque | quintus | quinquies |
| 6 | VI | sex | sextus | sexies |
| 7 | VII | septem | septimus | septies |
| 8 | VIII | octo | octavus | octies |
| 9 | IX | novem | nonus | novies |
| 10 | X | decem | decimus | decies |
| 11 | XI | undecim | undecimus | undecies |
| 12 | XII | duodecim | duodecimus | duodecies |
| 14 | XIV | quattuordecim | quartis decimus | quattuor-decies |
| 15 | XV | quindecim | quintus decimus | quindecies |
| 20 | XX | viginti | vicesimus | vicies |
| 50 | L | quinquaginta | quinquagesimus | quinquagies |
| 100 | C | centum | centesimus | centies |

# Appendix 5
## Systems of weights and measures

*A. J. Winfield*

## Introduction

In 1960 the Système International d'Unités (SI system), based on the metric system, was adopted as the standard. Since 1969 all prescriptions in the UK have been dispensed in this system. The older Imperial and Apothecary systems are still found in older books and formularies. This appendix outlines the three systems for weight and volume.

## UNITS OF WEIGHT

### Metric (SI) system

The basic unit is the kilogram, which is the mass of the International Prototype Kilogram.

| Name of unit | Abbreviation | Relationship |
|---|---|---|
| Kilogram | kg | |
| Gram | g | 1/1000 (0.001) kg |
| Milligram | mg | 1/1000 (0.001) g |
| Microgram | μg (or mcg) | 1/1000 (0.001) mg |
| Nanogram | ng | 1/1000 (0.001) μg |
| Picogram | pg | 1/1000 (0.001) ng |

To avoid confusion between mg, mcg and ng it is advisable not to use these abbreviations in dispensing.

### Imperial system

The pound (avoirdupois) is the basic unit.

| Name of unit | Abbreviation | Relationship |
|---|---|---|
| Pound | lb | |
| Ounce | oz | 1/16 lb |
| Grain | gr | 1/7000 lb |
| | | 1/437.5 oz |

## Apothecary system

The grain is the basic standard and is the same as the Imperial grain.

| Name of unit | Abbreviation | Relationship |
|---|---|---|
| Grain | gr | |
| Scruple | | 20 gr |
| Drachm | | 60 gr |
| Ounce (Apoth.) | | 480 gr |
| | | 8 drachms |

*Note:* the Imperial and Apothecary ounce are not the same weight.

## VOLUME

### Metric (SI) system

The basic unit is the litre which is defined as 1 cubic decimetre.

| Unit | Abbreviation | Relationship |
|---|---|---|
| Litre | l | |
| Millilitre | ml | 1/1000 (0.001) l |
| Microlitre | μl | 1/1000 (0.001) ml |

### Imperial system

The basic unit is the pint.

| Name of unit | Abbreviation | Relationship |
|---|---|---|
| Pint | pt | |
| Fluid ounce | fl. oz. | 1/20 pt |

## Apothecary system

The minim is the basic unit.

| Name of unit | Abbreviation | Relationship |
|---|---|---|
| Minim | m | |
| Fluid drachm | fl. dr. | 60 m |
| Fluid ounce | fl. oz. | 8 fl dr |
| | | 480 m |

## FURTHER READING

Wade A (ed) 1980 The pharmaceutical handbook, 19th edn. The Pharmaceutical Press, London (This book contains useful tables of conversion factors, including the accepted equivalents for dispensing non-metric prescriptions)

## AMOUNT OF SUBSTANCE

The basic unit is the mole which is the amount of substance containing as many formula units as there are in 12 g of carbon-12. The formula units may be atoms, molecules, ions, etc.

| Name of unit | Abbreviation | Relationship |
|---|---|---|
| Mole | mol | |
| Millimole | mmol | 1/1000 (0.001) mol |
| Micromole | µmol | 1/1000 (0.001) mmol |

## CONCENTRATION

Concentration can be expressed as g per l (g per $dm^3$) or mol per l. In dispensing, the former is normally used for drug concentration. Electrolyte concentration may be expressed as amount of substance (mol per l). In medical records and literature, mol per l is normally used.

## LENGTH

The metre is the basic unit.

| Name of unit | Abbreviation | Relationship |
|---|---|---|
| Metre | m | |
| Centimetre | cm | 1/100 (0.01) m |
| Millimetre | mm | 1/1000 (0.001) m |
| Micrometre | µm | 1/1000 (0.001) mm |
| Nanometre | nm | 1/1000 (0.001) µm |

When expressing quantity, it is important to avoid the risk of error or misinterpretation. To reduce this it is best to avoid decimal fractions where possible. Thus, it is better to use 50 mg rather than 0.05 g. Where a decimal point is used, it should be preceded by a 0, thus it should be 0.1 g rather than .1 g.

# Appendix 6
## Homoeopathy and other complementary therapies

*S. L. Hutchinson*

## Introduction

Public demand for complementary medicines over the last few years has increased. This has resulted in pharmacists being involved in stocking complementary medicines in community pharmacies, advising customers on their appropriate use, over-the-counter (OTC) prescribing and dispensing of prescriptions for homoeopathic remedies. This appendix gives information which pharmacists may require when dispensing a prescription for homoeopathic medicines or giving the appropriate advice when OTC prescribing is required. The information given will concentrate on homoeopathic medicines but will also give a brief outline of Bach flower remedies, herbal medicines and aromatherapy.

## WHAT IS HOMOEOPATHY?

In 1796, Dr Samuel Hahnemann, a German physician, discovered a different approach to curing people who were ill. He called it homoeopathy (from the Greek, meaning 'similar suffering'). Like Hippocrates in 460 BC, Hahnemann recognized that there were two ways of treating ill health, the way of opposites and the way of similars. By a process of observation, proving and testing he developed homoeopathy as we recognize it today. He studied the action of cinchona bark (from which quinine is derived) in the treatment of fever, by using himself and members of his own family to test his remedies. He took some quinine himself and found that he experienced malaria symptoms that rapidly disappeared when he stopped taking the quinine.

Hahnemann repeated his work using other healthy volunteers known as 'provers'. From his work, he was able to show that by some natural law, a remedy which was effective against disease could be used to produce symptoms resembling those of the disease in a healthy individual. Hahnemann continued his work by testing a whole range of substances on his healthy volunteers. He used a range of dilutions and discovered that dilution of the remedy appeared to increases its ability to cure the condition. In his work he was able to use substances which, in high doses, could be poisonous but, in the dilute form, had good medicinal properties.

In 1810, Hahnemann published *The Organon of the Healing Art* detailing the medicines he had 'proved' and how the remedies work. Many of the original medicines 'proved' by Hahnemann have been 're-proved' over the years and subsequent work has endorsed the accuracy of Hahnemann's work.

Additional medicines have also been 'proved' since Hahnemann's time and they are documented in the *Homoeopathic Materia Medica*. There are now over 2000 homoeopathic medicines available.

There are three basic principles of homoeopathy as proposed by Hahnemann:

1. A substance which in large doses could produce symptoms of a disease state could be used in a more dilute form to treat such symptoms in someone who is ill.
2. Dilution of a homoeopathic remedy can increase its curative properties and avoid undesirable side effects.
3. Homoeopathy has a holistic approach, treating the individual as a whole not just the illness.

Despite the death of Hahnemann in 1843, the use of homoeopathy continued to spread throughout the world. The 19th century saw the setting up of the British Homoeopathic Society (1844) and the foundation of homoeopathic hospitals. With the setting up of the NHS in 1948, existing homoeopathic hospitals were incorporated into the NHS. Today there are five homoeopathic hospitals in the UK. Homoeopathy is still available on the NHS and well over 2000 GPs in the UK are recommending the use of homoeopathic medicines for patients or referring them to a homoeopathic hospital.

## HOW ARE HOMOEOPATHIC REMEDIES MADE?

Homoeopathic remedies are prepared by removing active ingredients from an animal, vegetable or mineral source and dissolving them in a mixture of ethanol and water. This produces the concentrated starting solution known as the 'mother tincture' (symbol ø). The quality of source materials required for homoeopathic remedies is defined in the *British Homoeopathic Pharmacopoeia* (1993). The method of preparation used still adheres to the techniques laid down by Hahnemann in the late 18th century. From the mother tincture a series of dilutions is made using ethanol or water to give the required 'potencies' seen on prescriptions.

Homoeopaths believe that simple dilution is not sufficient and that the vigorous shaking at each stage of dilution is essential to the whole process. This is known as 'succussion'. The suggestion is that some form of energy release or development takes place that contributes to the properties of the resulting product. Dilution is normally by factors of 10, 100 or 1000. Homoeopaths believe that potency increases with dilution. Potencies are denoted by a letter which identifies the degree of dilution carried out, for example 'x' for a 1 in 10 dilution (referred to as the decimal potency). Table A6.1 shows other dilutions available.

Insoluble substances can be ground down (triturated) with an inert powder such as lactose and the trituration repeated to provide a powder which can then be dissolved in a liquid medium. The resulting solution is then diluted again with vigorous shaking at each stage to produce the required potencies.

## HOMOEOPATHY ON PRESCRIPTION

Pharmacists are obliged, under their conditions of service, to supply homoeopathic remedies prescribed on an NHS prescription, even if they decide not to stock homoeopathic remedies for OTC sale. Dosage forms prescribed on NHS prescriptions include tablets, powders, granules and tinctures. Most homoeopathic remedies are classed as general sales list (GSL) medicines. However, there are some exceptions: 'mother' tinctures, substances which

| Table A6.1 | Latin terms used in homoeopathy |
|---|---|
| ø or Tm | Mother tincture or basic tinctures |
| x or D | Preceded by a number referring to the dilution and decimal potency (1 in 10 dilution) |
| c | Preceded by a number referring to the dilution and centesimal potency (1 in 100 dilution) |
| M | Preceded by a number referring to the dilution (1 in 1000) |
| SL | Saccharum lactis (sugar of milk) lactose |
| **For solid dosage forms** | |
| 1 g | corresponds to 10 tablets |
| 7 g | corresponds to 50 tablets |
| 14 g | corresponds to 100 tablets |
| 25 g | corresponds to 200 tablets |

have a starting material which is a prescription-only medicine (POM) and certain formulations such as eye drops. Pharmacists dispensing homoeopathic prescriptions require knowledge of the terminology and Latin abbreviations used on homoeopathic prescriptions. Table A6.1 provides a list of commonly used abbreviations.

## Examples of homoeopathic prescriptions

Ignatia tablets 200c 7 g
1 o.d. for 10 days then p.r.n.

Ignatia is used to help people cope with bereavement. The prescription asks for 50 tablets (7 g), one tablet to be taken daily (o.d.) for 10 days then when required (p.r.n.).

℞ Nux vom. 6c 14 g
1 p.r.n. for heartburn

Nux vom. is used for heartburn occurring within 1–2 hours of eating food. 100 tablets (14 g) have been prescribed to be taken when required.

## THE WORK OF A HOMOEOPATHIC PRACTITIONER

Homoeopathy recognizes that the symptoms of ill health in an individual are expressions of disharmony within the whole person and that the patient needs treatment, not the disease. The holistic approach of homoeopathy means that a person attending a trained homoeopath would have a detailed patient history recorded. This would include details of symptoms experienced as well as personal characteristics and the health of the person's family both past and present. The aim of treatment is to select the medicine that most closely matches the symptoms observed in the patient. This is made possible by reference to recorded 'provings' which detail the appropriate medicines for the patient's symptoms. Following a consultation the patient could be prescribed one of several appropriate homoeopathic remedies. However, the pharmacist still has a role to play in offering advice and information regarding administration of such remedies.

Homoeopaths suggest that remedies available fall into several categories:

- *Specific*: medicines that have been proven to be most effective for a particular condition, e.g. Rhus tox for rheumatism. Such remedies are prescribed with a specific condition in mind.
- *Local*: remedies that are selected for a particular body organ, dependent on symptoms.
- *Fundamental* or *constitutional*: prescribed after recording patient details and considering the patient as a whole.
- *Polychrests*: remedies that are effective in a wide range of illnesses in anyone. Such remedies can be prescribed OTC by pharmacists, e.g. Arnica for bruising.

## OVER-THE-COUNTER PRESCRIBING OF HOMOEOPATHY

Stocks of homoeopathic remedies are available from a range of suppliers in the UK. Some suppliers provide self-treatment guides for patients to select their own remedies based on matching up their symptoms to appropriate remedies. For self-medication, homoeopaths recommend that a 6c potency is used and that administration is continued only until some improvement in the condition is seen. If no improvement is seen within about 24 hours, the choice of remedy may have to be changed. Appropriate questions and answers that a pharmacist should be aware of when dealing with homoeopathic remedies are detailed below.

## How do I take homoeopathic medicines?

Handle as little as possible. If tablets are being taken, tip the tablet onto a clean spoon or the cap of the container and transfer to mouth. Tablets can be sucked, chewed or allowed to dissolve under the tongue. Never swallow tablets whole. Homoeopathic tablets for children can be crushed to a powder before administration.

## Do I take homoeopathic remedies before or after food?

Take homoeopathic remedies approximately 15–30 minutes before or after food. Smoking, drinking strong-smelling liquids (including coffee or tea) or using toothpaste appear to affect the action of homoeopathic medicines (homoeopathic toothpaste is available).

## How often should homoeopathic remedies be taken?

Follow manufacturers' recommendations. In acute conditions, remedies can be taken every 1–2 hours, up to six times daily, reducing to three times daily as symptoms subside. Homoeopathic medicines can be given to children. Half the adult dose is recommended.

## How do I store homoeopathic remedies?

Store in their original container, away from direct sunlight, in a cool place. Store away from strong-smelling substances like perfume, aftershave and mouth fresheners.

## Will I experience any side effects when taking homoeopathic remedies?

Occasionally some people feel their symptoms become slightly worse at first but these feelings rapidly subside as the body's natural defence mechanisms begin to work.

## Can homoeopathic remedies be taken with conventional medicines?

Yes. Often homoeopathy is used to complement conventional medicines. However, it is important to let your own doctor know all the medicines you are taking including any homoeopathic remedies. Never stop taking prescribed medicines without consultation with your doctor. Aromatherapy oils are said to inactivate homoeopathic medicines; hence they should not be used while taking homoeopathic medicines.

## Are homoeopathic remedies safe to take in pregnancy?

Yes. Homoeopathic medicines have been used safely

during pregnancy and childbirth for a number of years. Remedies are available that can be used to treat conditions in pregnancy such as morning sickness and constipation. Homoeopathy can also be recommended for emotional and physical healing after childbirth and during breast-feeding.

## OTHER COMPLEMENTARY THERAPIES

Apart from homoeopathy, several other complementary or alternative therapies are available. Therapies that have a holistic approach to health are Bach flower remedies, herbal remedies and aromatherapy. Each will be discussed briefly in this section.

### Bach flower remedies

Such remedies are made from wild flowers, trees and bushes. Dr Edward Bach, a homoeopath, bacteriologist and doctor, identified 38 species of wild flowers that are today known as Bach flower remedies. The source material is placed in spring water and exposed to direct sunlight for several hours. The resulting solution, which is believed to take on the properties of the plant source, is then diluted to half strength with brandy to form a stock solution. Each remedy contains a few drops of the stock solution further diluted with brandy and water. The preparations available are recommended for use in treating a variety of negative emotional states and personality problems. Patients are required to honestly assess their emotional and mental state, habits and behavioural patterns in order to select a suitable remedy. There are seven categories of remedies available that are selected by patients themselves on a 'self-prescribe' basis. Categories listed are as follows: those who 'have fear', 'suffer uncertainty', 'suffer loneliness', 'are oversensitive to influences and ideas', 'suffer despondency and despair', 'lack of interest in present circumstances' and 'over-care for others' welfare'. The remedies can be used individually or in combination. Rescue remedy is an example of a combined preparation which contains five different ingredients. It is said to be useful for dealing with stressful situations in life – such as exams! Remedies are taken by diluting two drops of the stock solution in about 30 ml of boiled water. A few drops of this are taken in a teaspoon of water at least four times daily. For people who have difficulty in swallowing medicines, the remedy can be rubbed onto the lips, temples, wrists or behind the ears. Bach flower remedies are not believed to interact with prescribed

medicines and are safe to give during pregnancy and to children. Diluted preparations are said to remain stable for up to 3 weeks and should be stored away from direct sunlight. Bach flower remedies are available from UK suppliers and can be stocked in pharmacies for sale to customers.

### Herbal medicines

The source of herbal medicines is from whole plants or part of the plant, usually roots, leaves and berries. Herbal medicine as it is known today dates back to Galen who, in the second century AD, classified herbs by essential qualities: hot or cold, dry or damp. Herbalists today choose appropriate remedies on the basis of Galen's classification. Remedies are said to have 'heating' or 'cooling' properties. Heating remedies can be used to increase blood flow or metabolic rate. Cooling remedies allow increased digestion or absorption. Some cooling remedies can have sedative properties.

Herbal practitioners, like homoeopathic practitioners, have a holistic approach to treatment. They consider emotional and psychological symptoms as well as the patient's medical condition. Treatment can involve the use of a remedy that contains more than one herbal preparation to ensure that the whole condition is treated. In certain circumstances, advice may be given to modify the diet and to avoid substances such as alcohol and caffeine. Vitamin supplements may also be recommended.

Without consulting a herbal practitioner, several herbal preparations are available OTC in pharmacies and can be selected on a self-selection basis or on the recommendation of a pharmacist. Commonly used preparations include:

- Garlic for colds and as a general circulation stimulant
- Mint for constipation, flatulence, nausea and vomiting
- Camomile for digestive problems
- Fennel for insomnia, nausea and vomiting.

It should be noted that several herbal medicines should not be used in pregnancy as they can act as uterine stimulants. Examples of such medicines include Cinchona, Golden Seal, Juniper and Rosemary. A medical practitioner should always be consulted prior to taking any herbal medicines during pregnancy. Some herbal medicines can cause problems for people with underlying medical conditions. Examples are given below:

- *Diabetes mellitus.* Cowberry, Billberry and

Fenugreek can cause hypoglycaemia. Angelica has a high sugar content and must be avoided in diabetics.

- *Cardiovascular conditions.* Ma Hung should be avoided by people with hypertension and coronary thrombosis. Feverfew, Cowslip and Primrose can interfere with warfarin clotting time. Golden Seal, Ginseng and Liquorice should not be used by people with hypertension.

## Aromatherapy

This involves the use of essential oils distilled from plants to improve physical and emotional well-being. Oils can be applied to the body by using compresses, or added to a bath, massage or steam inhalation. There are no official doses for aromatherapy oils. The amount used in each case is based on individuals' experience and preference. Their use includes treatment of skin conditions such as eczema and psoriasis, minor infections such as thrush and cystitis, prevention of stress and anxiety and in relieving muscle and joint pain. However, caution should be exercised when recommending aromatherapy to women who are pregnant. It is advisable to recommend that pregnant women should consult a qualified practitioner prior to using aromatherapy oils.

The use of aromatherapy in conjunction with orthodox medicines and treatments appears to be common and no contraindications are documented. However, aromatherapy oils are believed to inactivate homoeopathic medicines and the two should, therefore, not be used in conjunction.

# Appendix 7
## Sources of information

*D. Stewart*

## Introduction

Pharmacists must be familiar with many different sources of information. This appendix outlines the scope of selected major pharmaceutical publications and other sources of information.*

## PHARMACOPOEIAS

### British Pharmacopoeia (BP)

This text details standards of purity and strength for medical substances, products and dressings, together with official assays. Products suitable for extemporaneous dispensing are fully described.

### European Pharmacopoeia (EP)

This was created to permit free circulation of drugs within the European Community. Monographs of the EP are reproduced in the current BP and certain official procedures are performed according to EP methods.

### Martindale: the Extra Pharmacopoeia
(Reynolds 1996)

This is perhaps the most widely used information source on drugs and medicines in the UK. It provides information on nomenclature, physical and pharmaceutical properties, adverse effects, actions and uses of drugs. A new edition is published every 3 years. It is also available as an on-line database which is updated frequently.

---

*Much of this material is based on the UK Drug Information Pharmacists' Group *Drug Information Procedures Manual* 1992, Leeds, with permission.

## THERAPEUTICS

### British National Formulary (BNF)

The BNF is produced jointly by the British Medical Association and the Royal Pharmaceutical Society of Great Britain. The content is determined by a joint formulary committee of consultants and pharmacists and is revised twice yearly. General guidance on prescribing is provided together with special requirements of children, the elderly, pregnant and breast-feeding women, and patients with renal or hepatic impairment. The main text contains notes on drugs and preparations, detailing information on indications, contraindications, cautions, side effects and doses. Drug interactions and their clinical importance are also covered in a separate section. An electronic BNF is now available on line.

### Clinical Pharmacy and Therapeutics
(Walker & Edwards 1994)

This text aims to help pharmacy students, pharmacists and other health care professionals understand clinical disorders and promote the safe, appropriate and effective use of drugs. Each therapeutic section contains case studies designed to encourage application of therapeutic principles.

### Goodman and Gilman's the Pharmacological Basis of Therapeutics
(Goodman et al 1996)

This is an American text which provides detail on the pharmacology behind the therapeutic application of drugs, but does not always reflect practice in the UK.

## Avery's Drug Treatment: Principles and Practice of Clinical Pharmacology and Therapeutics (Speight & Halford 1996)

This offers a disease-orientated approach to therapeutics. It is very useful in providing a review of the treatment of disease, but gives less detail on individual drugs.

## Applied Therapeutics – the Clinical Use of Drugs (Young & Koda-Kimble 1995)

This is also an American text which covers all aspects of the clinical use of drugs. The format is of a case presentation with questions relating to the case with fully referenced answers. This presentation can sometimes make specific information difficult to locate.

# ADVERSE DRUG REACTIONS AND DRUG INTERACTIONS

## Meyler's the Side Effects of Drugs (Dukes 1996)

This is the standard reference on adverse effects. It is published every 4 years and presents monographs on major drugs and their pharmacological groups.

## The Side Effects of Drugs Annuals

These offer a world-wide yearly survey of new data and trends, with much of the material presented having been published in the preceding 2 years.

## Drug Interactions (Stockley 1996)

This is the standard reference source on drug interactions listing mechanisms of drug interactions, clinical importance and management.

# PROPRIETARY MEDICINES

## Association of British Pharmaceutical Industry (ABPI) Data Sheet Compendium

This is produced annually by the Association of British Pharmaceutical Industries and contains copies of the data sheets of all participating companies. The information to be included in a data sheet is specified by the Medicines (Data Sheet) Regulations 1972. Information is given on drug presentations, uses, dosage, administration, contraindications, warnings and pharmaceutical precautions. This is an essential source of information on manufactured medicines but is limited in that data sheets are only included if companies are members of the ABPI.

## Monthly Index of Medical Specialities (MIMS)

This is designed as a reference and prescribing guide and is produced monthly. It lists proprietary preparations that can be prescribed or recommended.

## Patient Information Leaflet Compendium

This is produced yearly by the ABPI and includes copies of patient information leaflets found in proprietary medicine packs. It is intended to indicate to doctors and pharmacists the nature of such leaflets.

## Chemist and Druggist Guide to OTC Medicines

This is produced mainly for community pharmacists and is regularly updated. Data are presented in therapeutic categories giving general advice followed by monographs detailing directions for use, cautions and costs. There are also useful sections detailing herbal and homoeopathic products.

## OTC Directory

This is produced yearly by the Proprietary Association of Great Britain and is similar to the Chemist and Druggist Guide but is also aimed at general practitioners.

## Non-prescription Drugs (Li Wan Po 1990)

This is a useful information source for non-prescription drugs and the conditions for which they are used. It is primarily aimed at pharmacy students and pharmacists. It covers the underlying background to each condition, products available for use and cautions to be observed.

## Symptoms in the Pharmacy (Blenkinsopp & Paxton 1995)

Also aimed at pharmacy students and pharmacists,

this text covers those therapeutic categories particularly important for responding to symptoms. It has a very practical approach, determining appropriate questions to ask, significance of possible answers, when to refer and appropriate treatment.

## CHILDREN'S DOSES

Particular care is required in the calculation of doses suitable for children, yet such specialist information is not always available. The following are recommended information sources for drug use in young children. Much of the data are, however, based on clinical experience and do not always reflect manufacturers' recommendations.

### Alder Hey Book of Children's Doses

This lists doses of drugs in common use.

### The Paediatric Vade Mecum (Insley 1992)

This provides a range of prescribing data.

## REGULATIONS AND RESTRICTIONS

### Medicines, Ethics and Practice – a Guide for Pharmacists

This is a practical guide to the legal classification of medicinal products incorporating the 'Code of Ethics' and the 'Guide to Good Dispensing Practice' It is updated twice yearly and distributed with *The Pharmaceutical Journal*.

## ABSTRACTING SYSTEMS

### Medline

This is an on-line version of Index Medicus. It is produced in the USA by the National Library of Medicine, scanning over 3200 journals. Some areas of drug information, including *The Pharmaceutical Journal*, are not covered but the database is updated weekly.

### Iowa Drug Information Service

This abstracting system is produced by the Iowa Drug Information Service and concentrates on journals relating to human drug therapy.

### Pharmline

Produced by input from NHS drug information specialists, this abstracting system covers drugs and professional pharmacy practice.

### International Pharmaceutical Abstracts

This system covers journals with a greater emphasis on pharmacy-orientated subjects than any other system. It is produced by the American Society of Health-System Pharmacists and is updated monthly.

## OTHER INFORMATION SOURCES

There are occasions when insufficient published information can be found. In these circumstances, information may be obtained from the following:

### Drug information centres

These have been described in Chapter 36.

### The Royal Pharmaceutical Society

The Royal Pharmaceutical Society has two libraries: one, in Edinburgh, specializes in quality control; the second, in London, offers information on all aspects of pharmacy and is particularly useful in identifying foreign drugs.

### The National Pharmaceutical Association

This offers an information service which is intended mainly for its members, and is a useful source of information on proprietary products.

### The pharmaceutical industry

All large companies will provide information on their products which, particularly for new products, may not be available from any other source.

# BIBLIOGRAPHY

ABPI Compendium of data sheets and summaries of product characteristics, current edn. Datapharm Publications, London

ABPI Patient information leaflet compendium, current edn. Datapharm Publications, London

Alder Hey Book of Children's doses 1994 6th edn. Liverpool Area Health Authority, Liverpool

Blenkinsopp A, Paxton P 1995 Symptoms in the pharmacy. Blackwell Scientific Publications, Oxford

British National Formulary, current edn. British Medical Association and Royal Pharmaceutical Society of Great Britain, London

British Pharmacopoeia 1993 HMSO, London

Chemist and Druggist Guide to OTC Medicines. Miller & Freeman, Tonbridge

Dukes M N G (ed) 1996 Meyler's the side effects of drugs. Elsevier, Amsterdam

European Pharmacopoeia 1996 3rd edn. Maisonneuve S.A., Saint Ruffine, France

Goodman L S, Gilman A, Hardman J G (eds) 1996 Goodman and Gilman's the pharmacological basis of therapeutics. McGraw-Hill, New York

Insley J 1992 Paediatric vade mecum, 12th edn. Lloyd-Luke, London

Li Wan Po A 1990 Non-prescription drugs, 2nd edn. Blackwell Science, Oxford

Medicines, Ethics and Practice – a guide for pharmacists, current edn. Royal Pharmaceutical Society of Great Britain, London

Monthly Index of Medical Specialities (MIMS). Haymarket Medical, London

OTC Directory, current edn. Proprietary Association of Great Britain, London

Reynolds J E F (ed) 1996 Martindale: the extra pharmacopoeia, 31st edn. Pharmaceutical Press, London

Side Effects of Drugs Annuals. Elsevier, Amsterdam

Speight T M, Halford N H G (eds) 1996 Avery's drug treatment: principles and practice of clinical pharmacology and therapeutics. Adis International, Auckland

Stockley I H 1996 Drug interactions. Pharmaceutical Press, London

Walker R, Edwards C (eds) 1994 Clinical pharmacy and therapeutics. Churchill Livingstone, Edinburgh

Young L Y, Koda-Kimble M A 1995 Applied therapeutics – the clinical use of drugs. Applied Therapeutics, Vancouver

# Appendix 8
## The development and organization of pharmacy in the UK

*A. J. Winfield*

## DEVELOPMENT OF PHARMACY IN THE UK

By the time of the Norman conquest of Britain, there was little more than the use of materia medica. There was a need to import many of the plants used within the UK. This was undertaken by the spice merchants, of whom there were two types – the pepperers and the spicers. The former tended to operate in ports, whilst the spicers were also in inland towns. Modern day equivalents are the importers and wholesalers (pepperers) and retail traders (spicers). There are also records indicating the existence of a group called apothecaries, who appear to have been merchants who dealt with drugs. A trade Guild of Pepperers was founded in 1180, which may also have included spicers. The guilds, amongst other things, controlled the professions. In the case of the apothecaries, this required a 7-year apprenticeship in 1310!

The distinction between pepperers, spicers and apothecaries gradually disappeared. The 'Fraternity of St Anthony' was originally formed in the mid-14th century, consisting of all three groups. The term 'grocer' came to be used in place of spicer and pepperer, whilst the term 'apothecary' continued in use.

During the Tudor period, the roles of grocers and apothecaries began to divide. Apothecaries became more scientific in their approach and the Society of Apothecaries was formed. Apothecaries and physicians worked together, the latter using apothecaries shops. Thus apothecaries were coming under the power of physicians. This was consolidated by an Act of 1553 which gave physicians powers to inspect apothecaries, to fine them and to destroy drugs which were considered inferior. This power was not withdrawn until 1875.

A number of developments dating from this period still continue. Thus weights and pharmaceutical symbols were devised. The term 'Recipe', nowadays R, was used. Tensions began to develop between 'prescribing apothecaries' and 'dispensing physicians'. This came to a head when, in 1703–4, the 'Rose case' was heard. In it, physicians took court action against William Rose, an apothecary, for supplying a medicine which had not been prescribed by any physician. They won the case, but on appeal to the House of Lords, Rose won on the grounds that it was in the public interest for apothecaries to give and supply medicine. Thus, whilst they could only charge for the medicine, apothecaries had virtually become medical practitioners. Many people see a parallel between these events and the debates which are taking place at the close of the 20th century.

By the start of the 18th century, new names were being widely used – 'druggist' or 'chymist and druggist'. During the course of the century, there was a gradual erosion of training. As a result, by the start of the 19th century there was urgent need for reform. This was enacted in 1815 by the Apothecaries Act which made the Society of Apothecaries responsible for training and registration of medical practitioners. This Act did not affect the chemists and druggists, who could continue to practice without specific requirements for training or education. In effect this Act represents the division between medical practitioners and pharmacists. The apothecary became the medical practitioner – the name was abolished in 1820 and again in 1873 (following its revival during the Crimean War).

In 1850 Jacob Bell was elected a Member of Parliament where he moved the Pharmacy Bill in 1851, which became the Pharmacy Act 1852. This Act, amongst other provisions, gave the protection to the names 'Pharmaceutical Chemist' and 'Chemist and Druggist' which still exists. Figure A8.1 illustrates the chronology of the evolution of pharmacy as a profession.

Pharmacists nowadays work in three main branches of the profession: hospital, community and indus-

498

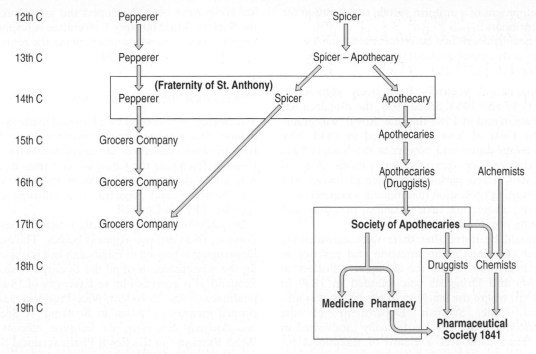

**Fig. A8.1**  An outline of the development of pharmacy.

trial practice. In addition there are many other roles in which pharmacists are placed, for example in academia, as pharmaceutical advisors, as community facilitators. Members of the general public are only likely to encounter pharmacists in the community pharmacy or on a hospital ward, although they may come across them in a residential home or making a visit to a patient's private home as part of their community pharmaceutical service. However, the health care which patients receive will also include input from pharmacists working as part of the health care team. In hospitals this will involve pharmacists working closely with doctors, nurses and others, as well as on their own. In the community, pharmacists are increasingly working with general practitioners, nurses, health visitors and others who come in regular contact with patients.

## THE PHARMACEUTICAL SOCIETY

During the first part of the 19th century the chemists and druggists were not well organized. It became obvious that some formal organization was required. In 1841, the apothecaries proposed a Bill which, if it had become law, would have put chemists and drug-

gists out of business. This stimulated two individuals – William Allen and Jacob Bell – to coordinate opposition to the Bill and to set up a permanent organization. On 15 April 1841 a general meeting of the chemists and druggists was held in the Crown and Anchor Tavern in the Strand, London. This meeting was chaired by William Allen who became the first President of the Pharmaceutical Society, which was founded at that meeting. Headquarters premises were rented at 17 Bloomsbury Square, London, where the Society remained until they moved to their present headquarters at 1 Lambeth High Street, London, in 1976. As a private enterprise, Jacob Bell established a journal in 1841. When it was handed over to the Pharmaceutical Society in 1859 'The Journal' was established as the main link between the Society and its members. A School of Pharmacy was established in 1842. This became the School of Pharmacy of the University of London in 1848. Membership of the Society rose from about 600 in 1841, to about 2000 by 1842. It stood at over 40 000 in 1996.

The Royal Charter of Incorporation was granted in 1843. This Charter lists four objects of the Society:

- the advancement of chemistry and pharmacy
- development of the protection of the business interests of chemists and druggists

- development of a uniform system of education for practitioners
- the establishment of a benevolent fund for the relief of distressed members, their widows and orphans.

Supplemental Charters have been granted in 1901, 1948 and 1953. Since 1937, the monarch has been Patron and in 1988 the title 'Royal' was granted. The Coat of Arms was granted in 1844. The constitution, duties and powers of the Society have been changed or extended by various Acts of Parliament. These have consolidated pharmacy as a self-governing profession maintaining a register of its members, inspecting their business premises and exercising disciplinary control.

It should be noted that there were considerable regional variations in organization and practice in the 18th century. Thus, for example, a Society of Chemists and Druggists was founded in 1839 in Aberdeen, where the teaching of pharmacy was also initiated. The Scottish Department of the Pharmaceutical Society was formally established in 1851. That same year a Board of Examiners for Scotland was established and a library was founded the following year. However, it was 1884 before the present headquarters at 36 York Place, Edinburgh were purchased to allow the creation of the laboratories. These are still in use by the Department of Pharmaceutical Sciences.

## The function and structures of the Royal Pharmaceutical Society of Great Britain (RPSGB)

The RPSGB has a number of functions, some of which are specified in law. They may be summed up as 'safeguarding the public with respect to the dispensing and distribution of medicines and regulating and promoting the profession of pharmacy'. Two important functions are to maintain the Register of Pharmaceutical Chemists and the Register of Premises. In order to become a registered pharmacist, a person must graduate from an accredited School of Pharmacy and, having completed a suitable period of postgraduate training, pass a registration examination. There are other arrangements for overseas pharmacists. The Society also has responsibility for controlling the conduct of pharmacies and for the sale and provision of medicines and poisons. To assist with this it has a number of Inspectors. They visit to ensure that the law is being followed and also offer advice and assistance to pharmacists. In order to maintain standards in the profession, eth-

ical codes have been developed and are enforced by the Society. The Statutory Committee is responsible for this, their ultimate sanction being the removal of a pharmacist from the Register.

### The Council and its committees

The Society is governed by a Council made up of 24 people. 21 are elected by the members (for a 3-year term of office) and three are appointed by the Privy Council. Each year the Council elects from its members a President, a Vice-President and a Treasurer. The Secretary and Registrar is a full-time official appointed by the Council.

In addition to the Council, which is based in London, there are two regional bodies. The Scottish Department is housed in Edinburgh and is responsible for the administration of all the Society's business in Scotland. It is governed by an Executive of 18 elected pharmacists, the President, Vice-President and any council members resident in Scotland. A Secretary and Assistant Secretary are full-time officials. The Welsh Executive of the Royal Pharmaceutical Society was formed in 1976 and is responsible, under the authority of the Council, for Society affairs in Wales. The Executive has 12 elected members plus the President, Vice-President and council members resident in Wales. The Secretary to the Welsh Executive is appointed by the Council and is a full-time official.

The Council operates through a series of committees. A representation of these is shown in Figure A8.2. Each of the main committees feeds business to the Council and many have sub-committees. Details of the responsibilities and membership of these bodies are given in the *Pharmacists' Directory and Yearbook*, which is published annually by the RPSGB.

In broad terms, the work of the Society is divided into a number of Departments. The main areas of responsibility are briefly outlined below.

- *Professional development.* This includes the Education Department, which deals with all matters to do with pharmaceutical education, including accreditation of undergraduate courses, postgraduate and continuing education, pre-registration training and the registration examination, careers, the British Pharmaceutical Students' Association, the Academic Pharmacy Group and research awards and fellowships. The Practice division supports the Practice Committee in developing policy on practice in all sectors of the profession. It also liaises with other health professions on practice issues and NHS policy. Various membership groups – Community

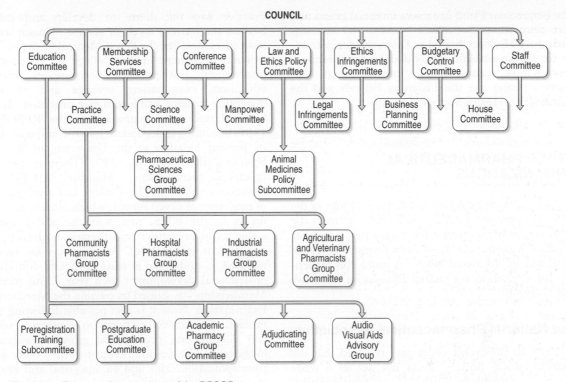

**Fig. A8.2**   The committee structure of the RPSGB.

Pharmacists, Hospital Pharmacists, Agricultural and Veterinary Pharmacists – are administered by this division.

- *Law Department*. This supports the work of the Law and Ethics and the Legal and Ethics Infringements Committees. The 26 inspectors work for this department to enforce the law on retail sale and supply of human and animal medicines. The inspectors also operate the NHS scheme for testing drugs and appliances. The Statutory Committee is an independent body which can be asked to consider breaches of the code of professional ethics. The Statutory Committee has the power to reprimand or remove from the Register pharmacists who fail to meet the required standards.

- *Department of Pharmaceutical Sciences*. This promotes the pharmaceutical sciences through a wide range of activities. These include the Information Centre (library, technical information service and museum), Medicine Testing Laboratory and Pharmaceutics Division, Scientific and Technical Services Division and the *Journal of Pharmacy and Pharmacology*.

- *Publications Department*. The Pharmaceutical Press has a wide range of titles the two most important being *Martindale: the Extra Pharmacopoeia* and

the *British National Formulary* (published jointly with the British Medical Association). Other titles include *The Pharmaceutical Codex*, *The Veterinary Formulary*, *The Handbook of Pharmaceutical Excipients*, *Drug Interactions* and *Clarke's Isolation and Identification of Drugs*.

- *Public relations*. An essential part of any professional organization is to maintain effective links with the public, politicians and the media. The Society retains the services of two Members of Parliament to act as consultants and a channel of communication.

- *Overseas activity*. The Society represents the profession on a number of bodies in the European Union. World-wide it has links with the International Pharmaceutical Federation (FIP) and administers the Commonwealth Pharmaceutical Association (CPA). The Adjudicating Committee deals with the eligibility of overseas candidates for registration in the UK.

Apart from these activities, the Society undertakes other functions. For example it has an annual conference – the British Pharmaceutical Conference – which has been hosted by various branches around the UK since 1864. A further objective is to help pharmacists who are facing difficulty or hardship.

The Benevolent Fund can make financial grants and offer counselling on welfare benefits and housing. Birdsgrove House, situated in Derbyshire, is a country retreat for pharmacists and their dependents in need of rest, recuperation or convalescence. Two newer schemes are the Listening Friends and the Pharmacists' Health Support Schemes.

## OTHER PHARMACEUTICAL ORGANIZATIONS

Despite the wide activities and responsibilities of the RPSGB, there are strict limits. In order to meet the other requirements within the profession, a number of other organizations have been formed. A few of these will be discussed below. A more comprehensive list is given in the annual *Pharmacists' Directory and Yearbook*.

### The National Pharmaceutical Association

In 1920 an important court case resolved that the Pharmaceutical Society could not act as a trade union for its members. That is, it could not negotiate terms of service or levels of remuneration. This was known as the Jenkin Judgement after the pharmacist who instigated the action in order to clarify this and some other issues.

It was as a direct consequence of this ruling that the National Pharmaceutical Association (NPA) was formed in 1921. The Scottish Pharmaceutical Federation (SPF) is the equivalent body in Scotland. The NPA provide a wide range of expert advice on pharmaceutical, legal, financial and commercial matters. They also offer a range of business and dispensary equipment and design consultancy. In addition they operate training courses for assistants and dispensing technicians, have a very comprehensive information department, publish a number of books and leaflets, operate a clearing house to help paying bills and run national advertising campaigns to promote community pharmacy. A successful example of this was the 'Ask your pharmacist – you'll be taking good advice' campaign in the early 1990s. Links enable them to supply insurance and other financial services to members.

### The College of Pharmacy Practice

The RPSGB has a responsibility to maintain the quality of pharmaceutical services. The motivation behind the foundation of the College of Pharmacy Practice was the desire to develop and extend beyond the current levels of service. Thus it would have a function like the Royal Medical Colleges. The Mission Statement of the College is 'To promote professional and personal development through education, examination, practice and research, benefiting patients and health care provision'. It was founded under the patronage of the RPSGB in 1981, becoming independent in 1986 and moving to its present location at the University of Warwick Science Park, Coventry, in 1991. There are two categories of membership – Members (MCPP) and Associates (ACPP). The College has a programme of professional development, which reflects developments in the NHS, new scientific and technical advances in preventive and therapeutic health care and patient involvement. All members are recommended to undertake at least 30 hours' continuing professional development each year. Until recently Membership was gained by passing the Membership Examination. Now it is also possible following submission of a satisfactory portfolio of practice, which will demonstrate professional growth, awareness, judgement and commitment, together with good communication skills and an analytical and evaluative approach to practice.

### Organizations for the pharmaceutical industry

The pharmaceutical industry ranges from small manufacturers through to large-scale multinational companies. Their products range from highly specialized, prescription-only products through to over-the-counter medicines. There are two main trade organizations. The Association of the British Pharmaceutical Industry (ABPI) represents the manufacturers of prescription medicines. It was founded in 1930 with the main functions of:

- maintaining and improving the reputation of the industry and its contribution to the health and economic welfare of the nation
- assisting contact between companies and government, professional, scientific and trade organizations and other similar bodies
- acting as a channel of communication
- putting into practice collective decisions.

Amongst other publications, the ABPI produces the *Compendium of Data Sheets* and the *Patient Information Leaflet Compendium* annually.

The Proprietary Association of Great Britain (PAGB) represents the manufacturers of medicines intended to be used without a prescription. It was formed in 1919 and is involved in all matters which affect the marketing and use of non-prescription medicines, including dealing with government departments about legislative changes (such as the POM to P re-regulations). It also has similar dealings with the European Union and the World Health Organization. In order to maintain standards it has adopted a strict Code of Standards. Amongst other things, this requires that all labels, leaflets and advertising are acceptable to the Association before they can be used. The PAGB publishes the annual *OTC Directory*.

The Proprietary Articles Trade Association (PATA) involves manufacturers, wholesalers and community pharmacists. It was founded in 1896. Its main function is to ensure that pharmacists receive fair remuneration for their services through the operation of resale price maintenance. Resale price mainentance was abolished by the Resale Prices Act 1964. However, in 1970, after a lengthy court case led by the PATA, medicines were exempt from the Act. At the time of preparing this chapter, medicines remain the only articles exempt from RPM and the issue is again under debate.

## THE UK NATIONAL HEALTH SERVICE

In 1946, the National Health Service Act was passed by Parliament. The NHS began on 5 July 1948, with the objective of providing health care to all, irrespective of their ability to pay. In its early days, the main emphasis was on the development of the hospital service. It was not until the 1966 General Practitioners' Charter that incentives were provided to broaden care and raise the quality of care in the community. Health centres began to emerge, involving health visitors, district nurses and other care workers in addition to doctors. By the mid-1970s, closer links between community and hospital care were developing. Over the last quarter century there have been many major changes, which will be briefly reviewed. It should be noted that there are differences in Scotland, which will be dealt with separately.

The 1974 reorganization removed the special status of the teaching hospitals, so that hospitals and health centres came under the same health authority, although general practice medicine remained separate. Health Councils gave patients an independent voice and promoted the interests of special groups such as the mentally ill or elderly. Unfortunately, in 1976 the Treasury found it necessary to introduce cash limits on public spending. Within the NHS it was only the GPs who remained free from financial restrictions. The reorganization of 1974 had failed to secure all its objectives which included cost cutting.

The next major development was in 1982, when power was transferred down from Regional Health Authorities to newly created, smaller, District Health Authorities. However, the financial constraints continued, with the emphasis of budgetary control moving from inputs (such as doctors per 1000 of population) to performance indicators (such as waiting time for treatment). The Griffiths Report studied the management structures within the NHS. In 1982 a new structure was adopted which took away the power of veto which medical and nursing representatives had previously enjoyed. However, the measures did not greatly affect the decisions taken by hospital doctors. GPs still remained free of limits on expenditure and referral to hospital. The first restriction on GP prescribing came in 1984 with the introduction of a limited list of drugs – often called the 'Black List' – which they could prescribe. This and other measures slowed the rate of increase in expenditure on the NHS. However, it also caused a gradual build-up of need for additional funding.

A radical review by government led to the introduction of the 'internal market'. The concept was to mimic the benefits of competition seen in the private sector. To achieve this, the purchase of health care was to be separated from the provision of health care. Thus both hospitals and community services – the providers – would 'sell' their services. The purchaser would choose from whom to buy. Hospitals and community services became independent 'trusts'. GP practices with sufficient patients would also operate their own funds. Thus providers would be in competition to obtain contracts from the voluntary and private sectors. The belief was that this competition would lead to improving quality of service, whilst keeping costs under control.

### NHS trusts

The first NHS trusts were formed in 1991. Each trust is a self-governing organization with its own Board of Directors. They are free to organize their affairs, subject only to the contracts into which they have entered and the legal framework under which they operate. Each trust must produce an annual business plan in order to meet their responsibilities which are:

- breaking even financially
- earning a 6% return on capital

- operating within financial limits set by the Secretary of State.

Most NHS services are now run as trusts. At first it was anticipated that trusts would be directly accountable to the Secretary of State. However, it has been realized that this is not feasible, so the regional offices of the NHS Executive were created to provide this intermediate tier of management. Income to trusts is from contracts with health authorities, GP fund holders and other purchasers.

## GP fund holders

GP practices which hold their own funds are called GP fund holders. They are responsible for:

- outpatient services
- X-rays and laboratory tests
- some inpatient and day-case treatments
- medicines
- services provided to patients by staff employed by the practice, such as nurses and dietitians.

The long-term aim is that GP funding should be based on a funding formula. This may be based on the number of patients, adjusted to allow for factors such as age, sex or other relevant factors. At present, however, such a formula is not in place, so funding is based on past needs, such as referral patterns and drug bills. As with the trusts, so there is an annual cycle of applications for fund holding status. Not all practices are eligible for, or desirous of, obtaining such status. In such situations, payment is made by the NHS directly to the provider.

## White Papers

A series of White Papers were published in the late 1980s which have led to further changes. These include 'Working for Patients', 'Promoting Better Health' and 'Caring for People'. These were combined in the Community Care Act 1990. This included the following reforms:

- the introduction of a new system of contractual funding
- proposals to strengthen all levels of management
- measures to manage clinical activity more effectively
- new arrangements for allocating resources.

These had implications for pharmacy as will be seen later.

Modification of the structures within the NHS occurs from time to time. The most recent (at the time of writing in early 1997) was implemented in April 1996. The most significant change was the abolition of the regional health authorities (RHAs) and family health services authorities (FHSAs). The Secretary of State is responsible to Parliament for the running of the NHS. To assist, he has the Department of Health which includes the NHS Executive. The latter manages the services directly through eight regional offices and the health authorities. There are 100 health authorities in England. However, it should be noted that these do not have the same function as the earlier health authorities. Rather their role is one of monitoring and they have no operational management function. In Wales, where similar reorganization took place, there are five new health authorities.

## The NHS in Scotland

The NHS in Scotland is separate from that in England and Wales. The Secretary of State for Scotland is responsible to Parliament for its operation. It is administered from the Scottish Office Department of Health, with the local administration carried out by 15 health boards. The primary care services in Scotland are the direct responsibility of the health board, with no equivalent to the former family health services authorities (FHSA) in England.

There are 12 Chief Administrative Pharmaceutical Officers (CAPOs), one for each of the larger boards, who act as pharmaceutical adviser to the health board. The responsibilities of a CAPO may be summed up as:

- coordinating plans for the maintenance and development of pharmaceutical services
- providing advice to the board
- planning pharmaceutical services in hospitals and clinics
- developing a working relationship between the board and the pharmaceutical advisory structures – the Area Pharmaceutical Committee
- coordinating with bodies responsible for continuing education
- advising on the adequacy of the hospital and general practice pharmaceutical services in the board's area.

The CAPOs hold regular meetings and have taken a number of important initiatives in developing pharmaceutical services in Scotland in response to government requests. The position of CAPOs is currently in a stage of further development and the service will largely be provided in NE Scotland by pharmacy staff of the two Aberdeen universities.

## The NHS in Wales

The legislation for the NHS in Wales is the same as that for England, but the operation of the service is separate. The Secretary of State for Wales is responsible to Parliament for the conduct of the NHS in Wales.

## Negotiation of terms of service

The RPSGB may not act to negotiate terms of service and levels of remuneration for its members. The NPA, whilst supporting pharmacists in their business interests, also do not act as negotiators. This function is provided by the Pharmaceutical Services Negotiating Committee (PSNC) in England and Wales and the Scottish Pharmaceutical General Council (SPGC) in Scotland. Both bodies have similar functions:

- negotiating remuneration and terms of service
- representing pharmacist contractors in other discussions
- monitoring proposed legislation which may affect pharmacists
- checking and agreeing prices used in pricing NHS prescriptions and maintaining a central checking unit
- supporting individual contractors on matters relating to the NHS.

# INDEX